The Complete Recovery Room Book

FOURTH EDITION

Anthea Hatfield
Taranaki Base Hospital
New Plymouth, New Zealand

Michael Tronson
Box Hill Hospital
Melbourne, Australia

OXFORD
UNIVERSITY PRESS

OXFORD

UNIVERSITY PRESS

Great Clarendon Street, Oxford OX2 6DP

Oxford University Press is a department of the University of Oxford.
It furthers the University's objective of excellence in research, scholarship,
and education by publishing worldwide in

Oxford New York

Auckland Cape Town Dar es Salaam Hong Kong Karachi
Kuala Lumpur Madrid Melbourne Mexico City Nairobi
New Delhi Shanghai Taipei Toronto

With offices in

Argentina Austria Brazil Chile Czech Republic France Greece
Guatemala Hungary Italy Japan Poland Portugal Singapore
South Korea Switzerland Thailand Turkey Ukraine Vietnam

Oxford is a registered trade mark of Oxford University Press
in the UK and in certain other countries

Published in the United States
by Oxford University Press Inc., New York

A catalogue record for this title is available from the British Library

Data available

Library of Congress Cataloguing in Publication Data

Data available

Typeset by Cepha Imaging Private Ltd., Bangalore, India
Printed in Great Britain
on acid-free paper by
Ashford Colour Press, Gosport, Hampshire

ISBN 978–0–19–923268–0

10 9 8 7 6 5 4 3 2

Whilst every effort has been made to ensure that the contents of this book are as complete,
accurate and up-to-date as possible at the date of writing, Oxford University Press is not able to
give any guarantee or assurance that such is the case. Readers are urged to take appropriately
qualified medical advice in all cases. The information in this book is intended to be useful to
the general reader, but should not be used as a means of self-diagnosis or for the prescription
of medication.

Dedication

This edition is dedicated to the anaesthetists, surgeons and nurses of Box Hill Hospital who have had so many of their patients 'Trono-ed' in the pursuit of good recovery from anaesthesia.

Third Edition Dedicated To

The staff of St Vincent's Hospital, Melbourne.

Second Edition Dedicated To

Staff working in isolated environments especially in the hospitals of the South West Pacific.

First Edition Dedicated To

Pamela Deighton, Palega Vaeau and Grant Scarf – the first recovery room team to visit Samoa.

Contents

Preface

Constant vigilance is the price of safety.

Patients believe they are asleep during their operation: they are not asleep, they are in a drug-induced coma, and it takes them time to metabolize and excrete these drugs. During this time, they gradually recover consciousness, but remain unable to care for themselves and are at risk of coming to harm. This is a period of extreme physiological insults: pain, hypothermia, hypoxia, acid-base disturbance and shifts in blood volume. Not only do the recovery room staff have to adeptly manage comatose and physiologically unstable patients, but also deal with the early postoperative care of surgical patients and attend to drips, drains and dressings.

The recovery room is a *critical care unit* where necessary skills and equipment are gathered in the one place. Here the care of patients passes safely from the intensive monitoring in the operating theatre to the wards. Before recovery rooms became available, more than half the deaths in the immediate postoperative period occurred from preventable conditions such as airway obstruction, aspiration of stomach contents, and haemorrhagic shock.

We wrote this book to help you to manage day-to-day problems that occur in recovery rooms. In teaching and specialist hospitals there are people around to ask for help or advice. But, at times in most hospitals, you will need to make difficult decisions on your own. This book should help you make these decisions. We have not covered the management of recovery from super-specialist surgery such as neurosurgery, cardiac surgery or procedures on sick children.

Begin to read the book anywhere. Each chapter is written to stand alone. Reading the chapters covering basic science which precede the practical sections will be worthwhile. Once you understand basic physiology and pharmacology it is easier to make sense of clinical disorders, anticipate problems and develop plans to avoid them.

The recovery room is one part of *perioperative practice*. In some sections the preoperative and operative procedure are described in detail, because what has happened before the patient reaches you is relevant to their management.

In this edition we have expanded sections on anaesthetic practice and the prevention of infection. There are new sections on *risk assessment* and *quality control*. If carried out properly, *evidence based practice* makes your recovery room safer.

In the recovery room most drugs are given intravenously. Once injected, you cannot retrieve them. The prescribed drug doses are those suitable for a fit 40 year-old man. You may need to increase or reduce the doses according to the circumstances. Never give a drug unless you fully understand its properties.

To comply with international standards, many drug names have changed from the older British Accepted Nomenclature (BAN) to the newer *recognized International Non-proprietary Names* (rINNs). Most of the new names are commonplace in the USA.

Words in *italics* are technical words or jargon. You are probably familiar with most of them. To stop unnecessary explanations cluttering the text we have made a compromise; relevant concepts are explained close by, otherwise the terms are amplified in a glossary at the end of the book.

The glossary also contains some other common terms you may encounter.

Short aphorisms are scattered through the text, to jog your memory long after the reasoning behind them has evaporated.

The opinions expressed in this book are our own. For the most part they are based on *best evidence* and use *principles of best practice*, but we also counsel common sense and humanity. There are no randomized blinded trials to prove that cuddling crying children comforts them. Not everyone agrees with the way we do things. This is a guidebook, not a rulebook. In places we suggest further reading. You must look elsewhere for theoretical analysis and closely reasoned arguments.

We hope you pick up this book and read the more difficult sections in your quiet times. Thoroughly absorbing the information here should enable you to look after your patients in an intelligent and thoughtful manner, and give you much personal satisfaction.

Seek help from colleagues to understand fully what is happening to your patient.

Acknowledgements

We thank all those people who have helped us wittingly or unwittingly. Over the years we have accumulated notes, listened to lectures and presentations at conferences, picked up brochures, found tips on recovery room notice boards, read journals and texts, searched the Internet, and absorbed information in operating theatre tea rooms. Many of the sources of this information are lost, but to these, our unknown teachers and advisors, we express our most grateful thanks.

Special acknowledgements to the fourth edition

Peter Amrosy for help with risk management.

Nursing staff in CSSD and Infection Control at Maroondah Hospital, Ringwood East, Victoria, Australia for help with infection control.

Carmella Corrello, Deputy Director of Pharmacy, Box Hill Hospital, Melbourne, Australia for help with pharmacology.

David Ernest, Director of ICU at Box Hill Hospital, Melbourne, Australia for help with resuscitation.

Jane and Arch MacDonnell of Inhouse Design, Auckland, New Zealand for their tireless attention to detail.

Richard Tronson for his skillful and patient help in proof reading and checking our English expression and grammar.

20 Golden Rules

'There is nothing more lethal than ignorance – or more frightful than a wilfully closed mind.' Johann von Goethe 1749–1832.

If you are in any doubt ... ask somebody!

1. The confused, restless and agitated patient is hypoxic until proven otherwise.
2. Your patient may be hypoxic even though the oximeter reads 98%.
3. Never turn your back on a patient.
4. The blood pressure does not necessarily fall in haemorrhagic shock.
5. Never ignore a tachycardia or a bradycardia; find the cause.
6. Postoperative hypertension is dangerous.
7. Never use a painful stimulus to rouse your patient.
8. Nurse comatose patients on their side in the recovery position.
9. If your patient is slow to wake up, or continues to bleed, consider hypothermia.
10. Noisy breathing is obstructed breathing, but not all obstructed breathing is noisy.
11. Let patients remove their airways when they are ready to.
12. Cuddle crying children; hold the hand of crying adults.
13. The opioids do not cause hypotension in stable patients.
14. When giving drugs to the elderly, start by giving half as much, twice as slowly.
15. If you do not know the actions of a drug, then do not give it.
16. Treat the patient, not the monitor.
17. Cold hands are a sign of a haemodynamically unstable patient.
18. Pain prevention is better than pain relief.
19. Do not discharge patients from the recovery room until they can maintain a 5-second head lift.
20. If confused read rule number 1!

Recovery room routines

In this chapter we will follow patients from the operating theatre to the recovery room, outline their care, describe routine procedures, and finally their discharge and transport to the ward.

The recovery room is the most important room in the hospital, for it is here that a patient is at most risk from inadvertent harm. Patients are in an unstable physiological state where critical events can develop rapidly. Most critical events are preventable, but detecting and treating them relies on skilled and vigilant nursing staff who can give constant and total care.

Immediate care

Things to check before the first patient arrives

Sign the recovery room's log book to confirm that:

- resuscitation trolleys are properly stocked;
- drug cupboards are restocked;
- disposable items are replaced;
- sharps and rubbish containers are empty and ready;
- suction equipment is ready, clean and working;
- oxygen supply is connected and working properly;
- Mapelson's C breathing circuit is connected;
- adequate supply of airways;
- monitoring equipment is all available and working;
- blood pressure machines and appropriate cuffs are available;
- intravenous drip hangers are ready;
- clean blankets and other linen are available;
- sufficient blankets in warming cupboard;
- working area is clean and uncluttered;
- alarm bells are working.

Recovery room step down

Stage 1 recovery

Patients who need Stage 1 recovery are those who are physiologically unstable, or who potentially may become so.

Patients in *Stage 1 recovery* must be attended by specialist staff proficient at advanced cardiac life support. (Advanced cardiac life support includes all the other skills, procedures and equipment needed to deal instantly with a deteriorating cardiorespiratory status, or arrest and including defibrillation.) Resuscitation equipment must be instantly available.

If you have any doubt about a patient's status then they should remain in Stage 1 recovery. Patients in Stage 1 recovery include those who are comatose; or require airway support, or continued frequent monitoring of their respiratory, cardiovascular, neurological or muscular function; or evaluation of their mental status; or assessment or management of core temperature, pain, nausea and vomiting, surgical drainage, blood loss or urine output. Patients transferred to the intensive care unit (ICU) remain in Extended Stage 1 recovery.

Whether a patient is likely to become physiologically unstable cannot be quantified, but experienced staff readily recognize those patients at risk.

While there is risk of harm
the patient remains in Stage 1 recovery.

Stage 2 recovery

At this stage the patients are conscious and fully able to care for their own airways. They are within the physiological limits defined by their preoperative evaluation. These patients must be attended by staff who are proficient at basic life support (this includes the basic ABC of resuscitation: maintenance of a clear airway, support of breathing and external cardiac massage). At this stage patients are fit to return to the ward, which by definition is Extended Stage 2 recovery and remains so for the whole period the patient is in the hospital. For *day case procedures* it refers to those who are waiting in a supervised area for discharge.

Stage 3 Recovery

Following day procedures patients can be discharged into the care of a competent and informed adult who can intervene should untoward events occur. The carer may have no skills in life support, but must be capable of recognizing problems and know what to do about them. Stage 3 recovery also applies to patients who are discharged home from the ward, even after days or weeks in the hospital. Patients remain in Stage 3 recovery until they have completely recovered from their operation, and no longer need hospital care in any form (even as an outpatient).

How to transport the patient to the recovery room

You need at least three people to gently move the patient from the operating table on to a specially designed recovery room trolley. Staff need to adapt their techniques if the hospital has a no-lift policy. It is the anaesthetist's responsibility to look after the patient's head, neck and airway.

The trolleys must be capable of being tilted head up or down by at least 15°, and carry facilities to give oxygen and apply suction, and a pole to hang drains and intravenous fluids. As you move the patient take care not to dislodge catheters, drains and lines.

Position patients on their sides in the *recovery position* with their operation site uppermost. Put the trolley sides up. Wheel patients feet first to the recovery room. The anaesthetist walks forward (never backward) maintaining the patient's airway. Put the trolley's sucker under the patient's pillow ready to use immediately if needed.

Figure 1.1 The recovery position

How to admit the patient to the recovery room

First check the patient is stable

The instant a patient is admitted to the recovery room, check that they are lying in an appropriate position, check they are breathing quietly, put on an oxygen mask, check their pulse and blood pressure: only receive the handover when you are satisfied the patient's condition is stable. There are two handovers: the nurse's and the anaesthetist's.

Nurse watching airway and chest movement

Note position of hands lifting lower jaw

Low flat pillow

Tilting trolley

Sucker under pillow

Figure 1.2 Attention to the patient's airway

The nurse's handover

The nurse's handover includes:

- surgeon's and anaesthetist's name;
- checking the patient's name against their medical records, and identity bracelet;
- care and placement of surgical drains;
- problems with skin pressure areas;
- organizing the patient's records;
- ensuring the correct charts and X-rays accompany the patient;
- care of the patient's personal belongings such as dentures, and hearing aids.

The anaesthetist's handover

The anaesthetist handover includes the:

- patient's name and age;
- indications for surgery;
- the type of operation;
- type of anaesthetic;
- relevant medical problems;
- conscious state;
- blood pressure;
- pulse and respiratory rate.

  Additionally the anaesthetist reports:

- untoward events occurring before and during surgery;
- analgesia given and anticipated needs;
- vascular monitoring lines;
- blood loss, and details of what intravenous fluids to give next;
- urine output during the procedure; and the expected output for the next few hours;
- drain tubes;
- patient's psychological state;
- what continuing monitoring is needed in recovery room;
- how much oxygen, and how to give it;
- orders for any further investigations;
- and provides a recovery room discharge plan.

Before the anaesthetist leaves the recovery room the patient must be breathing, have good oxygen saturation, a stable blood pressure and pulse rate. Anaesthetists should tell the nursing staff where to find them if necessary, and they must remain close by while the patient is in the recovery room.

Maintain the patient's airway during the handover.

Initial assessment

Immediate steps

Once the patient is transported to the recovery room, immediately apply an oxygen mask. First note the patient's conscious state. Then have an assistant

Figure 1.3 Outline of patient care plan on admission

attach the monitoring devices while you gain control by doing things in the following order of priority: A, B, C, D and E.

A Airway

B Breathing

C Circulation

D Drips, drains and drugs

E Extras

A = Airway

- Make sure patients have a clear airway, are breathing and air is moving freely and quietly in and out of their chest. Briefly, put one hand over their mouth to feel the airflow and the other hand on their chest to feel it rise and fall in synchrony.
- Begin administering oxygen with a face mask at a flow rate of 6 L/min.
- Attach a *pulse oximeter* to obtain a baseline reading.
- If necessary gently suck out the patient's mouth and pharynx. Be gentle otherwise you may provoke *laryngospasm*.
- If the patient is still unconscious make sure an airway is properly located between the teeth and tongue, and the lips are not in danger of being bitten.
- If the patient has clamped his teeth shut and you are unable to insert an airway into the mouth, then gently slide a lubricated nasopharyngeal airway along the floor of the nose.

Hint

Tidal air exchange is best felt in the palm of your hand as you support the chin; now you can feel every breath taken. Do not remove the oxygen mask for more than a few breaths.

B = Breathing

- Check the chest is moving, and you can feel air flowing in and out of the mouth.
- Just because patients fog up their face masks, does not mean that they are moving adequate amounts of tidal air.
- Listen for abnormal noises as the patient breathes: wheezes, rattles, gurgles; or snoring or crowing noises called *stridor*.

- Look at the strap muscles in the patient's neck; they should not tense with breathing. If they are contracting it suggests the patient is working hard to breathe. Check that the airway is not obstructed, and the patient is not wheezing. Airway obstruction is dangerous: notify the anaesthetist immediately.
- Look for signs of *cyanosis*. Cyanosis is a bluish tinge of the lips or tongue. It is a sign of severe *hypoxaemia*. If you are uncertain whether the patient is cyanosed then squeeze the tip of the patient's finger to engorge it with blood, and compare it with the colour of your own finger tip.
- Note in the patient's record the reading on the *pulse oximeter*. If the reading is less than 95%, then search for a reason. Seek help immediately if it is less than 90%.
- Chest movement does not always mean that breathing is adequate.

C = Circulation

- Once you are sure your patient is breathing properly and well oxygenated, measure the blood pressure, pulse rate and rhythm and record them in the chart.
- Record the patient's *perfusion status* in the notes.
- Check the patient is not bleeding into drains or dressings, or elsewhere. Look under the sheets.

D = Drugs, drips, drains and dressings

- Note the drugs given in theatre, particularly opioids that may depress the patient's breathing.
- Check whether the patient has any drug allergies or sensitivities.
- Note the intravenous fluids in progress, how much fluid, and what types have been given during the operation. Make sure the drip is running freely and is not sited across a joint (where it may be obstructed) or in the back of the hand (where it can be dislodged). Replace any pieces of sticky tape encircling the arm because they will cause distal ischaemia if the arm swells for any reason such as the drip fluid running into the tissues. If the cannula is sited across a joint, splint it until it is re-sited in a safer place away from the joint.
- Check the patency of drains and tubing; how much, how fast and what is draining out of them. Make sure the urinary catheter is not blocked, urine is dripping freely, and note the volume of the collecting bag's contents.
- Check vacuum suction devices are functioning properly.
- Check their dressings and make sure blood or ooze is not seeping through them.

E = Extras

- Measure the patient's *temperature*. This is essential for babies and patients who have had long major surgery.
- Measure the blood glucose of diabetic patients with a finger prick.
- If the patient has a limb in plaster, check the perfusion of the fingers or toes. Gently squeeze blood out of the tip of a finger or toe. It will turn white. If it does not turn pink again within three seconds of releasing the pressure then the limb is ischaemic; notify the surgeons. If the fingers or toes are congested and blue, this indicates venous obstruction; notify the surgeons immediately.
- Check peripheral pulses following vascular surgery.
- Check the circulation to graft sites.

Perfusion status

As the heart pumps blood to the tissues it must do so at sufficient pressure to ensure perfusion. There are two parameters involved: cardiac output and blood pressure. We do not usually measure cardiac output, but we can estimate whether it is adequate from monitoring other variables such as blood pressure, peripheral perfusion, urine output, pulse oximetry and where necessary, acid base status and central venous pressures.

Measuring perfusion status

Poor peripheral perfusion is sometimes called *peripheral shutdown*, because circulation to the hands and feet is almost absent, the patients' hands are blue or even white and cold, and their radial pulse may be feeble or absent. Perfusion status is graded according to Table 1.1.

Table 1.1 Perfusion status

Observation	Adequate	Poor	No perfusion
Conscious state	Alert, oriented in time and place	Obtunded, confused, anxious or agitated	Unconscious
Skin	Warm, pink, dry	Cool, pale, clammy, sweating	Cool/cold, pale +/– sweating
Pulse	60–100/minute	Either < 60/minute or > 100/minute	Absent or feeble pulse
Blood pressure	> 100 mmHg	< 100 mmHg	Unrecordable

Other signs of poor perfusion include:

- poor capillary return in fingernail beds;
- peripheral or central cyanosis;
- ischaemic changes on the electrocardiogram (ECG).

A useful way of testing perfusion is to press firmly for a moment on a patient's fingernail. When you let go the blood should blush back within a second or so. If the *capillary return time* (CRT) takes more than 2 seconds, your patient has poor peripheral perfusion.

During longer operations patients often cool down. This causes their skin perfusion to slow, so that when they first come to the recovery room their perfusion status is not a reliable indicator of how well their cardiopulmonary unit is functioning. In this case look at the perfusion inside their lips, rather than their fingertips. Even cold patients should not have central cyanosis, or a tachycardia.

Good records are eloquent evidence
of your competence.

Observations

There are no agreed criteria on how often to take patients' *vital signs* in the recovery room because it depends on the patient's clinical state. As a guide, if patients are stable, record their vital signs every 5 minutes for the first 15 minutes after their admission, and then every 10–15 minutes during their stay. If patients' vital signs are unstable then measure them at least every 5 minutes.

Recovery room records

The recovery room records are a direct continuation of the anaesthetic record. Keep them on the same chart.

Medical and legal responsibilities

Scrupulous and detailed records are your only medical and legal defence if problems should occur. If you do not write it down then it did not happen – it is a case of no record, then no defence. Remember that you may be called to a courtroom to account for an *adverse event* many years hence. Record only what you see and hear, and do not pass opinion unless it is directly applicable to the situation. 'The patient appears to me to be irrational' is an acceptable comment, but 'the patient is irrational' is passing a judgement you may not be able to substantiate years later.

Keep it legible, keep it relevant, and keep it factual. Only use abbreviations approved by your hospital and sign off on each entry.

The minimum information to document

Document your evaluation of the patient on their admission to the recovery room.

- Record the time the patient comes to the recovery room.
- Vital signs and levels of consciousness at specified times and intervals.
- All drugs given, including the dose and route.
- Amounts and types of intravenous fluids given.
- An ECG rhythm strip if one was taken.
- All unusual or untoward events.
- Certify the vital signs are stable.
- The patient can sustain the 5-second head lift test.
- Details about planned follow-up of the patient.
- Sign and date your entry.

Records and quality control

If you enter the recovery room scoring system on a standard spreadsheet computer program you can collect data and analyse it later. Use this data to identify potential problems, provide objective evidence about workloads, and help deploy staff effectively. Good data collection is an essential part of risk assessment and quality control.

Emergence from anaesthesia

Anaesthesia consists of three elements: coma, muscle relaxation, and abolition of unwanted *reflexes*.

Coma

A principal component of a general anaesthetic is a drug-induced and maintained coma. A useful definition of *coma* is a state of consciousness where the eyes are closed, and the patient does not respond to verbal or tactile stimuli. Practically, this means if the patient does not open their eyes when you gently shake them by the shoulder, and call their name, then they are by definition *comatose*.

But coma is more complex than this. To be conscious requires an intact *brainstem reticular activating system* (RAS), and intact cerebral hemispheres (or at least part of a hemisphere). As the RAS is sequentially suppressed, the coma deepens. A person can suffer extensive brain damage, but unless the reticular activating system is affected they will not lose consciousness. This is the reason why many patients with quite large strokes merely lose the movement of part of their body without becoming unconscious.

> *The reticular activating system continually prods the cortex to keep it awake.*

In the 1930s Dr Francis Guedel described four distinct stages of an ether anaesthetic, tracing the sequence of events as the reticular activating system was suppressed.

The stages are not as easily identified with modern volatile anaesthetics as they were with ether because they happen so quickly, but the stages are more obvious (in the reverse order) as patients emerge from anaesthesia.

Assessing the level of coma

Figure 1.4 demonstrates a simple way to assess the levels of a drug-induced coma. For example, a patient with periodic breathing, divergent gaze and reactive pupils who responds in a semi-purposeful way to a firm squeeze on their triceps muscle is in a level 1 coma, and about to emerge from their anaesthetic.

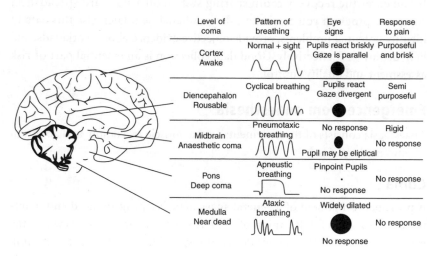

Level of coma	Pattern of breathing	Eye signs	Response to pain
Cortex Awake	Normal + sight	Pupils react briskly Gaze is parallel	Purposeful and brisk
Diencepahalon Rousable	Cyclical breathing	Pupils react Gaze divergent	Semi purposeful
Midbrain Anaesthetic coma	Pneumotaxic breathing	No response Pupil may be eliptical	Rigid No response
Pons Deep coma	Apneustic breathing	Pinpoint Pupils No response	No response
Medulla Near dead	Ataxic breathing	Widely dilated No response	No response

Figure 1.4 Levels of coma

Stages of emergence

Stage 1 – coma

Coma is one of the elements of a general anaesthetic. Patients do not respond to any stimuli. You cannot awaken patients from a coma. Be patient. Never use painful stimuli to try to rouse your patient.

Stage 2 – responsive

As patients emerge from coma, they start to respond to stimuli. Although not awake their pupils constrict in reaction to light, but the direction of their gaze diverges. Then, a few moments before waking, their pupils suddenly dilate, and patients move their limbs, and perhaps begin to shiver or shake. Their pulse rate and blood pressure rise.

Stage 3 – awake

Although now awake and responding appropriately to commands, their conscious state remains clouded. Later they will remember little, or nothing, about this stage. During this stage, some patients become confused, restless, disoriented and possibly fearful, and you will not be able to reason with them. This *delirium* usually passes within a few minutes. If the delirium persists then exclude hypoxia and hypoglycaemia as a possible cause.

Stage 4 – alert

The patient is fully conscious but may well have difficulty in concentrating or making complex decisions. This fuzzy thinking normally resolves within 48 hours, but occasionally subtle changes in the patient's mental processes persist for months. This *postoperative cognitive disorder* is more likely in older people having major surgery.

How the patient views emergence

Hearing is the first sense to return. Voices are very loud, distorted and sometimes alarming. Louder noises, such as a telephone, can be frightening. Because their pupils are dilated, the lights seem unduly bright and vision is blurred. Their arms and legs feel heavy. Pain may be excruciating. Finally, their sense of locality and memory will return. The patient may feel disoriented, giddy and often asks: 'Where am I?'

What the patient worries about

In a study patients voted for the following outcomes that they preferred to avoid.[1] Ranked in order from worst to best they are:

- vomiting;
- gagging on an airway;
- pain;
- nausea;
- recall without pain;
- residual weakness;

- shivering;
- sore throat;
- being drowsy and unable to think coherently.

Ongoing care

Why give oxygen?

Some drugs depress breathing

Opioids such as fentanyl and morphine given during the anaesthetic depress the brainstem's sensors for carbon dioxide and may cause shallow or slow breathing.

Volatile anaesthetic agents, such as isoflurane, sevoflurane, and especially desflurane, depress oxygen-sensitive chemoreceptors so that they do not respond to falling oxygen levels in the blood. As a consequence the chemoreceptors will be unable to stimulate breathing.

Other reasons to give oxygen

Diffusion hypoxia occurs after general anaesthesia as nitrous oxide washes out of the blood into the lungs to displace air oxygen-containing air.

Shallow breathing, resulting in *hypoventilation*, causes carbon dioxide to build up in the lungs to displace oxygen containing air.

In patients who shiver or shake oxygen consumption may increase seven to tenfold. To supply oxygen to the shivering muscles the heart must increase its cardiac output substantially. If patients with heart disease are unable to meet the extra demand they will become hypoxic.

Patients who have had either spinal or epidural *neuroaxial blocks* have vasodilated extremities. Normally the heart maintains the blood pressure by pushing blood against the *resistance* to flow offered by arterioles. If the arterioles dilate, then the heart has to pump harder to keep the blood pressure up. A hard-working heart needs more oxygen.

How to give oxygen

Low-dose oxygen

Low-dose oxygen is given by facemask. Different types of mask deliver different concentrations of oxygen. At flow rates less than 4.5 litres a minute some *rebreathing* occurs. Rebreathing occurs when the patient inspires a portion of their expired air, as you would do if you breathed into and out of a paper bag.

High-dose oxygen

In an unintubated spontaneously breathing patient the only way to give high-dose oxygen is with a mask and reservoir bag. This will achieve an inspired oxygen concentration of about 85% ($FIO_2 = 0.85$). In the comatose patient high-dose oxygen can also be given through an endotracheal tube or a laryngeal mask.

Table 1.2 Oxygen masks

Flow rate (L/min)	FIO_2*
1	0.24
2	0.28
3	0.32
4	0.36
5	0.40
6	0.44
10	0.50

* These figures are approximate because different types of mask deliver different concentrations of oxygen at the same flow rates.

Signs of hypoxia

Hypoxaemia is defined as an arterial partial pressure of oxygen (PaO_2) less than 60 mmHg (7.89 kPa). An otherwise well person with an oximeter reading of 90% or less is hypoxaemic.

In contrast, *hypoxia* occurs when the tissues are so deprived of oxygen that they produce *lactic acid* from anaerobic metabolism. This can be measured, either as *pH* or lactic acid levels, or indirectly by checking the *anion gap*.

Table 1.3 Severe or critical hypoxia

Organ	Severe	Critical
Central nervous system	Agitation, restlessness, confusion	Seizures, coma
Cardiovascular	Hypertension, tachycardia, extrasystole	Hypotension, bradycardia
Skin	Cyanosis	Pallor, sweating
Urine output	10–30 ml/hr	< 10 ml/hr
Oxygen saturation	86–90%	< 85%

Types of masks

Most oxygen masks use a venturi principle to entrain air; these are known as are *high airflow oxygen entrainment masks* (HAFOE).

HAFOE masks will not deliver the intended oxygen concentration if the patient is breathing deeply. In this case, turn up the flow to 10–14 L/min. Use masks made of clear plastic so you can see the colour of the patient's lips and the fog that forms as the patient breathes. Coloured masks obscure cyanosis. Masks can be washed and used again, but melt if you autoclave them.

If the patient does not like wearing the oxygen mask cut off the top third, including the metal bar, with scissors. Do not use nasal prongs in the recovery room. Patients recovering from anaesthesia tend to breathe through their mouths.

Early hypoxia

Early hypoxaemia can be difficult to detect clinically, but usually patients have a rising pulse rate, a decreasing perfusion status, and are unable to concentrate.

Monitors save lives

In the recovery room, about half of the life-threatening situations that occur are picked up by monitors. Monitors allow you to follow trends in blood pressure, pulse, heart function and other parameters, but they can fail to alert you when things go wrong or give false alarms. The best monitors are attentive staff.

Treat the patient, not the monitor.

Blood pressure

When the patient is first admitted to recovery room, take the blood pressure and then take it at 5-minute intervals for the first 15 minutes and then every 10 minutes after that. If you have given a drug intravenously then measure the blood pressure immediately and then every 5 minutes for the next 10 minutes. Non-invasive blood pressure monitors (NBP) give inaccurate readings if the pulse is irregular, such as with *atrial fibrillation* (AF). Do not rely on a non-invasive blood pressure reading if the systolic blood pressure is greater than 160 mmHg, or less than 80 mmHg. If you are not happy with the initial NBP reading check the blood pressure with a manual blood pressure machine. Keep at least one manual blood pressure machine in the recovery room.

Stir-up exercises

Once patients are awake encourage them to do simple stir-up exercises. These exercises reduce the incidence of postoperative chest infections and deep vein thrombosis.

Deep breathing exercises

The aims of deep breathing exercises are to inflate segments of lung that inevitably collapse during general anaesthesia. Encourage the patient to take 2–3 very deep breaths every 5 minutes.

Coughing exercises

Coughing explosively clears the airways of mucus and dried secretions. Sit patients up if possible. If they have an abdominal wound then show them how to support their wound when they cough. Holding a small pillow to the site is helpful. Coughing exercises must not be done after open eye, middle ear, intracranial, facial or plastic surgery, otherwise the cough may disrupt the surgery.

Leg exercises

Leg exercises help prevent deep vein thrombi forming. Get patients to move their feet up and down (to pump their calves), and to bend their legs at the knees (flex their quadriceps) and rotate their feet at least 20 times as soon as they are awake. Patients who are at risk from thromboembolism need good-quality compression stockings fitted before their surgery.

Most deep vein thrombosis begin in the recovery room.

Pulse rate and rhythm

A normal pulse rate should be between 50–80 beats/min. Although a *tachycardia* is defined as a pulse rate greater than 100 beats/min, recovery room staff should be concerned if an adult's pulse rate rises above 80 beats/min.

Babies and infants have higher pulse rates than children and adults. In babies, infants and very old people it is easier to feel their hearts' apex beat than their peripheral pulses.

Record the pulse rate, rhythm and volume. If the pulse is irregular, suspect an arrhythmia. Attach an ECG. In young people, the most common cause of an irregular pulse is sinus arrhythmia where the pulse speeds up as they breathe in, and slows down when they breathe out: this is normal.

In older people the usual causes of an irregular pulse are atrial fibrillation or ventricular extrasystoles. If a patient develops ventricular extrasystoles it is a valuable early warning of cardiac ischaemia. The most common reasons for cardiac ischaemia are hypertension or tachycardia, or both.

Respiratory rate

The normal adult *respiratory rate* is between 12–14 breaths/min. Measure it by feeling the chest rise and fall under your hand, and not merely by watching the patient breathe. A rising respiratory rate is an excellent early warning sign of heart failure, developing *pulmonary oedema*, aspiration, sputum retention or rising temperature. After trauma or neurosurgery, a change in the rate or rhythm of breathing may be the first sign of a dangerous rise in intracranial pressure. The commonest cause of a slowing respiratory rate is that the patient has received an opioid.

A change in the respiratory rate or pattern means the physiological state of the patient has changed.

Temperature

The normal *core temperature* range is 36.5° to 37.2°C. Patients are often cold, so have warm blankets nearby. If their temperature is below 36°C then warm them with a forced air convection heater such as a BairHugger™, or a WarmTouch™. Advise the anaesthetist if the patient's temperature exceeds 37.5°C, or falls below 36°C.

Patterns of breathing

You can gain a lot of information by simply monitoring the patients' breathing. Expose their chest. Put your hand on the sternum and feel it rise and fall. If there is mucus in the airways you will feel vibrations in the affected area. Listen to the tidal air exchange at the mouth for wheezes suggesting bronchial oedema, and the crackles of alveolar oedema. Sometimes *dyspnoea* is confused with a particular breathing pattern.

Kussmaul's breathing

Sometimes called *air hunger*, Kussmaul's breathing indicates metabolic acidosis. The patient breathes deeply, and feels breathless.

Cheyne–Stoke breathing

It is easy to recognize Cheyne–Stoke breathing (*periodic breathing*). The patient takes a series of breaths, and then slows or stops only to start again. In head injured patients, or after neurosurgery periodic breathing is often a sign of rising intracranial pressure. Warn the anaesthetist immediately. Periodic breathing may occur in older patients who have received an opioid.

Pleuritic pain

Pleuritic pain occurs where the lung's pleura have been breached at surgery, or the patient has a pneumothorax. As they attempt to breathe in an intense stabbing pain stops them. To avoid the pain patients breathe in shallow pants, and stop abruptly with a grunt as they feel the pain.

See-saw breathing

Normally the chest and the abdomen rise and fall together. *See-saw* breathing occurs life threatening airway obstruction. While trying to breathe against the totally obstructed airway the patient's chest falls, as the abdomen rises. See-saw breathing is also known as *paradoxical breathing*. Young fit patients who try to breathe against a closed glottis may generate such violent swings of pressure in their lungs that they develop *pulmonary oedema*.

Obstructive and restrictive defects

Obstructive lung disease imposes a pattern of slow deep breathing; in contrast, restrictive lung disease imposes a pattern of rapid shallow breathing.

Pulse oximetry

Put a *pulse oximeter* on every patient. Normal readings are between 96 and 100%. If the reading falls to less than 92% then seek a cause. At a reading of 90% patients are hypoxaemic. Pulse oximeters do not work if the patient has poor circulation to their hands, or is wearing nail polish.

ECG

At the end of the surgery the anaesthetists may give you some rhythm strips from their monitors. This is especially likely if the patient's rhythm has altered during surgery. Paste the strips into the patient's record.

When the patient arrives in the recovery room attach an ECG monitor, especially to those at risk of cardiac arrhythmias or ischaemic heart disease. Write the initial cardiac rhythm in the recovery room chart. If the rhythm is abnormal, or is different from the cardiac rhythm recorded during the anaesthetic, then paste a sample of the rhythm strip taken from your monitor on the chart too. Remember to label, and put the date and time on each strip.

When to alert the anaesthetist

Most reasons to call for assistance are obvious, but here are some subtle signs that give early warning of developing problems.

Notify the anaesthetist if:

- A previously stable blood pressure starts to decrease by > 5 mmHg or more over each of three successive readings.
- A previously stable pulse rate rises to > 100 beats/min.
- Pulse becomes irregular.
- Respiratory rate increases or decreases by more than 4 breaths/min.
- Pattern of breathing changes.
- Urine output falls to less than 30 ml/hr.
- Patient starts to sweat.
- Capillary return in their nailbeds slows.
- Conscious state deteriorates.

Recovery room scoring systems

Most recovery rooms use scoring systems for assessing and monitoring their patients to make sure they are safe to discharge and are comfortable.

Many scoring systems have been published, some are more useful than others. Choose your scoring system carefully. Many are complex, some are confusing, and others misleading. With some scores the patient can be hypertensive, hypoxic and at grave risk of myocardial ischaemia, yet still be rated as 'fit for discharge' from the recovery room.

The score sheet below is simple. Each component can be used as a stand-alone module. For instance the sedation score can be used to grade sedation during investigative procedures. The scoring system assesses two separate issues: first, is the patient safe to discharge from the recovery room, and second, whether they are comfortable? Notify the anaesthetist of any patient who does not score at least 10 out of 12 points after 30 minutes.

Table 1.4 Safety criteria

	Task	Score
Respiration	Needs assistance with ventilation	0
	Laboured or > 20 or < 10 beats/min.	1
	Normal rate: 12–15 beats/min	2
O$_2$ sats	< 90% even with oxygen	0
	> 90% but requires oxygen to keep it there	1
	> 95% on room air	2
Power	Unable to lift head or move limbs on command	0
	Moves limbs but unable to sustain a 5-second head lift	1
	Sustains head lift for full 5-seconds	2
Circulation	BP ± 50% preoperative levels; or pulse > 120 or < 40	0
	BP and pulse ± 20% preoperative levels	1
	Stable blood pressure and pulse with no changes in previous two sets of readings taken at 15 minute intervals	2
Sedation	Does not respond to shaking by shoulder	0
	Rouses when shaken by shoulder	1
	Awake, or awakes easily when spoken to, communicates coherently and coughs on command	2
Temp	Core temp < 35.5°C	0
	Core temp 35.5–36.5°C	1
	Core temp > 36.5°C and < 37.8°C	2
		Score out of 12

Table 1.5 Comfort criteria

	Status	Score
Nausea	Nauseated and vomiting	0
	Nauseated only	1
	Neither nauseated nor vomiting	2
Pain	Severe distressing pain	0
	Uncomfortable	1
	Pain free	2
		Score out of 4

Discharge from recovery room

How long should patients stay in recovery room?

Stage 1 recovery

Patients stay in the recovery room while they are in Stage 1 recovery, unless they are transferred to the ICU.

Adults

As a rough guide adult patients stay in the recovery room for about an hour after general anaesthesia, and half an hour after local anaesthesia. Unstable patients stay longer, but once patients' vital signs are stable and their recovery room scores are satisfactory they can be discharged to Stage 2 recovery.

Children

Observe healthy children for at least 30 minutes if they have received inhalational anaesthesia by mask or laryngeal mask. If they have been intubated observe them for at least an hour. It may take this long for laryngeal oedema with its accompanying noisy breathing to become apparent.

Following tonsillectomy, adenoidectomy, cleft palate repair, pharyngeal or other major intra-oral procedures observe the patient for 90 minutes. Infants less than 12 months of age and those who have received naloxone are best observed for a minimum of two hours.

The anaesthetist, or a member of the medical staff, needs to review and certify in writing that their patient is fit to be discharged, and that some other member of the medical staff is properly briefed, and ready to take over responsibility for the patient's medical care.

Fast-track recovery

In their quest for efficiency, some hospitals encourage *fast-track recovery* in selected patients who meet recovery room discharge criteria at the end of their procedure. These patients are transferred directly from the operating theatre to *Stage 2 recovery*; or after day case procedures, directly home (*Stage 3 recovery*). There is strong evidence that fast-tracking patients does not reduce nursing workload after ambulatory surgery,[2] and we worry about its safety.

Discharge to Stage 2 recovery

1. Minimum criteria for discharge to Stage 2 recovery are:
   - the patient has a stable pulse rate, rhythm and blood pressure;
   - the patient is conscious and able to lift their head clear of the pillow for 5 seconds on demand;
   - patients are able to take a deep breath and cough;
   - oxygen saturation greater than 93%;
   - patients are able to touch the tip of their nose with their forefinger;
   - pain has been relieved;
   - there is no excessive loss from drains or bleeding from wound sites;
   - observation charts are completed;
   - the patient is clean, dry, warm and comfortable.
2. Remove all unnecessary intravenous lines and cannulas.
3. Remove ECG dots, and check the diathermy pad is not still attached.
4. Check that the medical and nursing staff have completed all the charts and notes and send them back to the ward with the patient.
5. Ensure the patient's recovery room record is complete. The ward staff need an accurate record to quickly identify any later deterioration.
6. Allow 30 minutes to elapse between the last dose of opioid analgesia and the patient's discharge from the recovery room.
7. Mandatory minimum stays in the recovery room are no longer necessary providing discharge criteria are met.

Local or regional anaesthesia

Patients recovering from local or regional anaesthesia need the same standard of care as those who have undergone general anaesthesia. Those patients still affected by spinal or epidural anaesthetic can be discharged to Stage 2 recovery provided all their other signs are stable. Patients with peripheral nerve block can be discharged home (Stage 3 recovery) even if full sensation has not returned, provided that they can walk steadily and meet the other discharge criteria.

How to handover to ward staff

The recovery room staff must be certain that the ward nurse understands the patient's medical problems, and current physical status, and is willing and competent to accept responsibility for the patient's care. Record the details of the handover on the patient's chart. Make sure that the ward staff have clear written instructions about infusion pump settings including drug doses.

How to transport patients to the ward

A nurse must accompany the patient when they return to the ward. Every trolley needs to carry portable oxygen and suction. Keep an emergency box containing a self-inflating resuscitation bag, airways and a range of masks on the trolley.

To prevent motion sickness, do not give your patients a fairground ride by swinging their head in a wide arc when turning corners on their way back to their ward. Sit them up at 45°. Wheel them forward with their feet first. When going around corners swing their feet and keep their heads as still as possible. This common-sense manoeuvre reduces subsequent vomiting in the ward by about 50 per cent.

Stage 3 recovery

Patients discharged home either from day case procedures; or after days or weeks in the ward remain in Stage 3 recovery. All patients remain in Stage 3 recovery until they no longer need the care of the hospital (including follow-up outpatient visits) and their welfare can be fully taken over by their family doctor or clinic. Even after going home patients can have complications as a result of the surgery or anaesthetic. These include deep vein thrombosis, pulmonary emboli, myocardial infarction, wound infection, and psychological problems.

Criteria for discharge to Stage 3 recovery

The patient must have had stable vital signs for at least one hour prior to discharge,[3] and be able to identify the time, place and relevant people.
As well as:

- Adequately controlled pain.
- Have no untoward nausea.
- Be adequately hydrated and able to drink without adverse consequences.
- Have minimal bleeding or wound drainage.

Note in the patient's record that discharge criteria have been met.

Day case procedures

Discharge from day case procedures

The patient must fulfil the criteria for discharge to Stage 3 recovery.
In addition the following points are relevant:[4]

- The patient must be discharged into the care of a competent and responsible adult, who will accompany them home, and be able to report any untoward events.

- The patient should not be alone that night.

- The patient must have written instructions about diet, medication, acceptable physical activities, and a phone number to call in case of difficulties or emergencies. Bear in mind that about 15 per cent of the adult population cannot read even the simplest instructions. Staff should verify that the unit has the correct telephone number and address for a follow-up phone call. Usually this phone call is made on the evening of the procedure, and again the following day.

- In most cases it is not necessary for patients to have passed urine before discharge, or demonstrated the ability to drink and retain clear fluids.

Discharge to the intensive care unit

After any operative procedure patients discharged to the intensive care unit, or a high dependency unit after remain in Extended Stage 1 recovery.

Care of patients who come from ICU

The immediate postoperative care of patients who have come from ICU for surgery should be a collaborative effort of the ICU nurses who already know the patient well, and the recovery room nurses who know their recovery room and its facilities, equipment and procedures well. The care of the patient comes first, and who does what and when must not become a demarcation dispute.

Boarders from ICU

In some hospitals critically ill patients are managed in the recovery room when there are bed or staff shortages in ICU. As a rule, it is better that the patient is cared for by the ICU's medical and nursing staff, rather than the recovery room staff. The standard of medical and nursing care and the monitoring and other facilities available must be the same as it would be if the patient was in the ICU. Your protocols should include a specific plan to discharge the patient to a more appropriate area as soon as possible.

How to discharge a patient to ICU

If the patient is going to the intensive care unit send for the bed, and check it has the following equipment with it:

- a full cylinder of oxygen with flow meter;
- a portable battery-powered ECG monitor and defibrillator;
- a pulse oximeter;
- suction;
- emergency drugs, syringes, and needles in a closed sealed carrying box;
- an anaesthetist, or member of the medical staff, to accompany patients returning to the intensive care unit.

Who needs to go to intensive care postoperatively?

In many cases patients who need emergency surgery are gravely ill. Because of the urgency of their surgical condition there may not have been time to fully assess medical illnesses, and optimize their vital signs before their anaesthetic. This is one reason emergency cases have higher morbidities and are more likely to die than elective patients.

Other patients who may need intensive care include those:

- who are already in ICU but are having an operative procedure, such as a tracheostomy;
- patients who were not fully assessed before their emergency surgery and have significant comorbidities;
- patients having uncomplicated surgery, but with severe intercurrent medical conditions, such as unstable diabetes, myasthenia gravis or unstable angina;
- patients having a major surgery, such as oesophago–gastrectomy, liver or pancreatic surgery or prolonged plastic reconstructive surgery;
- patients where it may be anticipated complications will arise, such as head injured multiple trauma patients who are unable to protect their airway.

Elective postoperative ICU admissions

Patients who will have postoperative difficulties whatever their surgery, for example, the morbidly obese.

Families visiting the recovery room

In the past, apart from mothers of young children, it was thought unwise to allow visitors see patients recovering from anaesthesia. It was believed that visitors might become distressed if they saw a loved one disoriented, vomiting or in pain. More recently some hospitals have modified their practice to allow one visitor to see the patient in the recovery room. In many cases this humane practice seems to help the emotional welfare of both the patient and the visitor. Before surgery, thoroughly brief the visitor and the patient about what to expect. If you decide to adopt this practice you will need guidelines on how to ensure the patient's confidentiality and privacy (and that of other patients in the recovery room).

Death in the recovery room

Sooner or later a patient will die in your recovery room. Have protocols in place to deal with this event. Guidelines should be in place about how to inform relatives, who is to be present at the interview, and where to hold the interview. It is most important that the most senior medical and nursing staff initially tell the relatives. It is most unfair and quite improper, to delegate this sad task to junior medical or nursing staff.

Telephone the patient's relatives to ask them to come to the hospital. It is unwise to tell them about the death over the phone; simply say there has been a problem. Suggest that they bring someone with them. It is better that a friend drives them to the hospital. Road accidents have occurred because distressed relatives' concentration on their driving has wandered, or they have driven too fast.

Litigation usually arises when relatives believe they are being deceived. Many legal problems can be avoided if this difficult duty is done in a humane, honest, sincere and sensible manner by the senior staff responsible for the patient's care.

Expected death

Occasionally, a patient who is expected to die following their surgery is brought into the recovery room. Care for the person in an area away from other patients. Out of respect and kindness, never let a patient die alone behind a closed curtain. Once the person has died make provision so that relatives can see the patient, and be consoled afterwards.

Unexpected death

Sometimes patients die unexpectedly despite the best care. After the death the recovery staff may be upset, especially if the patient was young, or the circumstances distressing. Some staff may need counselling, especially if they feel that more could have been done to save the patient's life.

There are also legal responsibilities. If a patient dies, nothing should be touched. A death in the recovery room must be reported to the coroner and evidence must be preserved for the coroner's inquest. Each country or state has its own requirements and these must be included in your hospital's protocol for death in the recovery room. Drips must remain attached, and endotracheal tubes left where they are. All drug ampoules must be kept, and the area quarantined until an investigation is complete. Carefully document the events leading up to the death because these notes may be required in the coroner's court. They must be detailed enough to record events in a way that does not rely on memory even years later.

Notes

1. Macario A, Weinger S, Carney S *et al.* (1999) *Anesthesia and Analgesia* 89:652–8.
2. Song D, Chung F, Ronayne M *et al.* (2004) *British Journal of Anaesthesia* 93:768–74.
3. *Recommendations for the perioperative care of patients selected for day care surgery*, PS I5 Australian and New Zealand College of Anaesthetists Professional Standards 2006.
4. Marhsall SI, Chung F (1999) *Anesthesia and Analgesia* 88:505–17.

2
Recovery room procedures

Airway protection

- Airway control is an essential recovery room skill. Everyone caring for unconscious patients must be confident they can maintain the patient's airway, and recognize airway emergencies.
- Your most important tool is a high-capacity sucker, switched on and tucked under the patient's pillow where you can find it instantly.
- Have special trolleys (carts) ready and waiting for respiratory and other emergencies.
- Wherever possible nurse patients in the recovery position. Even conscious patients are safer in this position.

Those that look to heaven go to heaven.

Airways

Oropharyngeal airways

Oropharyngeal airways (*Guedel airways*) are inserted to stop patients clenching their teeth and obstructing their airflow.

- If an airway is in place, then leave it there, and allow the patient to either spit it out or remove it.
- In the elderly, especially if they have no teeth, try using a smaller rather than a larger size to maintain the airway.

Table 2.1 Airway sizes

Airway size	Indication
Size 4	For huge men
Size 3	For adult men
Size 2	For women, and men without teeth, and for children down to the age of 18 months
Size 1	For children under the age of 18 months
Size 0	Small for neonates
Size 00	Tiny

Nasopharyngeal airways

Have a range of nasopharyngeal airways available. They are useful in those adults whose airways are difficult to maintain. Size 5, 6 and 7 will cover most needs.

Commercially available nasopharyngeal airways are made of soft plastic with a flange to prevent them slipping in too far. They can, however, be made by cutting a 15 cm length of blue polyvinyl chloride endotracheal tube. Push a safety pin through the outer end so that the tube cannot disappear into the nose. Lubricate well and insert by pushing them gently straight back, parallel with the floor of the nose. Do not push them upwards.

Commercial   Improvized

Figure 2.1 Nasopharyngeal airways

Laryngeal mask airways

It is far easier to maintain an airway with a *laryngeal mask airway* (LMA) than with a normal rubber face-mask. Inserted through the mouth, laryngeal mask airways fit like a hood over the larynx. Inflating the cuff creates a loose seal in the pharynx to prevent air escaping.

Oesophagus

Trachea

Figure 2.2 Laryngeal mask

Advantages of laryngeal masks are that they:

- maintain a good airway, even in those who are difficult to intubate;
- are easy to use;
- do not traumatize or irritate the upper airway;
- are less likely to cause sore throats, coughing or bucking than an endotracheal tube;
- can be used to measure respiratory rate, minute ventilation and end tidal CO_2 levels;
- do not require muscle relaxants to insert;
- can be used again after they are cleaned;
- can aid to subsequent intubation by becoming a pathway for a bougie, endotracheal tube or fiberoptic bronchoscope;
- are used for the 'can't intubate, can't ventilate' protocol.

Disadvantages of laryngeal masks are that they:

- require constant skilled supervision;
- do not protect the airway when stomach contents are vomited or regurgitated;
- if you attempt to ventilate a patient through them they may fill the stomach with gas under tension;
- are unsuitable for fat patients, who frequently have hiatus hernias, and may regurgitate gastric contents;
- are unsuitable for patients with high airway resistance such as asthmatics or those with bronchospasm;
- are sometimes impossible to insert, do not sit properly in place, or they fail to preserve the airway;
- do not prevent regurgitation and must only be used in fasted patients.

Table 2.2 Laryngeal mask sizes

Size	Indication	Cuff inflation
Size 1	Neonate	2–4 ml
Size 2	Small child	10 ml
Size 2.5	Large child	15 ml
Size 3	Small adult	20 ml
Size 5	Large adult	30 ml

Hints

- Laryngeal masks can be left in place while patients are transferred from the operating theatre to the recovery room.
- Leave the cuff inflated unless the anaesthetist orders otherwise.
- Wait for patients to take out their own laryngeal masks.
- Use a 20 ml syringe to inflate and deflate the cuff.
- Patients emerging from anaesthesia are likely to clamp their jaws shut, biting the laryngeal mask and obstructing it. Support their airway by holding up their chin during this episode – it does not usually last long. If the patient is really struggling insert a nasal airway. This will sit behind the mask in the pharynx and allow oxygen to reach the lungs.
- Do not tie laryngeal mask airways in place because you must be able to remove them instantly if the patient vomits or regurgitates.
- Where practical recover patients lying in the recovery position.
- To give oxygen, attach a light T-Bag® to the mask.
- If they cough or gag on the laryngeal mask airway remove it. Do not deflate the cuff, because as your pull it out the inflated cuff will drag most of the mucus and secretions with it.
- Be careful not to rip the laryngeal mask on the patient's teeth.

Laryngeal masks do not sit well in babies, probably because they have short fat necks, and not much room in their pharynx. If the LMA keeps riding up, take it out and replace it with a Guedel airway.

How to clean and sterilize laryngeal masks

Put the dirty laryngeal mask straight into a bowl or jug of water. Dried secretions are difficult to wash off.

Soak the mask thoroughly in soapy water. Use a bottle brush to gently clean the lumen and rinse it thoroughly in clean water.

Do not use glutaraldehyde (Cidex®), formaldehyde or ethylene oxide.

Laryngeal masks may be autoclaved at low pressures and temperatures. Do not use the high-pressure high-temperature autoclave. To prevent the cuff from bursting as it is heated, deflate the mask almost completely before autoclaving.

Gas delivery circuits

T-Bag®

T-Bags are light disposable devices that are easily attached to endotracheal tubes or laryngeal mask airways. T-Bags® reliably give an oxygen supply of 70% at 6 L/min flow rate, and 50% at 3 L/min with no rebreathing of expired air.

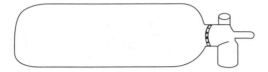

Figure 2.3 T-Bag

They are superior to T-piece circuits and outperform Hudson and other forms of high airflow entrainment masks.

Figure 2.4 Mapleson C circuit

Mapelson circuit

The Mapleson C circuit is frequently used in the recovery room to ventilate patients and to administer high concentrations of oxygen. Use fresh gas flows. In spontaneously breathing patients the Mapelson C circuit causes unacceptable rebreathing with CO_2 retention. If you do use it on a spontaneously breathing patient remove the bag, leave the corrugated tubing attached to the valve and turn up the fresh oxygen supply to 8 L/min. This converts the circuit into a useful T-piece type extension.

Do not use a Mapelson C circuit on a spontaneously breathing patient.

Self-inflating resuscitation bags

Self inflating resuscitation bags are portable and robust. The most commonly used are the Ambu® and the Laerdal Bag®. These bags are not easy to use; you may need to practice under supervision until you feel competent. They have a volume of about 1600 ml, but even with the biggest squeeze the maximum tidal volume you can deliver is about 1000 ml. Because they are self-inflating they automatically resume their shape after they have been squeezed, and do not depend on an oxygen or compressed gas supply.

If necessary they can deliver higher concentrations of oxygen by connecting them to an oxygen line. Attach a reservoir bag to increase the oxygen concentration of the inspired gas. Turn the oxygen on to a full flow of 10–15 L/min, using a flow less than this is no better than using room air.

Figure 2.5 Laerdal resuscitation bag

Practical summary of emergency airway care

1. Get help!
2. Keep a high-capacity sucker under the pillow.
3. Suck out the pharynx.
4. For laryngospasm consider 1.5 ml/Kg lidocaine IV.
5. Always try bag and mask ventilation first.
6. If you can't bag mask ventilate then insert a laryngeal mask.
7. If you still can't ventilate then prepare to intubate.
8. If you can't intubate and you can't ventilate then prepare to insert a cricothyroid airway.

Intubation

Intubation in the recovery room is always an emergency. As soon as you hear the possibility mentioned bring your intubation trolley to the bedside.

On the trolley

Keep the intubation trolley (cart) stocked and ready to wheel to a patient's side. Use the top shelf as a working area. On the bottom shelf keep everything you need for emergency airway management: laryngeal masks, cricothyroid puncture set, emergency tracheostomy kit, guide wires, bougies, and at least two spare working laryngoscopes.

Endotracheal tubes

Clear plastic tubes are preferable. You will need a range of sizes for different ages. Sizes are measured on their internal diameter. Children under the age of 10 usually do not require cuffed tubes, however above this age cuffs are needed for a good gas seal, and to prevent fluid entering the lower airways.

$$\text{The distance from the teeth to the midpoint of the trachea} = \frac{\text{height(cm)} + 2}{10}$$

add 3 cm to allow space to tie or fix the tube.

In the larger tubes a *Murphy eye*, which is a second hole near the distal end of the tube, prevents occlusion if the tip becomes obstructed.

Check the tubes you buy are non-irritant. They should have either 'IT' or 'Z 79' printed on the side of the tube. Use well-made tight-fitting plastic 15 mm connectors.

How to intubate a patient

You will learn more about the intubation by seeing it done by an anaesthetist than you will from reading books.

How to prepare the equipment

Connect an Air-Viva™ or black Mapelson's C circuit to the oxygen supply (most anaesthetists prefer the Magill circuit). Have a selection of oropharyngeal tubes, nasopharyngeal airways and masks nearby. Assemble at least two endotracheal tubes (ETT), one the expected size, and the other a size smaller. Men take 8.5–9 mm endotracheal tubes, and women size 7–8 mm.

Take an endotracheal tube and inflate the cuff with a 10 ml syringe to make sure it has no leaks. Keep your fingers away from its sterile end. Squeeze a glob of water-soluble lubricant such as KY-jelly™ on to a sterile gauze swab. Smear the endotracheal tube's cuff with jelly and put it in a sterile intubation tray where you can reach it later.

Check that all the equipment you need is on the close at hand:

- The patient is on a trolley that can be tipped quickly head down.
- A low pillow under the patient's head.
- A Yankauer sucker under the pillow, hissing and ready to use.
- A laryngoscope with a bright white light to inspect the larynx and vocal cords.

- A 10 ml syringe to blow up the cuff on the endotracheal tube.
- White cotton tracheostomy tape to secure the endotracheal tube.
- Magill forceps to remove chunks of matter in the airway or manipulate the endotracheal tube. Their handles curve out of the way so you can see what is happening at the tips.
- A lubricated gum-elastic *bougie* to railroad the tube along should there be any difficulty in getting the tip through the vocal cords.
- End-tidal CO_2 monitor to connect to confirm the tube is in the trachea.
- An intravenous infusion with warmed 0.9% *saline*.

Draw up the drugs and label the contents. Most anaesthetists prefer to do this for themselves. Do not throw away any ampoules; put them to one side. The usual drugs are an induction agent such as propofol, an ultra-brief muscle relaxant (succinyl choline or mivacurium), and a longer-acting muscle relaxant such as rocuronium. Other drugs the anaesthetist might need include atropine, midazolam, lignocaine, and ephedrine.

The anaesthetist preoxygenates, sedates and paralyses the patient. It takes three pairs of hands: the anaesthetist to do the intubation, a nurse or technician to apply cricoid pressure, and you to hand the anaesthetist the required equipment in the correct sequence.

Cricoid pressure

Cricoid pressure reduces the likelihood of aspiration of gastric contents into the airway. A nurse or technician applies cricoid pressure with one hand behind the patient's neck, and thumb and two fingers of the other hand firmly

Thumb and forefinger on
either side of the cricoid cartilage

Left hand supporting the
back of the neck

Figure 2.6 How to apply cricoid pressure

pushing the cricoid cartilage backwards so that nothing can come up the oesophagus into the pharynx. It must not be released until the anaesthetist says it is safe to do so. Accidents have happened because assistants have released cricoid pressure prematurely. The best way to avoid any chance of misunderstanding is for the anaesthetist to actually push the assistant's hand away once everything is secure.

How the head is positioned

The best position to view the larynx is with the neck gently extended and the face thrust forward into the 'sniffing the morning air' (or 'What's that awful smell?') position.

How to hand things to the anaesthetist

Offer the anaesthetist the laryngoscope in a clean kidney dish. The anaesthetist will open the blade, place it in the patient's mouth and sweep the tongue away to the left giving a clear view of the larynx.

Have the hissing Yankeur sucker ready for the anaesthetist to grab from your hand to suck out the pharynx. Have the lubricated endotracheal tube with the 10 ml syringe full of air already attached in the kidney dish ready to hand to the anaesthetist.

The intubation

The anaesthetist slides the tip of the laryngoscope blade along the tongue (A) and into the little valley between the epiglottis and the anterior pharyngeal wall. This flips up the epiglottis improving the view of the laryngeal opening.

The anaesthetist then pulls the handle of the laryngoscope moving the bottom jaw straight out (B) to reveal the vocal cords as a little white V with the

Figure 2.7 Positioning the laryngoscope

trachea disappearing like a tunnel beyond. The lubricated endotracheal tube is then slipped between the cords. To improve the view the anaesthetist may ask you to "pull the corner of the mouth down". To do this, put your gloved finger inside right side of the patient's mouth. Pull the cheek outwards and downward towards you. The person doing the cricoid pressure may be asked to move the larynx in a particular direction – usually either to the patient's right or left side.

To finish up

Once the tube is in place, hand the anaesthetist the catheter mount ('liquorice-stick') to connect the patient to the Air-Viva or Magill circuit. Not all anaesthetists will use this but have it available. Inflate the cuff and adjust the amount of air in the cuff until the leak just disappears. This usually takes 4–8 ml of air. Connect the endotracheal tube and the CO_2 monitor.

Hand the white tape to the anaesthetist who will use a clove hitch knot to secure the tape to the tube, being careful not to capture the pilot tube going to the cuff. Pass one end of the tape under the patient's neck.

Next the anaesthetist checks air entry into both sides of the lungs with a stethoscope. Note in the patient's record the size of the endotracheal tube, its length at the incisors (it should be between 19–21 cm and up to 24 cm for very tall people).

Never tape or tie a nasogastric tube to the endotracheal tube, because if something snags on the drainage bag it will dislodge the tube.

How to manage an intubated patient

About 5% of patients are still intubated when they come to the recovery room. Usually this is because they have *failed to breathe* adequately at the end of their anaesthetic and cannot be extubated safely at that time. Delayed extubation is more likely with prolonged operations, where the patient is hypothermic, in those with respiratory disease, in elderly patients and in sicker patients, or where the muscle relaxants have not yet reversed adequately. In this case, patients need to be ventilated until the muscle relaxant has worn off. Some patients may need to go to intensive care for further respiratory support, but in most cases the anaesthetist will extubate the patient later.

Is it safe to extubate your patient?

It is always the anaesthetist's responsibility to extubate their patient.[1] Before it is safe to extubate a patient they must fulfil three criteria:

1. They must be able to breathe adequately.
2. They must not be depressed by opioid or sedative drugs.

3. They must be able to able to protect their own airway against aspiration of material in their pharynx.

Can the patient breathe adequately?

It is unsafe to extubate patients who have sputum in their airways or whose oxygen saturation is below 93%. They must be able to take deep breaths on command through their endotracheal tube. If you are uncertain whether their tidal volume is adequate, then measure it with a respirometer. Before extubation the tidal volume needs to be 4–7 ml/Kg (about 500 ml) and the respiratory rate greater than 10 breaths/min. If you do not have a respirometer, then prime an anaesthetic machine with oxygen and attach it to the patient. When the patient takes a deep breath the black reservoir bag should deflate by more than 12 ml/Kg. This volume is about 800 ml for a normal adult. Gauge the volume with that of your fist. The volume of an adult's clenched fist is 350–400 ml.

Ten steps in extubation

1. Put the patient on high oxygen concentrations for 3 minutes before proceeding. Attach a *pulse oximeter*.

2. Check the larynx with a laryngoscope to make sure no foreign material is present, for example a throat pack, blood, or mucus.

3. Under direct vision gently suck out the pharynx. Check the nasopharynx up behind the soft palate is clear too.

4. Lay the patients preferably on their left side.

5. Remove the ties and tape securing the endotracheal tube and deflate the cuff slowly with a 10 ml syringe. Disconnect the catheter mount.

6. Pass a soft suction catheter down the tube. While applying suction ask the patient to take a big breath in. At the end of inspiration with one smooth movement, withdraw the tube and catheter together.

7. Give the patient oxygen at a flow of 6 L/min through a face mask.

8. Encourage a few deep breaths and cough.

9. Check the oxygen saturation.

10. Watch for signs of postoperative hypoxia or hypercarbia.

Coughing

Coughing sharply raises the blood pressure, intracranial pressure and intra-ocular pressure, causing venous congestion in the head and neck. Vigorous coughing can fracture ribs in the elderly, or disrupt surgical stitches.

Coughing is the commonest cause of a raised intracranial pressure. Following neurosurgery, it is critically important that patients' intracranial pressure does not rise. It may cause catastrophic intracranial bleeding. Those with a spiking pattern on their intracranial pressure trace are especially at risk.

After open eye surgery coughing raises the intra-ocular pressure, and can detach retinas and/or dislocate lenses. Any of these events may cause irreversible blindness.

How to prevent coughing

In neurosurgical cases, the anaesthetist usually gives a small dose of a short-acting muscle relaxant with a short-acting opioid or other sedative to prevent coughing or the *reflex* rise in blood pressure and pulse rate that occurs while sucking out the patient.

In other cases you can prevent endotracheal suction causing the blood pressure to rise, or the patient coughing by giving 3–5 ml of 1% lidocaine intravenously Before doing this check with the anaesthetist that it is appropriate.

How to prevent hypoxaemia

During tracheobronchial suction it is easy to overlook how quickly your patient can become hypoxaemic. Older patients, especially those with heart disease or unstable circulations, are more likely to have arrhythmias or become hypoxic. One excellent technique for timing suction is to exhale air from your own lungs, and then hold your breath. Now start sucking out your patient. After 15–20 seconds (about two passes) when you start to feel uncomfortable it is time to withdraw the catheter, and give your patient two minutes of 100% oxygen, and a chance to recover. Never allow your patient to strain and cough.

Note

1. Immediate Postanaesthetic Recovery (2002) *Position statement of a working party of the Association of Anaesthetists of Great Britain and Ireland.*

3

Monitoring and equipment

The best monitor in the recovery room
is an observant, informed and vigilant nurse.

Monitors warn of approaching problems, but they are not a substitute for carefully observing your patient. Do not automatically assume monitors give you accurate information. If you are concerned that the monitor is misleading you, then reassess the patient's condition: their colour, pulse rate, perfusion, and breathing. Measure their blood pressure manually and take their temperature.

Treat the patient, not the monitor.

Much modern equipment is so complex that it may confuse the most competent staff. Staff need to understand their monitoring equipment, know its limitations, and especially what can go wrong with it. Although well-designed monitors are intended to be used intuitively, it is easy to get lost in their hierarchical menus. It is worthwhile having a continuing education programme for newcomers, and to refresh the memory of more experienced staff. Keep the instruction manuals nearby.

Recovery room monitors should be compatible, and if necessary interchangeable, with the monitors used in the operating theatres.

For most otherwise healthy patients undergoing minor elective surgery a pulse oximeter, blood pressure monitoring and a record of temperature, pulse and breathing are all you need.

Routine monitoring

Making routine observations and collecting data helps you establish trends to assess whether your patient is improving, is stable, or is deteriorating. The data gives you an objective assessment – things that you can measure – of your patient's response to treatment.

All patients need certain parameters measured and recorded regularly. These involve:

- conscious state;
- pulse rate;
- blood pressure;

- perfusion status;
- oxygen saturation;
- respiratory rate;
- temperature.

Record the data at 5-minute intervals for 15 minutes; then if your patient remains stable every 10 to 15 minutes thereafter until the patient returns to the ward.

With sicker or unstable patients, the nurse, the surgeon and the anaesthetist should review their progress and make a comprehensive management plan for the following 24 hours before you discharge patients to the ward. This plan might include transferring the patient to the ICU or a high dependency unit.

Additional monitoring

Sicker or unstable patients, or those who have had long or physiologically stressful surgery need additional monitoring that may include:

- ECG;
- intra-arterial blood pressures;
- central venous pressures;
- pulmonary artery and wedge pressures;
- urine output;
- volume and nature of wound drainage;
- haematology;
- chemical pathology;
- blood gas estimation.

If your patient's observations deviate from the defined limits set by the surgical team, then seek help immediately. If in doubt, then play it safe: ask a senior colleague or the anaesthetist to review the patient and go over the data with you.

Pulse oximetry

Pulse oximeters are the most useful monitors in the recovery room. Correctly used on well-perfused skin they are reliable and accurate.

Pulse oximeters give an early warning of *hypoxaemia*. The device consists of a light-emitting diode and a photo detector applied to a fingertip or ear lobe. They measure the differential absorption by haemoglobin of two wavelengths of *pulsed* light: red and infrared, and then calculate the proportion of oxygen

Table 3.1 The saturation meter and its correlation with PaO$_2$

Oxygen saturation	PaO$_2$ at pH 7.25	PaO$_2$ at pH 7.40	PaO$_2$ at pH 7.55
60	36 < critical level	31	24
70	44	37 < critical level	28
80	53	45	34
81	55	46	35
82	56	48	36 < critical level
83	58	49	37
84	59	50	38
85	61 < danger level	52	39
86	63	53	40
87	65	55	41
88	67	57	43
89	69	59	45
90	72	61 < danger level	47
91	75	64	49
92	79	67	51
93	83	70	54
94	88	75	57
95	94	80	61 < danger level
96	102	87	66
97	113	96	73
98	129	109	83
99	157	134	101
100	241	204	155

Figures are calculated from Kelman modification of the Hill Equation for the oxygen dissociation curve.

saturated haemoglobin (SaO$_2$) in the capillaries, and display the result as a percentage on a screen.

Table 3.1 shows that, under some circumstances, a patient can be hypoxic with an oxygen saturation of over 90%. Hypoxia also depends on the pH of the blood.

Normal arterial blood is more than 97% saturated with oxygen. If the saturations fall to 90% or less, then the patient is hypoxaemic. Use an oximeter on every patient until they are fully awake, and have a consistent SaO$_2$ over 96%.

Table 3.2 Oxygen saturations

Status	Oxygen saturation
Normal	> 96%
Abnormal	< 96%
Hypoxaemia	< 90%

Do not discharge patients to the ward if their oxygen saturations are less than 95% without discussing it with the anaesthetist. If your patients have a persistently low oxygen saturation they need oxygen by mask during transport to the ward, and mandatory oxygen supplements in the ward.

You can use the pulse oximeter readings to estimate the arterial PaO_2, but to do this you must know the patient's *pH*. pH is a measure of hydrogen ion activity. Excessive hydrogen ion activity distorts the shape of haemoglobin, altering its ability to take up and release oxygen, and in so doing determines the pressure (PO_2) at which oxygen is pushed into the tissues.

Figure 3.1 Haemoglobin oxygen dissociation curve

You need to understand the graph in Figure 3.1 if you are to make sense of how oxygen gets into the tissues. The graph matches the haemoglobin's saturation with oxygen (on the vertical axis) to the pressure it exerts as it attempts to leave the haemoglobin (on the horizontal axis). For example if haemoglobin is 90% full of oxygen, the push oxygen exerts as it leaves the haemoglobin is about 60 mmHg (7.9 kPa). For oxygen to get into, and be used by the cells, it has to be delivered both in sufficient quantity and with enough pressure. The partial pressure of oxygen in capillaries provides the force to drive oxygen from the red cells into the tissues, then on through the cell membrane, through the cell's cytoplasm and into its mitochondria.

The shape of the curve changes with the pH of the blood, and the patient's temperature. Patients in recovery room are often moderately acidotic and hypothermic. Acidosis causes the arterial PaO_2 to be higher than normal at a given haemoglobin oxygen saturation. This is a good thing, as the extra pressure increases tissue oxygenation. On the other hand hypothermia decreases tissue oxygenation, but also reduces the tissue's oxygen consumption.

Once the saturation falls to 90% the signs and symptoms of hypoxia accelerate. A PaO_2 less than 60 mm Hg (7.9 kPa) is dangerous, and a PaO_2 less than 35 mmHg (4.6 kPa) is potentially lethal even in healthy people.

Purchasing a pulse oximeter

Points to check when purchasing a pulse oximeter:

- size, weight and portability;
- power: mains power or rechargeable batteries;
- display: easy to see from all angles and in all lights;
- alarms: easy to set;
- probes: robust, easy to repair or cheap to replace;
- finger probes: come in various sizes;
- ear probes are useful for babies and patients who are cold or have poor circulation.

Blood pressure

Physiology

Blood pressure is the force per unit area that the blood exerts on the vessel wall at right angles to direction of the flow. Arterial blood pressures are measured in millimetres of mercury (mmHg). Venous pressures are usually measured against column of water in centimetres of water (cm H_2O). Since pressure varies with the depth of the fluid, blood pressures are measured against a reference point called the *isophlebotic point*, which is at the same level as the right atrium. In a supine patient the isophlebotic point is located where the fourth intercostal space crosses the midaxillary line.

Blood pressure is maintained by a balance between the volume of blood ejected by the heart with each beat (*stroke volume*) and the *impedance* (resistance) the arterioles impose to blood flowing through the vascular bed.

Table 3.3 Normal blood pressures

Normal values of blood pressures	
Central venous pressure	0–7 mmHg
Pulmonary artery pressures	14–32 mmHg systolic 4–13 mmHg diastolic 8–19 mmHg mean
Wedge pressure	6–12 mmHg
Cardiac output	70–100 ml/Kg
Cardiac index	2.5–3.6 litres/min/m2
Pulmonary vascular resistance	700–1500 dyne-sec/cm5 77–150 kPa-sec/cm5
Systemic vascular resistance	20–120 dyne-sec/cm5 2–12 kPa-sec/cm5
Oxygen consumption	3.5 ml/Kg/min

By convention, we measure the peak or *systolic blood pressure* (when the heart contracts), and the trough or *diastolic blood pressure* (when the heart relaxes), however it is the *mean arterial blood pressure* (MAP) that determines tissue blood flow. For this reason, in the near future we will probably only record mean blood pressure.

As an approximation:

$$MAP = \text{systolic pressure} + \left(\frac{2 \times \text{diastolic pressure}}{3} \right)$$

Clinical aspects of blood pressure

Blood pressure (BP) is an important measure of a patient's physiological well-being. Blood pressure can be measured *non-invasively* with;

- a mercury sphygmomanometer;
- an anaeroid clock face device,
- an automated oscillotonometer; or *invasively* with an intra-arterial cannula attached to an electronic *transducer*.

Non-invasive blood pressure monitoring

Because blood pressure is such an important physiological parameter you must measure and record it accurately. The *gold standard* way to measure blood pressure in the recovery room is manually with a mercury-filled sphygmomanometer.

Anaeroid devices, unless calibrated regularly, are prone to lose their calibration and may become wildly inaccurate before anyone realizes it.

Non-invasive automated oscillotonometers are unreliable under certain circumstances.

Check the patient's first blood pressure reading manually, preferably with a mercury sphygmomanometer. This reading becomes your baseline measurement to use as a standard against which to gauge subsequent measurements by the automated device.

Manual blood pressure monitors

Mercury-filled sphygmomanometers

In most recovery rooms, the mercury sphygmomanometer is mounted securely to the wall. Choose a sphygmomanometer with an easy to read bright scale. Measure the blood pressure with the monitor at eye level to prevent parallax errors.

Unfortunately, staff often measure manual blood pressures inaccurately, either because they do not know how to use them correctly or their manometers are faulty.[1]

It takes some skill to get consistent results with a sphygmomanometer or an anaeroid device, so let us go step by step through the technique. Select the appropriate cuff size. Warn your patients what you are about to do. Check that their radial pulse is regular. Then with your finger on the radial pulse, quickly inflate the cuff to above the expected systolic pressure. Let the cuff deflate gradually.

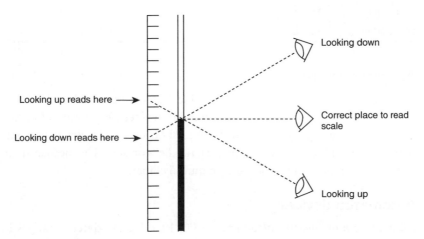

Looking down

Looking up reads here →

Correct place to read scale

Looking down reads here →

Looking up

Figure 3.2 The position of a mercury blood pressure machine may cause errors in the readings

Note the pressure at which the pulse returns. Now, having found the approximate systolic pressure, reinflate the cuff to above the previous reading. Listen with the diaphragm (but not the bell) of your stethoscope over the brachial artery in the cubital fossa. Deflate the cuff by no more than 5 mmHg per second. The systolic pressure is the point where you hear the first pulse. The diastolic pressure is the point where the sounds disappear completely (and not where they become muffled). Conventionally systolic pressures are measured to the nearest 5 mmHg, and diastolic pressures to the nearest 2 mmHg. The most common error is to allow the pressure in the cuff to plummet rapidly so that you miss the actual blood pressure between hearing adjacent beats.

Check the blood pressure in both arms if the patient is elderly, has vascular disease or diabetes because *pseudo hypertension* may deceive you. Here the cuff cannot compress the rigid calcified arterial walls to occlude blood flow, so that you can still feel the pulse even though the cuff is above systolic pressure.

Different sized cuffs are available: larger ones for obese adults and smaller ones for children. The best are wrap-around cotton ones. A local tailor can make replacements. The cloth cover should be 20% wider and longer than the rubber bladder. The inner rubber bladders perish quickly in the tropics. Keep a supply in an airtight container in a cool place.

Table 3.4 What is the correct cuff size?

	Cuff width (cm)	Cuff length (cm)	Arm circumference (cm)
Child	8–10	20–24	Up to 25
Adult	12–13	24	Up to 33
Large adult	13–15	35	Up to 38
Obese adult	15–18	35	Up to 42

Anaeroid devices

Anaeroid clock face devices are fairly reliable, but lose their calibration if they are not maintained regularly. These manual devices need to be calibrated against a mercury sphygmomanometer at least once a month. Before you start to measure the blood pressure, ensure the needle is on zero. The mechanism in some makes of anaeroid device rusts in humid climates.

Automated devices

Automated non-invasive blood pressure (NBP) devices detect changes in the pressure-wave form as it oscillates between systolic and diastolic pressure.

The result is fed into a microprocessor that calculates and displays the systolic, mean and diastolic blood pressures on a screen. The devices are popular because they measure blood pressure at regular intervals and give warnings if the blood pressure rises or falls beyond set limits, and free up staff to attend to other duties.

An NBP monitor is useful in most situations. Once the systolic blood pressure falls below 80–90 mmHg, these devices become unreliable. If they constantly recycle check the blood pressure manually. They are also likely to give misleading results if the pulse is irregular, patients are moving their arms about or the wrong-sized cuff is used. The mean pressure is most accurate. Wrinkled cuffs may bruise the skin. Repeated cycling can damage nerves or even cause ischaemic injury to the arm, especially in diabetics and those patients with vascular disease.

Invasive blood pressure monitoring

Arterial monitoring is used for haemodynamically unstable patients, or where infusions of vasoactive drugs are needed to control the blood pressure.

Invasive blood pressure (IBP) monitoring involves inserting a small cannula into an artery (usually the radial) and connecting it to a *transducer* with a plastic catheter. The signal is processed and the systolic and diastolic pressure, as well as the waveform, are displayed on a screen.

Check at least the first few readings with a manual blood pressure device.

One might assume that intra-arterial monitors measure blood pressure accurately, but if the fluid dynamics of the set-up are not properly balanced they are prone to errors of up to 70% or more. To avoid these errors, follow the manufacturer's recommendations and use properly matched catheters and cannulas, otherwise the pressure wave will not be faithfully transmitted to the transducer. Damping problems occur when pressure waves ricochet willy-nilly around inside the tubing (an *under-damped signal*) or are cushioned by pliant or excessively long tubing (an *over-damped signal*).

Keep the cannula patent by flushing it with one ml of 0.9% saline when your patient is first admitted to the recovery room. Usually a special valve trickles in saline at 3 ml per hour from a filled bag pressurized to 300 mmHg. Do not add heparin to the saline because it may cause *heparin-induced thrombocytopenia* (HITs).

Do not disturb the dressings around the arterial cannula. If a cannula accidentally falls out, then press firmly over the site with a gauze pad for at least 5 minutes. Arterial bleeding does not stop as readily a venous bleeding. Mark the arterial lines with red marker tags at both ends, and in the middle to ensure that so that drugs are not inadvertently injected into them.

Radial artery thrombosis after an arterial line occurs 2–15% of cases. To prevent this complication use arterial lines for as short a time as possible, especially if you are giving vasoconstricting drugs.

If your patient has an arrhythmia, then check the blood pressure manually.

Central venous pressure

Central venous pressure (CVP) is the pressure of the blood in the vena cava at the entrance to the right atrium. Central venous lines (CVL) are often used in acutely ill patients coming to surgery.

They are used:

- for measuring central venous pressure;
- as a guide to intravenous fluid therapy;
- for giving drugs that would injure peripheral veins; for example, adrenaline and nor adrenaline infusions, parenteral nutrition fluids, and 50% dextrose;
- to assess how effectively the heart is pumping.

The catheters are radio-opaque and about 20 cm long. There are single lumen and multiple lumen catheters available. With multi-lumen catheters, each lumen opens at a different point along the catheter: distal (at the tip of the catheter), medial (in the middle) and proximal (just inside the vein). In most multi-lumen catheters the distal lumen (brown port) has a wider bore for giving high volumes, viscous fluids, colloids or for measuring the central venous pressure. The middle lumen (blue port) is used for giving intravenous drugs, or parenteral nutrition. The proximal lumen (white port) is used for giving drugs or withdrawing blood.

Some types of catheters also have an on–off switch or clamping device to prevent air accidentally entering the system.

Inserting the catheter

Before inserting the catheter the patient is tipped about 10° head down, and the site prepped and draped. Inserting a catheter is a strictly aseptic procedure requiring gloves, gown, and mask. The anaesthetist usually inserts the catheter in the right internal jugular vein, but occasionally will use a subclavian approach. Each lumen is then flushed with 2 ml of normal saline. Once the procedure is over, the catheter is securely stitched in place, covered with a clear dressing so that you can see if the catheter becomes kinked, and its position is then checked with a chest X-ray. If the drip abruptly stops, then check that the catheter is not kinked where it enters the skin.

Measuring the central venous pressure

Measurements are made against one of two reference points: either at the *sternal angle*, or at the *isophlebotic point*. Once you have decided which point to use, then mark it with a waterproof pen so that staff know it is the *zero point*.

Unlike arterial blood pressure, which is measured in millimetres of mercury, central venous pressures are measured in centimetres of water using either a graduated fluid manometer, or a pressure transducer attached to an electronic monitor.

The new way of measuring central venous pressure is to use an electronic pressure transducer, which has been 'zeroed' to the reference point, and attached to your electronic monitor.

The old way of measuring the central venous pressure with a fluid-filled manometer is used in many hospitals. First, establish a zero point on the manometer with either a spirit level, or a loop of plastic tubing partially filled with coloured water. The aim is to make sure the *reference point* on the patient is exactly at the same level as the zero mark on the manometer. Fill the manometer from a bag of intravenous fluid. Close the three-way tap to the IV bag and

Isophlebotic point at the level of the right atrium in the mid axillary line

Figure 3.3 Measuring central venous pressure with reference to the isophlebotic point allow fluid from the manometer to run into the patient until it stops. At this point, the top of the column of fluid should swing up and down slightly as the patient breathes. Record the halfway point as the fluid swings. This is the *mean central venous pressure.*

The normal central venous pressure lies between 0 to 5 cm H_2O at the angle of the sternum, or between 5 to 10 cm H_2O at the isophlebotic point in the midaxillary line.

Complications

Complications during insertion include:

- pneumothorax when the lung is punctured;
- haemothorax where a major vessel or the heart is perforated;
- *chylothorax* if the lymphatic duct is damaged. This duct carries milky-coloured lymph back to the circulation;
- cardiac dysrhythmia if the catheter irritates the myocardium;
- accidental arterial puncture causing haemorrhage into the soft tissue around the site;
- nerve damage to the brachial plexus.

Complications during use include:

- air emboli;
- pulmonary emboli from sleeve clots or clots forming on the catheter tip;
- infection.

How to interpret central venous pressures

Table 3.5 How to interpret the central venous pressure

Problem	Central venous pressure	Arterial blood pressure
Blood loss	Low	Low
Cardiac failure	High	Low
Cardiac tamponade	High	Low
Over hydration	High	High

In adults and children the normal blood volume is about 70 ml/Kg. For a 70 Kg person this amounts to about 5 litres of blood. Of these 5 litres (at any given moment) 1 litre of the blood is in the heart and lungs, 2 litres are in the arteries and capillaries, and 3 litres are in the veins.

The *great veins*: the vena cava and the larger veins in the limbs are *capacitance vessels*. They act as collapsible reservoirs of blood. Unlike the arteries whose volume remains more or less constant, the volume of blood in the great veins increases or decreases as the total blood volume rises or falls. Once blood loss exceeds 500 ml the pulse rate starts to rise, however the central venous pressure does not alter until about 800 ml of blood is lost.

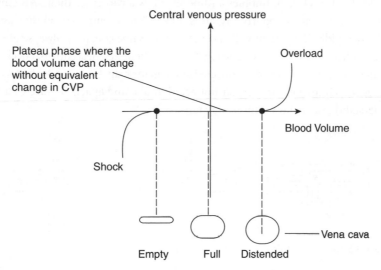

Figure 3.4 Cross-sectional shape of the great veins as they follow the blood volume.

If we transfuse blood into a normal person, the great veins expand to accommodate it. After receiving about 400 ml of blood they can expand no further, and at this point the central venous pressure begins to rise. We can use this phenomenon to work out whether the patient's hypotension is caused by hypovolaemia or something else.

A *CVP stress test* is done by quickly giving the patient 250 ml of colloid, such a 5% albumin or blood. If the central venous pressure does not rise by 5 cm of water or more then wait 5 minutes and give another 250 ml of colloid. You can cautiously repeat this, until either the blood pressure rises, or the central venous pressure rises by 5 cm H_2O.

Care of lines

Catheters are prone to set up havens for bacteria in the little clots that form at the tips of the lumens. These bacteria can leak out into the blood causing systemic sepsis, so take care to maintain sterility when you are injecting anything into a central line, and when changing infusions. Usually central lines are kept patent with a pressurized bag of 0.9% *saline* slowly dribbling through a valve at about 3 ml an hour. Do not use heparinized saline because you may cause a delayed immune reaction called *heparin-induced thrombocytopenia* (HITs).

> *Never inject anything into patients unless they are lying flat.*

Keep the lines free of bubbles and never allow air to enter them. Air emboli can be fatal. Given an opportunity, air is sucked into a central venous line astonishingly rapidly. If a patient with a central venous line collapses, always consider air embolism as a cause. Immediately tip the patient 20° head down, check that the lines have not become disconnected and call for help. Use Luer-locks on central venous lines so that they cannot accidental come apart. Be sure that you understand exactly how a three-way tap works.

Figure 3.5 Direction of flow in a three-way tap.

Special precautions

Do not give anything through a central venous catheter until a chest X-ray has confirmed the catheter tip lies 2–4 cm above the right atrium. On the chest X-ray this point is level with the *carina* at the junction of the left and right main bronchi.

Each lumen should be fitted with a *positive fluid displacement valve* (PFD). Infuse each fluid through its own lumen. Label the ports.

Pulmonary artery catheters

Some patients undergoing major surgery, especially those with heart disease, come to the recovery room with a pulmonary artery catheter in place. These catheters have several ports on them to enable you to measure pressures in the superior vena cava, pulmonary artery and pulmonary capillaries. Pulmonary artery and *wedge pressures* are used to diagnose various forms of shock (haemorrhagic, cardiogenic, septicaemic or combinations of these). Analysing the pressures allows us to distinguish between *high-pressure cardiogenic pulmonary oedema* and *low-pressure non-cardiogenic pulmonary oedema*. They can guide the use of cardiac ionotropes, vasodilator drugs, fluids, or diuretics.

Pulmonary artery pressure

Inflating a small balloon near the tip of the catheter allows it to float into one of the larger pulmonary arteries and become wedged there. This allows the back pressure exerted by the pulmonary capillaries and pulmonary vein to be measured. These wedge pressures reflect the pressure (*preload*) stretching the left atrium. The normal wedge pressure is about 1–3 mmHg. If the pulmonary wedge pressure rises beyond a critical pressure of about 24 mmHg in a healthy lung, the excessive pressure drives fluid from the capillaries into the lungs causing *pulmonary oedema*. In septicaemia, bacterial *endotoxins* are released into the blood stream. These endotoxins damage the linings of the capillaries so that they leak much more easily. Consequently, a pressure sufficiently high to cause pulmonary oedema may be much lower than normal, perhaps as low 10–12 mmHg or even less.

Cardiac output

Another port in the pulmonary artery catheter allows you to rapidly inject a small quantity of saline *coolth* (as distinct from *warmth*) into the pulmonary artery. A *thermistor* on the tip of the catheter measures the duration and temperature profile as this wave of coolth passes by. From this data, a microprocessor calculates the rate of blood flow through the pulmonary artery, and hence estimates the cardiac output.

Problems with pulmonary artery catheters

As with central venous catheters, there is a risk of puncturing the lung, major blood vessels, the lymphatic duct, or damaging nerves.

- Being such long catheters they can kink or even knot inside veins.
- The balloon can burst, or if inflated inadvertently inside a small vessel, it may rupture it.
- The catheter can irritate the heart causing arrhythmias, especially right *bundle branch block* (RBBB).
- The tricuspid valve and pulmonary valve shuts around the catheter more than 100 000 times a day. This continuous friction can damage the valves.
- Sleeve clots around the catheters harbour micro-organisms, or cause pulmonary emboli when the catheter is pulled out.
- Bleeding or air embolism can occur if the catheter becomes accidentally disconnected.

Table 3.6 Typical pressures measured by a pulmonary artery catheter

Site	mmHg	KPa
Right atrium	−1 to 7	0.13–0.93
Right ventricle	22/0	2.92 /0
Pulmonary artery	22/8	2.92/1.06
Pulmonary artery mean	15	1.99

Monitoring respiration

Clinically, the best way to monitor patients' breathing is to place your hand on their chest, count the rate and feel what is going on. The normal respiratory rate is 12–14 breaths/min for adults, and slightly faster for children. Seek advice if the respiratory rate exceeds 20 breaths/min or falls below 8 breaths/min.

Feeling your patient's chest can give you a lot of information. You can gauge the rate and rhythm as the chest rises and falls: normal inspiration should be half the length of expiration. You can feel whether their intercostal muscles are contracting (they should not). Furthermore, you may be able to feel the fine vibrations of wheeze, or the coarser vibrations of loose sputum rattling in the airways.

Modern recovery room monitors sense the respiratory rate from the changes in voltage of the ECG. Sensory pads are available that detect apnoeic periods in babies under 12 months of age. It is still better to routinely feel the patient's chest move with your hand.

Respirometers

Respirometers (also called *anemometers*) measure gas flows. You can attach them to a tight-fitting facemask, laryngeal mask, or endotracheal tube to measure tidal and minute volumes on patients in the recovery room. There are two main types of mechanical devices: the Wright's respirometer® and the Dragermeter®. The Wright's respirometer is the more sensitive of the two, but it is also delicate. Never blow into a Wright's respirometer because you will shred the gears and tear the vanes. The more robust Dragermeter® can be autoclaved if necessary. Electronic anemometers are also available.

Capnography

Capnography is useful to monitor ventilation in intubated patients. With each breath, capnographs measure carbon dioxide concentrations in the expired air. During expiration, the last little bit of air expelled from the lung comes from the alveoli. This *end-tidal CO$_2$* gives a good estimate of the *partial pressure* of carbon dioxide ($P\text{A}CO_2$) in the lungs, and reflects the partial pressure of carbon dioxide in arterial blood ($PaCO_2$).

Arterial blood gases

Arterial blood gases (ABG) measure the partial pressure of oxygen in arterial blood, the partial pressure of carbon dioxide, and the pH of the blood. From these measurements other parameters are calculated including the standard bicarbonate, and base excess.

Arterial blood gases are best taken from an arterial cannula, or failing that the radial or femoral artery. Do not use the posterior tibial or dorsalis pedis arteries except in *neonates*. Brachial or femoral artery punctures in patients with diabetes of vascular disease may dislodge an atheromatous plaque, which if it lodges in a distal vessel, may infarct the limb causing gangrene. Avoid the using the ulnar artery because it provides the collateral circulation to the hand, and never take blood from arteriovenous fistulae in patients on renal dialysis.

To collect arterial blood you need a blood gas syringe, an alcohol swab, 23 gauge needle, a pressure bad, protective eyewear and non-sterile gloves, a patient identification label, and a sharps disposal container within reach.

Commercial kits of needles and syringes are available to collect blood gases. If you do not have these, then lightly smear the inside of 5 ml glass syringe

Allen's test

Use a modified *Allen's test* to check the patency of the collateral ulnar artery's blood supply to the hand before inserting a cannula or needle into the radial artery. You will need an assistant to help you do this test. Where possible, take blood from the patient's non-dominant hand. Ask your assistant to curl the patient's hand into a tight fist to expel blood from the patient's hand. Now prevent blood from flowing into the patient's hand by using your forefingers and middle fingers to occlude both their radial artery and ulnar artery just proximal to the skin crease at the wrists. Then ask your assistant to open the patient's fist. With no blood flowing into it, the patient's palm should be pale. Now release the pressure on the ulnar artery, but keep the pressure applied to the radial artery. If the hand flushes pink, then the ulnar artery is supplying the hand. Repeat the test, but this time release the radial artery is first. If the patient has blood flowing into the hand from both arteries it is safe to puncture the radial artery. If not, then choose another site. Since the Allen test is not infallible, it is better to collect your sample from the patient's non-dominant hand.

with heparin. Attach a 23 gauge needle to collect the blood. Once you have collected the blood press firmly on the puncture site with a pad for 5 minutes by the clock. Remove the pad, and check that the bleeding has stopped. Reapply the pressure if necessary. It is better not to tape a cotton-wool swab over the site; simply leave it uncovered so that you can periodically check whether it is bleeding or swelling.

Things to check after performing an arterial puncture include: bleeding, bruising, swelling around the puncture site, nerve injury, impaired circulation to the hand or fingers, or pain.

Store the blood immediately in melting ice, and send it quickly to the laboratory for analysis. Unless the blood is processed within 10 minutes of collection, the results will be unreliable. Make sure the laboratory knows the patient's temperature and the inspired oxygen concentration so they can adjust their calculations to compensate.

Table 3.7 How to interpret blood gas results

	PH	PaO_2 mmHg (kPa)	$PaCO_2$ mmHg (kPa)	Standard bicarbonate mmol/L
Normal	7.35–7.42	90–10 (11.8–13.2)	35–42 (4.6–5.5)	22–26
Danger	< 7.25	< 60 (< 7.9)	< 45 (> 5.9)	< 16
Critical	< 7.12	< 35 (< 4.6)	> 60 (> 7.9)	< 12

Nerve stimulators

Nerve stimulators use an electrical pulse to stimulate a nerve (usually the ulnar nerve) to cause the hypothenar muscles to contract. With each stimulus the thumb moves toward the little finger. Ignore any movements in the other fingers. Nerve stimulators are used to assess the degree and type of paralysis caused by neuromuscular blocking drugs in intubated patients. Do not use them on conscious patients – they hurt.

If a nerve stimulator was repeatedly used during the anaesthetic patients may well complain of pins and needles – *paraesthesia* – around their little finger and down the inner aspect of their arm. The paraesthesia resolves in a few hours.

X-ray

Portable X-ray may be needed in recovery room in patients with:

- a suspected pneumothorax;
- respiratory distress;
- to check the position a CVP line or a pulmonary artery catheter;
- suspect aspiration;

- heart failure;
- renal surgery: where the pleural space has been breached.

Electrocardiography

Electrocardiography (ECG) is an essential monitor in the recovery room. It warns of arrhythmias and myocardial ischaemia, but not hypoxaemia, or hypercarbia or hypotension.

The ECG monitor gives a continuous picture of the heart's electrical activity. Apart from screen monitors, the recovery room needs at least one machine capable of taking a full 12-lead ECG and printing out a hard copy of the trace. Electrodes placed at strategic points on the skin track the passage of myocardial *action potentials* as they pass through the heart. Each electrode views the potential from a different vantage point. As the current passes towards an electrode it causes an upward (*positive*) wave on the trace, and when travelling away it causes a downward (*negative*) wave. By studying the amplitude and form of the waves at each electrode an experienced observer can build up a three-dimensional picture of the where, when and how the current is travelling.

Who to monitor?

Myocardial ischaemic and arrhythmias commonly occur in patients in the recovery room, particularly if they have pre-existing risk factors. So use ECG monitoring with all patients who have, or are at risk of having cardiac instability, or who have had major surgery, but especially in those at risk of ischaemic heart disease.

Table 3.8 Monitor patients with these risk factors

Age > 50 years	Smoked for > 10 years
Family history	Hypertension
Diabetes	Dyslipidaemia
Depression	Peripheral vascular disease
Cerebrovascular disease	Chronic kidney disease

About 40% of patients with ischaemic heart disease have a normal preoperative resting ECG, but *postoperative adverse cardiac events* (PACE) only occur in 2% of these patients. However, in those patients with an abnormal preoperative ECG, about a quarter will have adverse cardiac events (arrhythmias, ischaemia, or hypotension) either while they are in the recovery room, or later in the ward.

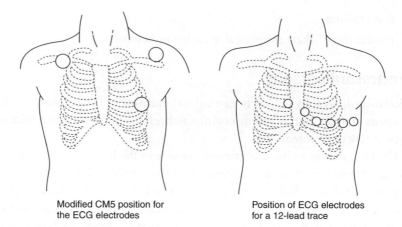

Modified CM5 position for
the ECG electrodes

Position of ECG electrodes
for a 12-lead trace

Figure 3.6 Where to put the electrodes

It is important to detect ECG abnormalities in the recovery room because arrhythmias or signs of ischaemia forewarn of cardiac problems in the coming days. These patients will need careful surveillance in the ward.

ST-depression or elevation are hallmarks of ischaemia, but the absence of ST changes on the ECG does not guarantee that there is no ischaemia present. Most modern cardiac physiological monitors can detect ST changes and warn you as they occur. Make a note in the patient's records of any arrhythmias or ST changes – even if they are only transient.

If arrhythmias or signs of ischaemia occur, notify the anaesthetist, and do a 12-lead ECG. Give a hard copy to the anaesthetist, and save another copy for the patient's notes. Compare the hard copy to the preoperative one.

How to apply the electrodes

Put a diagram on the wall so that every one knows exactly where to put the sticky ECG electrodes. The red electrode on the upper part of the manubrium, the yellow electrode on the left shoulder, and the black electrode over the heart's apex beat, which is usually near the anterior axillary line between the fourth the fifth rib. Now select lead II. This arrangement is called the CM5 lead, and it is the most useful single lead to pick up arrhythmias, and most ST depression. Sometimes you may not be able to use the normal electrode positions, in which case place the electrodes anywhere as long as they roughly form an equilateral triangle around the heart. If necessary, you can put the red electrode on the forehead, the yellow on the left arm and the black electrode over the lower back.

A single lead CMV5 trace detects about 75% of ischaemic episodes. In contrast, if your monitor can display a three-lead trace with lead II, lead V4 and lead V5 then you can detect 98% of ischaemic events.

How to get a good trace

To get a good trace the electrodes must have excellent contact with the skin. You may need to shave the area, but always clean the skin with an alcohol wipe. Poorly applied electrodes cause noisy ECG traces, especially when the patient moves.

The ECG leads may also pick up other noise such as electromagnetic interference ('AC hum'). If the leads are lying across power cables, or are in contact with metal AC hum may blur the trace. Move the leads away from nearby electrical devices. Plugging the ECG monitor and other nearby electrical apparatus into the same power socket (*general power outlet*) usually eliminates the problem. Still having trouble? Try loosely coiling the ECG cable to stop it acting as an aerial.

ECG monitors

To make servicing and maintenance easier, buy all your ECG monitors from the same company as your other equipment. The better ECG monitors have a clear display, easily read from 2–3 metres away, audible pulse monitoring and pulse rate display. There should be a cascade mechanism to view the last 30 seconds of trace and a screen freeze function to analyse a pattern. You will need a paper printout to record arrhythmias for later analysis. Printouts must be properly calibrated. On the vertical axis 1 cm = 1 millivolt; and on the horizontal axis 1 large square = 0.2 seconds.

Most modern monitors have the facility to measure multiple parameters including blood pressure and oximetry, as well as the ECG. Keep all the manufacturer's instructions and electronic technicians' phone numbers, in a convenient place.

ECG leads are easily damaged, so treat them gently. Store spare cables and sensors loosely coiled in a dry dark place. If you are in a tropical climate, seal the storage unit against moisture.

Glucose monitors

Measure the blood sugar of diabetic patients as soon as possible after they arrive in the recovery room. Every recovery room must have a glucose meter (*glucometer*) on hand. These small cheap electronic devices measure blood glucose concentration by using a drop of blood from a finger or heel prick. Keep the instructions on how to use the device in the box with the instrument. Store the reagent strip in a cool dry place.

Hypoglycaemia, like hypoxia, quickly causes brain damage and kills unless it is detected in time. Those at risk of hypoglycaemia include: neonates and babies, diabetics, patients who drink excessive alcohol, or who have liver disease. Make it part of your protocols to measure the blood glucose in these patients as soon as they come to the recovery room. Notify the anaesthetist if the blood glucose is less than 3.8 mmol/L (*hypoglycaemia*) or greater than 12 mmol/L (*hyperglycaemia*). It is not well known that in patients with diabetes even brief episodes (as little as 20 minutes) of hyperglycaemia in the recovery room increases, by several fold, the risk of postoperative myocardial infarction and stroke.

Remember not to take blood from the feet or toes of diabetics or patients with peripheral vascular disease because they may get an infected ulcer at the site.

Monitoring temperature

When patients come to the recovery room routinely check their *temperature*. This is essential for babies who get cold on the operating table.

Humans tightly maintain their *core temperature* around a *set point* of 37±1°C. The core of the body, the heart, liver, kidneys, lungs and brain are warmer than the skin and limbs. Skin temperature depends principally on ambient air temperature; in contrast the metabolic rate determines the core temperature. Normally the skin temperature is about 33°C or 91°F, but this varies enormously from site to site. For this reason, axillary temperature is highly misleading. It does not reflect core temperature and should never be used in the recovery room.

How to measure temperature

Mercury thermometers are unsafe and should not be used in recovery rooms. Apart from being fragile, they do not register temperatures below 35.8°C. Clinical thermometers have been replaced by user-friendly *thermistor* electronic temperature probes.

The most popular electronic probe are hand-held devices (such as Thermofocus® and the Exergen Temporal Scanner®). When pointed towards the patient the device collects infrared emissions from the skin without actually touching it. The large temporal artery supplies the blood to the forehead, a convenient place to measure body temperature. Additionally the head, with its rich blood supply, is the first region of the skin to change temperature with fever.

Infrared tympanic thermometers reliably estimate core temperature. The tympanic membrane in the ear shares the same blood supply as the body's thermoregulatory centre in the *hypothalamus*. Be gentle when you insert a probe into the ear. They need to be placed precisely to get an accurate result.

Adult skin temperature sensors have small thermistors set in hypoallergenic sticky pads that can be placed anywhere on the body surface, but the only place to get a reliable estimate of the core temperature is over the temporal artery. If the patient becomes sweaty, the pads can fall off. Other forms of measuring skin temperature, such as thermoresponsive crystal sensors, are not as reliable.

Body temperature can also be measured with rectal, oesophageal or pharyngeal probes, or with a thermistor incorporated into pulmonary artery flotation catheters. Rectal temperature probes are not as reliable as once thought. They can be cooled by blood returning from the legs, or warmed by up to 1°C by heat generated by thermogenic bacteria in the faeces.

Hyperthermia

Hyperthermia is uncommon in the recovery room and is always serious. Causes include blood transfusion reactions, a pre-existing febrile state or a thyroid crisis. The most sinister cause is malignant hyperthermia. This condition is fatal if not treated quickly.

Hypothermia

Hypothermia is defined as a core temperature of 36°C of lower. About 60 per cent of patients arrive in the recovery room with a low body temperature. An even larger number who have had their chest or abdomen opened become hypothermic during surgery. Feel your patient's chest with the palm of your hand. If it feels cool to touch then recheck the patient's temperature.

Hypothermia is a gravely under appreciated problem. It is the principal cause of blood failing to clot after surgery; drug *metabolism* is delayed, and it is a major predictor of postoperative infection and wound breakdown.

Warming blankets

Convection warming blankets work by blowing warm air into a light plastic envelope enclosing the patient. They are highly effective in preventing further heat loss and help rewarm cold patients in recovery room. One of the most popular makes of warming blanket is the BairHugger™; it can increase the body temperature by 1.5°C per hour when set on high.

Air-warming devices are not without risk, they may contribute to cross infection and it is possible to cause burns if the blankets are not properly attached to the hose. You are likely to burn your patient if you simply place the hose under the sheet or blanket.

Note

1. Best Practice (1999) 3:1-6 published the Joanna Briggs Institute, Australia.

4

Pain

What is pain?

Pain is a subjective experience; its intensity depends on how one interprets what one is feeling. The intensity of pain is influenced by the neural stimuli received from damaged tissue, the memory of previous pain, the expected outcome; and psychological factors, predominantly anxiety.

Individuals perceive and respond to pain in different ways. It is not easily described in words and even less easily measured. For instance your splitting headache is not necessarily the same as my pounding headache. How can I possibly explain to you what I am feeling and how much it hurts? This problem remains unsolved.

Pain has survival value. This unpleasant sensation and emotion helps prevent further injury. A widely accepted definition of pain is 'a sensory and emotional experience from actual or potential tissue damage, or described in terms of such damage'. In more practical sense, pain is what the patient says hurts, and when the patient says it hurts – this is a most important concept to grasp. Pain is a combination of what your patients feel, and their emotional response to it.

Table 4.1 Various types of pain

Type of pain	Description
Clinical	
Somatic pain	Well localized, sharp, acute pain arising from skin, muscles, joints.
Visceral pain	Deep, diffuse, ill-localized arising from an organ.
Pathological description	
Neuropathic pain	Arises from injured nerves.
Nocioceptive pain	Occurs where inflammation stimulates pain receptors.

Why pain is harmful

Uncontrolled pain is harmful because it:

- causes restlessness, which increases oxygen consumption; this in turn, increases cardiac work, and can result in hypoxia;
- contributes to postoperative nausea and vomiting;
- increases the blood pressure, with the risk of precipitating cardiac ischaemia;
- decreases hepatic and renal blood flow, delaying the metabolism and excretion of drugs, and promoting fluid retention;
- prevents the patient from taking deep breaths and coughing, especially following thoracic or upper abdominal operations. This increases the risk of postoperative sputum retention and pneumonia;
- discourages patients from moving their legs, slowing blood flow through the legs. The venous stasis contributes to the formation of deep vein thrombi, and pulmonary embolism;
- increases the postoperative stress response, with greatly increased cortisol secretion. This delays wound healing, and predisposes to infection;
- increases metabolic rate, protein breakdown, and the catabolic effects of injury;
- delays the return of normal bowel function;
- impairs the bonding of a mother with her newborn child if the mother is in pain after Caesarean section, and
- demoralizes the patient, disrupts sleep, and causes distressing anxiety and despair.

Uncontrolled pain can delay healing,
and increase the risk of infection.

The greatest physiological risk of untreated pain is to frail patients, those with heart or lung disease, the very young and the very old, and those undergoing major procedures such as aortic, abdominal, or major orthopaedic surgery.

How we perceive pain

How we perceive pain involves two inputs: the injury that hurts (*noxious stimulus*) and the anxiety or fear (*affective feelings*) that goes with this. These interact in a complex way to form the sensation of pain.

If you stubbed your toe against a door, you would probably not feel very anxious about it. You know the pain will soon go away, and there should be no consequences. Your logical analysis involves experience, knowledge, memory and foresight.

If you were to wake suddenly in the night with a terrible abdominal pain you would rightly be alarmed, and your physiological and psychological response quite different. The emotional responses to pain can be harmful. Emotions may range through acceptance, apprehension, fear or even terror. Fear of physical deformity is particularly evident in patients who have been burnt, or who are undergoing disfiguring operations such as mastectomy or amputation. The young tend to be more fearful than older people. Sincere empathy, reassurance and skilled nursing reduce destructive emotional responses substantially.

Emotional stress activates the sympathetic nervous system: blood pressure rises, the heart beats faster and more forcibly and the brain becomes hypervigilant about its surroundings and what is happening to the body. If this stress remains unmodulated then enough cortisol is secreted from the adrenal gland to jeopardize wound healing and predispose to infection.

Pain physiology

Those organisms that can recognize they have been injured and then avoid further injury are far more likely to survive long enough to pass on this ability to their offspring. One billion years of evolution have refined this aptitude endlessly. We are the beneficiaries of eons of physiological adaptations by these survivors, our ancestors, and we have inherited their complex ways of recognizing and reacting to pain. The following description is the barest outline of this process, but should give you a feeling for its complexity, and how we can use this knowledge to modify the response.

Sensory nerves to the spinal cord and brain carry pain sensations. Here they are integrated and modified to produce a coordinated response and remembered for later analysis. 'What part of me is hurting?' 'Am I in danger?' 'How much does it hurt?' 'Have I felt it before?' and so on. Meanwhile the subcortical areas of the central nervous system recruit background responses such as an increase in blood pressure and heart rate, the amount of sweating and the size of the pupils.

Nociceptors

Inflammation causes pain

Pain receptors in the tissues are called *nociceptors*. Under a microscope nociceptors have no distinct structure, but appear as a woven network of free bare nerve endings distributed everywhere through the tissues; they are found in viscera, in periosteum, in connective tissue and around blood vessels.

Inflammation is ultimately the original cause of all pain. Where there is one, you will find the other: nevertheless, under some circumstances, when the inflammation resolves, the pain persists. This *neuropathic pain* can be unremitting and can eat away people's lives. The sad thing is that in most cases neuropathic pain is preventable if the original pain is treated early and vigorously.

Inflammation is caused by thermal damage, mechanical trauma, or chemical irritation. Surgery also damages tissue. The dead and damaged cells release pain-producing (*algogenic*) chemicals including eicosanoids, potassium ions, and bradykinins. The nerve endings also release *substance* P. All these biochemicals cause vasodilation, and oedema at the site of injury. Ischaemic injury does likewise, but adds hydrogen ions to the inflammatory soup. Soaked in inflammatory mediators, the capillary beds in the area leak protein-rich fluid (*exudate*) into the tissues. The exudate carries more bradykinins and other algogenic chemicals such as histamine, *serotonin* and noradrenaline into the area.

Macrophages and white cells flock to the site to mop up the damaged cells, to deal with invading micro-organisms and start the repair process. They send out distress messengers in the form of cytokines, histamine, serotonin, bradykinin, purines and many others. All these biochemicals further stimulate pain receptors.

Analgesics such as aspirin and the *non-steroidal anti-inflammatory drugs* (NSAIDs) impair the synthesis of some inflammatory mediators, and reduce pain and the inflammatory response.

Pain thresholds

What you feel depends on the type of sensory ending stimulated, and its connections to the spinal cord and the brain. The stimulus, such as a burn, a stab or a bite, must have enough strength (*to exceed threshold potential*) to trigger a response; in contrast a signal of insufficient strength is said to be *sub-threshold*. A mosquito bite is subthreshold and passes unnoticed, in contrast a dog bite certainly exceeds the threshold potential.

Nociceptors fire more easily, at a lower threshold, if they are exposed to repeated high-intensity stimulation, or irritated by inflammatory biochemicals. This process is called *sensitization*. If anyone has slapped your sunburnt back you will recognize sensitization. *Allodynia* is the name for the pain where a stimulus that does not normally cause pain, begins to do so.

Peripheral nerves

First-order neurons carry sensation from skin, muscle, bone and the organs to the spinal cord. If you have ever burnt your hand on a hot stove you might, with dispassionate analysis, have noticed two sorts of pain. First a fast onset pain that only last for a short time and pricks, stabs or lances. Large myelinated A-delta nerve fibres carry this pain sensation. Second, a slower onset pain is duller, and lasts longer. Small unmyelinated C fibres carry this pain impulse. Both these first-order neurons carry impulses from the periphery to the spinal cord.

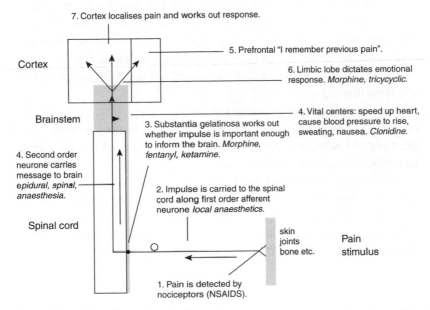

Figure 4.1 Neural pathways involved in pain

Substantia gelatinosa

Once a painful stimulus exceeds the threshold level, the impulse is carried to the substantia gelatinosa (SG) in the dorsal horn of the spinal cord. The substantia gelatinosa crudely analyses the intensity and quality of the pain. Like a gatekeeper it acts to control which impulses are important enough to pass and where to pass them. Are you wearing a watch? Normally you are unaware of it, but once your conscious self (in your *cerebral cortex*) interrogates your substantia gelatinosa it will direct attention to the appropriate wrist, and allow a previously subthreshold stimulus to pass back to your consciousness.

If you touch a hot stove you will immediately pull your hand away – a *withdrawal reflex* – about 0.6–0.8 seconds before you consciously know anything has happened, and hopefully before too much damage is done.

The *substantia gelatinosa* in the spinal card instantly recognized the supra-maximal stimulus, and directed an impulse down your motor nerves to get your hand out of the way of danger. This simple *reflex* response avoids wasting about 1.8–2 seconds needed to pass messages back and forth to obtain directions from your conscious self.

An experiment

Without having to actually burn yourself, you can demonstrate the effects of the fast (A delta fibres) and the slower (C fibres) neuronal transmission. Take your Achilles' tendon at the back of your heel between your forefinger and thumb. Now, quickly squeeze it hard. You will feel two pains; the first is sharp, well-localized and brief, and the second dull, deep, diffuse, persistent, and uncomfortable.

Consider walking barefoot along a stony path. The substantia gelatinosa, receiving impulses arising in the prefrontal region in the brain, readjusts the threshold potential in the SG to tolerate jabs and pricks on the sole of your foot. Now, if you stand on a thorn, the adjusted threshold stimulus is exceeded and the withdrawal reflex pulls your foot out of the way.

To some degree you can consciously override a response to pain, such as when you make a grab to pull the plug out of a sink full of hot water. Although the pain threshold is exceeded, you expected the pain, and for that moment you can override the withdrawal reflex.

Endorphins

All these responses to pain are regulated by local neurotransmitters, which open and close neural gates in the substantia gelatinosa. Open gates allow pain impulse to pass, and closed ones do not. Inhibitory neurotransmitters close the gates and excitatory ones open them. One of these inhibitory substances is a member of a group of naturally occurring opioids called β-*endorphin*. This acts on opioid μ-receptors near pain *synapses*. hyperpolarizing the neuronal cell membrane so that it takes a bigger stimulus to make them fire. Opioids, given with epidural or spinal anaesthetics, mimic β-endorphins and impede the passage of pain impulses to the brain.

Ketamine blocks the effects of an excitatory neuropeptide, *glutamate*, in the substantia gelatinosa. This slams the gate shut to stop pain impulses reaching the central nervous system. Ketamine also profoundly affects how the brain perceives pain.

Second-order neurons

Once through the gate, the pain impulses are relayed to second-order neurons that splay out in the spinal cord to carry information to the brain. Some impulses pass up to the *thalamus* in easily identifiable contralateral spinothalamic tracts. Others enter the diffuse spinoreticular tracts that connect with *vital centres* in the brainstem's reticular formation. These vital centres coordinate innate responses such as heart rate, blood pressure, sweating, pupil size, respiratory rate and depth.

Thalamus

Astride the top of the midbrain sits the *thalamus*. It acts as the body's administrative head quarters coordinating the body's automatic functions such as temperature control, respiration, and blood pressure maintenance. In the spinal cord the *spinothalamic tracts* lie laterally and the paleospinothalamic tracts lie medially. The neospinothalamic tract passes up the spinal cord to the posterior thalamus to carry and process information about the location, duration and intensity of pain. The paleothalamic tract sends its fibres to the medial thalamus and is associated with the autonomic and emotional aspects of pain.

Third-order neurons

In the medial thalamus the quality of the pain touches consciousness for the first time. Messages pass on through third-order neurons to the prefrontal lobes (foresight and previous experience) and the limbic lobe (emotion) where we analyse the memory and the emotional implications of the pain. In other words 'I have felt this before, it hurts – it's a burn.'

Meanwhile messages from the lateral thalamus pass on to the postcentral gyrus in the sensory cortex, where we integrate all the messages to discover 'my left hand is burning'. Now we know our hand is burnt we can organize other appropriate and complex behavioural responses such as finding water to cool it.

How pain is modified

We are genetically programmed to forget some types of acute pain. This is fortunate, otherwise a woman would never go through childbirth for the second time.

Sometimes we need to cope with, or even ignore, pain. In the brainstem the periaqueductal grey matter (PAG) monitors emergencies. If roused it blocks pain impulses on their way to the brain. This is why people injured in war, or on the sports field, often do not feel pain until after the drama is over.

When the thalamus perceives the situation is an emergency it induces the hypothalamus and pituitary gland to secrete β-endorphin. These endogenous opioids impede inward-bound pain impulses through the PAG so that they are not passed on to consciousness.

Plasticity and wind-up

Plasticity

Once barraged by pain, stimuli sensory nerves recruit help from their neighbours by producing neuropeptides including substance P, neurokinin A, and calcitonin gene-related peptide (CGRP). These substances also pass up the axon to the cell body, which then remodels its connections in the substantia gelatinosa.

With repetitive painful stimuli nerves establish more peripheral pain receptors, send out new dendrites to their neighbours, and increase the number of receptors in the post-synaptic endplates in the substantia gelatinosa. At the distal end of the nerve the overall effect is to increase local sensitivity to inflammation, while at the proximal end in the substantia gelatinosa the nerve radically improves its communication with the central nervous system.

Now alerted to the problem, the neurons in the central nervous system establish new connections, allow others to lapse, and then increase their production of peptide neurotransmitters (*glutamate*, *aspartate*, and *substance* P). All this ability to change, to remodel, nerve connections and to adapt biochemical responses according to need is termed plasticity.

Plasticity does not only occur with pain. Just studying this book will actually remodel parts of your brain. Repetition reinforces the process; hence the observation that practice makes perfect.

How wind-up leads to chronic pain

Continuous severe pain changes the structure and function of sensory nerves. If the neural circuits in the substantia gelatinosa are barraged with pain impulses then calcium channels in the nerve membranes become jammed open. Calcium ions flood into the nerve cells and stimulate certain genes to act (express themselves). The genes programme the microsomal protein factories to produce many more neuropeptide transmitters, new receptors and cell membrane pumps. With all this new equipment for detecting pain, the cell now responds massively to stimuli that would previously have passed unnoticed.

With good pain relief we can prevent a catastrophe: unrelieved severe pain can cause so much calcium to enter the nerve cells of the dorsal horn that they die. Once this happens the neural gate mechanism in the substantia gelatinosa is permanently jammed open. Pain becomes entrenched so that even a minor stimulus now causes a massive response. Unhappily this response continues long after the precipitating injury has healed. An example of this phenomenon is the severe pain of post-hepatic neuralgia following an attack of shingles.

Ketamine prevents chronic pain

We can predict that some injuries, such as pelvic fractures or surgery like rib resection, will be so painful that *wind-up* is likely to occur. In such cases ketamine is useful for preventing the onset of chronic pain syndrome.

*Unrelieved severe pain can evolve
into permanent chronic pain.*

Ketamine blocks polysynaptic reflexes in the spinal cord and functionally dissociates the thalamus so that it cannot pass on impulses from *limbic system* (which recognizes pain) to the cortex (where the pain impulses are consciously analysed). This means the pain never reaches a conscious level.

5

Postoperative pain

It is not only distressing to emerge from anaesthesia in agony, it is harmful. Pain is physiologically damaging, and mostly preventable. In the recovery room pain control has improved by the simple *paradigm* shift of titrating opioids intravenously, instead of giving them intramuscularly.

10 Pain principles

1. Pain has two principal elements: hurt and fear. You need to treat both.
2. Treat pain it before it occurs (pre-emptive *analgesia*).
3. Attack pain at more than one point on its path from the tissues to consciousness (multimodal analgesia).
4. Do not allow uncontrolled *acute pain* to develop into disastrous chronic pain.
5. Cuddle crying children.
6. Opioids do not cause hypotension in stable patients.
7. If the patient's pain seems inappropriate call the surgeon or anaesthetist. There may be a cause such as a tight plaster, or a different drug may be more appropriate.
8. If you do not know all the actions of a drug, do not use it.
9. In elderly patients, use small doses more frequently.
10. The cause of pain might not be surgical.

Misunderstandings about pain

Patients tend to assume:

- pain is inevitable after surgery; or
- that modern surgery is absolutely pain free;

- pain is simply something they have to put up with;
- pain is not hazardous merely uncomfortable;
- staff know when they are in pain;
- if they wait a while it will get better.
- if they complain, they will be thought to be making a fuss.

Acute pain service

Many hospitals have an acute pain team to take over pain management once the patient has left the recovery room. These specialist teams provide consistent and superior pain management when compared to less disciplined means of treating it. You may find it appropriate to refer some of your more difficult patients to this team.

How to manage pain

Although pain is a complex phenomenon, acute pain is relatively easy to assess and treat. First, ask patients whether they are in pain, and then give enough analgesic to alleviate it. The recovery room is the logical place to assess, plan, organize, and start the treatment of coordinated postoperative pain management.

C – Cause of pain.

A – Assess the amount of pain.

R – Reassure and comfort your patient.

E – Effective and appropriate analgesia.

R – Reassess.

C = Causes of pain

Tissue damage causes pain, but how the pain is interpreted depends on psychological factors.

Tissue damage

Postoperative pain is initially caused by the inflammatory response associated with tissue damage, but not all pain is due to the surgery. The severity of acute surgical pain is determined by the site of incision, the mass of tissue damage, and the type of operation. Long incisions cutting through bone, muscle and nerves (for example thoracic and abdominal incisions) are more painful than short incisions elsewhere. Little incisions are one of the reasons that laparoscopic surgery is less painful. Orthopaedic, facio-maxillary and especially perineal incisions are more painful. Donor sites for split-skin grafts are surprisingly painful.

Sharp well-localized (somatic) pain comes from the skin and muscle incision, and deep poorly localized gnawing (visceral) pain comes from the deeper structures.

Psychological factors

Tissue damage is only part of the story. Pain is always a subjective experience, and so depends on how patients interpret what they are feeling. It is not only determined by the neural stimuli from the damaged tissue, but also the patients' expectations and other psychological factors, of which anxiety is easily the most predominant.

Most people feel pain in an equivalent way but they react to it differently. Fear potentially exacerbates pain. Some people are more stoical than others; for example older people tend not to complain as much as the young. Some cultures expect a stiff upper lip while in others it is fine to scream one's head off.

Individuals respond differently to analgesics. Young healthy people usually require higher doses than older people, and Caucasians need more opioids than Asians (or those with red hair) to achieve the same effect.

Pain is less likely to be distressing if the patient:

- expects pain;
- knows how long it will last;
- feels it is less severe than expected;
- has been involved in deciding the options for pain management;
- has been taught relaxation methods before surgery;
- and most importantly is not anxious about the outcome of the surgery.

Pain control is likely to be good if the staff:

- understand how patients perceive pain;
- know the profound damage uncontrolled pain can cause;
- do not consider complaints about pain to be a psychological weakness in the patient;
- know the properties of the drugs they are using;
- use pre-emptive analgesia;
- know how to treat respiratory depression and hypotension;
- are not worried that the patient may become a drug addict;
- formulate a sound plan for continuing analgesia.

Non-surgical causes of pain

Not all postoperative pain is caused by surgery. Pain is an important sign that something is wrong. Ask the patient to point to where it hurts.

Consider non-surgical causes of postoperative pain.

- Sore throat from endotracheal tubes, laryngoscopy or metal suckers.
- Headache is particularly common after a general anaesthetic.
- Myocardial *ischaemia* or *infarction* is serious.
- Pressure on peripheral nerves during the operation.
- Stretched ligament caused by poor positioning on the operating table.
- Tight bandages or plasters.
- Muscle shearing caused by the use of succinyl choline.
- Poor position on the operating table causing severe back or joint pain.

Myocardial ischaemia

One important cause of pain that may occur in the recovery room is myocardial ischaemia. This can present as an ill-localized pain or more often aching discomfort, anywhere above the umbilicus. It does not have to be retrosternal, and may be in the jaw, neck, back or even the top of the head.

Use the PQRST system

P = Pain. Does the patient have pain?

Q = Quality of pain. Is it well-localized, or diffuse? Is it sharp or dull?

R = Radiation. Does the pain go anywhere else? After laparoscopy pain may radiate to the shoulder tips.

S = Severity. How severe is the pain?

T = Time course of the pain. Is it constant? Does it come and go? Are there spasms?

A = Assess the severity of pain

Subjectively, if the patient says it hurts, then they are in pain. The only humane way to assess and manage pain is to believe what the patient tells you.

Objectively, it is difficult to measure pain, because there are no biochemical tests to confirm its presence.

Severe pain may cause crying, splinting, grimacing and hypertension; while agonizing pain may cause bradycardia, hypotension, nausea, vomiting, dilated pupils, pallor and loss of bowel and bladder control. It is to be hoped we never allow patients to enter these realms.

Gauge the severity of pain

Attempts to quantify pain have produced many ingenious pain scales, but none do the job perfectly. The best technique of all is to simply ask whether your patient is in pain, and if so whether it hurts a little, a lot, or is terrible.

Visual analogue pain scale

Adult patients report the most useful way of scoring pain is the *visual analogue pain scale* (VAPS). They are especially useful in those who cannot speak English, or have trouble with numeric scales. This scale takes into account both the pain and the anxiety component of the patient's feelings. The scale is simply a 10 cm long line drawn on a piece of paper. The right-hand end of the line is labelled 'worst pain ever', and the other end 'no pain'. It is called an analogue scale because it has no units marked on it, and therefore patients need not fret about the numerical magnitude of their pain.

There is no point in trying to explain a visual analogue scale for the first time to a patient in recovery room because they will not be able to concentrate sufficiently to understand it. Unless the scale is explained to patients before they come to theatre, the scales are almost useless.

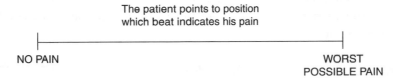

Figure 5.1 Analogue pain scale

There should only be two descriptors: one at each end of the scale. If you use the straight line visual pain analogue the patient needs to point at it with their finger. The visual pain analogues can also be used to assess other subjective phenomenon such as nausea and anxiety.

The visual pain analogues may be inaccurate in patients who have no education, because they have never learned to prioritize items or to think in a linear manner.

Numeric scales

Many recovery rooms use numeric scales to assess pain. With these scales staff ask the patients to rate their pain using a 1 to 10 scale. If you do elect to use a numeric scale then aim for a pain score of less than 4 out of 10. Numeric scales do not deserve their popularity, because they require the patient to be educated, and have the ability to understand and reason. Furthermore they assume the patient is numerate, understands English, is not deaf, or has impaired vision and has no cognitive disorder. It is not surprising that patients in pain who are often sedated and distracted by other unfamiliar sensations find abstract intellectual tasks difficult.

What to document

Pain assessment includes location of the pain, its intensity using a pain score, verbal descriptions (sharp, burning, aching), physical signs (hypertension, sweating, tachycardia, pupillary dilation), clinical signs (limitation of breathing or moving, abdominal rigidity or guarding), affective emotional response (distressing, annoying, irritating), psychological response (acceptance, anxiety, fear), and biochemical response (hyperglycaemia).

Pain charts

Some hospitals, especially those with pain teams, use *pain indicator and assessment charts* (PINDA) to record a standardized assessment of the patient's pain. PINDA charts are useful for pain audits and include details of the analgesic agent, the method of delivery, the effect of the analgesia using a pain score, whether nausea and vomiting are a problem, a sedation score, and how pain limits patients' normal activities. Sometimes PINDA charts are started in the recovery room.

How to assess pain in the elderly

It is difficult to assess pain in elderly patients who have cognitive impairment or who cannot communicate well. Elderly people cannot process the standard pain scores, but are easily able to tell you whether their pain is 'very bad', 'bad', 'moderate', 'just a little', or 'no pain'; and whether their pain is better after an analgesic. Even the terms 'severe' and 'minimal' are too complicated for some demented patients to understand after their anaesthetic.

Behavioural pain assessment

Patients who have had strokes, or have major intellectual impairment, or are too sedated or sick to respond will not be able to tell you that they are in pain.

In this case you need to assess their body language. If you stroke the patient and they scream or wince then you know they have pain. If you like working to tables here is one you can try.

Table 5.1 The CALMS scale

	0	1	2
C Comfort	Responds quietly when touched	Reassured when hand is held, or brow stroked	Difficult to comfort
A Activity	Deep breathes, cough and moves limbs freely	Reluctant to deep breathe, cough or move limbs	Moves only minimally when asked
L Looks	Relaxed or sleeping	Grimaces only when moved	Screwed up face and clenched jaw
M Moves	Relaxed	Tenses muscles when moved	Continuous clenched grasp, or rigid, may writhe around
S Speaks	Quiet	Moans only when moved	Continually grunts or whimpers
Score out of 10			

How to assess pain in the intellectually impaired

Assessing pain in an intellectually disabled patient is the same as it is for a child of similar mental capabilities, or an elderly patient with dementia. Some intellectually impaired patients, especially those with Down's syndrome, may have a lower tolerance for drugs such as the benzodiazepines and opioid analgesics. Start with a half dose of analgesic based on their lean body mass.

How to assess pain in neonates

Even the most premature *neonates* respond to pain. Diagnosing pain in neonates is easy if they cry, but sick neonates may be too weak to cry. Look for a furrowed brow, flared nostrils, and an open mouth with a taut tongue. Their chins may quiver and their tongue may protrude.

There is overwhelming evidence that pain does great harm to the newborn, and because of the plasticity of the developing nervous system, there are likely to be adverse long-term consequences. Neonates mount a qualitatively much greater neurohumoral response than adults. Cruel procedures, such as circumcision without anaesthesia, disturb bonding, disrupt feeding patterns and cause behavioural changes that persist for days or weeks and can even affect development of the central nervous system permanently. In some cases very painful procedures have been known to cause a neonate's blood pressure to rise high enough to cause an intracranial haemorrhage.

How to assess pain in children[1]

It is also difficult to assess pain in children, and no single method works every time. Many children are comforted by their 'security blanket': a familiar and loved toy or object. You can use such toys to assist with explaining things and assessing how the child feels.

Toddlers

Children over the age of 2 years will tell you it hurts and where it hurts. Toddlers often express pain by rubbing the affected part; or by kicking, biting and hitting at staff (*combative behaviour*) in an attempt to escape the situation. They also cry and seek comfort from people they trust.

Children from 3–5 years

Even pre-school children will reliably tell you when something hurts and where it hurts, but unlike toddlers they can tell you how much it hurts – 'a little bit', or 'a lot'. Believe what they say. If they say they are not in pain then you can believe that too. Sometimes younger children play down their pain because they are afraid of the needle, and have difficulty in connecting the idea that an injection will relieve the pain in 15 minutes time.

Children from 6–9 years

School age children are able to tell you more about the quality and intensity of their pain. It feels 'sharp like a knife' or 'dull' like after someone has punched you'. They will also be able to tell whether the pain is worse or better than it was previously. They should be able to grade the pain into 'hurts a lot', 'hurts a bit', and 'doesn't hurt at all'.

Older children

Older children can be assessed in the same way as competent adults.

R = Reassure the patient

Patients who have had disfiguring operations, or those with cancer, are far more likely to focus on the site of surgery and suffer more pain. Anxious patients suffer more with pain than those who are calm. A recovery room nurse can give a patient in pain two great gifts. The first is empathy; (the ability to respond with genuine compassion to your patient's reality), while the second is effective analgesia.

Almost all patients at or beyond middle age fear cancer. Many men and women affectionately remember the recovery room nurse who held their hand briefly, and told them everything went well. The patients say that with those few words their pain simply went away.

E = Effective analgesia

There are four main ways of controlling postoperative pain:

1. Parenteral drugs.
2. Regional or neuraxial local anaesthetic blockade.
3. Infiltrating the wound with local anaesthetic.
4. Oral analgesia.

It is best to use drugs intravenously. If drugs are given subcutaneously or intramuscularly they may be absorbed erratically, and act unpredictably. Giving drugs by mouth requires the patient to drink, swallow, not to vomit, and for the medication to be absorbed reliably.

Why various analgesics are used

Visceral pain

Visceral pain is diffuse, deep, aching pain arising from injury to an internal organ such as bowel. Patients localize it with the flat of their hand. Visceral pain responds best to opioids.

Somatic pain

Somatic pain is sharp, *acute pain* arising from skin, muscles, bone, joints, connective tissue and parietal pleura. Patients can accurately localize it with the tip of their fingers. Somatic pain responds best to NSAIDs.

Spasmodic pain

Spasmodic pain occurs when patients have operations on tendons or have diseases like muscular sclerosis. If opioids are not giving relief the anaesthetist may ask you to give diazepam. There are suppositories available that are useful in children.

Colic

Colic will respond to pethidine or diclofenac if morphine seems ineffective.

Pre-emptive analgesia

Experienced recovery room nurses know that once pain is established far more opioid is needed to relieve it than if the opioid is given before the pain starts.

This observation is the basis for the 'get in first' approach of pre-emptive analgesia. Local anaesthetic techniques used during surgery substantially reduce the amount of opioids needed to control pain in the recovery room. Even under general anaesthesia surgical pain causes changes in the way neurons in the spinal cord behave, and the way these neurons relay pain impulses to the brain.

Once the changes become established, it is difficult to suppress this hyperexcitable state with analgesics.

A single dose of pre-emptive analgesia given before the incision provides no more analgesia than the same dose given after surgery,[2] but repeated doses of opioids used during surgery certainly have a good effect.

Multimodal analgesia

Advances in receptor pharmacology have identified exactly where in the pain pathway various drugs work. The rationale of *multimodal analgesia* is to block the pain at more than one point on its path from receptor to consciousness. For example, a patient who has had a radical nephrectomy might have a combination of a thoracic epidural, or intercostal blocks, to treat the *somatic pain* from muscle and skin; as well as morphine to control the *visceral pain* from the peritoneum and an NSAID to quieten the inflammatory response at the site of injury.

R = Reassess

Never send a patient back to the ward in pain. Adequate pain control means the patient can move with ease about the trolley or bed, take deep breaths, cough effectively, and feel comfortable. Just before discharging the patient to the ward record your assessment of their pain in their medical record.

Day surgery patients

Several hours after their procedure, day surgery patients are discharged into the care of a responsible adult. Because the day surgery patient is in hospital for so little time, their discharge needs to be planned at the time they are first assessed for their anaesthetic. The plan should include how to control pain, and what to do about potential postoperative problems. Often patients need a few analgesic tablets, paracetamol is usually sufficient, to take home with them to tide them over the next day or so.

Patients may ask if they will be fit to go back to work the next day. Reassure patients that most people do not go to work the following day, and that they should only return to work if they feel fit to do so.

Notes

1. RCNI (1999) *Clinical Guidelines for Recognition and Assessment of Acute Pain in Children. Recommendations.* London, Royal College of Nursing.
2. Moiniche S, Kehlet H, Dahl JB (2002) *Anesthesiology* 96: 725–41.

6

Analgesics

Analgesics are drugs used to relieve pain

Three principal groups of drugs are used for parenteral pain relief:

1. Opioids.
2. Non-steroidal anti-inflammatory drugs (NSAIDs).
3. Adjuvants.

Opioids

Opioid analgesics include morphine, diamorphine, pethidine, fentanyl, codeine, oxycodone, methadone, buprenorphine, and tramadol. To use opioids effectively we need to know their properties thoroughly. Opioids are the best parenteral drugs we have to control moderate to severe pain. They are most effective against constant dull deep-seated (visceral) pain, and not as effective against sharp, well-localized intermittent pain, spasmodic pain or colic.

Buprenorphine and tramadol are not typical opioids. Although they are analgesics, many of their properties differ from other opioids. Most significantly they do not suppress the undesirable emotional aspects of pain and may increase feelings of anxiety and unease.

Pharmacology of opioids

Opioids (once called *opiates*) are analgesic drugs that work on the same receptors as our own intrinsic pain-killers called β-*endorphins*. Endorphins are a group of naturally occurring opioid *peptides* synthesized in the hypothalamus. When people are in pain, their hypothalamus releases β-endorphin into the cerebrospinal fluid, and the pituitary gland releases it into the circulation. β-endorphin latches on to opioid receptors in the spinal cord and brain. In the spinal cord, β-endorphin inhibits pain impulses passing through the *substantia gelatinosa* to reach the brain. In the brain opioid receptors are found in the periaqueductal grey matter (involved with the subconscious gauging of the level of pain), in the thalamus (where the decision is made whether or not to alert 'the conscious you' about the pain) and the limbic system (responsible for our emotional response to pain). Opioid receptors are also scattered through-out the gut (causing constipation) and *adrenal medulla*. They are widely spread in tissues, on lymphocytes and associated with pain receptors where they have anti-inflammatory activity.

Pharmacodynamics

Opioids work by binding to receptors on nerve cell membranes where they pull a series of biochemical levers to restrain nerves from reacting to incoming pain stimuli.

The opioids are classified by how they act on the various opioid receptors. There are three main groups of opioid receptors: mu (μ), delta (∂) and kappa (k). The mu receptor is named after morphine, the kappa receptor after the only known pure *agonist*, ketocyclazone; while the delta receptor is so named because it was first found in rat vas deferens.

The mu receptor is the most effective for pain relief, but unfortunately it is also the one responsible for respiratory depression. Importantly, the mu receptor gives opioids their wonderful ability to dissolve anxiety. As anxiety dissipates, patients report that although they still feel the pain, it doesn't hurt anymore.

Although delta and kappa receptors give *analgesia*, stimulating them has unfortunate effects. Stimulating delta receptors causes vomiting; while stimulating kappa receptors causes feelings of profound unease. These proper-ties are not desirable in an analgesic. So it is hardly surprising that the effective pain relieving morphine, diacetylmorphine, and pethidine are highly effective stimulators of mu receptors. Unfortunately their ability to temporarily wipe away the cares of this world makes them candidates to become drugs of addiction.

On the other hand, kappa receptor analgesic drugs (such as buprenorphine) or those with low mu receptor affinity (such as tramadol) are unlikely to cause addiction, and as they stimulate feelings of unease and cause vomiting, they are unpopular with patients (and opioid addicts too).

Pharmacokinetics

Once an opioid is injected into a vein it is first rapidly carried to regions of the body that have a good blood supply: this process is called uptake. The opioid concentration in the blood then falls away in an exponential fashion as the drug is distributed through less well-perfused body tissue compartments. Meanwhile the liver and the kidneys start to eliminate the drug from the body. Only a tiny fraction of the dose of opioid gets through the blood–brain barrier to act on receptors in the central nervous system and spinal cord.

Clinical properties of the opioids

All the opioids have common properties, but there are also important differences. One opioid is not superior to another, but some opioids are better suited to some patients and procedures. Adverse effects are dose related: the more you give, the more likely problems will occur.

Effective dose

The effective dose of an opioid varies greatly from patient to patient, and can vary as much as fourfold in any particular age group. This variation is greatest in the elderly.

> *Patients in pain are unlikely to experience severe respiratory depression.*

Opioids depress respiration

Respiratory depression causes either the patient's rate or depth of breathing, or both, to lessen. Opioids may slow the rate of breathing from 12–14 breaths/min to 8 breaths or fewer per minute. Initially, as the respiratory rate slows, the patient takes bigger breaths, but eventually breathing becomes shallow. Given enough opioid, a patient will stop breathing altogether. Addicts who die from heroin overdose usually just stop breathing. Combining an opioid with a benzodiazepine, such as diazepam or midazolam, compounds respiratory depression.

Given normal doses of opioids patients in pain are unlikely to develop respiratory depression. There is, however, a trap where a patient in severe pain has received a large dose of an opioid and subsequently is given a local anaesthetic block. Unopposed by pain, the opioid is likely to cause severe respiratory depression.

In patients who are not in pain even low doses of opioids suppress the innate desire to take a breath. People affected by opioids can voluntarily hold their breath long enough to become cyanosed.

Equi-analgesic doses of all the opioids tend to cause about the same amount of respiratory depression.[1] All the potent opioids with the suffix '-nil or nyl' (fentanyl, alfentanil, sufentanil, and *remifentanil*) potently suppress breathing even in small initial doses. The less potent analgesics, morphine and pethidine, suppress breathing if higher doses are used.

On arriving in the recovery room many patients, although rousable, seem to forget to breathe, only taking a breath when reminded to do so. This phenomenon is called *Ondine's Curse*. For a short time you can help a patient over this hurdle of respiratory depression, by simply waking them and reminding them to take each breath. This helps avoid the risks of giving naloxone.

Respiratory depression, if it is going to occur, takes place within the first 3–5 minutes after giving an intravenous opioid. Carefully observe the depth of breathing, count the respiratory rate and do not turn your back on your patient during this period. Sedation and respiratory depression occur in parallel. Once a patient becomes drowsy they have had enough opioid, but watch for developing respiratory depression with a decline in respiratory rate. Patients who become drowsy with lower doses of opioids in the recovery room need lower doses of opioid, and a longer interval between doses in the ward.

Respiratory depression is more likely to occur in patients who are:

- asthmatics;
- diabetics;
- heroin addicts;
- elderly, frail, and feeble;
- neonates;
- obese;
- trauma patients affected by drugs or alcohol.

or who have:

- heart failure;
- lung disease;
- liver disease;
- renal impairment;
- neuromuscular diseases;
- Asian ethnicity;
- obstructive or central sleep apnoea.

With respiratory depression the $PaCO_2$ rises, and this causes:

- raised intracranial pressure;
- raised intraocular pressure;
- drowsiness (but not confusion);
- peripheral vasodilation;
- hyperglycaemia;
- respiratory acidosis.

With respiratory depression accumulating carbon dioxide spills over into the lungs, displacing oxygen to cause hypoxaemia. If you are giving the patient an opioid always give supplemental oxygen, and ensure the oximeter reading is at, or above, 95%. Send patients who are at risk of respiratory depression back to the ward on supplemental oxygen by mask.

If you are using an opioid then also give oxygen.

Opioids and blood pressure

Opioids do not significantly alter a stable, well-perfused patient's blood pressure, although they may cause the heart rate to slow. You cannot blame opioids for hypotension without excluding other causes.

Hypotension occurs when an opioid lessens the sympathetic response to some other insidious problem such as hypovolaemia, *cardiac failure*, hypoxia, or septicaemia. Postoperatively, the most common reason for a falling blood pressure is hypovolaemia.

Hypotension? Exclude hypovolaemia.

Even sick patients tolerate small doses of morphine given cautiously and slowly intravenously. Start with a low dose, say morphine 2 mg diluted in saline slowly intravenously, and wait 5 minutes to gauge the results.

Opioids, such as morphine and fentanyl, do not cause significant myocardial depression or hypotension and do not predispose to arrhythmias; but pethidine is an exception to this rule. Pethidine, being a vasodilator and myocardial depressant, often drops the blood pressure when given intravenously. If pethidine unmasks hypovolaemia or cardiac failure the blood pressure will fall, within a minute or two.

Neonates and infants may drop their blood pressure with morphine, and almost certainly will do so with pethidine.

The short-acting opioids fentanyl (and its daughter sufentanil, and son alfentanil) cause bradycardia and profound respiratory depression and their pain-relieving qualities are short-lived. They are useful for patients on a ventilator, but not for spontaneously breathing patients in the recovery room.

Opioids sedate patients

Opioids cause drowsiness. Patients tend to lie quietly and not move much unless prompted. When asked what they are thinking about they report a non-dreaming sleep-like state, but they are aware of their surroundings. Time appears to pass more quickly. This inability to structure thoughts, to anticipate or plan, and the disinclination to move is called *psychomotor retardation*. Do not tell patients important information while they are under the influence of opioids. They almost invariably forget it. This includes instructions about their care after surgery. Obviously, while sedated with an opioid, they cannot sign legal documents such as consent or release forms.

Opioids cause nausea and vomiting

Twenty to thirty per cent of patients who receive opioids during their anaesthetic become nauseated, or vomit in the recovery room. Equivalent doses of all opioids trigger nausea in certain patients, but those with kappa effects (such as tramadol) do so more readily. Opioids make patients susceptible to motion sickness by increasing their sensitivity to inputs from the vestibular apparatus in their middle ear: they get giddy easily. Agonizing pain itself can cause nausea and vomiting.

Opioids dissolve anxiety

Opioids promote an overwhelming feeling of well-being. They make it difficult to worry about anything and anxiety melts away. As the threatening feelings of alarm and fear dissolve, so does the activity of the sympathetic nervous system: tachycardia, hypotension and the other metabolic effects all fade away. Pain becomes less threatening, and although it is often still present it does not cause the patient much concern. As one patient said, 'Yes, I still have pain, but it doesn't hurt any more.'

Opioid-induced itch

Opioids cause itchy noses, and patients sometimes rub them vigorously when emerging from anaesthesia. This becomes a problem after eye or nose surgery, and facial plastic surgery. A small dose of intravenous promethazine 0.3 mg/Kg usually solves the problem.

Opioids and urinary retention

Not only do opioids reduce the desire to pass urine, they cause the bladder's vesicle sphincter to tighten while relaxing detrusor muscle. In older men this can cause problems. Patience, encouragement and the sound of running water often help; failing that, they will need a catheter.

Opioids and pinpoint pupils

Pinpoint pupils (meiosis) are greatest with fentanyl, intermediate with morphine and least with pethidine. Meiosis does not abate as tolerance develops. A patient who is not tolerant to opioids, and who has meiosis after morphine, is unlikely to be in substantial pain.

Opioids can cause allergy

Like many low molecular-weight drugs, some opioids (but not the fentanyl group) displace histamine from mast cells. This is not an immune response, but it may cause the patient to develop an itchy rash near the site of injection. This resolves within a few minutes. True allergic (IgE- or IgG-mediated responses) to opioids are rare, but not unknown. Usually morphine is the culprit. In theory morphine may precipitate bronchospasm in asthmatics, but in the recovery room this is not a problem provided the morphine is given slowly.

Tolerance and addiction

There are two groups of patients where opioids may cause problems in the recovery room: patients with cancer pain who are on long-term opioids, and narcotic-dependent people such as heroin addicts.

Patients with disseminated cancer presenting for surgery are frequently taking long-term opioids, usually fentanyl patches or oral morphine solutions, and occasionally both. Because they develop tolerance they may need up to ten times as much opioid as a normal patient to control their postoperative pain. Consult with the oncology staff for guidance about their opioid requirements.

Tolerance and the opioids

With frequent administration opioids gradually lose their effect, and larger and larger doses are needed to achieve the same response. This tolerance to opioids takes a few days to develop. Tolerance is a problem in patients presenting for repeated painful procedures, such as debriding or grafting burns, or those with cancer pain.

It is cruel to withhold opioids because you fear a patient may become addicted to them. Patients in pain rarely become psychologically dependent (*addicted*) to opioids.

How to manage heroin addicts

Heroin addicts, and opioid-dependent patients, need proper analgesia, just like anybody else. In 'recovering addicts' there is no evidence that opioid analgesia will trigger a relapse, but many would prefer not to receive opioids for analgesia, because they fear the consequences.

Heroin addicts on a methadone programme are already taking an opioid and will have cross-tolerance with other opioids. Addicts on a methadone programme need their usual dose of methadone on the day of surgery. Do not attempt to withdraw their drugs before surgery.

The dose of methadone taken daily is equivalent to the same dose of morphine taken 4-hourly; thus methadone 30 mg per day is equivalent to 30 mg of morphine taken 4-hourly. The best option is to simply maintain their baseline methadone regime, and use other options to control their pain such as NSAIDs, or regional anaesthesia. If you do elect to use opioids, simply add a normal dose of opioid to their baseline methadone requirement. Do not use tramadol or buprenorphine.

How to manage patients taking buprenorphine

Buprenorphine is a partial opioid mu *agonist* sometimes used to control persistent pain in patients with chronic painful diseases and to treat drug addicts and alcoholics. Sometimes patients taking long-term buprenorphine come to surgery.

Buprenorphine is a potent long-acting drug – the effects last for 8 or more hours. Its elimination half-life is 20–72 hours. Because it is metabolized in the liver there is little risk of accumulation in patients with renal impairment or in the elderly. If a patient is taking long-term oral buprenorphine, using additional opioids for pain relief may have unpredictable effects. Respiratory depression caused by buprenorphine is not reversed by naloxone.

Some patients may come to the recovery room wearing low-dose transcutaneous patches impregnated with buprenorphine. These are applied once a week to provide analgesia for low back pain or osteoarthritis of hips and knees. Sometimes patients forget to take them off. Because the buprenorphine trickles into the circulation so slowly, it has less than 15 per cent receptor occupancy. This means that 85 per cent of the opioid receptors are still unoccupied. Consequently, for these patients, you can use normal doses of morphine or other opioids for postoperative analgesia.

Opioid withdrawal syndrome

In the recovery room, if you give naloxone, or even a partial agonist such as tramadol, to patients taking long-term opioids (including heroin addicts) you will precipitate *withdrawal syndrome*. In its severe form this causes sweating, shaking, shivering, a runny nose, abdominal cramps, headache, nausea, and dilated pupils. Although unpleasant, it is rarely fatal, unlike alcohol. Mild withdrawal usually brings on nothing more than a headache, and an itchy nose. Some patients feel apprehensive, shaky and jittery. Signs of opioid withdrawal in the neonate include convulsions, excessive crying, and hyperactive *reflexes*.

How to use opioids

Intravenous administration is best

In the recovery room the only reliable and predictable way to give drugs is intravenously. After surgery the muscles are usually poorly perfused, consequently intramuscular drugs are unreliably absorbed and may take more than 30 minutes to work. This unacceptable delay aggravates the physiological and emotional stresses caused by pain.

Intravenous opioids are safe even with unstable or shocked patients. Small increments of well-diluted opioids given intravenously start to have an effect within 2–3 minutes, and measures can be taken instantly to compensate for changes in blood pressure. On the other hand it is risky giving large irretrievable doses of opioid into poorly perfused muscle where the absorption and uptake is erratic. In this case unwitnessed respiratory depression may occur back in the ward many hours after the patient has left the recovery area.

How to give an opioid

Start by putting your patient on 35% inspired oxygen by mask. Make up 10 mg of morphine to 10 ml in saline. To build up effective blood levels, load the patient with a slow intravenous injection of 2 ml of this solution over a 5-minute period. Use the pain algorithm set out in this chapter to guide you. Wait 5 minutes for the drug to be distributed through well-perfused tissues and then continue to give the opioid until the pain is either relieved, or the patient becomes drowsy with droopy eyelids and pupils about 2–3 mm in diameter. Stop giving the opioid if the respiratory rate drops to 8 breaths/min or less. In adults, the age of the patient is better predictor of opioid requirements than weight, but the response varies widely so that some patients need larger doses.

What to do next

Once the loading dose is effective make some judgements about when to give the next dose. The answer is to wait until the patient begins to complain of pain once more. The interval between the first dose and this time gives an indication of the *context-sensitive* duration of action of the drug. Since this next dose of opioid is simply a booster, it only needs to be a half to a third of the first dose.

Do not wake patients to ask if they are in pain.

Table 6.1 Duration of effect of the opioid analgesics

Opioid analgesic	Duration of action in hours
Morphine	3–4
Pethidine	2–3
Diamorphine	3–4
Oxycodone	4–6
Tramadol	5–6

What to do if opioids do not relieve pain

Opioids are powerful analgesics. They are excellent at removing the anxiety component of pain, especially deep visceral or bone pain, but they are relatively ineffective against pain originating in skin, or with some forms of headache: in this case use either paracetamol or a NSAID.

Try clonidine

For restless patients, especially if they are hypertensive, a small dose of clonidine 150 μg in 10 ml of saline given in 2 ml increments, that is clonidine 30 μg is often effective. Because clonidine causes the blood pressure to fall, measure the blood pressure after each increment.

Consider a surgical cause

If pain persists despite normal amounts of an opioid, consider a surgical cause for the pain. Persistent pain after a *laparoscopy* or colonoscopy may be the first sign of a perforated bowel, or pain after an arthroscopy may be a sign of bleeding into a joint. Pain following manipulation of a fracture under anaesthetic (MUA) means the plaster might be too tight. Inform the surgeon about any persistent pain.

Persistent pain? Consider a surgical cause.

Special precautions with opioids

Patients who eliminate opioids slowly

Some patients eliminate opioids slowly. This is likely if they have chronic kidney disease, liver disease, are elderly, or are less than 2 years old; or if they have been hypovolaemic at any stage before or during their surgery. Opioid requirements can vary by up to tenfold in elderly people. Some elderly patients tolerate morphine well and consequently may receive inadequate pain relief.[2] The message is give it slowly, use incremental doses, and watch for the effects.

Enzymes in the liver convert codeine to morphine. About 12 per cent of Caucasians and most Chinese lack the necessary enzymes and consequently may receive no analgesia at all from codeine or tramadol.

Opioids in shocked patients

It is safe to use small doses of morphine in shocked patients. Morphine does not usually depress myocardial contractility, but pethidine most certainly does.

It is hazardous to give large irretrievable doses of opioid into poorly perfused muscle where the absorption and uptake is erratic, and adverse reactions may occur hours after patients leave the vigilance of the recovery area.

Opioids in children

Neonates, and especially premature babies up to the gestational age of 22 months, or those with neurological or pulmonary abnormalities, have a high risk of respiratory depression and apnoea if given opioids. Apnoea and respiratory depression are dose-related. If opioids are used in these children then once they leave the recovery room they must go to an area where they can be monitored with apnoea alarms for at least 24 hours.

Babies require lower doses and longer intervals between doses. As with the elderly, it is best to give small doses incrementally. Infants under the age of 3 months need about a quarter of the dose per kilogram recommended for older children.

Opioids in pregnancy

Opioids are safe to use in pregnant patients, but excessive doses in labour may cause respiratory depression in the newborn.

Opioids and lactation

All the opioids, along with many anaesthetic drugs, enter breast milk and may be transferred to the baby. If the baby is tiny or vulnerable it is best for the mother to express her milk before surgery and store it in the refrigerator. She can also express and discard the first feed after surgery.

Opioids in hypothermic patients

Hypothermic patients metabolize and excrete opioids slowly, although opioid requirements do not seem to be affected by mild postoperative hypothermia.[3] Patients with temperatures less than 35.5°C may stop breathing if given normal doses of opioids. Use small doses intravenously with great caution.

When to avoid opioids

Avoid opioids in patients with chronic obstructive pulmonary disease, unstable asthma, cor pulmonale, and severe liver disease; also refrain from using opioids in those with suspected raised intracranial pressure; and in patients who have had neurosurgery, inner or middle ear surgery, and open eye surgery.

Consider alternatives to the opioids

Keep in mind that other techniques, and drugs apart from the opioids, can be used to *facilitate* pain relief: paracetamol, NSAIDs, cyclo-oxygenase Type 2 (COX-2) inhibitors, a regional nerve block, clonidine or ketamine.

Occasionally relaxation techniques are useful for acute postoperative pain, but the patient needs to be familiar with these before coming to the operating theatre.

Transcutaneous electrical stimulation (TENS) has been used to treat post-operative pain, but is not particularly effective.

Opioid drugs

Morphine

Advantages

Morphine effectively controls moderate to severe pain. It attaches to mu receptors and works better with deep-seated ill-defined (visceral) pain, than sharper well-localized (somatic) pain. Patients who only experience pain when they move are unlikely to get pain relief from morphine.

Morphine is a safe drug even in patients with heart failure. It is unlikely to cause hypotension and tachycardia, however if they do occur then you must find the reason (first eliminate hypovolaemia). Morphine suppresses the cough reflex. It is the only safe opioid to use to relieve the symptoms of acute *pulmonary oedema*. It is unlikely to have serious adverse reactions with other drugs.

What happens with a bolus dose

If we give a slow bolus of 15 mg of morphine intravenously to a fit young man who is in moderate pain (say after a stabilization of a fractured arm) we would observe the following:

Time	Effect
Immediately	Venous flare may run up the vein with a little stinging feeling.
2–5 minutes	Drowsiness with light-headedness.
5–8 minutes	Onset of pain relief.
8–10 minutes	Decline in respiratory depth and rate.
	Rate may drop below 10 breaths/min.
10 minutes	20% of patients report nausea.
30–45 minutes	Analgesia peaks.
3–4 + hours	Duration of effective pain relief.
4 hours	Pain relief wears off, but respiratory depression may persist.

Disadvantages

Morphine is slow to act. It makes little difference whether it is given intravenously or intramuscularly because the time to achieve satisfactory analgesia is about the same. It is said to cause more smooth muscle spasm than pethidine, which makes it less suitable for biliary, intestinal or renal colic.

Dose

Titrate the dose to the patient's needs. Younger adults need high loading doses than older patients. Patients in severe pain need doses at the higher end of the range. In fat patients calculate doses on their *lean body mass*, not their total body weight.

Table 6.3 Morphine dosing regimes

	Dose type	Dose
Neonate	Loading dose	10–20 µgm/Kg
	Infusion	10–20 µgm/Kg/hr
Child	Loading dose	100–200 µgm/Kg
	Infusion	100–200 µgm/Kg/hr
Adult	Loading dose	30–150 µgm/Kg
	Infusion	20–50 µgm/Kg/hr

1 µg = 1/1000 of a milligram.

For morphine infusions in both adults and children

Make up the infusion with 0.5 mg/Kg of morphine in 50 ml of 5% dextrose.

1 ml/hr = 10 µgm/Kg/hr

Normal morphine requirements range between 2–10 µgm/Kg/hr.

Useful information

For patients older than 20 years of age, the average 24 hourly intravenous morphine requirement is, approximately (100 – age in years) milligrams.

For single intravenous doses, take the average 24 hourly requirements, divide it by 8 and give it every 2 hours. For example a 52 year old would require 100 – 52 = 48 mg in 24 hours. A single intravenous dose would be 48/8 = 6 mg given every two hours intravenously.

Morphine 1–5 mg given into an intra-articular space after arthroscopy gives good analgesia for up to 48 hours.

Top-ups

In 4 hours time there is still quite a lot of morphine in the body; so a smaller dose is needed to bring the levels back to the effective (therapeutic) range. An appropriate top-up dose is morphine 7.5–10 mg slowly injected intra-venously over 10 minutes. Monitor for drowsiness, and a decrease in the rate and depth of breathing.

Going through this procedure every 4 hours is time-consuming. Instead we can use a computer-driven pump to allow patients to give themselves a small dose of intravenous opioid when they are in pain. This technique called *patient-controlled analgesia* is discussed in the next section.

If you give morphine to people who are not in pain many report nausea or dizziness especially if they move their head around. They have difficulty in concentrating, feel vague and uneasy (dysphoria), and they perspire. Objectively they are pale, with pinpoint pupils, they look sweaty and their rate and depth of breathing decreases. Most would prefer not to receive the drug again.

Liver disease

Where possible avoid opioids in patients with *hepatic impairment*. These drugs may cause hypoventilation, hypoxia and acidosis and precipitate liver failure. Although morphine metabolism is not overly prolonged in most patients with stable cirrhosis, it is best to start with 50% of the normal loading dose of morphine. For subsequent doses give only 50–75% of the initial dose, and increase the interval between doses by 50%. For instance for the first dose give 5 mg of morphine (instead of 10 mg) and for subsequent doses give 2.5 mg (instead of 5 mg) and give it 6-hourly (instead of every 4 hours). You can always give more morphine if necessary.

Chronic kidney disease

Morphine is metabolized to morphine 6-glucuronide (M6G), which itself is more potent than morphine. M6G is excreted by the kidneys and will accumulate in patients with chronic kidney disease. If the estimated glomerular filtration rate is less than 30 mL/min/1.73 m^2 then halve the loading dose and reduce subsequent doses by 75%. You can always top-up the dose in small increments if necessary.

Pethidine

Advantages

Although seldom used now pethidine (called meperidine in the USA) has many properties similar to morphine, but it also has some very important differences. Being a potent mu *agonist* it is useful for rapid control of moderate to severe pain. Given intravenously it works within 2–3 minutes, which is faster than morphine, but it causes more hypotension, and tachycardia. When surgery causes smooth muscle spasm, for example, on the Fallopian tubes, pethidine is more effective than morphine.

Disadvantages

Pethidine has a low *therapeutic index*. This means the toxic dose (which is a dose that exceeds 150 mg in an adult) is close to the therapeutic dose (50–100 mg).

Pethidine adversely interacts with many drugs and may precipitate the serotonin syndrome in patients taking:

- tramadol;
- SSRI inhibitors;
- tricyclic antidepressants;
- MAOI type A inhibitors (moclobemide);
- MAOI type B inhibitors (phenelzine or tranylcypromine).

What happens with a bolus dose

If we give 75–100 mg of pethidine over a 5-minute period to a fit young man in moderate pain we would observe the following.

Time	Effect
Immediately	A venous flare may run up the vein causing a little sting
30–60 seconds	Onset of drowsiness with light-headedness
2–5 minutes	Onset of pain relief
5 minutes	Decline in respiratory depth and rate. Rate may drop below 10 breaths/min
6 minutes	30% of patients report nausea
8 minutes	Analgesia peaks
2–3 + hours	Duration of effective pain relief
3 + hours	Pain relief wears off, but respiratory depression may persist

Do not give pethidine or tramadol to people taking psychiatric medication.

Dose

Titrate the dose of pethidine to the patient's needs. In some cases the effective dose can be high, especially if the patient has been on long-term opioids for the relief of cancer pain, or is a recovering heroin addict taking methadone.

In patients with chronic kidney or liver disease, pethidine is not as safe as morphine.

Top-ups

As with morphine, patients need a smaller dose to bring the levels back within the effective therapeutic range. An appropriate dose would be pethidine 75 mg slowly injected intravenously over 5 minutes while watching for drowsiness, and a decrease in the rate and depth of breathing.

Liver disease

Avoid opioids in patients with *hepatic impairment*, because any respiratory depression may cause liver failure. In patients with stable cirrhosis, after giving 50 per cent of the normal loading dose, reduce subsequent doses by 50–75% and increase the dosing interval by half.

Chronic kidney disease

Pethidine is metabolized to 6-pethidinic acid (6PA) which has no analgesic activity. 6PA is toxic and if it accumulates it causes agitation, muscle twitching, seizures, coma, and even death. 6PA is excreted by the kidneys and accumulates in patients with chronic kidney disease. Avoid pethidine if possible and certainly if the estimated creatinine *clearance* is less than 30 ml/min/1.73 m^2. If you must use it reduce the dose by 50% and double the interval between doses. In this case do not exceed a total cumulative of more than 3 mg/Kg.

Fentanyl

Fentanyl is a potent opioid working predominately on mu receptors. It is useful to treat severe pain in ventilated patients. Fentanyl is commonly used in epidural infusions, in this case do not give other opioids (including codeine) or the patient may stop breathing.

Advantages

Fentanyl is an excellent analgesic, quick acting and unlikely to cause hypotension (even in hypovolaemic patients). Metabolized entirely by the liver, and not depending on the kidneys for its elimination, fentanyl is safe to use in renal disease.

Disadvantages

Fentanyl is not a good analgesic for the recovery room, it is very short acting and the patient's pain scarcely settles down before another dose is required. Because it causes profound respiratory depression it can bring on Ondine's curse with a vengeance, where the patient is awake, but not breathing.

Fentanyl can cause unpredictable respiratory depression some hours after a patient returns to the ward. This is more likely in the elderly, especially after endoscopic procedures, where fentanyl sequestrated in muscle vascular beds is released back into the circulation when the patient begins to move about.

Occasionally higher doses of fentanyl cause glottal spasm making it impossible to ventilate a patient with a bag and mask. Until recently, chest wall rigidity was thought to cause this phenomenon.[4] In large doses fentanyl causes bradycardia.

Diamorphine

Although diamorphine (heroin) is an illegal drug in most parts of the world, it is widely used in the United Kingdom. In many ways it is the ideal opioid. It has a quick onset, is highly effective, and is unlikely to cause hypotension. It reputedly causes less nausea and vomiting than morphine. Dose is 0.015 mg/Kg intravenously. The liver quickly metabolizes diamorphine into an active metabolite, which may well be the principal analgesic.

Hydromorphone

Hydromorphone is a synthetic derivative of morphine. It is 7 to 10 times more potent than morphine. The typical adult dose of hydromorphone 1.5 mg acts for 4 to 5 hours. It is popular in some parts of the USA because it is said to cause less hypotension than other opioids.

Methadone

Methadone, a long acting opioid, is equipotent with morphine. It works for about 30 hours. This means a 10 mg dose of morphine given every 4 hours is equivalent to 10 mg of methadone give daily. Because of its long action, methadone does not allow for flexibility in dosing regimes.

Codeine

Codeine is a useful analgesic, especially when combined with paracetamol, but it does have some drawbacks. To act as an analgesic, codeine has to be metabolized to morphine by the liver's CYP 2D6 cytochrome *enzymes*. About 12 per cent of people of European origins lack this enzyme and consequently get no pain relief from codeine, while an additional 40 per cent of Caucasians have reduced levels of the enzyme. A typically effective dose of codeine is 30–60 mg orally. In contrast, some North Africans have many copies of the genes that code for the enzymes and quickly convert codeine to morphine.

Tramadol

Tramadol is an unusual opioid analgesic. Not only does its metabolite bind weakly to opioid mu receptors in the brain and spinal cord, but tramadol also inhibits the uptake of noradrenaline and *serotonin* into nerves. This gives it some of the properties of tricyclic antidepressants (which are sometimes used to manage chronic pain).

Unlike morphine, which has high mu activity, tramadol's affinity for the mu receptor is 6000 times less than morphine's. As a result tramadol does not have the anxiety-relieving properties of morphine or pethidine and it certainly is not as effective as morphine against acute severe pain. We feel that tramadol is not a good drug to treat acute postoperative pain after surgery. Although it relieves moderate to severe pain, many patients find that they feel awful, sweaty, restless, and nauseated. The combination of paracetamol 500 mg and codeine 30 mg orally, is equally effective, faster acting, and certainly less expensive than tramadol.

Tramadol is contraindicated in epileptics or those at risk of seizures (alcoholics, heroin or cocaine addicts, head injuries, liver disease and possibly diabetics). Naloxone only partly reverses its effects, and may increase the risk of seizures.

Unlike morphine, tramadol adversely interacts with many drugs, especially almost all psychotropic medication (SSRIs, tricyclic antidepressants, and MAOIs) where there is an appreciable risk of the serotonin syndrome.[5]

Although many patients dislike tramadol's effects, it remains popular with clinicians who feel that, in contrast to morphine, people are unlikely to abuse tramadol.

Do not use pethidine or tramadol in patients taking psychotropic drugs.

Dose

Give tramadol 100 mg by slow intravenous injection over 3 minutes. Top-up doses 50–100 mg every 4–6 hours, up to a total daily dose of 600 mg. It takes effect in 12–15 minutes. Do not use tramadol in children.

Serotonin syndrome[6]

Serotonin is a monamine neurotransmitter in the central nervous system. (Serotonin is another name for 5-hydroxy tryptamine, or 5-HT). Many drugs have serotoninergic activity. Clinical depression is sometimes treated with selective serotonin *re-uptake* inhibitors (SSRIs). These include sertraline, citalopram, fluoxetine, paroxetine and fluvoxamine. Other drugs, such as pethidine, tramadol, venlafaxine and some tricyclic antidepressants, or monoamine oxidase inhibitors also release serotonin and noradrenaline in the brain. If these drugs are used concurrently with SSRIs then within minutes to hours the excessive serotonin in the patient's brain causes them to develop the *serotonin syndrome*.[7] They develop mental changes (becoming confused, agitated and mentally clouded); neuromuscular excitation (with jerky clonic muscle movements, abnormal muscle twitches and shakes); and autonomic stimulation (with hypertension, and tachycardia, and ventricular extrasystoles). Excessive muscle movement causes the body temperature to rise, with sweating and flushing.

Treat the serotonin syndrome by stopping the offending drug, treat each symptom as it arises. In severe cases it may be necessary to use serotonin antagonists such as cyproheptadine and methylsergide.

Newer opioid drugs

The quest for the ideal analgesic continues in the hope of finding a strong analgesic that is not addictive, not a respiratory depressant and is cardiac stable. New opioid drugs are introduced every few years, prescribed with enthusiasm, and then fall by the wayside. The drugs have included buprenorphine, pentazocine, dipipanone, meptazinol, nalbuphine and others.

Although morphine has unpleasant and annoying side-effects, inconvenient pharmacokinetics, needs to be locked away in a cupboard, and is a bad drug from many points of view; all the others are worse.

Opioid antagonists

Naloxone

Naloxone is a highly potent opioid mu receptor antagonist. Given intravenously it rapidly (within 1 to 2 minutes) reverses respiratory depression, but it also reverses all the analgesic and *narcotic* effects of the opioid (and the patient's own endorphins too). Usually patients are catapulted into agonizing pain and their blood pressure may rise abruptly. The hypertension in turn may cause myocardial ischaemia, and the first sign might be the onset of *Ventricular premature beats* on the ECG monitor. Naloxone works in an 'all or none' manner.

The sudden onset of agony can result in a strong adrenergic jolt, which is severe enough to cause the pulmonary vascular pressures to surge abruptly resulting in acute *pulmonary oedema*. Patients start to wheeze, and their oxygen saturations fall. Naloxone has caused sudden death in this manner.

Naloxone reverses the respiratory depression caused by opioids for about 35 minutes, and then its effect wears off. If, after this period, patients still have effective levels of the opioid in their brain they will relapse into respiratory depression. After a single dose of naloxone continue to observe your patients for about an hour to ensure that they do not relapse. If you have given naloxone and the patient does not respond, then there is probably another cause for their respiratory depression or altered mental state.

If the patient does not respond to naloxone then you may need to use the non-specific stimulant doxapram, or if this fails the patient may need to be ventilated. We feel that assisted ventilation is the safest option, and gives time to reassess what might have gone wrong.

Naloxone does not reverse myocardial depression caused by pethidine or tramadol, nor the bradycardias caused by fentanyl, or the seizures caused by norpethidine or tramadol.

Opioids

1. Diamorphine is the best analgesic of all.
2. Morphine is good for deep diffuse poorly localised pain.
3. Pethidine works faster, but can be toxic.
4. Best to use opioids intravenously in recovery room.
5. Tramadol is inferior.
6. Avoid naloxone if possible.
7. If patients are over 55 years and receiving opioids, then give supplemental oxygen.

Patient-controlled analgesia

Since only the patients know how much pain they have, it seems reasonable to allow them to control their own *analgesia*. *Patient-controlled analgesia* infusion devices use a minicomputer to give a bolus dose of an opioid when the patient presses a button. This is followed by a lock-out time where no further drug is given no matter how often the button is pressed. Patients will not press the button if they are drowsy, asleep, or not in pain.

Patient-controlled analgesia has proved an effective and safe way to administer opioids, while keeping opioid doses to a minimum. The technique has fewer complications than intermittent intramuscular injections of opioids.

PCA is a maintenance technique;
it is not useful for delivering a loading dose.

Some devices give a background maintenance infusion. We firmly believe background infusions are hazardous. There is no evidence that they are helpful, and there are many reports of respiratory depression. A constant background infusion does not reduce the night-time demands for analgesia, nor ensure better sleep.

Table 6.5 Advantages vs. disadvantages of PCA

Advantages of PCA	Disadvantages of PCA
Patient feels in control	Drowsiness, nausea and itching
Frees up nursing staff	Costly equipment
Respiratory depression less	Nurses need training in its use
Fewer sleep disturbances	Ties patient to bed with the IV line
Lower doses of opioid used	No use in demented patients
Can be used in children > 6 years	May mask pain warning of postoperative complications such as angina, pulmonary embolism, too tight plasters, or full bladder

Elderly patients often have difficulty using PCA, but in those elderly patients who can cope, it causes much less postoperative confusion than in those receiving intramuscular opioids.

Start patient-controlled analgesia in the recovery room. The staff can give the first few loading doses, and they have the training to recognize adverse effects and gauge the drug's efficacy.

Morphine is the best drug for patient-controlled analgesia. Pethidine is not a safe drug to use for patient-controlled analgesia, because it has a low *therapeutic index* and there is a risk of norpethidine toxicity.

Patient-controlled analgesia is useful and appropriate for patients with a history of opioid dependence (whether legal or otherwise), but they require on average three times as much opioid as a non-dependent person to control their pain. These patients are not tolerant to the sedative effects of the opioids, so adjust dosages according to their sedation score and respiratory rate, rather than pain relief.

How to reduce mishaps

There have been many reports of accidents and mishaps with automated patient-controlled analgesia devices: they are good, but not foolproof. Monitor your patients carefully. There are many different makes of PCA device on the market, so make sure you are familiar with the devices available in your hospital.

Age is the best predictor for opioid requirements. In the elderly double the lock-out time to start with. You can always increase the doses later if more is needed.

The best way to avoid problems is to use a standard protocol and a standard order form in every ward. Most slips occur when setting up the infusion, such as prescription errors, errors in administering the drug, and patient factors.

Prescription errors

Prescription errors include wrong dose, wrong lock-out time, and wrong infusion rate.

The prescription sheet should clearly set out:
- drug dose and dilution;
- dose increments (the dose given when the patient presses the button);
- allowable number of doses per hour;
- lock-out time;
- maximum amount of drug allowable in any 4-hour period;
- how often nurses need to make observations;
- acceptable limits of blood pressure, and respiratory rate.

The protocol should include details about:

- who is responsible for setting up the infusion;
- disposal of unused solutions;
- how to treat side-effects;
- where to find medical support staff (pager and telephone number).

Administration errors

Simple mistakes in setting up the apparatus are the source of most problems. These include preparing the wrong concentration of drug, not reading the prescription form accurately, setting up the equipment incorrectly, and accidentally injecting drug while changing the infusion apparatus.

- Make sure your hospital uses only one type of PCA device so that every ward uses identical devices.
- Have a checklist (just like an airline pilot) and go through it step-by-step with another member of staff.
- Design your forms to be clear. A common source of error is where doses can be either written as milligrams or millilitres. Design your patient-controlled analgesia form to eliminate this error. The orders need to be written exactly as they appear on the machine.
- Use a dedicated intravenous line. Opioids infusions need their own separate intravenous line; nothing else should run through this line. Piggy-backing it on another line risks the drug being pushed backward if the cannula becomes blocked. When the cannula is unblocked the large dose that has backed up in the line will run into the patient.

Do not start PCA in patients who are still having opioid infusion into their *epidural space*. In this case respiratory depression is almost inevitable.

Patient factors

Sick or confused patients are unable to use PCA.

Occasionally problems occur because visitors and staff press the button for the patient. One variation on the theme of PCA is parent-controlled analgesia where an anxious parent, worried their child is in pain, unnecessarily presses the button. Some patients, especially those with a dependent or anxious personality, dislike PCA; so respect their wishes.

Sleep apnoea

Many obese patients have a sleep apnoea syndrome. If they receive opioids, they sometimes simply stop breathing, often in the early hours of the morning when the ward is 'nice and quiet'. Patients with sleep apnoea have less active respiratory drives, and opioids turn down the response even further. Sedated with morphine, propped up on pillows, and becoming even drowsier as their $PaCO_2$ rises, their head lolls forward to quietly obstruct their upper airway. A couple of attempted gasps, and it is all over. The nurse finds them an hour later – dead. *Ondine's curse* strikes again.

Continuous opioid infusions

Fortunately continuous opioid infusions are no longer widely used in adults. We have seen many incidents and heard of a number of deaths with this regime. Oximeters do not guarantee safety.

In a fully supervised area, with properly trained nursing staff and meticulous monitoring, continuous opioid infusions are useful for children when used with apnoea alarms and pulse oximeters.

Anti-inflammatory drugs

Inflammation, with its biochemical mediators, causes nearly all pain. Inflammation is a result of tissue damaged by trauma (including surgery) or infection. The COX (cyclo-oxygenase) enzymes use *arachidonic acid* (which is in part derived from the *phospholipids* in damaged cell membranes) to produce a whole zoo of biochemical inflammatory mediators collectively called *eicosanoids*. These biochemicals stimulate pain nerve-endings to send pain signals to the brain and are also responsible for producing fever.

Non-steroidal anti-inflammatory drugs (NSAIDs) inactivate COX enzymes, and in doing so dampen the inflammatory response, reduce pain and decrease fever.

COX-2 inhibitors

COX-2 inhibitors have largely had their heyday. They are certainly effective, but have serious side-effects in a tiny minority of patients.

There are two principal isoforms of COX enzymes in the tissues: COX-1 and COX-2. The isoform COX-1 does useful things: it produces certain *prostaglandins* to dilate bronchi, protect the stomach against its hydrochloric acid, and dilate arterioles in the kidney. In contrast, COX-2 produces another separate set of prostaglandins to turbo-charge the inflammatory response.

Conventional NSAIDS, such as aspirin, diclofenac, ibuprofen, naproxen, indometacin (indomethacin), and piroxicam, inactivate both the isoforms of COX enzymes. Apart from taking the pain out of the inflammatory response they also aggravate asthma, peptic ulcers, and renal impairment.

This led to the development of highly selective COX-2 inhibiting drugs: celecoxib (Celebrex®) and meloxicam. These drugs did not cause as many peptic ulcers, or impair platelet aggregation, but did have adverse effects on renal blood flow.

Paracoxib, an injectable form of a COX-2 inhibitor, is occasionally used in the recovery room, but not in patients with ischaemic heart disease, or following coronary artery bypass surgery. This parenteral COX-2 inhibitor is given intramuscularly or intravenously as a once only dose. It is moderately effective for acute pain having a ceiling effect equivalent to 4 mg of morphine. When combined with a low dose of opioid it is a useful analgesic.[8] It has no effect on blood clotting. The intramuscular dose is 40 mg by deep slow injection. Do not use in patients who are sensitive to aspirin, or are likely to have renal impairment. Curtailing its use are reports of an increased incidence of postoperative myocardial infarction, stroke, and pulmonary embolism.

Non-steroidal anti-inflammatory drugs (NSAIDs)

Advantages of NSAIDs

NSAIDs (pronounced 'enn-sade') are popular for the management of mild to moderate postoperative pain because they do not cause respiratory depression, sedation or tolerance. They also reduce fevers, and make patients feel better. They are not effective as the sole agent after major surgery, but they do reduce opioid requirements and improve the quality of opioid analgesia.

Disadvantages of NSAIDs

Reduce kidney blood flow

All the NSAIDs can seriously jeopardise renal blood flow; especially in the elderly or in patients who are, or have recently been, hypovolaemic. Young people are not necessarily immune to this effect. Depending on the half-life of the NSAID the effect can persist for hours or days after the drug has been stopped. Do not use them in patients whose preoperative *estimated glomerular filtration rate* (eGFR) is less than 60 mL/min/1.73 m^2.

Impair blood coagulation

NSAIDs block prostaglandin production and *thromboxane* synthesis, and consequently the ability of platelets to aggregate to form a clot. It is unclear to what extent NSAIDs aggravate bleeding, but many surgeons prefer to stop them at least 4 days before surgery where bleeding may be a problem. For most

NSAIDs platelet aggregation returns to normal after 3 to 4 half-lives have elapsed. Aspirin. however, permanently destroys platelets' ability to function for the whole of their 10-day life span; and it takes at least 4–6 days before the bone marrow can manufacture enough platelets to restore blood clotting to normal.

Aggravate asthma

Some patients, particularly those who have a hypersensitivity to aspirin, are likely to get severe bronchospasm if given an NSAID. Again this is due to their ability to block the production of bronchodilating *prostaglandins*. NSAIDs are better avoided in asthmatics. Asthma may be aggravated by any of the NSAIDS, but aspirin, naproxen, indomethacin, and ibuprofen are particularly bad offenders. Paracetamol does not cause a problem.

Cause peptic ulcers

Parietal cells in the stomach mucosa produce quantities of strong hydrochloric acid. All NSAIDs inhibit the production of prostaglandins that protect the gastric mucosa from the damage caused by hydrochloric acid. Avoid them in patients with peptic ulcer disease. If the patient is already taking proton pump inhibitors (PPIs) such as esomeprazole, and pantoprazole, then you can use an NSAID. PPIs partially alleviate the damage by preventing the stomach from making hydrochloric acid; in contrast the 5-HT3 inhibitors, such as ranitidine, are not so effective.

May cause hypersensitivity

NSAIDs cause hypersensitivity reactions in certain patients causing angioedema, rhinitis, and urticaria. These are not truly immune-mediated hypersensitivity reactions, but are caused by the overproduction of a group of inflammatory mediators produced by *lipoxygenase* enzymes.

Other precautions

NSAIDs should not be used in patients with pre-eclamptic toxaemia, hypovolaemia, suboptimally controlled *hypertension*, or abnormal clotting studies.

Only give NSAIDs to healthy patients having straightforward surgery.

Adverse drug interactions

Do not use NSAIDs in patients taking thiazide diuretics (such as hydrochlorthiazide, or indapamide); loop diuretics (furosemide); beta blockers (such as metoprolol, atenolol); and *ACE inhibitors* (end in '-pril' e.g. enalapril) or angiotensin receptor blockers (end in '-sartan' e.g. candesartan).

Varieties of NSAIDs

A large number of NSAIDs are available. Despite strong drug company promotion, no drug is demonstrably superior to the others; all have their problems. There is some early evidence that NSAIDs may impair bone healing, so some orthopaedic surgeons prefer not to use NSAIDs for postoperative pain relief in their patients.

Aspirin

Aspirin alone is used rarely in the recovery room. Aspirin in combination with paracetamol is effective against mild to moderate pain, and certainly more effective than paracetamol alone, or paracetamol and codeine for pain arising from joints or ligaments. The dose is 300–600 mg 4 to 6 hourly. It is contraindicated in children under the age of 17 years, and in breastfeeding mothers because of the remote risk of Reye's syndrome (encephalopathy and liver damage) in her infant.

Diclofenac

Diclofenac is most useful for the control of ureteric colic, pelvic gynaecological surgery and pain after the insertion of ureteric stents. It is sometimes used as eye-drops after eye surgery to suppress inflammation. It is rapidly absorbed from the gut and has a half-life of 1 to 2 hours.

Ibuprofen

Ibuprofen has the lowest incidence of side effects of any of the non-specific NSAIDs. It is an effective analgesic, but its anti-inflammatory effect is weaker.

Table 6.6 Duration of effect of NSAIDs

NSAID	Duration of effect in hours
Aspirin	4
Ibuprofen	8
Indometacin	8
Ketorolac	6
Meloxicam	18
Paracoxib	8
Naproxen	24
Piroxicam	24
Atypical NSAID	
Paracetamol	4

It is useful for the pain following dental extractions and *laparoscopy*. Give it preoperatively to allow it time to act. It is rapidly cleared with a half-life of 1 to 2 hours. The dose of ibuprofen is 200–400 mg 6 hourly.

Ketorolac

Ketorolac can be given intravenously or intramuscularly. It gives moderate pain relief, and remains popular in day-surgery cases because it does not cause the problems of opioids. Do not use repeated doses if there is any chance of surgical bleeding. Start with 0.2 mg/Kg and then use 10–30 mg 6 hourly. The maximum daily dose is 90 mg in those under 50 years and 60 mg in those between 50 and 65 years.

Avoid using ketorolac in children or those over the age of 65 years; or those with coagulopathy hypovolaemia, renal impairment, diabetes, peptic ulcer disease, or those who are older smokers. Anaphylaxis can occur with ketorolac, and it must not be used in patients who are sensitive to aspirin or any of the NSAIDs. There are reports they can cause renal failure even in young people.

Tips about using NSAIDs

- Ibuprofen is the drug with the least troublesome side-effects.
- Used as a sole agent, NSAIDs do not effectively control pain after major surgery, but may do so after minor surgery. They are more effective if combined with paracetamol.
- NSAIDs are best used in combination as one of the modes in multimodal analgesia. Add an opioid. You can then reduce the dose of the opioid by one-third, with the added benefits of decreasing nausea and respiratory depression.
- Paracetamol and NSAIDs are valuable components in multimodal analgesia.
- NSAIDs need time to work. They are more effective if given 3 to 5 hours before the pain is expected.
- NSAIDs are a useful pre-med for patients having laparoscopic surgery.
- Do not use NSAIDs in pregnant or breastfeeding women.
- NSAIDs are effective with biliary pain and renal colic.
- Avoid NSAIDs (particularly ketorolac) in patients who are likely to have renovascular disease such as diabetics, the elderly, smokers, and those with heart failure (especially if they have, or had, peripheral oedema).
- Do not use NSAIDs or aspirin in children under the age of 18 years;
- There is no advantage in using more than one type of NSAID.

- Intravenous NSAIDs (including the COX-2 inhibitors) are no more effective than the same drug given orally.
- Avoid NSAIDs in elderly patients who are taking drugs with a low *therapeutic index*, such as digoxin or aminoglycosides.

NSAIDs

1. Ibuprofen is best, but it takes 3 hours to act.
2. Paracetamol works if there is no inflammation, otherwise use ibuprofen.
3. Avoid COX-2 inhibitors for acute pain.
4. Do not use NSAIDs in people over 70.
5. Do not use NSAIDs in patients with chronic kidney disease.

Paracetamol

As a first choice, paracetamol (called acetaminophen in the USA) is the best and safest drug for mild acute pain. Paracetamol, especially when combined with codeine or NSAID, is an effective analgesia. Unlike other NSAIDs it has no anti-inflammatory properties. It does not aggravate asthma, disturb renal function or prolong bleeding. Larger doses can be hepatotoxic so use it cautiously in alcoholics or patients with liver disease. The optimal dose is 100 mg 4 to 6 hourly. Its ceiling effect means that increasing the dose does not increase its efficacy. To get better analgesia increase the frequency of dosing rather than the dose. It works better if taken regularly rather than when required (prn). The maximum safe dose for an adult is 4000 mg per day (8×500 mg tablets), but in this dose it may cause nausea. In overdose, it causes fulminating potentially fatal liver damage which requires expert treatment with n-acetyl cysteine infusion.

In children, suppositories of paracetamol 20–30 mg/Kg are effective, but in adults suppositories may not achieve effective *plasma* levels. Intravenous paracetamol is available in most countries and it is very effective in the recovery room where patients may be unable to take oral medication. It is more effective than oral paracetamol.

Adjuvants

Ketamine

Ketamine is a non-barbiturate, non-narcotic, dissociative anaesthetic agent that acts on the spinal cord and at many places in the brain. Its principal action is to prevent pain impulses being relayed to consciousness.

In anaesthetic doses

In anaesthetic doses, ketamine produces a *dissociative anaesthesia* where patients appear to be in a trance with their eyes wide open, but not responding to any stimulus (*catalepsy*). Their eyes may flick from side to side. Their muscle tone is increased slightly. Patients remember nothing of the procedure (amnesia). The blood pressure usually rises except in severely shocked patients. Ketamine causes a tachycardia.

Patients usually salivate profusely, and may develop transient *laryngospasm* and apnoea immediately after receiving the drug. It is prone to cause postoperative nausea and vomiting.

In analgesic doses

Given judiciously by infusion ketamine is superb for controlling agonizing postoperative pain.[9] It is useful to manage the pain after burns debridement, and amputations. It is also useful when phantom limb pain reappears during or after spinal anaesthesia, or with severe metabolic stress.

Used alone ketamine often causes unpleasant visual and tactile hallucinations. Patients see weird things, often in vivid colours, and occasionally feel strange things crawling over their skin. These hallucinations can be quite frightening. To prevent them many anaesthetists add a benzodiazepine (such as midazolam or diazepam). To achieve effective plasma concentrations, give a loading dose of 0.1 mg/Kg of ketamine and follow this with an infusion of 12 mg/Kg/hr. Good analgesia occurs within an hour, but if no loading dose is given, it takes about 48 hours for plasma concentrations to reach effective levels. Usually, at these doses, hallucinations and dysphoria are not a problem.

Ketamine reduces opioid requirements in opioid-tolerant patients.

Gabapentin

Gabapentin, an antiepileptic drug, is one of a new class of analgesics.[10] Given preoperatively it enhances the effects of morphine, does not depress breathing, however it may cause drowsiness.

Clonidine

Clonidine is a centrally acting alpha$_2$-agonist used occasionally to treat severe hypertension. It is becoming popular because it usefully potentiates the effects of other analgesics. It appears to work on the spinal cord. It can be given orally, intravenously, or as a skin patch. Most of these uses are *off-label*. Clonidine causes sedation, lessens anxiety, reduces shaking, nausea and vomiting in doses of 3 µg/Kg made up to 10 ml in saline and given intravenously in 2 ml increments. Being an anti-hypertensive drug it may cause hypotension.

Figure 6.1 Pain algorithm

Using a pain algorithm

This algorithm shows how to give incremental doses of morphine. To rescue a patient in severe pain you may have to use double the dose suggested by the algorithm for the first and perhaps the second dose. While patients are receiving intravenous opioids they remain in Stage I recovery. Abandon the pain protocol and seek advice from the anaesthetist if any of the following occur: their pain is not adequately controlled, their respiratory rate falls below 8 breath/min, they do not open their eyes when their name is called, or they are nauseated or vomit. Record each dose in both milligrams and millilitres of drug given in the patient's recovery room chart.

Notes

1. Stein C, Rosow C (2004) *Receptor Ligands and Opiate Narcotics in Anesthetic Pharmacology*, Churchill Livingstone Philidelphia USA.
2. Aubru F, Moncel S, Langeron O *et al.* (2002) *Anesthesiology* 96:17.
3. Persson K, Lundberg J (2001) *European Journal of Anaesthesiology* 18:679.
4. FL Scamman (2003) *Anesthesia and Analgesia* 62:332–4.
5. *Report of Australian Adverse Drug Reaction Advisory Committee*, March 2004.
6. Jones D, Story DA (2005) *Anaesthesia and Intensive Care* 33:181–7.
7. Isbister GK, Buckley NA, Whyte IM (2007) *Medical Journal of Australia* 187:361–5.
8. Malan T P, Gordon S, Hubbard R *et al.* (2005) Anesthesia and Analgesia 100:454–60.
9. Bell RF, Dahl JB, Moore RA (2005) *Acta Anaesthesiol Scand* 49:1405–28.
10. Eckhardt K, Ammon S, Hoffmann U *et al.* (2000) *Anesthesia and Analgesia* 91:185–91.

Postoperative nausea and vomiting

Nausea and vomiting are feared

Postoperative nausea and vomiting (PONV) is common. Its severity ranges from mild queasiness through to a distressing, prolonged, life-threatening event requiring resuscitation with intravenous fluids. Postoperative nausea and vomiting delays discharge from the recovery room, and increases nurses' workload. About 1 per cent of day surgery patients have to stay in hospital overnight because of uncontrollable nausea and vomiting; this makes it an expensive complication.

In many cases patients fear PONV more than pain. They are willing to accept drowsiness, increased pain and increased cost. The best prophylactic management only reduces the incidence of nausea and vomiting by 20–25 per cent. This means that in 100 patients who are at risk of vomiting, 75–80 per cent of them will do so no matter what we do.

Nausea

Nausea is an unpleasant feeling of the need to vomit. It may be accompanied by sweating, pallor, bradycardia, and salivation. The terminology is confusing. If patients are nauseated, it means that they feel as though want to vomit. On the other hand if patients are nauseous, it means that something about them is so vile and repulsive that they make you feel sick. Overall, patients are nauseated, and rarely nauseous. To remember this, think of the statement that people are 'poisoned but not poisonous'.

Vomiting

Vomiting (*emesis*) is an involuntary active protective *reflex* for evicting ingested toxins from the gut. The patient usually realizes a few seconds beforehand that they are about to vomit. Vomiting begins with a deep inspiration, the glottis closes, and diaphragm and abdominal muscles contract violently, ejecting the stomach contents.

Vomiting is hazardous because it:

- can cause pneumonitis if aspirated into the lungs;
- damages the cornea if it gets into the eyes;
- damages facial skin flaps;
- raises intra-ocular pressure;
- may tear suture lines;
- causes bradycardia in patients with ischaemic heart disease;
- causes hypotension in patients with peripheral vascular disease;
- leads to hypokalaemia and saline depletion if prolonged;
- may rupture the oesophagus in a few susceptible individuals.

Regurgitation

Regurgitation is a passive process where fluid matter refluxes up the oesophagus from the stomach. It occurs without warning, and can cause aspiration pneumonitis in a comatose or mentally *obtunded* patient.

Regurgitation is likely to occur in a patient with:

- hiatus hernia;
- obesity;
- distended abdomen;
- intestinal obstruction;
- ascites;
- pregnancy.

Aspiration

Mendleson's syndrome

Aspiration during pregnancy is called Mendleson's syndrome, although the term is now more widely used to cover all patients who have aspiration pneumonitis. All pregnant patients are at risk, and if it occurs in pregnancy the pneumonitis is peculiarly fulminant, and often fatal.

Pregnant patients are most at risk during induction of anaesthesia, but nausea at any time during their recovery, even after spinal or epidural anaesthetics, must be treated quickly to prevent this complication.

Aspiration pneumonitis

Aspiration pneumonitis is a severe inflammation of the lungs caused by inhaling gastric contents into the lower airways. Severe aspiration is said to occur in about 3 in 10 000 anaesthetics, but it is probably less than that. Even the longest fast does not abolish the risk of aspiration because the stomach is never empty. Water is cleared exponentially from the stomach; half is gone after 12 minutes, and about 60 minutes later it has all gone leaving only acidic gastric juice behind. A fasted stomach contains about 30 ml of fluid composed of hydrochloric acid and peptic *enzymes*, which are strong enough to blister skin. Subtle micro-aspiration in the recovery room soon after patients emerge from anaesthetic is probably responsible for many postoperative chest infections.

Nurse patients in the recovery position until they are fully conscious. Once they can touch their noses with the tip of their forefinger their co-ordination is good enough for them to care for their own airway, and they can sit up or change their position.

If aspiration occurs then patients need their respiratory function closely observed in ICU. Initially give them oxygen by mask, and if their oxygen saturation deteriorates then they may need intubation and ventilation. If the oxygen saturation is above 90% intubation can be avoided. An endotracheal tube abolishes the patient's ability to cough and deep breathe. X-ray changes revealing inflammation may take several hours to develop and usually first appear in the right lower lobe. Bronchial lavage, steroids and antibiotics are not useful in the early stages. If solid food has been inhaled then a bronchoscopy may be needed to remove the larger lumps.

Physiology

Vomiting

Vomiting is a *reflex* that evolved to eject ingested toxins, and the unpleasant nausea is a reminder not to ingest that toxin again. There are three components to the vomiting reflex: emetic detectors, coordinating centres, and motor outputs. Retching involves the same processes, but no stomach contents are ejected.

Input

The *vomiting centre* (VC) lies protected inside the blood–brain barrier in the brainstem. In contrast, the *chemoreceptor trigger zone* (CTZ) lies outside.

Processors

The centres coordinating vomiting in the brainstem have neural inputs from the stomach, the vestibular apparatus in the ear, emotional centres, in the cortex and from direct stimuli by toxins carried in the blood.

Figure 7.1 Brainstem centres involved in nausea and vomiting

The vomiting centre coordinates the control of the complex vomiting reflex. Rich in cholinergic receptors, it receives incoming signals from the pharynx, gastrointestinal tract and mediastinum via the vagus nerve; and from the vestibular portion of the eighth cranial nerve and the chemoreceptor trigger zone. It is interconnected with centres controlling various activities of the autonomic nervous system such as salivation, sweating, bradycardia, and blood pressure control.

The receptors

There are three principal types of receptors involved in stimulating nausea and vomiting. Once stimulated they relay information to the vomiting centre, which then initiates and coordinates vomiting.

Dopamine D_2 receptors are mostly found on afferent input pathways from the vagus nerve serving the abdominal viscera, pharynx and genitals. Anti-dopaminergic drugs, such as metoclopramide, and droperidol, partially block these receptors.

Cholinergic receptors are mostly found in the pathways from the vestibular apparatus. Anti-cholinergic drugs such as scopolamine, some antihistamines and prochlorperazine block them. Opioids tend to sensitise the vestibular apparatus, and essentially cause motion sickness.

Serotonin (5-HT$_3$) receptors are mostly involved in the final common pathway relaying information from the chemoreceptor trigger zone to the vomiting centre. They are blocked with 5-HT$_3$ antagonists such as ondansetron, or just as effectively by a far cheaper drug, cyclizine.

Recently research has uncovered a number of other neurotransmitters and neuropeptides including *neurokinin-1* (NK1) involved with vomiting. Drugs are being developed to counteract these biochemicals.

Toxins and impulses from nerves stimulating the chemo-trigger receptor zone are relayed across the blood–brain barrier to the vomiting centre which then coordinates all the processes needed for vomiting.

NSAIDs do not cause postoperative nausea and vomiting.

Output

Most vomiting is preceded by a feeling of nausea, however patients with raised intracranial pressure or acute gastric distension may simply vomit without warning.

Once the stomach is empty vomiting usually ceases unless it is caused by toxins in the gut. then dry retching occurs because the stimulus to vomit has not been removed.

Retching and vomiting involves violent contractions of the abdominal wall and diaphragm. The effort may be strong enough to fracture ribs in elderly patients with osteoporosis.

Causes of nausea and vomiting

Postoperative nausea and vomiting occurs in all types of patients, and with all types of operations and anaesthetics. There are, however certain groups of people, and certain types of procedures where vomiting is more likely.

Surgical factors

The following procedures are associated with more nausea and vomiting:

- intra-abdominal operations where the peritoneum is stretched, or the gut's perfusion or oxygenation is compromised;
- biliary surgery;
- breast augmentation surgery;
- thyroid surgery;
- gynaecological laparoscopic surgery;
- ophthalmic operations, especially squint surgery;
- ENT surgery; especially tonsillectomy and middle ear surgery;

- urological surgery; especially if the spermatic cord is involved;
- emergency surgery, especially for fractures.

Patient factors

Children vomit more frequently than adults. Women are more likely to vomit than men and elderly patients over 70 years do not often vomit. There is no evidence that obese patients are more likely to vomit than thin patients. Patients who get motion sickness are at high risk. There is also a strong psychological factor: those people who think that they are likely to vomit, or who have a history of doing so, are three times more likely to vomit after subsequent operations. Smokers are less likely to vomit than non-smokers, because they are already tolerant to exogenous noxious chemicals.

Supplemental oxygen helps prevent postoperative nausea and vomiting.

Anaesthetic factors

Opioids

Opioid drugs are a potent cause of nausea and vomiting. Opioids act directly on the brainstem centres, and are more likely to cause vomiting if the patient is moving around. They sensitize the vomiting centres to input from the vestibular apparatus. In effect opioids make patients sea-sick. Opioids given as premedication, and during operations more than double the incidence of vomiting. All opioids are approximately equivalent in this respect.

Anaesthetic agents

All the inhalational anaesthetic agents and many induction agents (thiopentone, ketamine, and particularly etomidate) cause nausea and vomiting.

Propofol decreases the risk of vomiting. Benzodiazepines and muscle relaxants have no effect on the incidence of nausea and vomiting. The best anaesthetic option to prevent the nausea and vomiting is total intravenous anaesthesia (TIVA) with propofol. Neostigmine given to reverse muscle relaxants at the end of surgery may cause vomiting on waking.

Type of anaesthetic

Patients who have a general anaesthetic with volatile agents are eleven times more likely to vomit than those who have regional anaesthesia. Patients who breathe spontaneously during the operation are less likely to vomit than those who are ventilated. This may be related to the greater use of opioids in the ventilated group.

Patients who are hypotensive during or after their anaesthetic are highly likely to feel nauseated and vomit. This is probably related to suboptimal oxygen supply to the gut. If the gut becomes hypoperfused or hypoxic, its neural network almost instantly releases serotonin ($5HT_3$) which initiates nausea. Even brief periods of hypotension quickly cause nausea and then vomiting. Giving higher concentrations of supplemental oxygen almost halves the incidence of PONV after major abdominal surgery.[1] The length of surgery has little effect on the amount of postoperative vomiting.[2]

Recovery room factors

In the recovery room nausea and vomiting may be induced by:
- severe pain, which tends to produce nausea rather than vomiting;
- hypotension;
- hypoxia;
- hypovolaemia;
- anxiety;
- early mobilization;
- swallowed blood;
- water intoxication syndrome.

Transport causes motion sickness

Moving patients around after giving them an opioid is a potent cause of nausea and vomiting postoperatively. When transporting patients on their trolleys sit your patients up, and face them forward. Turn the trolley from the foot end. Do not swing the head in a wide arc (as occurs in stomach-churning fairground rides) when turning corners. We have found these simple measures reduce vomiting in the first hour after returning to the ward by about half. This simple measure is more effective than anti-emetic drugs.

Nausea after epidural, or spinal anaesthesia?
Eliminate hypotension.

How to manage nausea and vomiting[3]

Identify those at risk

Not everyone is likely to vomit. Patients at risk of postoperative nausea and vomiting are frequently given anti-emetic drugs before they come to the recovery room.

Apfel's risk score [4]

Apfel's risk score predicts which patients will vomit. The use of volatile agents only makes a marginal difference to the sensitivity of this scale.

Table 7.1 Apfel score

Risk	Score
No risk factors	1
Females	1
History of motion sickness or previous PONV	1
Non-smoker	1
Give opioids	1
Total out of 5 =	

Prophylaxis against nausea and vomiting

With high-risk patients, strategies to prevent nausea and vomiting should begin long before the patient comes to the recovery room.

Prolonged preoperative fasting causes *dehydration*. If the patient is not well hydrated during or after anaesthesia they will become hypotensive, especially when you move them. Hypotension is a potent cause of nausea.

Although the optimal fasting period for solid food is 4–6 hours, most patients should be allowed to drink water until 2 hours before their surgery. Water is exponentially cleared from the stomach, half being absorbed within 12 minutes, and it is all gone within one hour, leaving behind normal stomach fluids. During the procedure the anaesthetists will give a base line infusion of 15–20 ml/Kg of crystalloid fluid, for example Plasmolyte®. If the anaesthetist has not given fluid, and your patient is nauseated, then give them an infusion of crystalloid before using anti-emetic drugs.

Once the patient comes to recovery room prevent nausea and vomiting by:

• avoiding hypotension;
• giving high concentrations of oxygen;
• treating pain;
• avoiding sudden movement.

Not all patients need PONV prophylaxis.

Immediate management

In semi-conscious patients who are about to vomit, roll them on to their side, take their pillows away, and turn their head so that the vomitus can drain from their mouth.

Once they have finished vomiting gently suck out their mouth and pharynx with a wide bore sucker. Be gentle, or you will stimulate further vomiting.

Patients who are expected to be susceptible to either regurgitation or vomiting after major surgery usually leave the theatre with a nasogastric tube draining freely. A nasogastric tube will not prevent regurgitation, nor reduce the risk of aspiration pneumonia. It may even predispose to regurgitation.

Children

Children usually only vomit once or twice and do not suffer nausea. They are susceptible to the dystonic side-effects from anti-emetic drugs so it is best to avoid treatment initially. If it is necessary to use an anti-emetic in children droperidol 50 µg/Kg is unlikely to cause problems. This drug often stops vomiting, and does not cause prolonged sedation.

The bad news

No matter how vigorously we treat vomiting we can only reduce the incidence by about a quarter. For instance if a patient has an 80 per cent chance of nausea or vomiting, then the most we can hope for using all our techniques is to reduce the risk to about a 60 per cent chance of postoperative nausea and vomiting. Nevertheless, with treatment, if they do vomit then the duration and severity of nausea and vomiting is reduced too.

The good news

Simple measures such as hydration, avoiding prolonged fluid deprivation, supplemental oxygen, and especially sitting your patient up and wheeling them feet first when transporting them back to the ward are surprisingly effective.

Anti-emetic drugs

Anti-emetics include several classes of drugs that relieve the symptoms of nausea and vomiting. There are many controlled studies of the efficacy of anti-emetic drugs, but they often contradict each other, the results are confusing, the trials are bedevilled by problems of *heterogenicity* and some studies are arguably fraudulent. This makes it difficult to arrive at valid conclusions.

The following facts, however, emerge:

- anti-dopaminergic anti-emetics seem to work best against inputs from the vagus nerve;
- anti-cholinergic drugs appear to work best against cholinergic input from the labyrinth (vestibular apparatus) in the ear;
- anti-serotonin (anti-5-HT$_3$) antagonists work well against both.

Table 7.2 Anti-emetic drugs

Group	Drug	Best for
Phenothiazines	Promethazine	Opioid-induced PONV
	Prochloperazine	Opioid-induced PONV
Antihistamine	Cyclizine	All PONV
5-HT$_3$	Ondansetron	Gut and gynaecological surgery
antagonist	Granisteron	Major tissue damage
Steroids	Dexamethasone	All PONV
Benzamide	Metoclopramide	Gut and gynaecological surgery
Butyrephenones	Droperidol	All PONV
Anti-cholinergic	L-hyoscine (scopolamine)	Opioid-induced PONV

Dexamethasone

Dexamethasone is a steroid related to cortisol. It reduces the incidence of postoperative nausea and vomiting while potentiating the effects of other antiemetics. It has no obvious side-effects. It is given as a single dose at the start of the anaesthetic and should not be repeated.

It probably inhibits *prostaglandin* synthesis and gives patients a feeling of well-being. The recommended dose is 150 µg/Kg for children and 4–8 mg for adults. Since it takes at least 2 hours to work, it is best given on induction of anaesthesia, rather than in the recovery room. Its effect persists for up to 24 hours.

If the anti-emetic you have given is not effective,
try one from another group.

Serotonin antagonists[5]

Serotonin (5-hydroxytryptamine) antagonists include ondansetron, granisetron, dolasetron, and tropisetron. Serotonin is a neurotransmitter involved in activating vagal afferent pathways, principally from the gut and reproductive organs. These drugs are all equally effective and equally safe. They are more effective when used at the end of the anaesthetic, and are the most effective drugs to give if the patient is actually vomiting. These drugs are expensive and overused. If cyclizine is available consider using it instead.

Repeated or higher doses of the serotonin antagonists are not any more effective. If this first dose is not effective then do not persist; instead use an agent from another class of anti-emetics such as promethazine 12.5 mg, or droperidol 0.625 mg.

Granisetron

Granisetron is probably the best of this group of drugs. It is equally if not more effective as ondansetron and has similar side-effects and disadvantages, but granisetron is much cheaper. Furthermore, because it is not metabolized by CYP 2D6 enzymes in the liver, granisetron is less likely to cause drug interactions than other 5-HT$_3$ antagonists. Usually granisetron 1 mg IV is given at the end of the anaesthetic, or if not then in the recovery room. Apart from an occasional annoying headache, granisetron has few side-effects, and it does not cause extrapyramidal syndrome.

Ondansetron

Ondansetron was the first of this group. Give ondansetron 4 mg IV over 90 seconds. Repeat after 5 minutes if necessary. Higher doses are not more effective, and are just more likely to cause headache, and disturbed liver function. Ondansetron is an expensive drug, but more than twice as effective as metoclopramide for treating postoperative nausea and vomiting in intestinal and gynaecological surgery.

Note: both tramadol and ondansetron are metabolized on the liver CYP 2D6 enzymes, if the patient has already taken one it may aggravate the effects of the other.

Cyclizine vs ondansetron

Cyclizine, a histamine receptor blocker, is more than one hundred times cheaper than ondansetron and at least equally as effective[6] but it is only available in some countries (not in Australia or the USA). The dose of cyclizine is 25–50 mg intravenously in adults and 1 mg/Kg IV in children.

Antihistamines

Antihistamines block H1 receptors, in the brain and periphery. Their anti-emetic effect is probably due to their anti-cholinergic blocking activity. Cyclizine and promethazine are two antihistamines without significant anti-dopaminergic activity.

Cyclizine (Valoid®, Marezine®) is a safe and most effective anti-emetic against opioid induced nausea and vomiting, and the dizziness associated with motion sickness (incurred during the trip back to the ward). It is a potent histamine receptor blocker. Cyclizine also has anti-cholinergic properties. It makes patients drowsy, but less so than either prochlorperazine or promethazine. Cyclizine deserves to be more popular.[7] The adult dose is 25–50 mg IM and it works for about 4 hours. Later, in the ward, it can be given as a tablet.

Promethazine (Phenergan®), an antihistamine (one of the phenothiazine group), is sometimes used to treat nausea and vomiting, but it makes patients drowsy, delays emergence, and can drop their blood pressure by causing peripheral vasodilation. It works mainly through its anti-cholinergic action on the chemo-trigger receptor zone. The adult dose is 12.5–25 mg IM, 4–6 hourly.

Phenothiazines

Phenothiazines are anti-emetics primarily because, as dopaminergic D2 antagonists they act on the chemo-trigger receptor zone. They are only slowly cleared as they are long acting with a half-life of more than 30 hours. In elderly or debilitated patients they are prone to cause hypotension, agitation, apprehension, and sleep disturbance.

Extrapyramidal syndrome

Children, young adults, and debilitated elderly patients are susceptible to extrapyramidal syndrome (dystonia and nystagmus). This is frightening for the patient, who develops muscle rigidity, and marked oscillations of the eyes, (nystagmus) known as an *oculogyric crisis*. With phenothiazines the incidence is about 0.3%, but a quarter of these reactions occur after a single parenteral dose. Treat this with benztropine (Cogentin®) 1 mg IV, and repeat in 10 minutes if necessary.

Prochlorperazine (Stemetil®) is effective for postoperative nausea and vomiting, particularly if the stimulus is coming from the vestibular apparatus in the ear. The dose is 0.1–0.2 mg/Kg IM, but it causes a dry mouth and its sedative effects make it unsuitable for day case surgery. It is long-acting, so do not repeat the dose in less than 6 hours.

Neuroleptic malignant syndrome

Neuroleptic malignant syndrome is a result of extreme dopamine blockade. It occurs when here is an excessive or abnormal response to metoclopramide, droperidol, and phenothiazines such as prochlorperazine, promethazine, and particularly perphenazine. It presents just like quick-onset Parkinson's disease. The patient starts to move slowly (bradykinesia) as their muscles stiffen up, they then become immobile and seem unresponsive. In reality they are locked-in because their vocal cords and voluntary muscles are too stiff to move. They also become febrile, their blood pressure rises and blood tests show muscle damage reflected in a raised plasma phosphokinase (CPK) levels. Neuroleptic malignant syndrome is treated with bromocriptine.

Anti-dopaminergics

Droperidol and metoclopramide are dopamine D_2 antagonists. Do not use them in patients who have Parkinson's disease because they will precipitate rigidity. Anti-dopaminergic drugs can cause an unpredictable *extrapyramidal syndrome*, particularly in children and young women. They also may cause *serotonin syndrome* in patients who are taking SSRIs. Do not use them in patients taking long-term psychotropic medication – such as lithium or any of the phenothiazines – because they have been reported to cause the *neuroleptic malignant syndrome* (NMS).

Droperidol

Droperidol (Droleptan®) has strong anti-dopaminergic activity, and blocks input to the chemoreceptor trigger zone. It is also an alpha-blocker, and larger doses cause *postural hypotension.*

Droperidol is among the most effective of the antinauseants, but in higher doses causes hypotension and often causes severe *dysphoria* and motor retardation so that the patient is unable to move voluntarily or even talk. The dysphoria makes patients feel as though they are locked inside their body where they feel agitated and frightened, yet are unable to tell anyone about it. This horrible effect may persist for 6 or more hours.

> *If the patient has had one dose of droperidol,*
> *do not repeat it.*

The most effective dose of droperidol is 10–20 µg/Kg. Droperidol 0.625 mg IV is often given at the end of the anaesthetic where it is effective for about 6 hours.

Droperidol's 'black box warning'

In December 2001 the American Food and Drug Administration (FDA) issued their highest grade 'black box warning' about the use of droperidol after some reports of deaths from the cardiac arrhythmia torsades de pointes when it was used in high doses. Some authorities convincingly argued this warning was based on flimsy hearsay evidence.[8] No report of an adverse cardiac event has ever been published in a peer-reviewed journal since its introduction for the management of PONV.[9,10] It is estimated that adverse cardiac events following the use of droperidol is about 74 cases in 11 million. Consequently, the FDA modified its warning to allow droperidol to be used in anaesthesia as an anti-emetic.

Metoclopramide

Many studies have shown that the standard dose of 10 mg of metoclopramide (Maxalon®, Reglan®) is no better than placebo for postoperative nausea and vomiting. If you think about its pharmacology and its effect on the vagus nerve, metoclopramide may have a place in treating nausea and vomiting where the bowel or uterus or ovaries have been manipulated; or after laparoscopy or where blood has been swallowed. The effective dose appears to be metoclopramide 15–20 mg slowly intravenously. In some patients it may cause bradycardia. If the initial 10 mg dose is ineffective it is safe to repeat it. Being anti-dopaminergic metoclopramide will precipitate acute Parkinsonism in patients taking anti-parkinsonian drugs such as L-dopa, or bromocriptine.

Other drugs

Anti-cholinergics

Anti-cholinergic drugs block the cholinergic muscarinic receptors in the brain, and in the periphery. Centrally acting anti-cholinergic drugs block input from the vestibular apparatus in the ear to the chemotrigger receptor zone; so they are effective against motion sickness. Anti-cholinergic drugs are seldom used because they have many adverse effects. Scopolamine is still occasionally used in children.

Ephedrine

Ephedrine is sometimes used in day case surgery. In many patients a dose of 0.5 mg/Kg IM is as effective as droperidol, but without the side-effects. It probably acts by preventing *postural hypotension* in ambulant patients, but there may be a central mechanism. If you keep your patients well hydrated, you probably will not need to use this drug.

Accupressure

Accupressure techniques are well worth trying for postoperative vomiting.[11] The pressure point (P6 or Neiguan point) is in the midline on the anterior aspect of the left forearm about a Chinese inch above the proximal skin crease of the wrist. (A Chinese inch is the length of the interphalangeal joint of the thumb.) Firmly probe about with the tip of your thumb between the tendens until you find a point of deep ache. It has to cause an ache to be effective. Press firmly here and the nausea may abate, let go and it will return. Instruct patients to find their own pressure points. Accupressure is ineffective once vomiting has started.

Figure 7.2 Accupressure

Complementary techniques

Aromatherapy with oil of ginger, isopropyl alcohol, and peppermint oil have been tried with varying degrees of promise.[12] Music therapy, therapeutic suggestion and guided imagery are probably no more effective than a placebo.

Rescue techniques

You have tried everything and your patient is still incapacitated by nausea or vomiting. First consider giving an additional 500 ml of Hartmann's solution. Then check what anti-emetic the patient received during their anaesthetic and give one from another group. Third, try droperidol, and as a last resort ephedrine.

Further reading

British National Formulary (BNF), 48, September 2004.
Martindale *The Complete Drug Reference*, 34th edition.
MMS New Ethicals Catalogue, Issue 1, May 2004.

Notes

1. Grief R, Laciny S, Rapf B, *et al.* (1999) *Anesthesiology* 91:1246–52.
2. Echbehart LH, Hogel J, Seeling W *et al.* (2000) *ACTA Anaesthesiology Scandinavica* 44:480–8.
3. Asraf S H, Tong JG (2004) *Canadian Journal of Anaesthesia* 51:341–62.
4. Apfel CC, Läärä E, Koivuranta M, Greim CA *et al.* (1999) *Anesthesiology* 91: 693–700.
5. Wilhelm SM, Dehoorne-Smith ML, Kale-Pradhan PB (2007) *Annals of Pharmacotherapy* 41:68–78.
6. Colwill JM, Wright W, Hobbs GJ (1999) *British Journal of Anaesthesia* 83:611–14.
7. Grimsehl K. Whiteside JB, Mackenzie N (2002) *Anaesthesia* 51;326–41.
8. Gan TJ, White PF, Scuderi PE (2002) *Anaesthesiology* 97:287.

9. Gan TJ (2002) *Journal of the American Medical Association* 287:1233–6
10. Habib AS, Gan TJ (2003) Anesthesia and Analgesia 96:1377–9
11. Rowbotham DJ (2005) *British Journal of Anaesthesia* 95:77–81.
12. Mamaril M, Windle PE, Burkard JF (2006) *Journal of Perianesthesia Nursing* 21:404–10.

Regional analgesia

Patients who have had regional anaesthesia, epidurals, spinals and various nerve blocks come to the recovery room. They may be awake and appear easy to care for, but problems may occur. This chapter will enable you to assist the anaesthetist to insert regional anaesthetics, monitor patients with regional analgesia, identify problems and deal with them.

The recovery room must be equipped to handle complications of regional anaesthesia.

Epidural anaesthesia

Advantages of epidurals

- Epidurals give excellent pain relief from pain in skin and muscle.
- Postoperative nausea and vomiting is minimized.
- Epidural blockade reduces the bad effects of postoperative stress syndrome.
- Wounds heal faster, wound infections are less prevalent, and the metabolic insults caused by surgery are less.
- Deep vein thrombosis and pulmonary emboli are reduced because the blood flow through the lower body and legs is increased.
- Epidurals reduce postoperative myocardial ischaemia.
- They improve blood flow to the legs following vascular surgery, and reduce the rate of graft occlusion.
- Dressings and other surgical manipulations can be done without causing pain or requiring additional analgesia.

Disadvantages of epidurals

- They may cause *postural hypotension*, in which case the patient will feel faint or nauseated when they try to sit up.
- They cannot be used in patients who have recently received *low molecular-weight heparins* (LMWH) or who are anticoagulated with warfarin and have an INR > 1.2.

- Low dose aspirin (<100 mg) daily is unlikely to cause problems with bleeding into the *epidural space.*
- Patients must have a urinary catheter, because they will not know when their bladder is full.
- Pressure sores can become a problem if the patient lies in one position for too long. You will need to help adjust the patient's position to relieve pressure areas every 30 minutes.
- Continuous epidural infusions need specifically designed pumps.
- Patients must receive supplemental oxygen.
- The patient must have an intravenous drip running.
- Epidurals may confine the patient to bed.

Inserting an epidural in the recovery room

Consent

The patient must give consent for epidural analgesia before surgery is commenced: check that this fact is clearly documented in the medical record. Valid consent cannot be obtained in the recovery room from a patient who is affected by residual anaesthetic drugs, or is under the influence of opioids.

Precautions

Double-check that the patient has not received anticogulant medication preoperatively. The risk of haemotoma from bleeding in to the epidural space is real.

Ensure the patient has secure intravenous access before the anaesthetist commences the block.

Where to site epidurals

Epidurals can be inserted in the thoracic, lumbar or caudal regions. Thoracic epidurals provide postoperative analgesia for upper abdominal operations. They are particularly useful for long subcostal incisions like radical nephrectomy, and for patients donating a kidney. Sensibly sited catheters allow the patient to move around.

Lumbar epidurals are easier to insert than thoracic epidurals. They give pain relief for incisions below the umbilicus including operations on the lower limbs. They are particularly useful to control pain after abdominoperineal resections, major intra-abdominal vascular surgery, and hip replacement surgery.

A caudal block is used for operations around the perineum such as haemorrhoids. Inserted through the caudal canal in the sacrum, it gives useful pain relief for perineal surgery in adults and circumcision in babies. Caudal pain relief is also very effective after surgery on babies' feet.

Inserting an epidural

Inserting an epidural is a strictly sterile procedure requiring gloves, gown, drapes and mask. Use special precautions and especially allow three measured minutes for the antiseptic skin prep to work. Use chlorhexidine solutions for skin preps, because they are more effective than iodine containing ones.

Position the patient comfortably on their left side with their legs tucked up. It is not usual to sit patients up to insert epidurals in the recovery room, although the anaesthetist may find it easier to insert epidurals in obese patients if they are sitting up.

Drugs can be given as one-shot bolus dose without a catheter, or through a catheter to give intermittent bolus doses, or more effectively a continuous infusion. Once the local anaesthetic is injected, carefully monitor the patient so that you can react promptly if an adverse reaction occurs.

Test the segmental efficacy of the block with ice (never a pin-prick). If the patient cannot feel the cold then that dermatome is anaesthetized. If there are painful skip areas then the anaesthetist may withdraw the catheter a centimetre or two.

Looking after a patient with an epidural

If your patient starts to feels nauseated, it probably means they are becoming hypotensive. Increase the rate of the IV infusion. Give oxygen. Check their blood pressure and pulse rate. Lift their legs on to pillows; but never tip them head down.

Nausea warns of hypotension.

Epidural opioids sometime cause nausea and vomiting. This usually responds to cyclizine preferably, or ondansetron. In contrast, metoclopramide is ineffective, and promethazine and prochlorperazine are sedating.

Dermatomes

Dermatomes are areas on the skin innervated by a spinal sensory nerve originating in a single posterior spinal segment. They are labelled sequentially: cervical C1–5, thoracic T1–10, lumbar 1–5, and sacral S1–4. As they enter the spinal cord, each sensory nerve trunk usually contains separate fibres that spread out to enter their own spinal segment. Dermatomes overlap considerably at their edges, as shown in Figure 8.1.

Useful landmarks

Useful dermatome landmarks are S1, which is the groin area; T10, which is the level of the umbilicus (think of it as the 0 in T10); and the tip of the xiphisternum is at the level of T6. Once the local anaesthetic reaches T5 it starts to affect the sympathetic outflow to the heart, which may cause the blood pressure to fall. The intercostal muscles necessary for coughing are served by motor fibres from T1–10, the muscles and skin in the arms from C5–8, while C3, 4, and 5 'keep the diaphragm alive' (the phrenic nerve).

If a spinal or epidural is causing tingling or weakness in your patient's arms or hands it has reached the cervical level. Monitor them carefully, because they may complain they are finding it difficult to breathe.

Figure 8.1 Dermatomes

Problems with high blocks

Local anaesthetic is soaked up by nerves in much the same way as ink is soaked up by blotting paper. The initial spread of local anaesthetic in the *epidural space* is affected by the position of the patient. If the patient is sitting up, then most of the local anaesthetic solution will sink to the bottom of the *epidural space*, affecting the dermatomes in the lower part of the body.

*If a patient with an epidural can not cough effectively
then notify the anaesthetist immediately.*

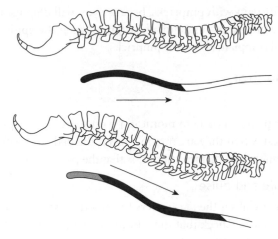

Figure 8.2 How posture affects the spread of local anaesthetic

Now, if you immediately lay the patient flat, the local anaesthetic moves along the epidural space towards the nerves serving the upper body. Fortunately the spine is S-shaped, and the local anaesthetic is unlikely to rise up the thoracic curve. However, should you tip patients head down, the local anaesthetic progressively anaesthetizes the intercostal muscles making it more and more difficult for the patient to breathe. Once it reaches T4, it blocks the sympathetic outflow to the heart so that the cardiac output falls, and should it reach the upper cervical region the patient will be completely paralysed and unable to breathe.

Anaesthetists adjust the dose of local anaesthetic they inject into the space to catch the nerves to the painful area. After a single shot of local anaesthetic, it takes about 10 minutes for the anaesthetic to fully soak into the nerves. Warning signs the block is too high are that the patient finds it hard to take a deep breath; or more alarmingly their arms become weak or their little fingers go numb.

*Do not tip patients with an
epidural head down.*

How to test the level of block

Use ice to test the level of a block because the sensations of cold travel in the same nerve pathways as pain. Put a piece of ice in a disposable glove and touch your patient's forehead with it so that they know what to expect. Then starting at T2, just under the clavicle, slowly move the ice down until the patient says the sensation has changed – this is the level of the block.

Never test for pain with pinpricks, because you will damage the skin and may introduce infection – and quite justifiably, when the epidural wears off the patient will complain about the pinpricks.

What to monitor

Pain score

Use the linear pain analogue to monitor a pain score. Check pain when the patient is at rest, when they are moving about the bed, and when they deep breathe and cough. The therapeutic aim is that the patient has no pain at rest.

Blood pressure and pulse

The anaesthetist will set the parameters for blood pressure and pulse on the epidural order sheet. Check that these limits are still appropriate before discharging the patient to the ward.

Level of the block

Unless the block is sufficiently high the patient will experience breakthrough pain. For most abdominal operations this level is about T6 and for surgery below the waist about T8.

Motor power

Record the patient's ability to bend each their legs at the knee, and waggle their feet up and down. Any deterioration of this ability may be an early warning sign of a developing epidural abscess or haematoma.

Sedation score

There are many sedation scores, but the most useful is the one used on the recovery room assessment score sheet.

How to rescue breakthrough pain

If the patient is in pain, the first priority is to rescue the patient. With breakthrough pain it may be possible for the anaesthetist to give a 5 ml bolus of 2% lidocaine, and increase the infusion rate in increments of 4 mls up to a maximum of 20 ml/hr. If this fails the anaesthetist may elect to use an alternative block, or otherwise treat pain with paracetamol or diclofenac. If the patient has received epidural opioids they must not have parenteral opioids or they may have a respiratory arrest. Remind the ward nurses to put a sign on the bed warning: "EPIDURAL – NO OPIOIDS".

Problems with epidurals

When to notify the anaesthetist

The local anaesthetic may extend beyond the intended area, or the opioid may cause respiratory depression. Both events can cause problem, notify the anaesthetist if the patient:

- block reaches T4 level – the nipple line;
- complains of weakness in their arm or numbness in their hands or little fingers;
- has difficulty in taking a deep breath or coughing;
- blood pressure falls by more than 20%;
- pain remains unrelieved, or skips certain areas;
- respiratory rate falls to 10 breaths/min or less.

Hypotension

The local anaesthetic blocks the sympathetic outflow serving the lower body. The consequent arteriolar vasodilation will cause the blood pressure to fall. Once the local anaesthetic reaches thoracic T4 level it will totally block the sympathetic outflow to the heart. When this occurs the heart cannot increase its output to prevent the blood pressure falling.

Avoid epidurals in patients with aortic or mitral stenosis, hypertrophic obstructive cardiomyopathies, cardiac *tamponade*, or restrictive pericarditis because they will become alarmingly hypotensive.

Do not overlook other causes for hypotension such as bleeding or volume depletion. If the patient has cold hands this is a highly suspicious sign of another cause for the hypotension. If the patient's blood pressure falls by more than 20 mmHg when you sit them up at 45° then suspect they are bleeding or hypovolaemic.

Nausea is an early warning sign that the blood pressure may be falling. Check the blood pressure. Lay your patient flat. Lift their legs onto a pillow. DO NOT TIP YOUR PATIENT HEAD DOWN. Increase the intravenous infusion rate and prepare to give a dose of ephedrine.

Nausea is one sign of hypotension.

How to manage hypotension

Hypotension usually occurs within 10–15 minutes of a top-up.

If the patient's blood pressure falls by more than 20 mmHg then lay the patient flat, and lift their legs on to pillows. Never tip the patient head down.

Give oxygen and infuse 250–500 ml of colloid such as gelofusin.

If the blood pressure does not rise give ephedrine. Dilute ephedrine 30 mg in 10 ml of sterile saline and give 3 mg (1 ml) increments every 2 minutes until the blood pressure returns to a safe level.

Monitor the blood pressure every 5 minutes to ensure the hypotension does not recur.

Respiratory depression

Respiratory depression can occur when the patient has received an opioid in their epidural. The incidence of respiratory depression is about 0.2–0.4%. It can occur within 30 minutes, or be delayed for any time up to 24 hours. Typically, the patient's respiratory rate falls slowly to 6–8 breaths/min (or even less) over an hour or more. The patient becomes drowsy, sweaty, and may even become cyanosed. Respiratory depression usually outlasts the analgesia. Respiratory depression may develop up to 2 hours after a single dose of fentanyl. Keep patients under close supervision for at least 3 hours after epidural fentanyl.

Use smaller doses of opioid where there is an increased risk of respiratory depression, such is in the elderly, the very frail or in patients with significant chronic obstructive airway disease. If the patient is receiving opioids into the *epidural space* never use intravenous or intramuscular opioids, because the patient may stop breathing.

Epidural opioids exclude the use of systemic opioids.

Delayed respiratory depression is more likely with morphine than more highly lipid soluble opioids such as fentanyl. Instead of quickly binding to opioid receptors in the spinal cord, morphine remains in solution in the *cerebrospinal fluid* (CSF). As the CSF slowly circulates, the dissolved morphine moves up to the brainstem where it may depress the respiratory centres.

Once the patient's respiratory rate falls to 10 beats/min, attach a pulse oximeter, and check for signs of hypoxia. Treat respiratory depression if the respiratory rate falls below 8 beats/min or the oxygen saturations fall below 94%. Naloxone 100–200 μg intravenously will usually cause an immediate improvement, but it only lasts for 30 minutes. For established opioid induced respiratory depression use a naloxone infusion: it will require about 10 μg/Kg/hr intravenously. This dose reverses the analgesic effects of morphine, but not necessarily the analgesia of epidural fentanyl.

Postdural puncture headache

The dural membrane can be punctured if the epidural needle is advanced too far. Once punctured, the CSF continues to leak into the epidural space, putting tension on blood vessels around the brain and spinal cord causing a severe headache. Accidental dural puncture occurs in 1–2% of epidural blocks, but is less common with an experienced anaesthetist.

Large bore needles are more likely to cause headache than smaller ones. Typically the patient gets an excruciatingly severe frontal headache, which gets worse when he moves, or tries to sit up. Diagnostically, it is relieved when the patient lies flat. Other features include photophobia, nausea and even vomiting.

If the headache does not resolve with simple measures such as hydration and analgesia within four hours, then it may be necessary to stop the leak with a *blood patch*.

Blood patch to control headaches

Although dural puncture during epidural anaesthesia is uncommon in experienced hands, there is an overall incidence of 1–4%. To plug the hole in the dura 10–20 mls of blood is taken from the patient's arm and injected into the epidural space at the level of the skin hole. Lay the patient flat for 2 hours. The blood will clot over the hole to block the leak. In most cases the headache eases almost immediately.

The procedure needs two operators; one takes blood from the patient's arm, while the other locates the epidural space. Use the strictest of sterile precautions. Infection of the clot in the epidural space risks abscess formation and irreversible paraplegia may follow.

Do not use a blood patch if the patient has unexplained neurological symptoms; any sepsis or chance of sepsis (such as immediately after urological or bowel surgery or draining an abscess), or localized sepsis near the site of injection.

Patchy epidurals

Sometimes epidural analgesia skips segments, yet everything around the area may be numb. The block may extend beyond the intended dermatomes.

In some people the epidural space is broken up into compartments by thin membranes which causes erratic spread of the local anaesthetic. Furthermore patients who have had previous epidurals may have the scars from old blood clots in their epidural space that prevent the local anaesthetic spreading correctly.

If the local anaesthetic does not diffuse uniformly enough to soak into the nerve roots within the 5 minutes, then sometimes simply rolling the patient so that the unblocked side is downwards often fixes the problem.

One-sided blocks

Occasionally a *unilateral block* occurs where one side of the affected area is analgesic and the other side not adequately blocked. Usually this is caused by septa or scarring inside the epidural space. Simply rolling the patient so that their unaffected side is downwards often solves the problem. Gravity encourages the local anaesthetic to flow down to reach the nerves.

Bloody tap

Sometimes the needle penetrates an epidural vein. Blood then comes back into the syringe. In this case the needle is withdrawn and the epidural re-attempted in an adjacent space.

Itch

Morphine and diamorphine commonly cause itching. If you use fentanyl this is less of a problem.

How to manage anticoagulated patients

Epidural and spinal anaesthesia is contraindicated if the patient is anticoagulated, or has an INR greater than 1.2. Nevertheless, deep vein thrombosis (DVT) prophylaxis with a low molocular weight heparin (LMWH) is considered safe providing sufficient time has elapsed since the last dose. Epidurals and spinals must not be inserted, or epidural catheters withdrawn within 12 hours of the administration of a standard dose of the LMWHs enoxaparin or dalteparin; or within 4 hours of a dose of unfractionated heparin (UH), or within 2 hours of a heparin infusion being turned off. In the case of the heparin infusion, check the activated pointial thromboplastin time aPTT is normal beforehand.

Be particularly careful if the patient has been taking the anticoagulant clopidogrel, because this drug's effects persist for 7 to 10 days. You will need to take special precautions in those who will receive heparin or LMWH perioperatively.

Risks of epidurals

Nerve damage

Although some patients complain of patchy areas of skin numbness for up to 6 weeks after an epidural anaesthetic, major neurological sequelae are rare. The big risk of neurological damage occurs with epidural haematoma or infection, or in attempts to place an epidural in a patient who has already had a laminectomy where the *epidural space* no longer exists.

Backache

Backache is common after spinal and epidural anaesthetics. Recovery room staff can help prevent this by supporting the lumbar arch with a small pillow, or a rolled-up towel to prevent the arch sagging and unintentionally stretching the interspinous ligaments. The lumbar spine has a natural lordotic arch. Once the epidural takes effect the muscles sustaining the arch lose their protective tone, the arch sags and stretches these ligaments.

Support the lumbar spine to prevent
stretching of the ligaments

Figure 8.3 How to prevent post-epidural back pain

Although you are unlikely to encounter it in the recovery room, always remember that back pain is also a sign of potentially disastrous epidural haematoma or infection.

Epidural haematoma

Bleeding into the epidural space is a grave but fortunately rare complication. Alarmingly, with the introduction of the newer anticoagulants the incidence of epidural haematomas is increasing.

Haematomas are more likely in elderly women undergoing hip or knee replacements, but particularly if they have been given low molecular-weight heparins such as enoxaparin or dalteparin as prophylaxis against deep vein thrombosis.

The epidural space is not empty; it is filled with an engorged network of venous plexuses and scattered fatty tissue. Continued bleeding into the confined space will compress the spinal cord and unless this is recognized and treated the patient will become paraplegic. To have a reasonable chance of complete or partial neurological recovery, surgical decompression must be performed as soon as possible and certainly within 8 hours.

Spinal cord compression is an emergency.

The signs and symptoms of spinal cord compression are:

- the onset of new, severe or persistent back pain;
- tingling or persistent numbness in the legs;
- muscle weakness in the lower limbs;
- urinary or faecal incontinence.

A recently reported sign of a developing haematoma is that the patient's sensory block alters to become denser, this is soon followed by a progressive motor block leading to a point where the patient cannot move their legs.

It is critically important to notify the anaesthetist immediately if you notice any back pain, or any deterioration in the patient's motor or sensory function. Your hospital's epidural protocols must have provision to 'red flag' these events and automatically obtain an urgent MRI or CT myelogram and immediate neurosurgical referral.

Unfortunately these signs of a developing haematoma are absent in 20 per cent of cases.

Table 8.1 Complications of neuraxial blocks

Risk	Approximate incidence
Transient low back pain	16:100
Dural puncture headache	1:100
Temporary paraesthesia	1:1000
Total spinal anaesthesia	1:10 000
Permanent nerve damage	1:14 000
Epidural haematomas	1:15 000
Paraplegia	< 1:30 000
Epidural abscess	< 1:20 000

Epidural infections

Infection is a rare but devastating complication. If bacteria, especially staphylococci or streptococci, get into the space they can produce an abscess. The signs are similar to epidural haematomas with the added sign of a possible fever and raised white cell count.

Epidural abscesses are more likely in diabetics, immunocompromised patients, those on steroid therapy, where the patient has already been in hospital for more than 48 hours before the catheter was placed, and where the catheter is to be left in for longer than 3 days. You may need to start appropriate antibiotic prophylaxis in the recovery room in patients with these risk factors.

Total spinal

If the tip of the epidural needle is advanced too far it will pierce the dura mater, and cerebrospinal fluid will gush back into the syringe. If this dural tap is not recognized, and more than a few millilitres of local anaesthetic is accidentally injected into the cerebrospinal fluid it causes total spinal anaesthesia. The patient abruptly collapses, loses consciousness, becomes unresponsive to pain, develops widely dilated pupils, profound hypotension, and stops breathing. With urgent intubation, ventilation and ionotropic support dopamine to maintain the blood pressure, and with suitable care the patient usually recovers with no sequelae within 24 hours. Fortunately total spinal anaesthesia is rare, and at worst most dural taps cause a postdural puncture headache.

Table 8.2 Signs and treatment of toxicity

Stage	Signs	Treatment
1.	Numbness of face, visual disturbances, confusion	Give oxygen by mask; encourage deep breathing; summon help
2.	Coma	Turn into coma position; clear airway, assist breathing; attach oximeter and ECG; check pulse and BP
3.	Convulsions	Thiopentone 1–3 mg IV
4.	Hypotension	Give IV fluids, ionotropes

Local anaesthetic toxicity

There is a risk of toxicity if local anaesthetic is injected into an epidural vein. Should enough local anaesthetic reach the heart or brain it will rapidly cause coma and cardiac failure. The patient's blood pressure falls and they lose consciousness. Bupivacaine in particular may cause "stone heart" where the heart simply stops and remains unresponsive. This may respond to intravenous infusion of lipid emulsions[1] (Intralipid®), however if this fails cardiac bypass may be required for several hours.

The earliest feature of systemic toxicity is numbness or tingling of the tongue and around the mouth. The patient may become light-headed, anxious, or drowsy, with slurred speech or complain of tinnitus.

Epidural infusions

Patients find continuous epidural infusion highly effective to control acute pain after surgery to the chest, abdomen, pelvis or lower limbs.[2]

Once an infusion is established measure the vital signs: blood pressure, pulse and respiratory rate, and oxygen saturation every 10 minutes for the first hour. Watch carefully for any trends in patients' respiratory rates especially if they have been given epidural opioids. Once patients are pain-free encourage them to deep breathe and cough. Record the neurological signs of pupil size and reaction to light, and the level of consciousness.

With specifically trained nursing staff, clear protocols, and anaesthetic staff on duty in the hospital epidural analgesia can be continued quite safely in the ward.

Although epidural infusions are general safe, there is always the possibility of adverse events including respiratory depression, hypotension, epidural haematoma or abscess. When you transfer a patient with an epidural to the ward ensure that:

- there are clearly written protocols. Your hospital should have a standard form, with precise limits for vital signs and infusion rates. The form needs clear instructions on what to do if the limits are exceeded;
- your handover to the ward staff follows the guidelines;
- if opioids are used then a stat dose of naloxone is ordered in the drug chart;
- the epidural system is completely closed and must not be breached;
- the epidural lines are clearly identified with the yellow marker tag;
- there are always suitably trained nursing staff on the ward to monitor the patient closely;
- the ward has facilities for resuscitation, and that there a resuscitation team available at all times;
- suitably trained medical staff are on-call and nearby.

How to remove an epidural catheter

- Wait until at least 12 hours have elapsed since the last dose of enoxaparin or dalteparin.
- Ease the catheters out gently.
- If you meet resistance, then call for skilled assistance. These fine catheters can occasionally break off in the epidural space while being removed.
- Once you have removed the catheter make sure it is intact, and record this fact in the patients notes.
- Apply a dressing over the hole.
- If a piece of catheter is left behind usually it causes no problems, but the patient must be warned in writing, because it can become a focus for infection at any time in the future.

Drugs used for epidural analgesia

Local anaesthetic drugs anaesthetize the somatic nerves as they leave the spinal cord, and the opioids interrupt the transmission of pain impulses within the spinal cord itself. This gives analgesia for the incision, the nearby skin, and muscle, and will almost completely relieve postoperative pain. Ill-defined deep visceral pain from the organs may persist, because visceral pain impulses are transmitted through the vagus nerve, and do not travel in the spinal cord.

The choice of drugs used for analgesia depends on the indication for the epidural. Bupivacaine and epidural opioids are the agents most frequently used drugs. Lignocaine is too short-acting to be useful for postoperative analgesia.

To avoid the inconvenience of continually having to top up the epidural use a volumetric pump to infuse epidural opioids when the patient returns to the ward.

Bupivacaine

Bupivacaine hydrochloride is an amide local anaesthetic. Compared to lidocaine it has a relatively slow onset, but a long action. In a single shot it lasts 3–4 hours for epidural block, and may last 12–24 or more hours with brachial plexus and some other nerve blocks. It is more cardiotoxic than lidocaine or ropivacaine. The maximum dose is 2 mg/Kg.

Ropivacaine

Ropivacaine is an amide local anaesthetic chemically closely related to bupivacaine, but it is less lipid soluble, less toxic and less potent. It is cleared from the body 40 per cent faster than bupivacaine. The maximum safe dose is about 3 mg/Kg and therefore it does not act for as long as bupivacaine.

Levobupivacaine

Levobupivacaine is a derivative of bupivacaine and has the same properties as bupivacaine, but is less neuro- and cardiotoxic. It is not yet widely used.

Dose of local anaesthetic

The dose of local anaesthetic needed for effective analgesia depends on the where the tip of the epidural catheter lies. For a catheter inserted in the lumbar region the dose is 8–12 ml and between 3–8 ml for catheters inserted in the thoracic region. If the local anaesthetic is injected rapidly it will spread further, but this is difficult to do through a fine catheter and a bacterial filter.

Opioids

Epidural opioids do not interfere with motor function or cause hypotension, allowing the patient to move about. Opioids are ten times more potent when used in the epidural space than when used intravenously. The combination of epidural local anaesthetic and an opioid improves analgesic effect and reduces the dose required for both drugs.

Fentanyl

Fentanyl is the most commonly used opioid in epidural anaesthesia. It comes in pre-prepared packs in concentrations of 2–4 µg/ml infused at 5–15 ml/hr with one or other of the local anaesthetic agents. Since it does not cause a motor block it allows the patient move around after surgical procedures, and deep breathe and cough. Because fentanyl causes neither sympathetic blockade nor peripheral vasodilation, it should not cause hypotension. Profound respiratory depression, however, can occur as much as 2 hours after a single dose of epidural fentanyl. Patients should be under close observation for at least 3 hours after a dose of epidural fentanyl.

Diamorphine

Diamorphine 50–100 µg/ml infused at 5–15 ml/hr is used in the United Kingdom but not elsewhere.

Morphine

Morphine is rarely used because it causes itch.

Other blocks

Intercostal blocks

Intercostal blocks give pain relief after upper abdominal operations such as cholecystectomy and thoracotomy. The patient lies with the side to be blocked uppermost and 2–3 ml of local anaesthetic with adrenaline are infiltrated behind each rib into the neurovascular groove. The two main dangers are accidental puncture of the pleura causing a pneumothorax, and intravascular injection of local anaesthetic causing toxicity.

Thoracic paravertebral blocks

Thoracic paravertebral blocks are useful to relieve the pain of thoracotomy. A catheter is placed in the paravertebral space and may be left in for up to 5 days. The risk of infection is less than a catheter in the epidural space.

Brachial plexus blocks

Brachial plexus blocks are useful for upper limb surgery. There are two approaches, the axillary and the supraclavicular. Both are effective, but the supraclavicular approach carries a high risk of pneumothorax and nerve damage. With fully successful blocks patients lose all muscle power in their arms. Since biceps flexion is sometimes spared, warn patients not to bend their arm or try to look at their hand, because it might fly out of control and hit them in the face. If the patient has a plaster on their arm, they can break their nose. Bupivacaine may cause the block to last for 18 hours or more. Use long-acting local anaesthetics only if such a long-lasting effect is required.

Intra-articular local anaesthetics

Arthroscopies can be painful and bupivacaine injected into the joint space provides effective analgesia. Patients should not be discharged until one hour after intra-articular injection of bupivacaine, because peak plasma levels are delayed by slow absorption from the joint, and any side-effects may take this long to become apparent.

Spinal anaesthesia

Spinal anaesthetics are rarely inserted in the recovery room, but many patients will have them for their surgery, and come to the recovery room still affected by them.

Spinal (intrathecal) anaesthesia has many features in common with epidural anaesthesia, but there are some differences. Epidurals can be topped up whereas spinals cannot. Spinals are used for many operations below the waist and provide good conditions for painful procedures. It is the anaesthetic of choice for elective Caesarean sections, and transurethral prostate resection. Spinal anaesthesia is sometimes used for surgery on premature babies and reduces the incidence of life-threatening apnoea.

Spinal anaesthesia is safe, and complications are few. As with epidural anaesthesia backache may be a problem, and mild pain can last for a week or so after the injection. The principal reason for backache, as it is with epidural anaesthesia, is inadequate support of the lumbar arch during and after surgery.

Criteria for discharging a patient after a spinal

It is not always possible for recovery rooms to keep otherwise stable patients until their spinal block has worn off. Because the sensation of cold and pain are carried in similar neural pathways you can easily test the level of sensory block with a piece of ice. The patient can be discharged to the ward if the level of sensory blockade is below T10 (the umbilicus) and the patient's cardiovascular and surgical state is otherwise stable and adequate. The nurses on the ward must be experienced in looking after patients with a spinal anaesthetic, and must know how to respond to various complications that might arise.

Obviously if the patient is going home the spinal block must have worn off and the patient must be able to walk and void. In most units this means in most day case surgery spinal anaesthetic is only used for morning cases.

A protocol for ward care of the patient after spinal anaesthetic

Standard post-anaesthetic observations

Sensation should return within 4 hours. If after 4 hours the patient remains numb, and there are no 'pin-and-needles' sensations, notify the anaesthetist immediately because delayed return of feeling is a warning sign of epidural haematoma.

Analgesia. Severe pain may return suddenly once the spinal block has worn off. Give analgesia at the first complaint of pain.

Fasting. Fasting is not necessary unless it is a surgical requirement, such as after abdominal operations.

Posture. It is not necessary to lie the patient flat for 24 hours. The patient should be able to sit up as soon as the analgesia has worn off.

Ambulation. If not surgically contraindicated, the patient may get out of bed 2 hours after the return of normal sensation, but only with assistance. Before getting the patient out of bed, sit him up slowly and check his blood pressure. If the systolic blood pressure falls more than 20 mmHg, of if the patient feels faint, dizzy or nauseated, then lie the patient down, and notify the anaesthetist.

Potential complications

Postural hypotension. Lie the patient in bed, and notify the anaesthetic registrar on duty who will increase the fluid intake.

Urinary rentention. Encourage the patient to void urine when sensation returns. If the patient has not voided within 4 hours, or his bladder can be palpated, he will require a catheter.

Notes

1. Soltesz EG, van Pelt F, Byrne JG (2003) *Journal of Cardiothoracic and Vascular Anesthesia* 17:357–8.
2. Royal College of Anaesthetists, The Royal College of Nursing, The Association of Anaesthetists of Great Britain and Ireland, The British Pain Society, and the European Society of Regional Anaesthesia and Pain Therapy (2004) *Good practice in the management of continuous epidural analgesia in the hospital setting.* A joint publication.

9

Special problems

Allergy

Allergy is an immunological response to foreign molecules. It is marked by urticarial rash (hives), oedema of the face, wheeze, and if severe, hypotension. Allergic responses are not common in the recovery room, but may be serious when they do occur. The most severe manifestation of allergy is anaphylaxis.

Types of allergic response

There are three types of allergic response: immediate, intermediate and late.

Immediate response

Onset 0–1 hour: anaphylaxis and anaphylactoid response are the most severe. They present with hypotension, laryngeal oedema causing stridor or hoarse voice, wheezing, urticaria and hypotension.

An immediate allergic response is a medical emergency.

Intermediate response

Onset 1–72 hours: urticaria, angio-oedema, laryngeal oedema with stridor, and wheezing.

Stridor is an emergency.

Late response

Onset after 72 hours: morbilliform rash, haemolytic anaemia, thrombocy-topenia, neutropenia, and interstitial nephritis. Variations of this late response are called the Stevens–Johnson syndrome, and serum sickness.

How to avoid problems

Many drugs cause allergic responses including morphine, codeine, radio-contrast media, muscle relaxants and blood, blood products or colloidal plasma expanders.

Give intravenous drugs cautiously and slowly. Watch the patient's face and breathing. If the patient gasps or coughs this may forewarn of a developing allergic response. Although this sign is not present on every occasion, it is a useful warning. If there is any hypotension or wheezing after a patient has received a drug then consider anaphylaxis. In this case notify the anaesthetist.

Many drugs given intravenously cause a red flare to run up the vein. This is usually just a local reaction, but if the patient develops a motley or hive-like rash then consider allergy.

Penicillin allergy

Many patients report they are allergic to penicillins. The actual prevalence is difficult to establish, but deaths from penicillin allergy are rare.

Patients' reports of penicillin allergy are unreliable, and usually arise from some vaguely remembered incident in the past. Often it was simply an unpleasant reaction, such as pain at the site of the injection, or nausea, or feeling faint or bowel upsets. This of course is not allergy, but from then on the patient is labelled 'allergic to penicillin', which may unnecessarily deprive them of this life-saving group of drugs. One in twenty patients who are truly allergic to penicillin, are also allergic to cephalosporins.

Latex allergy

Latex allergy is a major occupational health problem among exposed people. Allergy to natural rubber latex (NRL), commonly referred to as latex, was an uncommon occurrence before 1980. Since then latex allergy has become a major occupational health problem to those who work in hospitals.

Latex is ubiquitous in the domestic and hospital environment. In hospitals latex is found in gloves, infusion ports on intravenous sets, caps on drug vials, mattress covers – the list is long, varied and seemingly endless.

It affects up to 10 per cent of exposed workers and about 2.5 per cent of the general population. The symptoms of latex allergy range from mild local skin erythema after wearing latex gloves, through the range of reactions of urticaria, conjunctivitis, angioedema, and asthma, to a full-blown anaphylactic reaction.

Sensitized workers must have a safe environment. Non-sensitized people should use low allergen powdered gloves, or better still use only powder-free latex gloves or gloves made from non-latex material.

It is important your recovery room and operating theatres have a carefully researched protocol on how to manage patients and staff allergic to latex. Establish a database of known latex-free products, and keep a stock of these in the operating theatre suite.

How to manage patients with latex allergy

- Clearly identify patients and staff with latex allergies.
- Remove all latex products from the vicinity of affected patients.

- Use only latex-free products.
- Tightly enclose equipment known to contain latex with plastic sheeting.
- Have a tray with suitable drugs available to treat any reaction should it occur.

Delayed emergence

Some patients take a long time to fully emerge from their anaesthetics. There are many reasons for this; most are benign, but a few are serious.

Why patients have postoperative apnoea

Hyperventilation-induced apnoea

The residual effects of intraoperative opioids, volatile agents and sedatives (such as midazolam) can all suppress patients' ventilation, but the commonest cause of postoperative apnoea is the inadvertent hyperventilation of the patient during the anaesthetic. Volatile agents raise the *apnoeic threshold*; this means that patients' medullary respiratory centres do not respond to rising arterial pressures of carbon dioxide ($PaCO_2$).

To treat hyperventilation-induced apnoea the anaesthetist may simply ventilate the patient at a lower tidal volume until their $PaCO_2$ increases enough to stimulate breathing again. This may take 15 to 20 minutes. Never leave the patient apnoeic, because they may become hypoxic. Furthermore the brain, having little capacity to buffer abrupt pH changes, will be affected by a rapidly rising $PaCO_2$.

Hypothermia

Hypothermia increases the effects of the volatile agents, antagonizes the reversal of muscle relaxants, and delays drug *metabolism*.

Hypercapnea

In a hypoventilating patient as the $PaCO_2$ rises above 70 mmHg (9.21 kPa) the patient becomes increasingly comatose.

Prolonged action of other drugs

Some patients are very sensitive to anaesthetic drugs. If the patient is cold, or has liver or renal disease, they will be slow to metabolize or excrete anaesthetic drugs.

Patients should progressively lighten from their anaesthetic in an orderly sequence. Look at the patient's eyes. Initially their pupils will not react to light and be about 2 mm in diameter. They may be eccentrically set in the iris. Next the pupils will start to react to light. Then the direction of gaze becomes divergent, and finally just before the patient wakes, the pupils dilate slightly. The process may take anywhere from a few minutes to 45 minutes or so. If the progress stops, then consider the more serious causes of delayed emergence.

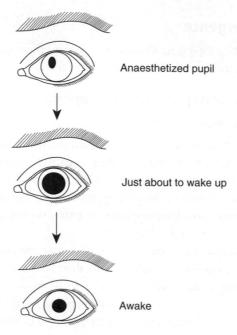

Anaesthetized pupil

Just about to wake up

Awake

Figure 9.1 Eyes' signs on emergence

Practical point about delayed emergence

1. Everyone who is not brain damaged, will wake up – eventually.
2. The fewer drugs you use to achieve this, the safer it is for the patient.
3. Never use painful stimuli rouse the patient, because they are not asleep, they are in a coma.
4. Nerve stimulators hurt. Do not use them on conscious patients.

Check the history for drug interactions that may delay emergence; for instance erythromycin prolongs the effect of midazolam for many hours; droperidol prolongs the effect of benzodiazepines (especially diazepam).

Naloxone rapidly reverses the effects of opioids. Proceed cautiously because you may well precipitate agonizing pain. Start with a dose of 1.5 μg/Kg and repeat it in 2 minutes if necessary. Naloxone works for about 30 minutes. Once it wears off the remaining opioid may re-exert its respiratory depressant effects.

Benzodiazepines

Benzodiazepines have varying *half-lives*. The effect of diazepam 10 mg lasts as long in hours as the patient's age in years, so for an 80-year-old the diazepam would still affect their mental processing 80 hours after the dose. This does not necessarily mean the patient is sedated, but it certainly means their conditioned reflexes are affected to the extent they should not drive a car. Smaller doses are cleared more quickly.

Midazolam is cleared 10 times faster than diazepam. Midazolam has an elimination of half-life of 1 to 3 hours. Men metabolize it more slowly than women, but older people metabolize midazolam at the same rate as younger people.

Flumazenil reverses benzodiazepines. It only works for 35–45 minutes, so it may need repeating, because most of the benzodiazepines, such as diazepam, have a longer action. Give flumazenil 3–5 µg/Kg intravenously over 15 seconds. Be careful, because in susceptible people this drug may cause convulsions. Susceptible people include those with epilepsy, head injuries, cerebrovascular disease, or who are febrile.

Brain damage

A serious complication, and sometimes a cause of delayed emergence from anaesthesia is neurological damage caused by hypoxia, stroke, fat or gas emboli, or intraoperative hypotension. Water overload after prostate surgery or uterine endoscopic procedures can cause coma or hemiparesis. Consider occult head injury or alcohol poisoning in trauma patients who are slow to wake up. A stroke following a carotid endartectomy requires immediate re-operation.

How to tell if there is brain damage

If a comatose patient does not move one side of their body, or is rigid only on one side, has an asymmetrical face with their mouth drooping in one corner, or has a dilated or non-reacting pupil only on one side, then these lateralizing signs indicate brain damage. Seek help immediately. Occasionally you will need to give a painful stimulus to evoke a lateralizing sign. An effective way to this is to take the skin over patient's triceps muscle between your thumb and forefinger and squeeze firmly. This should evoke a withdrawal response. Do not rub your knuckles up and down their sternum, squeeze their ear, or press on their orbital ridge, because you will bruise your patient, and certainly cause their intracranial pressure to rise.

Other signs of possible brain damage are a change in the rate or pattern of breathing, especially if it becomes deep and sighing. A bilateral up-going plantar response is normal in patients emerging from anaesthesia, but if one toe goes up, while the other goes down, then you have a lateralizing sign.

Lateralizing signs suggest structural brain damage.

Residual relaxant

Anaesthetists use neuromuscular blocking drugs to paralyse skeletal muscle so that the surgeon can get at the surgical site, and also to make it easier to ventilate patients. Deep anaesthesia achieves the same result, but also depresses the cardiac output.

The effects of muscle relaxants sometimes persist or recur in the recovery room. The best sign that patients' muscle relaxation is reversed adequately is their ability to lift their head from the pillow, and hold it up for 5 seconds (5-second head lift test). They must be able to do this before you discharge them from the recovery room. If you are concerned about residual relaxation straight leg lift, coughing and a firm handgrip (but only offer the patient two of your fingers otherwise you may be hurt) are all tests of recovered muscle power.

Although commonly used, asking patients to "Stick out your tongue" is a useless test of muscle power, and of no help in assessing airway competence.

If patients are still partially paralysed their arms flop and jerk like a rag-doll when they try to move, and they may complain of double vision. You will see tracheal tug as their larynx jerks downward every time they attempt to breathe in. You may see the strap muscles in their neck contract as they recruit them to breathe in. Fortunately, respiratory muscles are the last affected by muscle relaxants. Most patients can breathe adequately even though their skeletal muscles are floppy, and they are unable to cough effectively.

If patients are struggling to breathe, or starting to panic, then support their breathing with a bag and mask, attach an oximeter and an ECG, and summon the anaesthetist.

Why muscle relaxants persist

There are many reasons why muscle relaxants fail to reverse properly.

These include:

- over-dosage of relaxant drug;
- hypothermia;

- liver or renal disease delaying their excretion;
- hypokalaemia;
- concurrent use of certain antibiotics such as gentamicin or neomycin;
- or intercurrent diseases affecting nerves and muscles such as myasthenia gravis, carcinomatous or alcoholic myopathy or motor neurone diseases.

What to do

The anaesthetist may elect to use a half-dose of neostigmine 0.625 mg and atropine 0.3 mg intravenously. Before repeating the half-dose, consider the consequences. Excess neostigmine will potentiate the neuromuscular block, may disrupt bowel anastomoses, cause bronchorrhoea and bradycardia.

Nerve stimulators do not help

Residual paralysis is not an emergency, but it can easily become one. If a patient is distressed, struggling to breathe or starts to become alarmed because of residual paralysis there is little point using nerve stimulators to diagnose the type of block. Safe treatment remains the same. Never allow the patient to struggle on. If a single small dose of neostigmine and atropine does not relieve the situation within 5 minutes, then the safest option is to sedate, re-intubate and ventilate the patient. The anaesthetist may elect to insert a laryngeal mask and use this to support the ventilation. Do not try to use additional doses of cholinesterase inhibitors of whatever type.

All muscle relaxants wear off eventually, and most within an hour. It does not matter what agent is causing the residual paralysis. We have encountered respiratory arrests, and some fatalities, where this rule has been circumvented. Residual paralysis is not the time 'to wait and see' what happens.

Plasmacholinesterase deficiency or "Sux apnoea"

Occasionally, a short-acting muscle relaxant, succinyl choline (also called suxamethonium), causes prolonged relaxation. This phenomenon is colloquially known as *sux apnoea*. Patients may come to the recovery room needing a short spell on a ventilator.

Normally, a circulating enzyme called *plasma cholinesterase* (once called pseudocholinesterase), breaks down succinyl choline within 3–5 minutes. In people with a congenital or acquired *plasma cholinesterase deficiency*, succing choline may continue to act from between 10 minutes to an hour or more. In this case the only option is to sedate, re-intubate and ventilate the patient until the succinyl choline wears off. No drugs safely reverse this sort of block.

Agitation and confusion

Emergence delirium

As they emerge from anaesthesia about 5 per cent of patients become agitated, bewildered,[1] or even combative needing restraint. This phenomenon is called *emergence delirium*. It tends to occur in younger patients, drug or alcohol abusers, and especially where the patient was anxious before surgery. Patients seem not to know where they are, or what is going on around them, and are unable to concentrate sufficiently to obey simple commands. Usually the delirium settles within a minute or two as their conscious state improves. If it does not resolve quickly then eliminate other causes for delirium, especially hypoxia or hypoglycaemia because these will quickly maim or kill.

The principal causes of delirium are:

- residual effects of anaesthetic drugs during emergence;
- intraoperative complications;
- pre-existing confusional states;
- hypoxia;
- hypoglycaemia;
- pain;
- awareness during the anaesthetic.

Why emergence delirium occurs

The neurophysiology involved in emergence delirium is not fully understood. It probably occurs because various parts of the brain emerge from anaesthesia at different rates. For example, delirium occurs when the cortex 'wakes up' before the frontal lobes are able to moderate its behaviour. It is certainly worse if the patient has received additional psychoactive drugs such as hyoscine, atropine, ketamine or a phenothiazine (such as prochlorperazine used as an anti-emetic).

Alcoholics sometimes wake in a dream-like state. They may sit up, peer around and yet not respond when spoken to. If you forcibly try to restrain them, take care, because they may lash out. Guide them to lie down.

Emergence delirium is common after nasal surgery, especially if it is cosmetic surgery. Patients are distressed to wake and find their noses blocked by packs.

Emergence delirium in children is common, affecting approximately 13 per cent of those under the age of 15 years. If babies or toddlers go to sleep crying, they often wake crying (and some sob gently all through their general anaesthetic). There are reports of the newer inhalational agents, sevoflurane and desflurane, causing more emergence delirium in children than halothane or isoflurane.[2] Poor intraoperative pain control is probably another major factor causing delirium. Children aged 2 to 5 years may wake agitated, combative and inconsolable. A dose of 1 mg/Kg of pethidine quickly settles them.

Delirium

1. If the patients have clouded consciousness, but are not excitable and they know where they are, then consider hypothermia, hypercarbia, or psychoactive drugs used during the anaesthetics.

2. If patients are excitable and agitated, and do not know where they are, then consider the early stages of hypoxia, or hypoglycaemia.

3. Children and those who were anxious or agitated before surgery are tenfold more likely to have emergence delirium.

4. Review the anaesthetic notes for hints about the cause: psychoactive drugs used during or before the operation, periods of hypotension, or gas or fat embolism.

5. Occasionally midazolam or other benzodiazepines can cause paradoxical excitement. This is reversed with flumazenil.

6. Pain is a potent cause of delirium in semicomatose patients.

Intraoperative complications

Intraoperative complications include air or particulate embolism, cerebral ischemia, intracranial haemorrhage, hypoxic encephalopathy, or hypotension. These complications may cause delirium, but are far more likely to present because 'the patient won't wake up'.

Pre-existing confusional states

If a patient has dementia, or a cognitive disorder, before their anaesthetic then it is not surprising that they are confused afterwards. Never simply assume that their cognitive disorder is the sole reason for their delirium. They are as much at risk of other causes of delirium as any patient.

Hypoxia

Severe hypoxia or hypoglycaemia causes irreversible brain damage within minutes. Suspect impending hypoxia if the pulse oximeter reading is 94% or less. Give oxygen; review the patient's record to identify risk factors for hypoxia.

If, during the anaesthetic, the patient has had a transient hypoxic episode, such as a period of hypotension, then they may well wake up confused even if they are not hypoxic when the delirium is first recognized.

The cause of cerebral hypoxia can be subtle. Hypoxia can involve one or more of a combination of factors including inadequate inspired oxygen, airway or lung disease, anaemia, and cardiac failure. Each additional factor amplifies the effect to aggravate hypoxia; for example, anaemia amplifies hypoxia caused by lung disease.

Hypoglycaemia

As with hypoxia, hypoglycaemia can cause brain damage in minutes. Review the patient's record to establish risk factors for hypoglycaemia, check their blood glucose levels with a portable glucose meter, and get help. Hypoglycaemia is a particular risk in alcoholics who have fasted, and more predictably in diabetics receiving insulin.

Pain

While emerging from anaesthesia pain or especially discomfort from a full bladder makes patients extremely restless.

The violent patient

Occasionally a patient will warn you they have become violent while emerging from previous anaesthetics. Take their warning seriously. They may become a danger to themselves or staff. Sometimes they rip out their drips and become combative. If you have no intravenous access, then give ketamine 1.5 mg/Kg into any muscle mass you can find. It will rapidly bring the patient under control, but you will now have a fully anaesthetized patient to care for. Paradoxically benzodiazepines, instead of sedating these patients, makes some of them more aggressive. If you cannot manage the patient you should call for help before anyone is hurt.

What to do for emergence delirium

- Give 100% oxygen.
- Reassure and orient patients as to where they are, and what has happened.
- Eliminate hypoxia and hypoglycaemia.
- Gently restrain the patient lest they fall from the trolley and hurt themselves.
- Notify the anaesthetist.

- If the patient has not improved within 5 minutes then consider causes for delayed emergence.

Crying patients

Occasionally patients sob after emerging from their anaesthetic, particularly if they have been given propofol. Often they do not know why they are crying. It does not necessarily mean they are in pain.

Unpremedicated patients, and those anaesthetized for short procedures, are more likely to cry, especially if the procedure is for a sad reason such as a termination of pregnancy. Patients with anxiety or depression are more likely to cry as well, as are children and elderly demented patients. Sit with them; hold their hand. Do not try to comfort them with reassurances. Crying is a useful natural tranquillizer and a good way of resolving emotional stress. Others who may weep are those who have had mastectomies, lost a limb, or were involved in accidents.

Awareness

Some people are more resistant to the effects of anaesthetic drugs, and while paralysed with muscle relaxants and unable to move, may be consciously aware during their operation. Postoperatively, these patients are often upset and crying and restless. Awareness is more common in women having Caesarean sections under general anaesthesia, the very ill, trauma surgery, and during open-heart surgery. The incidence of recall is estimated to be about 0.5 per cent. Even under seemingly adequate general anaesthesia memories can be laid down, and the patient may subconsciously remember what has gone on. Hearing is the last modality lost. The experience may range from merely a fleeting impression of voices, through to the horrendous calamity of being completely conscious, in agony and unable to move or tell anyone about it. Those who experience awareness also range from those who are mildly interested, and not at all upset by the incident, through to those who develop post-traumatic stress disorder (PTSD). This is especially likely if the patient was in pain.

Post-traumatic stress disorder is characterized by flashbacks. These are like emotional malaria with intrusive memories, which recur again and again when the person is awake, or are relived in their nightmares. It may be all so awful that the patients hide it in a dark corner of their mind, and forget about it; but they become changed people: irritable, anxious, jumpy, depressed, and constantly on their guard. These patients need debriefing over many sessions with a psychiatrist – this is not a job for amateurs.

Explicit awareness

Explicit awareness occurs where the patient is consciously aware of what went on during surgery. They may or may not have felt pain.

Implicit awareness

Implicit awareness is more common. There are vague memories, but they are jumbled. This is more likely in the very old, the very ill, those undergoing emergency surgery, and especially during Caesarean section under general anaesthetic where the incidence can be as high as 3 per cent.

Pseudo-awareness

It is common for patients to recall wearing an oxygen mask in recovery room. If they have not been forewarned of this, some interpret this event as awareness. Some have even sued. It is always prudent to tell patients several times that their surgery is over, everything went well, and not to take off their oxygen mask because they might get a headache.

What to do

- Recognize that how you handle your patient may determine whether or not they are affected for years to come. This is a potent cause of a prolonged Stage 3 recovery.
- Reassure and comfort your patient but never negate the claims.
- Empathize with the patient, acknowledge their feelings and reflect them back to the frightened person. If it is appropriate, hold their hand. Allow them to cry.
- Notify the anaesthetist.
- Record your observations in the patient's unit record – what you see, hear and measure – but not your opinions.

Headache

About 30 per cent of women get postoperative headaches after surgery, but men are less often affected. Many factors contribute to postoperative headache including dehydration from excessive fasting, nuchal spasm (especially in patients who get tension headaches), and caffeine withdrawal. Place a cool wet towel on their forehead, and keep bright lights out of their eyes. Start with simple analgesics such as paracetamol. You may occasionally need to resort to pethidine, but avoid morphine because it tends to make headaches worse.

What are the serious causes of headaches?

Postdural puncture headaches occur after the dura mater is punctured tap with a spinal or epidural anaesthetic. The headache is exacerbated when the patient sits up, and relieved when they lie down. The patient may need a blood patch to relieve it.

Severe hypertension may cause headache, photophobia, vomiting, visual disturbance and clouding of consciousness. This malignant hypertension must be treated early before it causes a haemorrhagic stroke. Malignant hypertension may occur abruptly when the blood pressure exceeds 220/120 mmHg.

Water intoxication after urological surgery or hysteroscopy causes cerebral oedema, which presents with a headache.

Extravasation and arterial injections

Extravasation

Extravasation occurs when, during infusion, intravenous fluid leaks from the vein into the surrounding tissues. Some drugs are highly toxic to tissues and may cause horrific tissue damage, killing muscle, skin, tendon and nerves and requiring disfiguring and destructive debridement. Toxic drugs include dopamine, adrenaline, 50% glucose, sodium bicarbonate, calcium chloride, potassium chloride, chemotherapeutic agents and some antibiotics.

The amount of damage depends on the type of drug, the amount extravasated, and how quickly it is recognized. Often the tissue damage is not immediately obvious, and can take days or even longer to become apparent.

Those most at risk are the elderly with delicate skin and fragile veins. Patients who are emerging from anaesthesia may not report pain before substantial damage occurs.

Where there is pain there is tissue damage.

Extravasation is easier to prevent than treat. If you are about to infuse something which could cause tissue damage, then it is prudent to set up the new infusion at a fresh site in a different vein. Give drug infusions into the largest possible vein. Avoid siting a cannula in the back of the hand, or a vein crossing a joint. Use clear plastic dressings so you can see the puncture site and surrounding skin. Do not cover the site with bandages.

Replace painful drips.

How to tell if the drip has tissued

Colloquially, extravasation has occurred when the drip has 'tissued'.

One or more of the following occur:

- the patient complains of pain over the drip site or up the vein;
- the infusion begins to run slowly;
- you cannot aspirate blood from the cannula;
- the tissues around the cannula start to swell.

If you press on the vein a few centimetres above the cannula and the drip does not slow or stop, then it is probable that the fluid is running into the tissues. Another test is to place one finger on either side of the tip of the cannula and press gently down on the tissues. If the drip slows or stops, then chances are the drip has tissued.

What to do about extravasation

- Stop the infusion immediately.
- Leave the cannula in place.
- Aspirate as much of the drug or fluid as possible.
- Outline the affected area with an indelible marking pen.
- Apply a warm compress on the site. This may not help prevent tissue damage, but it is comforting to the patient.
- Elevate the limb and notify the anaesthetist.
- Make clear and careful notes in the patient's record.

When to use specific interventions

It is best to use the following techniques as early as possible, but they can be used with decreasing effect up to 12 hours later.

For substances that cause tissue damage with increasing concentrations, hyaluronidase (an enzyme) reduces the extent of tissue damage following extravasation of parenteral nutrition solutions, concentrated glucose solutions, electrolyte infusions, antibiotics, aminophylline, mannitol and chemotherapeutic agents. Some anaesthetists dilute hyaluronidase to 15 units/ml and inject 1 ml of the solution through the catheter or sometimes subcutaneously around the site.

Extravasation of a vasoconstrictive agent, such as dopamine, dobutamine, adrenaline, or noradrenaline, can cause severe ischaemic tissue damage. Phentolamine, an alpha-adrenergic antagonist, reduces both arterial and venous vasospasm. Inject a dose of 10 mg in 5 ml of 0.9% saline through the catheter or subcutaneously around the site.

Inadvertent intra-arterial injection

Whenever you give an intravenous injection, always check that bright red blood does not pulse back into the needle. Accidental injection of a substance into an artery usually occurs when intravenous injections are attempted in the antecubital fossa, but may occur anywhere, even on the back of the hand. In almost every case the patient immediately reports intense pain in their fingers or a site distal to the injection, and many will report soon thereafter sensory disturbances such as tingling, burning or paraesthesia. The consequences can be catastrophic, but it may take hours and sometimes up to a week or more before the full extent of the tissue damage becomes apparent. Within the first 2 hours you may see nailbed pallor and decreased capillary refill in the fingertips.[3]

What to do

- Stop the injection.
- Keep the arterial line in place.
- Aspirate, flush and inject procaine 0.1 ml/Kg into the arterial line.
- Start a slow intravenous infusion of 0.9% saline.
- Give pain relief if necessary.
- Notify the anaesthetist.
- Seek the advice of a vascular surgeon.

Further steps

- Stellate or brachial plexus blocks may help.

- Phentolamine 1 mg diluted to 10 ml in 0.9% saline injected into the artery over 10 minutes is useful to relieve vasospasm, Papaverine with heparin has been used successfully[4] but it is not known whether the eventual outcome is changed.

Eyes and pupils

Unconscious patients do not blink. It only takes a few moments for ulcers to form once the cornea dries out. Keep their eyes closed. Use a lubricating ointment such as methylcellulose to protect them. Do not use chloramphenicol ointment because of the slight risk of serious bone marrow depression. Recent evidence suggests that placing polyethylene sheeting (Gladwrap®) over the eyes is more effective than lubricating drops or gels.[5]

The patient may complain of sore gritty eyes if they have been open during the operation. In this case, make a note in the record whether their eyes were taped shut during the procedure. If you are concerned then use fluorescein stain to reveal corneal or scleral damage. Irrigate the eye with saline, tape it shut, and consult an ophthalmologist.

When plaster of paris is used to splint fractured noses, fragments easily enter the eye. Gently wash these out with 0.9% saline.

Pupils

Dilated pupils occur with:

- hypoxia;
- severe head injury – this sign signals a poor prognosis;
- homotropine, used in eye surgery to dilate pupils.

Pinpoint pupils occur with:

- pilocarpine eye drops used to treat glaucoma;
- *narcotic* overdose;
- pontine (brainstem) haemorrhage.

An oval pupil may indicate early brainstem compression. A fixed unilateral dilated pupil indicates severe brainstem compression. If this develops after neurosurgery, notify the neurosurgeon and the anaesthetist immediately.

A unilateral constricted pupil on the affected side occurs in Horner's syndrome. This occurs when the cervical sympathetic nerves are paralysed after surgery on the neck or thorax, or brachial plexus blocks.

Irregular pupils occur for a few minutes when the patient is emerging from a general anaesthetic where volatile agents were used. If you test the patient's plantar reflexes at this time, you will find they are up-going. This phenomenon lasts only about 10 minutes.

Hiccups

Hiccups frequently occur after laparoscopy, or more rarely after open abdominal procedures where something is irritating the diaphragm. Usually patients respond to gently stimulating their oral pharynx with a soft sucker. If hiccups persist they usually disappear with a low dose of metoclopramide, or ephedrine. Tell the surgeon about persistent hiccups, because it may indicate blood accumulating under the diaphragm.

Nerve injuries

Nerve injuries are the commonest reason for patients taking legal action against their anaesthetists. Nerve injury is more common in diabetics, smokers, alcoholics and those with disseminated cancer, possibly because these patients are already susceptible to peripheral neuropathies. Nerve damage is usually caused by improperly positioning the patient on the operating table or the recovery room trolley. Sometimes, even with the most scrupulous care, injuries still occur. The physiological reason for this remains a mystery.

In the recovery room the patient may complain of numbness or tingling, or loss of power in a limb. Notify the anaesthetist immediately should you encounter this problem.

Brachial plexus

Brachial plexus damage causes weakness in the hand with wrist drop. Brachial plexus nerve blocks are the commonest cause of plexus damage in the operating theatre. They may occur if the head is rotated in the opposite direction to the arm that is adducted on the operating table's arm board. About 20 per cent of brachial plexus injuries occur when the arm is dropped while moving a comatose patient where the sudden jolt stretches and tears the plexus. This can occur in the recovery room if the patient's arm falls off the trolley.

Ulnar nerve

Damage to the ulnar nerve causes numbness along the ulnar side of the arm and the hand. It is the commonest problem, and five times more likely to occur in men than women. It usually occurs in the arm that was adducted on the arm board away from the operating table. The ulnar nerve can be damaged in the medial superficial groove at the elbow (the 'funny bone') during transport to, or in the recovery room. Check that the patient's elbow is not resting against anything that could damage it, such as the trolley's cot sides, and pad it if necessary.

Median nerve

The median nerve is prone to damage where intravenous injections of drugs are attempted in the antecubital fossa. It causes numbness in the palm of the hand and weakness of the fingers.

Common peroneal nerve

The common peroneal nerve can be damaged if it is compressed against the head of the fibula in the lithotomy position when stirrups are used during surgery. The patient develops foot drop and paresthesia in the lower leg. This may present in the recovery room.

Facial nerve

Damage to the facial nerve occurs if it is crushed against the mandible. This can happen when you are trying to maintain a difficult airway. The facial nerve passes through that little notch you can feel if you run your finger along the bony edge of the mandible just in front of the angle of the jaw.

Optic nerve

Hypotension or increased intraocular pressure may jeopardise blood flow to the retina. Patients most at risk are those with glaucoma who have either been hypotensive during surgery, or where a facemask has inadvertently pressed on their eyeball. This may occur when you are ventilating a patient with a bag and mask.

Shaking, shivering and rigidity

Shaking and *shivering* are quite different phenomenon. Shivering is a reflex response to cold. Treat this by warming your patient.

In contrast shaking is a central nervous system response to unmodulated neural inputs into the brainstem and tectum. Usually this is triggered by an excessive adrenergic stimulus, such as we might experience after a big fright.

About 35 per cent of patients shiver or shake after a general anaesthetic, but fewer do after spinal or epidural blockade.

Shaking is worse where higher levels of adrenaline are circulating such as in the young, after long general anaesthetics; where the patient has breathed spontaneously for longer than 30 minutes on a volatile agent; if analgesia has been inadequate; or they have been hyperventilated during the procedure. This usually resolves within a few minutes as their circulating adrenaline levels declines. The shakes are accompanied by vasoconstriction, goose-bumps (*piloerection*), clonus, increased spike activity on an electroencephalograph (EEG), increased oxygen consumption and a rise in intra-ocular pressure.

Oxygen requirements increase up to sevenfold with shivering and shaking. Those with cardiopulmonary disease may become severely hypoxic and suffer the consequences of myocardial ischaemia, arrhythmias, and even a mild to moderate lactic acidosis.

What to do

- Take care to prevent patients hurting themselves.
- Protect their airway.
- Give oxygen.

- A small dose of intravenous pethidine 25 mg usually stops the shaking immediately. It is effective in more than 75 per cent of cases, but if it fails, and the shaking continues to cause problems, such as after delicate plastic surgery, then use doxapram 0.25 mg/Kg intravenously.

Figure 9.2 Management of shivering or shaking

Shaking after "dirty" surgery

Shaking (rigor) is an early sign of a septic shower. Bacteria *endotoxins* enter the circulation when an abscess is drained, or during urological surgery. They cause tissue and white blood cells to release chemical distress signals called *cytokines* to alert the body to the invasion. One of the body's first-line responses is to raise the body temperature in an attempt to prevent the bacteria replicating. Alerted by cytokines, the hypothalamus signals the adrenal medulla to produce adrenaline, and the thermoregulatory centre to increase body temperature. The consequent rigors increase body temperature, while vigorous muscle activity increases oxygen consumption several fold.

Start oxygen therapy in anticipation of the increased metabolic rate, and take blood cultures. During surgery showers of bacteria can enter the blood that may progress to septicaemia within a few hours. When surgery involves a potentially septic field then prophylactic antibiotics help prevent this complication.

Rigidity

Patients sometimes pass through a phase of transient muscle rigidity when emerging from their anaesthetic. They may clench their teeth tightly. This phenomenon of trismus can be dangerous because patients may catch their tongue between their teeth with the risk of partially amputating it; dislodge expensive dental caps, crowns and bridges; or patients may obstruct their airway.

Guedel airways have a metal flange to prevent the lumen being crushed. You can make patients open their mouths by inserting a soft catheter through their nose until it touches the posterior wall of the nasopharynx. This usually makes them shake their heads from side to side, grimace and then open their mouths.

Keep patients' lips, and tongues out of the way
of their teeth until they wake up.

Anti-emetics can cause the extrapyramidal syndrome with rigidity, dystonia and nystagmus. It is more common in children, young adults, and the debilitated elderly. The incidence is about 0.3 per cent, and a quarter of these occur after the first dose. The culprit drugs include prochlorperazine, metoclopramide, and droperidol. The symptoms can be alarming; the patient becomes rigid, unable to move, their eyes are flickering from side to side and they can only speak through clenched teeth. This rigidity responds rapidly to benztropine 1 mg IV. You may need to repeat the dose in 10 minutes.

Persistent rigidity is a warning sign of malignant hyperthermia.

Skin, nails, hair and joints

Bruising

If you do not apply firm pressure to a puncture wound after you withdraw the needle the patient will get a bruise. Venipunctures stop bleeding after one minute of firm pressure. Do not merely tape a piece of cotton wool over the site and assume the job is done. Underneath the cotton wool a hidden painful haematoma might develop.

After arterial punctures you must press firmly on the site for at least 5 minutes, timed by the clock. To be sure there is no bruising or swelling check the site again in 5 minutes time.

Pallor

Pallor warns that an activated sympathetic nervous system is causing cutaneous vasoconstriction. The main reasons for this noradrenergic response are hypoxia, shock, bleeding, pain, hypoglycaemia, angina, and nausea. Other causes include anaemia and drugs such as pethidine, oxytocin, vasopressin and desmopressin.

Pressure areas

Pressure injury is a localized area of tissue damage caused by direct sustained pressure on the skin and underlying tissue. Sometimes they are called pressure sores, pressure ulcers or bed sores. Pressure injuries develop very quickly, progress rapidly and are difficult to heal.

Sustained pressure cuts off the circulation to vulnerable tissue. Normal skin can withstand about 30 minutes of moderate pressure without long-lasting damage, but if sustained over a long period it causes localized ischaemia and tissue death.

Initially stage 1 pressure injury appears as a persistent area of red warm inflamed skin, or in people with darker skin, appears to have a blue or purple hue. At this stage the injury quickly resolves. The next, stage 2, presents with a breach in the skin, an open sore that gets infected easily and is slow to heal. The final stage 3 injuries are deep necrotic ulcers with a large amount of underlying tissue damage.

Postoperative pressure sores are a major cause of postoperative morbidity[6] and huge economic burden to health services.[7] Timely intervention in the recovery room can prevent much morbidity later in the ward.

Those at greater risk of pressure injury are the elderly with their fragile thin skin, those with malnutrition or recent weight loss, the cachectic, and those patients with connective tissue diseases such as rheumatoid arthritis. It also affects people with vascular disease (especially smokers) and those who cannot move easily such as quadriplegics. Patients who are longer than an hour on the operating table are at higher risk.

The mattresses on most operating tables are firm and flat so that a patient's body weight is not evenly distributed, and some points such as the skin over the sacrum, hips, or heels, carry more than their fair share of weight. It does not take long for the skin over these pressure areas to become ischaemic: tissue death follows and then pressure ulcers become inevitable.

When patients come to the recovery room after a long operation, examine their pressure areas: their sacrum, heels, shoulder blades and thoracic spine. These are all areas which may have received excessive pressure. Also check tourniquet and blood pressure cuff sites, and the sites where the diathermy plate has been attached. If the erythematous skin on a pressure blanches when you press on it, then the skin is unlikely to break down, but if it is does not blanch or worse still is white, then expect an ulcer to form. Do not massage the area, because you will increase the risk of damage.

Even slight adjustments in the patient's position give some relief of pressure on the area. Once the patient is settled in the recovery room, alter their position to take the weight off their pressure areas. Moist skin is more at risk than dry skin so make sure the affected skin is clean and dry. If the patient is incontinent consider inserting a catheter to protect the skin.

The principle behind protecting pressure points is to distribute the pressure over as wide an area as possible. Gel pads are very effective, but rolled towels and foam pads are much less so.

Skin can also be damaged by friction or shearing forces. It is easy to tear or bruise elderly patients' skin. Be careful not to drag elderly patients across their bed sheets, because the friction may damage their skin. Be careful too when removing adhesive surgical tape. Ease it off; otherwise you may rip the skin.

Your hospital should have protocols for identifying patients at risk of pressure injury, and educating staff and patients, and management plans.

Shoulder tip pain

Shoulder tip pain is likely to occur after laparoscopic procedures. If the diaphragm has been irritated by carbon dioxide used to inflate the peritoneal cavity during laparoscopy then the pain will be referred to the shoulder tip. More ominously, shoulder tip can occur after the perforation of the bladder, bowel or uterus during endoscopic procedures. Occasionally it is a sign of angina.

Sweating

Sweating is sometimes called *diaphoresis*. Sweating, especially when associated with pallor, is a sign that something is very seriously wrong. It is associated with hypoxia, hypotension, hypoglycaemia, and cardiac failure, overt or silent myocardial ischaemia or if the patient is nauseated.

Management

- Give oxygen by mask and attach a pulse oximeter.
- Check the vital signs: pulse rate and rhythm, blood pressure, perfusion status and tympanic membrane (or rectal) temperature.
- Check the blood glucose levels.
- Check for chest discomfort.
- Is the patient able to take a deep breath comfortably?
- Notify the anaesthetist.

Fingernails

If a patient with long fingernails rests them on her chest, the nails quickly damage the skin.

Hair

Coagulated dry blood occasionally remains on the hair after head and neck surgery. Dried blood is difficult to get out, and putrefies if left. Wash and comb the hair with aqueous cetrimide being careful not to get it in their eyes. Rinse with ample water.

Mouth and airway

Hoarse voice

A hoarse or croaky voice is likely in patients who were intubated, but it usually resolves over the next couple of hours.

Following thyroidectomy it may be a sign of recurrent laryngeal nerve damage; in this case notify the surgeon. Characteristically the patient will not be able to say "eeeee" in a high-pitched squeak.

Infants and children with a hoarse voice are at risk of developing laryngeal oedema and obstruction in a few hours time. They must never be sent home, but admitted and observed carefully for the development of stridor.

Teeth

Damaged teeth are a common reason for patients take legal action against their anaesthetists. Many patients' teeth are in poor repair with caries, and especially gum disease, while prolonged illness makes teeth fragile and brittle. Teeth can be chipped or dislodged during intubation, or when the patient develops masseter spasm (trismus) in the recovery room. Before placing an oropharyngeal airway check their teeth are stable enough to withstand biting on the airway. Move the airway to one side to avoid precarious teeth. Some recovery rooms stock special mouthguards to protect teeth. Make a note in the patient's record if you find loose, chipped, or other damage to teeth.

Thirst and dry mouth

One of patients' most vivid memories is their dry mouth and thirst in recovery room. They forget the pain, but remember their thirst. Dry mouths can make patients restless. Give them small sips of water, or ice (frozen grape juice is especially appreciated) or wet gauze to suck. Glycerine-based lipsalves dehydrate epithelium, causing painful cracks later.

Do not use glycerine-based lip salves.

After minor day surgery patients are sometimes given something to drink and eat before leaving the hospital. Check with the anaesthetist and surgeon first though.

Sore throat

If asked, about half of the patients complain of a sore throat. The causes are dry anaesthetic gases, which desiccate the mucosa; damage during intubation;

pharyngeal packs; insertion of nasogastric tube after bronchoscopy. Their sore throat usually resolves in 24–36 hours.

Urinary retention

A full bladder causes restlessness in a patient emerging from a general anaesthetic.

Opioids tighten the bladder's vesical sphincter, while relaxing its detrusor muscle. They make it difficult for older men to know when their bladder is full, and then to pass urine. Patience, encouragement, privacy and perhaps the sound of running water help overcome the problem.

Patients under spinal or epidural anaesthesia cannot pass urine, because they do not know their bladder is full; and even if they did, they cannot voluntarily contract their muscles to empty it. Serious future bladder and continence problems occur if the bladder becomes over-distended. Aim to suspect, detect, and treat it early. Once the bladder extends above the pelvic brim it is severely damaged; in this case you will feel a bladder as a small firm dome just over the symphysis pubis.

If urinary retention is likely, the surgeons will insert a catheter while the patient is in the operating theatre. In contrast, some orthopaedic surgeons are reluctant to catheterize patients with joint replacements, because they fear a urinary superinfection may migrate to the operation site. In this case, the surgeon may allow you to pass a catheter, empty the bladder and then withdraw the catheter.

Notes

1. Van der Walt JH, Webb RK, Osborne GA, Morgan C, Mackay P (1993) The Australian Incident Monitoring Study: recovery room incidents in the first 2000 incident reports. *Anaesthesia and Intensive Care* 21:650–652.
2. Veyckemans F (2001) *Current Opinions in Anesthesiology* 14:339–43.
3. Sen A, Chini E, Brown MJ (2005) *Mayo Clinic Proceedings* 80:783–95.
4. Arquilla B, Gupta R *et al.* (2000) *Journal of Emergency Medicine* 19:139–43.
5. Joyce N (2002) *A systematic review no. 21.* The Joanna Briggs Institute for Evidenced-Based Nursing.
6. Royal College of Nursing, London (2001) Press ulcer risk assessment and prevention-recommendations."
7. Allman RM, Goode PS, Burst N et al (1999) Advances in Wound Care 12:22–30.

10

Pharmacology

Pharmacology is the study of the uses, modes of action and effects of drugs. To administer drugs confidently in the recovery room staff need to understand how they work, and how they interact with anaesthetic agents and other drugs.

Most drugs given in the recovery room are administered intravenously. Once given drugs act rapidly, and they cannot be retrieved if something untoward should happen. Unless recovery room staff have a basic knowledge of pharmacology it is easy to harm patients. Never give a drug unless you understand what the likely effects are, and what to do if there is an abnormal reaction.

Drugs are substances given intentionally either to enhance, or to suppress normal physiological activities of the body with the aim of achieving a beneficial effect. Drugs cannot force a cell do something it normally would not do, for instance drugs cannot make nerve cells contract or muscle cells secrete thyroxine.

Surgical and anaesthetic stresses unmask many medical problems, some of which you will need to treat urgently. It is prudent to keep a wide range of drugs in the recovery room to treat pain, and medical emergencies.

Problems with drugs

- the incorrect dose is used;
- interactions with other drugs;
- adverse drug reactions;
- allergic responses.

Ignorance about drugs can be lethal.
If you are in any doubt ... ask someone!

The potential for adverse effects

Many elderly patients do not take their medication either regularly or appropriately, and toxicity is common.[1] About 30 per cent of patients over the age of 50 years are taking non-prescribed complementary and alternative medicines (CAMs), which they have concealed from their doctors. Many CAMs such as St John's wort, ephedra, and garlic concentrate, are potent drugs in their own right, and far from harmless.

Some patients are taking medication that may interact adversely with drugs used in the recovery room. The most potentially serious of these are psychoactive drugs such as selective serotonin reuptake inhibitors (SSRIs), *tricyclic antidepressants*, and *monamine oxidase inhibitors* (MAOIs), which can have lethal interactions with pethidine and tramadol. Patients occasionally and inadvertently present for major surgery still taking warfarin, clopidogrel or other anticoagulants.

Drugs are often chemically incompatible with each other, and strange things happen if you mix them, or dilute them with the wrong fluid. Most, but not all, drugs are stable in 0.9% saline or 5% dextrose. Do not add drugs to blood, blood products, fat emulsions, parenteral nutrition fluids, or albumin solutions and plasma expanders. Read and follow the manufacturer's instructions, or check with your hospital's pharmacist if you are in doubt about how to use a drug. Paste into a book the detailed instructions, which come in the drug packages, to use as a reference. Although drug information is available on the computer it is still useful to keep a good pharmacology reference book in your recovery room.

Drugs to keep in the recovery room

You may need to treat the problems listed in Table 10.1, so keep the appropriate drugs either in the recovery room or close by.

Table 10.1 Recovery room emergencies

Adrenal crises	Allergic reactions
Anaphylaxis	Bronchospasm
Cardiac arrest	Cardiac arrhythmias
Coagulopathies	Hypertension
Hypoglycaemia	Hypotension
Pulmonary oedema	Raised intracranial pressure
Respiratory depression	Uterine atony
Residual paralysis	Cardiac failure
Seizures	Violent patients

Prepare protocols about how to treat each of these crises including the drug doses, and importantly what to do next if what you have just done did not work. Some recovery rooms keep all the necessary drugs to treat a particular crisis in dedicated boxes; for instance, a 'Residual Paralysis' box might contain atropine, glycopyrrolate, neostigmine, physostigmine and diazepam, and a 'Violent Patient' box might contain haloperidol, diazepam, midazolam, and ketamine (which works almost immediately when injected into any accessible muscle).

Store drugs safely

Even though recovery rooms are areas of restricted access, drugs must be stored safely. Opioids and other scheduled drugs of addiction or dependence must be kept in an appropriate locked cupboard. A box with drugs that may be needed in an emergency should be stored on or close to an *emergency trolley*. Other drugs can be stored in alphabetical order on shelves in a cupboard, which is easily closed and locked when the room is unattended.

Recent name changes

Generic names

In 2004, drug regulatory authorities in the UK, and Europe changed the generic names of many drugs to conform to a uniform standard coordinated by the World Health Organization. For the most part this meant abandoning the British Approved Names (BAN) and following the terminology used in the US. European and UK legislation requires the packaging, labelling and pre-scribing of drugs to follow recommended International Non-Proprietary Names (rINNs). Australia and New Zealand regulatory authorities are finaliz-ing an agreement to conform to the new standards.

In line with the Medicine Commission's (UK) advice, the terms *adrenaline* and *noradrenaline* are being retained rather than the USA's epinephrine and norepinephrine. Pethidine has not yet been changed to the US name meperidine.

Syringe labelling

In 2003 the UK authorities recommended adopting the International Colour Code for Syringe Labelling, which was already widely used in North America and Australasia.

Below is a table of drugs commonly used in the recovery room with their old and new names.

Table 10.2 Drug names

Obsolete British approved name	New rINNs
Adrenaline (retained)	(Epinephrine in USA)
Amoxycillin	Amoxicillin
Benzhexol	Trihexphenidyl
Chlorpheniramine	Chlophenamine
Frusemide	Furosemide
Indomethacin	Indometacin

Table 10.2 (continued) Drug names

Obsolete British approved name	New rINNs
Lignocaine	Lidocaine
Noradrenaline (retained)	(Norepinephrine in USA)
Suxamethonium	Succinyl choline
Thiopentone	Thiopental

Beware of administering drugs from unlabelled syringes.
Draw up a new ampoule if you are unsure.

Table 10.3 Syringe labels

Agent	Colour of label
Anticholinergic agents	Green
Hypnotics, e.g. midazolam	Orange
Induction agents	Yellow
Local anaesthetics	Grey
Muscle relaxants	Warm red
Narcotics	Blue
Vasopressors	Violet
Other agents	White

Pharmacokinetics

Pharmacokinetics is the study of drug absorption, distribution, metabolism, and excretion. Pharmacodynamics is the study of the effects of drugs, whether these are wanted (*therapeutic*) or unwanted and harmful (*side-effects*).

Absorption

In the recovery room most drugs are injected either intramuscularly, where they are absorbed and released slowly into the bloodstream, or intravenously where they are quickly carried to every tissue in the body. Most oral drugs pass through the liver, which may modify them, before they reach the general circulation.

Distribution

Once the drug reaches the circulation it is distributed to the organs and tissues. Cardiac failure slows the distribution of drugs. Some drugs soak into the tissues (especially fat or muscle tissue). Only a small amount of drug remains in the bloodstream, and its concentration is low. If you measure the concentration of drug in the blood it usually appears to be diluted in a larger volume than you would otherwise expect. This calculated volume, which may vary from a few litres to many hundreds of litres, is called the *volume of distribution*.

Following an appropriate loading dose; repeated smaller amounts will maintain the drug at a *therapeutic level*. The dose of drug needed to keep a constant therapeutic level is called the *maintenance dose*. To sustain a clinical effect the drug must be given at the same rate at which the body eliminates the drug.

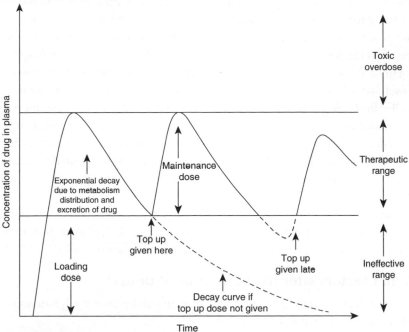

Figure 10.1 Exponential decay of drugs in blood

Elimination and excretion

Once a drug is distributed the body immediately starts eliminating it by:

- metabolizing it in the liver;
- excreting it through the kidneys;
- using *enzymes* to break it down;
- storing it;
- or a combination of two or more of the above.

Some drugs are eliminated from the body in a minute or two (such as remifentanil and succinyl choline), while others take months (such as amiodarone).

The time taken to eliminate half the given dose is called the *elimination half-life*. The *context-sensitive half life* is the time is half the time it takes for the clinical effects of the drug to fall below its therapeutic range.

Pharmacokinetics describes how the body handles the drug.
Pharmacodynamics describes what the drug does to the body.

Pharmacodynamics

Once the drug reaches its site of action it causes an effect. Most drugs act on special structures called *receptors*, either on the cell membrane, or within the cell, while others alter cellular *metabolism* in other ways. The drug's effect depends on how much is given. All drugs are *toxic* if given in too great a dose, and ineffective if the dose is too small. The right dose is called the *therapeutic dose*. With many drugs it is necessary to give enough to build up the concentration to a level that will achieve the desired effect. The dose of drug needed to do this is called the *loading dose*. The dose range between the ineffective dose and the toxic dose is called the *therapeutic margin*. Safe drugs have a wide therapeutic margin.

A drug's *potency* is the amount you need to give to achieve the desired effect. For instance one-thousandth of the amount of fentanyl is required to achieve the same level of analgesia as pethidine. Fentanyl is 1000 times more potent than pethidine.

Sometimes, despite a therapeutic level of a drug in the blood, the clinical effect begins to wear off. This phenomenon is called *tachyphylaxis* if it occurs over minutes or hours and *tolerance* if it occurs over days or weeks.

What factors alter the behaviour of drugs?

Clinical factors altering the pharmacokinetics and pharmacodynamics of a drug given in the recovery room are:

- cardiac failure delays their distribution;
- bleeding or shock alters their distribution;
- interaction with residual anaesthetic drugs;
- hypothermia delays drug metabolism and elimination.

In people with cardiac failure, give intravenous drugs twice as slowly as you would in a normal patient and monitor its effects as you do so. If you give intramuscular or subcutaneous injections to patients who are shocked, or have a poor perfusion status, the drugs will stay in the tissues waiting to be absorbed when the blood supply is restored. If the patient has received opioids during their anaesthetic, their tissues will already be partly saturated with the drug, so they may need a smaller dose when in the recovery room.

Drug doses

Drug doses are calculated on *ideal body weight* (IBW). For patients over the 150 cm in height this equates to:

$$\text{IBW (Kg)} = \text{height (cm)} - 100 \text{ (for men)}$$
$$= \text{height (cm)} - 105 \text{ (for women)}$$

For example A man who is 184 cm tall would have an IBW of 184–100 = 84Kg.

If a patient weighs less than their ideal body weight, then the dose is calculated on their actual weight. In patients less than 150 cm tall, the drug doses are calculated in the same way they are for children.

Drugs and the elderly

The elderly, with their multiple ills, are often taking many drugs, and frequently over the counter 'alternative' therapies as well. This increases the chance of drug interactions and unwanted effects. An elderly patient taking more than seven medications has a high chance of having drug conflicts, or taking inappropriate medication, or taking medication inappropriately.

Failure to adjust drug doses appropriately is the most important reason that the elderly have more adverse drug reactions than younger people.

Of all the factors that affect the behaviour of drugs in the aged, the most important is the decline in renal function that occurs with age. This delays the excretion of drugs and their active metabolites and prolongs their effects.

One of the reasons that an elderly person needs proportionally smaller doses of drugs is that their body contains more fat and less muscle than a younger person. Fat tissue contains about 10 per cent water; in contrast muscle is 60 per cent water. This means older people have less body water than young people, so that the same dose of a water-soluble drug is more concentrate in the elderly.

In the elderly drugs take longer to reach their target, because their cardiac output is lower and their circulation time is slower. The onset of fast-acting drugs is delayed; for instance, in the elderly intravenous naloxone may take 3 or more minutes to work, whereas in a young person the effect would be seen in less than 90 seconds. It is easy to give an overdose of fast-acting drugs if this point is not understood.

When using drugs in the elderly, give half as much, twice as slowly.

The elderly cool down quickly on the operating tables. Hypothermia delays the metabolism and excretion of many drugs. This becomes an important cause of adverse drug reactions if operations last more than an hour.

Bleeding associated with aspirin and other NSAIDs is more common in the elderly, and the consequences are more severe. The risk of postoperative bleeding is accentuated further if SSRIs are taken concurrently with aspirin, or anticoagulants.

Chronic benzodiazepine use

Some older patients have been taking one or more of the *benzodiazepine* drugs for many years. If a benzodiazepine is abruptly withdrawn in these patients it can cause *withdrawal syndrome*: acute unease, agitation, or even convulsions. Long-acting benzodiazepines, such as diazepam, nitrazepam and oxazepam, tend to cause problems some days after withdrawing the drugs, but the shorter-acting ones, such as temazepam or flunitrazepam, may cause symptoms within a day or so, and consequently problems may arise in the recovery room. Agitation in benzodiazepine-dependent patients settles quickly with a small dose of diazepam. The problem of their dependence on benzodiazepines can be addressed later.

Older patients are at less risk of opioid tolerance than young patients, and those over the age of 60 years rarely need the progressively increasing doses to maintain analgesia that those under the age of 50 years require.[2]

Delayed respiratory depression

Fentanyl is a short-acting intravenous opioid analgesic often used during anaesthesia. It is extremely potent and may cause delayed and profound respiratory depression. The typical story is that of an elderly female patient, following a minor procedure such as a colonoscopy. She is awake and alert in the recovery room with no signs of respiratory depression. She returns to the ward, chats to the nurses, and is found an hour or two later – dead.

Fentanyl has a peculiar double camel-hump (biphasic) decay curve. When it is first injected most of it binds to skeletal muscle cells. In the recovery room the elderly woman is awake, but not moving much. The liver rapidly breaks down and inactivates any circulating fentanyl, and there is no sign of respiratory depression.

Then back in the ward, when she starts to move her limbs again, the increased muscle blood flow washes the bound fentanyl back into her circulation. Fentanyl is not very sedating but her breathing slows. Sleep dramatically increases the ventilatory depressant effects of the opioids. She dozes off, stops breathing, and silently dies. Warn the ward staff to watch for slow or shallow respiration when patients over the age of 70 years have received more than 75 μg of fentanyl.

Drugs and the obese

To avoid overdosing your obese patients calculate their drug doses on their estimated ideal body weight and not their actual weight.

To guarantee drugs reach the circulation, where possible give them intravenously. If you are giving drugs intramuscularly you may have to use special long needles to make sure they reach the muscle, and you are not injecting into poorly perfused fat tissue.

Drugs and children

Children under the age of 12 years do not respond to drugs in the same way that small adults of the same weight do. For this reason it is better to calculate children's drug doses on their body surface area; but it is still common practice to give drugs based on their body weight. As children in industrialized nations become fatter, there is the risk of a child receiving a greater than appropriate dose. If a child is under 15 years of age or 150 cm tall and weighs more than 50 Kg then prescribe drugs according to their age and ideal body weight.

Preventing slips and mishaps

There are hundreds of drugs on the market: all have side-effects, and all interact with one or more other drugs. Most adverse events with drugs occur because staff do not fully understand the pharmacology of the drugs they are using.

All drugs are potentially hazardous.

Common slips include:

- wrong drug;
- wrong dose;
- wrong dosing interval;
- failing to anticipate predictable drug interactions;
- using trade names to prescribe drugs, instead of generic names.

Always use generic names, when prescribing a drug.

Common mishaps include:

- adverse reactions;
- unpredictable or rare drug interactions;
- allergic reactions.

Drug interactions

Drug interactions occur when two or more drugs given concurrently, result in increasing the effects (*synergism*), decreasing the effects (*antagonism*) or produce *adverse effects*.

Drug interactions can be expected, predictable or obscure.

Expected interactions occur if two or more drugs are given that have the same effect or act on the same receptors. For instance diazepam and midazolam will potentiate each other to produce additive sedation; while metoclopramide will antagonize dopamine used to support blood pressure.

Predictable interactions occur when two drugs are eliminated by the same pathway, produce similar clinical effects, or block a compensatory response. For example: volatile agents slow the breakdown of ketamine because volatile agents reduce liver blood flow. NSAIDs and warfarin exacerbates bleeding, and erythromycin or ketoconazole prolongs the action of midazolam by many hours.

Obscure interactions occur when the mechanism of the interaction is not well described. For example; low molecular-weight heparins can cause hyperkalaemia in patients taking *angiotensin-converting enzyme (ACE) inhibitors*, and droperidol can cause a fatal encephalopathy when give to patients taking lithium.

Gentamicin inactivates penicillin

Solutions containing penicillin chemically inactivate gentamicin. For this reason, do not combine gentamicin and penicillin in intravenous injections or infusions. The problem is especially likely in patients with renal failure, because they maintain a high level of penicillin for a longer time. If you are using both gentamicin and penicillin in patients with chronic kidney disease, then separate the infusion of each drug by at least 3 hours.

Always give gentamicin and penicillin separately.

Adverse events

An adverse drug reaction occurs when a drug, given in normal doses and at normal intervals, has an unintended effect. The effects can be life-threatening (anaphylaxis), debilitating (prolonged vomiting), irritating (itchy rash), or merely annoying (sedation).

Adverse drugs reactions are more likely in the elderly, the sick and the frail. Because of their smaller size, and different distribution of body fat, women are more susceptible to mishaps than men. Higher doses of drugs are more likely to cause problems than lower doses. There are marked genetic differences in the way some people metabolize and excrete drugs; for instance Asians tend to be more susceptible to respiratory depression when given opioids than Caucasians. About one person in eight of Caucasians descent cannot metabolize codeine to its active forms, and so derive no benefit from it.

How to avoid problems

- Always use a drug's generic name.
- Do not use a drug unless there is a clear reason to do so.
- Never use a drug unless you know its effects, the dose and what can go wrong.
- Check the patient's record to know what drugs are already in the patient's system. Also check for over the counter complementary and alternative medications (herbal remedies).
- As far as possible, avoid giving drugs to pregnant patients.
- Never accept an illegible, altered or doubtful order for drugs.
- Discourage telephone orders for drugs.
- Check the patient's record and allergy bracelet before giving a drug.
- Check the drug, its dose, and the route of administration with a second person.
- Many slips occur because staff misread orders (illegible handwriting contributes too).

Correct	Incorrect
Insulin 40 units	Insulin 40 u
Morphine 5 mg	Morphine 5.0 mg

- Query a prescription if it is difficult to read, or you have any doubt at all about the way it should be given.
- Give intravenous drugs slowly while monitoring the patient for adverse reactions.
- Reduce the dose in the elderly and frail.
- Obese patients do not need larger doses of drugs. Calculate the dose of most drugs on the patient's ideal body weight.

Injections

In the recovery room, drugs are usually given injected intravenously, and sometimes intramuscularly. If patients are fully awake they can have an oral analgesic.

Give deep intramuscular injections only into the upper (outer) lateral quadrant of the thigh. Adults of normal weight and muscle mass can tolerate a maximum of 5 ml of fluid injected. Patients less than 45 Kg can tolerate no more than 2 ml injected into muscle. In obese people, make sure your needle

Figure 10.2 Safe area for intramuscular injections, on the upper outer lateral quadrant of the thigh

is long enough to reach the muscle. Unlike muscle, which is well perfused, fat is poorly perfused and drug absorption will be delayed. Apply skin prep to the site, and wait until it dries. Grasp the injection site firmly and insert your needle at 90° to the skin. Dart the needle in, aspirate slightly to make sure you are not in a blood vessel, and press the plunger slowly to avoid painful distension of the muscle. Do not massage the injection site, but encourage the patient to move their leg around.

Never give intramuscular injections into the buttocks of children because you might accidentally inject a drug into the sciatic nerve and permanently damage it causing the leg to become paralysed. Avoid injections into the deltoid muscle in children and young adults because you may damage the circumflex nerve.

Bad places to site cannulas

It is tempting to put drips and infuse drugs into the large veins in the back of the hand; but this is a bad place for a long-term infusion. Inflammation here may cause patients months of pain. If this happens, particularly to older people, they suffer every time they try to flex their fingers. If drugs extravasate in the back of the hand the consequences can be disastrous. The tendons that serve the fingers run close by; and a corrosive sloughing ulcer here may permanently damage tendons (or their sheaths) and cripple their hand.

Do not be tempted by those fragile little veins on the anterior aspect of the wrist, because the cannula will cut out in the next few hours. Beneath those veins are the flexor tendons to the hand as they enter the carpal tunnels. Extravasation here can cause permanent damage.

Do not put drips in the cubital fossa. Lying very close to that large cubital vein are the brachial and radial arteries, and the median and radial nerves. Damage to these could mean impaired function of the patient's hand.

Anaesthetic drugs

Anaesthesia is derived from the Greek and means 'without feeling'. The history of anaesthesia is colourful, poignant and racy. In April 1857 Queen Victoria, courageously, and to demonstrate a point, because she certainly did not need an anaesthetic, gave birth to her eighth child (Leopold) under chloroform anaesthetic. The method of *chloroform à la reine* soundly rebuffed those people who believed the biblical injunction "in sorrow shall thou bring forth children"[3], and was a big step towards making anaesthesia acceptable for surgical procedures.

Anaesthesia has three aims: to prevent the patient experiencing pain, to keep the patient safe from harm, and to provide the surgeon with the best possible operating conditions.

Anaesthetists use a variety of drugs, to induce *coma*, maintain it, and then reverse it at the end of the operation. Anaesthesia consists of three components: coma, muscle relaxation, and abolition of unwanted *reflexes*. Using drugs the anaesthetist can vary each these three components quite independently of each other.

Analgesia is omitted from this triad, because deeply comatose patients do not respond to pain, and in the lightly comatose pain causes unwanted reflex response. Furthermore the accepted definitions of pain do not allow the patient to be "unaware" of it.

Induction

Coma is usually induced with propofol. The effects of this drug lasts for a few minutes. During this period the patient may be intubated using a short-acting muscle relaxant, or stabilized while spontaneously breathing on a volatile agent.

Maintenance

Coma is maintained with:

- a volatile halogenated hydrocarbon such as isoflurane, sevoflurane, or desflurane; or
- continuous intravenous anaesthesia with propofol.

Muscle relaxation is achieved with:

- Short-acting muscle relaxants such as succinyl choline, and mivacurium.
- Longer-acting muscle relaxants such as vecuronium, atracurium, cis-atracurium, pancuronium, and rocuronium.

Unwanted reflex responses are managed with a variety of drugs according to need. For instance a fentanyl and propofol induction often causes *bradycardia*, which responds to atropine. Good analgesia modifies unwanted reflexes.

Analgesia is achieved with:

- Opioids such as morphine, fentanyl, alfentanil, and *remifentanil*.
- Ketamine.
- Nitrous oxide.

Emergence

At the end of the anaesthetic the anaesthetist may reverse the effects of:

- muscle relaxants with neostigmine;
- opioid-induced respiratory depression with naloxone;
- sedative effects of midazolam with flumazenil.
- usually the anaesthetist prefers to select the drugs in such a way that they have worn off by the end of the anaesthetic.

Notes

1. Bedell SF, Jabbour S, Goldberg R *et al.* (2000) *Archives of Internal Medicine* 160:2129-34.
2. Spurgeon D (2005) *British Medical Journal* 330:1230.
3. *Holy Bible*, King James Version, Genesis 3:16.

11

Mothers and babies

Pregnancy

Pregnant women come to the operating theatre for the usual elective and emergency operations, as well as those specific to their pregnancy. They present special challenges for those who look after them in the recovery room because their physiology is altered from the non-pregnant state.

Physiological changes during pregnancy

As pregnancy progresses the women's physiology:

- is affected by hormonal changes – principally involving progesterone;
- adapts to accommodate the mechanical effects of an enlarging uterus;
- adjusts to the increasing metabolic demands of a growing foetus;
- compensates for the low pressure arteriovenous shunt in the placenta; and
- simultaneously prepares her for birth.

Changes in the cardiovascular system

Under the effects of progesterone in early pregnancy, the arterioles dilate decreasing peripheral vascular resistance. Having less *resistance* to push against, the heart needs to increase its output by 30 per cent merely to maintain the blood pressure. As pregnancy progresses the cardiac output increases by 30 per cent from about 4.5 L/min to about 6 L/min by the 17th week. The increase in stroke volume accounts for 40 per cent of the increase in cardiac output, while the remainder is due to a rise in pulse rate of about 15 beats/min. Because of the decreased peripheral vascular resistance the diastolic blood pressure falls, but the increase in cardiac output allows the systolic pressure to remain almost unchanged. Mean blood pressure is lowest at mid term and rises toward the non-pregnant level as the 37th week approaches.

Blood volume increases by 40 per cent, reaching a peak at 37 weeks. Pregnant women have a relative anaemia because the red cells are diluted in the increased blood volume, however they actually have a greater mass of red cells. Non-pregnant women have haematocrit 40–45%; and during pregnancy this drops to about 35%. Because of this dilution the blood viscosity is lower, and blood flows more easily through the microcirculation.

Because of these physiological adaptations, any alteration in cardiac output or peripheral vascular resistance will cause larger changes in blood pressure than in non-pregnant women. Despite this adaptation, blood loss is better tolerated by the mother but it may be fatal for the foetus.

Supine hypotensive syndrome

About 11 per cent of pregnant patients who lie on their backs experience a fall in blood pressure of up to 30 mmHg. This supine hypotensive syndrome is caused by the pregnant uterus pressing on pelvic veins and delaying blood flow back to the heart. If a pregnant woman feels uncomfortable lying on her back, gently tilt her to her left side. The hypotension may be severe enough to cause foetal hypoxia and loss of consciousness of the mother.

Changes in the respiratory system

As the uterus grows larger, the work of breathing increases. Both mother and foetus need extra oxygen. Higher levels of the *hormones* progesterone and oestrogen stimulate the mother to breathe more deeply.

As the enlarging pregnant uterus pushes up the diaphragm, the lungs' functional residual capacity decreases. By full term the functional residual capacity is reduced so much that perfectly healthy women feel breathless at times. This is aggravated if the woman has an epidural during labour. As the abdominal muscles relax under the epidural the abdominal contents push the diaphragm up even further. Any increased demands for oxygen, such as shivering or severe agitation, will rapidly cause hypoxaemia that could compromise the foetus.

Changes in gastrointestinal function

As the uterus enlarges it pushes up the stomach, displacing the oesophageal sphincter and allowing reflux gastro-oesophageal contents to cause heart burn. Gastric emptying is delayed. All pregnant patients coming to surgery should be treated as though they have a 'full stomach'. Nausea and vomiting is common. Because gastric emptying is slow it takes longer for drugs to reach the small intestine delaying the onset of drugs absorbed there, such as paracetamol. Opioids, such as pethidine, further delay gastrointestinal emptying.

Kidneys work more efficiently

Renal blood flow and the glomerular filtration rate increase with the rise in cardiac output. This enhances excretion, secretion and reabsorption of substances during pregnancy. Wastes are eliminated more efficiently so that plasma and creatinine concentrations decrease by almost half. Rising aldosterone secretion increases the reabsorption of water and sodium. Tissues tend to become oedematous as pregnancy progresses.

Blood coagulation increases

Pregnant women are specially adapted so that they do not bleed excessively after delivery. Although the mother's blood has a lower viscosity, it clots more easily. Deep vein thrombosis is always a risk. Fit graduated elastic stockings before surgery, and encourage leg exercises in recovery room. Heparin does not cross the placenta and is safe during pregnancy. Warfarin causes fatal foetal abnormalities if used in during the first trimester, and may contribute to bleeding if used within a month of term.

Surgery for obstetric conditions

In many older hospitals the obstetric operating theatre is in a different part of the hospital to the main operating suite. If this is the case in your hospital make sure that the recovery room is meticulously equipped, staffed and maintained to the same standards as the main operating theatres. Resist the temptation to relegate older equipment to this area.

Surgery in obstetric patients can be usefully grouped as follows:

- before 24 weeks of gestation;
- between 24 and 30 weeks of gestation;
- after 30 weeks of gestation.

Before the 24th week

Before 24 weeks the most common operations are dilation and curetage (D&C), circlage, and surgery for *ectopic pregnancy* and termination of pregnancy.

Dilatation and curettage

Dilatation and Curettage (D&C)s are performed for spontaneous, missed, or incomplete miscarriages. No attempt is made to save the foetus. Blood loss is sometimes enormous, especially if the pregnancy has progressed beyond the 12th week. Resuscitation for bleeding may begin before they reach the operating theatre.

After their admission to the recovery room watch for any vaginal bleeding. This is usually treated with ergometrine, or 8 prostoglandin F_2 alpha, or misoprostol. If these drugs cause nausea, give an antiemetic such as cyclizine. Many women are distressed by the loss of their baby. If practical allow her partner or mother to come and sit with her.

Cerclage

Cervical incompetence, with threatened abortion, is the final common pathway of a chorioamnionitis, and placental abruption.

Sometimes a cervical stitch (Shirodkar) to close the cervix is inserted in an attempt to forestall the threatened miscarriage. It is also used for women who repeatedly abort during the second trimester. This operation is sometimes called cerclage.

If the woman starts to bleed in the recovery room, it indicates she is either bleeding from the suture line, or is loosing the foetus. Notify the obstetrician immediately. Either salbutamol or nifedipine is used to slow premature labour. Once the situation is under control the patient will be given steroids.

Painful uterine contractions often occur after cerclage. These do not necessarily indicate premature labour, but they will worry the patient. Tocolysis is now routinely used during and after the procedure, and will be continued in the recovery room. As a precaution against possible sepsis, make sure the antibiotics have been ordered before the woman leaves the recovery room.

Tocolysis

Tocolytics are drugs used to suppress premature labour. For example, the calcium channel blocker nifedipine is sometimes combined with the beta agonist, salbutamol, (this combination is highly likely to cause hypotension). These drugs are required initially to gain control of the contractions. The patient is then given steroids. Tocolytics are not used in cases of placental abruption, chorioamionitis or where there is foetal death *in utero*, or after the 34th week of pregnancy.

Ectopic pregnancy

An *ectopic pregnancy* is one that has formed outside the uterus, usually in the Fallopian tube. After about 10 weeks from conception the enlarging foetus ruptures the Fallopian tube causing bleeding. This is an emergency with a potentially massive blood loss. Usually surgeons excise the Fallopian tube, but if they attempt to repair the tube, the procedure can take some hours.

In recovery room the patient may be cold, and anxious. Record her temperature, and warm her with a BairHugger®. The anaesthetist will order her intravenous fluids, which may include blood transfusion.

Termination of pregnancy

The surgical procedure is similar to D&C. The women's emotional response to having their pregnancy terminated ranges from relief, to heart-rending grief. Occasionally they are in a lot of pain, which responds to incremental doses of 20 mg of pethidine. If the termination occurs after the 12th week, the patient may require an oxytocin infusion to prevent bleeding. The usual dose of oxytocin is 30 units in 500 ml of 0.9% normal saline given at 85 ml/hour. Attach this as a side arm to the main intravenous infusion.

Watch for vaginal blood loss. If she soaks more than one perineal pad then notify the obstetrician.

From the 24th to the 30th week

From the 20th week to 26th week is the optimum time for doing unavoidable intra-abdominal surgery.

Between the 24th and 30th week the likely reasons for surgery are:

- antepartum haemorrhage;
- severe early onset pre-eclampsia requiring urgent delivery by Caesarean section;
- premature labour with breech or twin pregnancy facing unavoidable delivery.

Antepartum haemorrhage

Keep a close watch on the vaginal pads, and the bed sheet below the woman's buttock for excessive blood loss. Notify the obstetrician if the blood loss continues or you need to replace one or two pads.

Monitor

Blood pressure, pulse rate, ECG, oximetry, urine output, perfusion status, and external blood loss.

Laboratory

Haemoglobin, packed cell volume, platelet count, aPPT, INR, fibrinogen and fibrinogen degradation products. Cross-match four units of blood and notify the haematologist on duty.

Suspect disseminated intravascular coagulation if:

- the platelet count is less than 70 000 /mm^3;
- there is increased INR or partial thromboplastin time (aPPT);

- the fibrinogen levels are less than 0.15 gm/L;
- there are increased levels of fibrin degradation products.

Make sure the patient has a wide bore needle in both arms, capable of conveying freely flowing infusions. Should disseminated intravascular coagulation occur, then be prepared to give a massive blood transfusion. These patients are highly anxious; it is probable their baby has died, so they need a lot of comfort and emotional support.

From 30 weeks to term

Pre-eclampsia

Pre-eclampsia is a serious condition which can develop during pregnancy. It is associated with hypertension, proteinuria and fluid retention causing oedema. Complications can lead to death from cerebral haemorrhage, pulmonary oedema, gastric aspiration, and hepatorenal failure. Although delivery of the foetus usually terminates the disease it does not always. In some cases it may take up to six weeks to resolve completely.

In severe, early onset pre-eclampsia some form of coagulopathy is almost always present. It most commonly presents with thrombocytopenia with a platelet count less than 100 000 /mm^3. Pre-eclamptic women behave as if they are volume depleted with an excess noradrenergic drive pushing up their blood pressures. Their decreased blood volume is associated with decreased renal blood flow. This may progress to renal failure.

Before coming to the operating theatre the patient should be stabilized on an intravenous infusion of magnesium sulfate. It suppresses convulsions, controls hypertension, stabilizes cardiac rhythm, and improves renal blood flow. The usual infusion rate is about 1.5 mg/Kg/hr. Other drugs including hydralazine, labetalol and methyldopa are also used to control the blood pressure and also phenytoin, and diazepam as the risk of convulsions is high. Make sure you have detailed written protocols about how to care for these infusions.

In recovery room woman with pre-eclampsia should be kept very quiet. Avoid bright lights. Seizures can be stimulated by noise or light.

Vomiting remains a grave risk, even after a spinal or epidural anaesthetic for Caesarean section. Because magnesium sulfate is sedating, the women will be drowsy, and remain at risk of aspiration pneumonitis. Never turn your back on these women, because they can quickly get into difficulties. Nurse them in the recovery position and not on their back. Make sure you know how to tip the trolley head down.

Usually there is urinary catheter in place. Note the urine output every 30 minutes, and report if it falls below 30 ml/hr. Monitor her blood pressure every 5 minutes for the first 30 minutes. If she has had a Caesarian section watch for excessive vaginal bleeding more than one sooked pad or ooze from the suture line

Eclampsia

Haemolysis, Elevated Liver enzymes and a Low Platelet count constitutes the *HELLP syndrome*. This indicates that pre-eclampsia is progressing towards eclampsia. A diastolic pressure greater than 110 mmHg needs immediate treatment with labetalol or hydralazine or nifedipine.

Patients who have a seizure or who lose consciousness have progressed from pre-eclampsia to eclampsia. Women who already show signs of toxaemia, such as hypertension, proteinuria, oedema, hyperreflexia, muscle twitching, headache, proteinuria, or thrombocytopenia may deteriorate in the recovery room. These women need close monitoring for at least 48 hours, and preferably longer.

Delivering the foetus is not the terminating event in eclampsia – or pre-eclampsia.

If the woman starts to wheeze, then suspect encroaching pulmonary oedema. This is usually caused by over-enthusiastic fluid replacement, or less commonly by cardiac failure. An oxytocin infusion will aggravate the problem because it raises pulmonary artery pressures pushing fluid into alveoli. The best sign of impending *pulmonary oedema* is an increasing respiratory rate, and feelings of shortness of breath. A chest X-ray will confirm the diagnosis.

Check that anti-epileptic drugs have been ordered before she leaves the recovery room. All pre-eclamptic patients must go to a supervised area such as labour ward or high dependency unit (HDU)for at least 24 hours post-delivery.

Premature labour

If the mother comes into premature labour, whether it is a single or multiple birth, she may well be anxious about the smallness and vulnerability of her babies. Be supportive and reassure her where it is appropriate.

Often the woman will have been receiving *tocolytic therapy*, such as nifedipine or salbutamol, before her delivery. Nifedipine increases the risk of postpartum haemorrhage and hypotension. If she starts to bleed the loss can become overwhelming – be prepared for a *massive blood transfusion*.

The mother will also be receiving steroids to help prevent the baby developing *neonatal respiratory distress syndrome*.

Obstructed labour

Patients in obstructed labour are often well behind in fluid replacement. During their fruitless labour large fluid losses are caused by: over-breathing, sweating, nausea, vomiting, and the inability to retain fluids by mouth. Furthermore, and especially in remote regions, the woman may have been like this for many hours. By the time they come to the recovery room these fluid deficits should be corrected. The patient must have a urinary catheter, and it is important that her urine output is at least 60 ml/Kg/hr. The urine output is an excellent guide to fluid status.

Caesarean section

Traditionally Caesarean sections are only performed to deliver a baby who would otherwise be in jeopardy, or because the mother has an intercurrent medical or physical problem that makes it impossible to deliver her child safely. Increasingly, Caesarean sections are performed in otherwise healthy women who are capable of normal vaginal delivery, for reasons of convenience, or fear of medical litigation.

Both the mother and baby undergo huge physiological changes in the first few hours after delivery. For this reason they need one-on-one nursing care for a short time.

Common intercurrent morbidities in the mother include obesity, diabetes, asthma and anaemia. Lifestyle illnesses such as drug or alcohol and nicotine addiction affect both mother and baby. Sometimes religious beliefs or social pressure impinge on the care of the woman: for instance blood transfusion in a Jehovah's Witness patient who refuses blood transfusion.

Let the mother have the baby as soon as she is fully conscious. Position the mother on her left side with the baby beside her.

You may need to give psychological support to the woman or her partner, especially as the normal maternal–child bonding process may have been circumvented. Normal bonding takes longer after Caesarean section than after normal birth.

Watch the baby carefully, and monitor it continually.

Monitor

Perfusion status including pulse, blood pressure, oximetry, and urine output. Feel the uterine fundus; it should feel like a large orange just below the umbilicus. If it feels soft, like a loaf of bread, tell the obstetrician. A soft doughy uterus is likely to bleed later. Clots may prevent the uterus contracting. Ask the obstetrician to review the patient.

Check that the indwelling catheter is patent: a full bladder prevents the uterus from contracting.

Check that the intravenous line runs freely.

Oxytocinon (Syntocinon®) is given to contract the uterus after delivery.

Check for bleeding into the perineal pad, and look for pooling under the patient's buttocks. The normal vaginal blood loss is about 100 ml, or one saturated vaginal pad. If the blood loss exceeds this then tell the obstetrician.

If the patient continues to bleed from her vagina she may require an oxytocinon infusion. Oxytocinon 30 units is added to 500 ml of saline given at a rate of 80 ml/hr.

Record the blood pressure every five minutes for the first 30 minutes, and then every 10 minutes. If the pulse rate exceeds 100 beats/min, or the systolic blood pressure falls below 100 mmHg, then assume the patient is bleeding. If bleeding persists the patient will need to return to the operating theatre to be examined under anaesthetic to see whether the bleeding is coming from the uterus (retained products) or a torn cervix.

Caring for the baby

'At-risk' babies are usually taken straight to the neonatal nursery. The babies who come with their mother to the recovery room are usually well, but remain vulnerable. They get cold easily. Keep them wrapped warmly. Often the mother is drowsy even if she has had had a spinal anaesthetic. She will find it difficult to care for the baby by herself. Let her hold her baby, and allow her to breastfeed once your initial observations are completed.

Prolonged labour

If the labour has been long the woman's pain relief might include multiple doses of pethidine or epidural infusions of local anaesthetics and diluted opioids. Her requirements for continuing postoperative pain relief and the liveliness of her newborn child will be affected by this preoperative medication. Continuing pain relief after the Caesarean section is not really a problem in recovery room. Make sure adequate prescriptions have been written for the ward.

Never turn your back on a woman holding a
newborn baby in recovery room.

Breech deliveries

Premature breech presentations and footling presentations often have Caesarean section. With a vaginal breech deliver there may have been a period of great urgency, which the mother interprets as panic. If she was given an urgent general anaesthetic without much preliminary explanation, she might wake in a state of extreme anxiety. Have all the information about the baby ready to show her. If the baby is unwell it is the obstetrician's duty to explain what has happened. Do not attempt this yourself.

Uterine muscle stimulants

Oxytocin is given to contract the uterus after delivery. Normally the oxytocin infusion contains 30 units in 500 ml of 0.9% saline. The usual rate is about 85 ml/hr. Oxytocin can sometimes drop the blood pressure because it reduces peripheral resistance, so check the blood pressure every 5 minutes.

Additionally, sometimes, intravenous ergometrine 5–10 mg is given to help contract the uterus. This causes nausea or vomiting. Give an anti-emetic such as metoclopramide.

Prostaglandin F2 alpha, called Carboprost®, is sometimes used for postpartum haemorrhage that does not respond to ergometrine. This must be given by deep intramuscular injection, and it may have unpleasant side-effects such as bronchospasm, nausea, vomiting, diarrhoea and flushing. Excessive doses have caused uterine rupture. Check the dose with another member of staff before giving it.

Primary postpartum haemorrhage

One of the most common causes of maternal death is inadequately managed postpartum haemorrhage. Primary postpartum haemorrhage is where more than 500 ml of blood is lost within the first 24 hours after delivery. One reason reason is retained products of conception (a stray piece of placenta). In the absence of a coagulopathy, the empty contracted uterus should not bleed. If the woman is receiving blood when they arrive in the recovery room, then warm the intravenous fluids. Intra-arterial monitoring and a central line may be needed. The patient may require ICU care once stabilized.

Other postoperative problems

Other postoperative problems that may arise are: air embolism, aspiration pneumonitis, amniotic fluid embolism, and post-spinal headache.

Air embolism

Air emboli occur surprisingly often during Caesarean section. These small emboli seldom do harm, but may account for the feelings of alarm and restlessness that occur in patients having Caesarean sections under regional blockade. Occasionally air embolism is sufficient to cause hypotension, breathlessness and chest pain, which persists into the recovery room.

Aspiration pneumonitis

All pregnant patients are at risk of aspiration pneumonitis (Mendleson's syndrome). This is particularly fulminant and often fatal in obstetric patients. Following general anaesthesia, the anaesthetist will personally supervise her care until the woman is fully awake and has competent reflexes.

Patients who have had their operation under spinal or epidural blockade are also at risk, especially if they become hypotensive, which causes nausea, or are sedated. Nurse them in the recovery position until they are fully conscious and can both touch the tip of their nose with the tip of their index finger, and mount an effective cough.

If aspiration has occurred in the operating theatre, the patient will remain intubated, and be transferred to intensive care for continuing management. In a fully resourced unit the woman will be given a trial without intubation and ventilation. This has the advantage that she will be able to deep breathe and cough on her own. She will require high oxygen flows, and if she cannot maintain her oxygen saturations above 90% or develops a tachycardia or signs of hypoxia she may require intubation and ventilation. Steroids, bronchial lavage, and prophylactic antibiotics are no longer warranted in the early stages of aspiration pneumonitis. If lumps of food have been vomited then she may need a bronchoscopy to remove the foreign material. Chest X-ray changes do not show up for several hours.

Amniotic fluid embolism

Amniotic fluid embolism is fortunately an uncommon complication of labour and Caesarean section. It occurs when amniotic fluid enters the circulation, and is more severe if the foetus has been distressed *in utero* and produces meconium to soil the fluid. The incidence of amniotic embolism is thought to be about 1:50 000 deliveries. It is characterized by sudden collapse at the time of delivery, hypotension, cyanosis, disseminated intravascular coagulation and continuing haemorrhage. There are no specific tests available to confirm the diagnosis, even though foetal cells can sometimes be isolated from the mother's blood. The patient will require ventilation in the intensive care unit with ionotrope support of her blood pressure, antibiotics and management of the coagulopathy. The mortality exceeds 80 per cent.

Post-spinal headache

Post-spinal headache occurs in about 1–2 per cent of patients who have had either an epidural or a spinal anaesthetic. Excessive cerebrospinal fluid leaks into the *epidural space* causing traction on the meninges in the brain. This produces a fearful headache which is exacerbated by sitting or standing and relieved by lying flat. Using pencil point spinal needles lessens the risk. Good hydration helps prevent spinal headache and eases the symptoms if they occur. Most patients will require a blood patch.

Incidental surgery in pregnant women

About 1.5 per cent of pregnant patients need surgery during their pregnancy for non-obstetric reasons. Appendicectomy is the most common emergency operation during pregnancy, and usually erupts in the third trimester.

Less common operations are cholecystectomy, ovarian cystectomy, and a procedure for strangulated haemorrhoids. If they are elective operations then they are usually performed between the 14th and 24th week of gestation. Since the women are mostly young, fit and otherwise healthy their recovery should be straightforward, however they remain at risk of aspiration.

Nurse the patient in the recovery position to reduce the risk of aspiration. Give supplemental oxygen by mask to prevent hypoxaemia affecting either the mother or her foetus. Make sure that any drugs you give are safe in pregnant patients.

Laparoscopic surgery

Carbon dioxide insufflated during laparoscopic cholecystectomy can cause problems. Carbon dioxide embolism is more likely during pregnancy because of the increased vascularity of the vessels in her abdomen. Carbon dioxide causes capillaries to dilate increasing the risk of postoperative ooze into the peritoneal cavity.

Following appendicectomy, systemic sepsis may be a great risk to the baby. Women having an appendicectomy will need prophylactic antibiotics; usually with a combination of a cephalosporin and metronidazole.

Major surgery

If the woman is having major surgery then consult the labour ward staff about monitoring the foetus to detect signs of foetal distress such as bradycardia or persistent tachycardia. Usually the labour ward staff will come to the recovery room to help you with this.

If foetal distress occurs then do everything possible to improve uterine perfusion and foetal oxygenation. Keep the mother on her left side, give supplemental oxygen, and ensure the maternal perfusion status is optimal – her skin is warm and her urine output exceeds 1 ml/Kg/hr. Use colloids, such as Gelofusion solutions to restore vascular volume.

About 20 per cent of women having surgery in the second or third trimester will go into labour in the following week. This is treated with nifedipine or salbutamol.

It is good practice to check the maternal blood glucose levels in pregnant women in the recovery room because surgery increases the levels of stress *hormones*, to cause hyperglycaemia.

Pre-eclamptic patients coming for incidental surgery may need magnesium sulfate infusions.

Should a pregnant patient need an X-ray in the recovery room, then shield her uterus and her baby from stray X-rays.

Options for pain relief

After surgery

Pain relief after surgery during pregnancy is managed in the same manner as pain relief after surgery in patients who are not pregnant.

Opioids

Although most clinicians believe pethidine to be the safest opioid in obstetrics, this has never been substantiated by controlled trials. Many studies suggest that pethidine is no better, and sometimes is worse than other narcotics. Indeed a single maternal dose of pethidine 50 mg caused significant depression in newborn babies. Placental cord concentrations reach two-thirds of the concentration in the mother's blood. Morphine seems somewhat better. Morphine and diamorphine are cleared very quickly in labour and the concentration of morphine in the newborn is almost undetectable.

After Caesarean section

Most mothers are not overly concerned by pain after Caesarian section and they are distracted by their babies. If they have been given opioids as part of their anaesthetic these may still be effective.

Frequently a small dose of fentanyl is added to the spinal anaesthetic to provide analgesia that lasts a few hours after the block wears off. Adding morphine to spinal anaesthesia provides long lasting postoperative analgesia but can cause annoying itch. After receiving spinal morphine, the mother's respiratory rate needs monitoring when she returns to the ward.

Many obstetric units routinely give paracetamol intravenously in theatre, or orally in the recovery room. If severe wound pain is anticipated, then long acting oral morphine can be used. Patient controlled anaesthesia (PCA) is favoured by some units. If so, then PCA should be started before the effects of the spinal anaesthetic wear off. Sometimes the anaesthetist will give a loading dose of intramuscular opioid before the patient leaves the theatre. It is extremely distressing for a patient to have spinal block wear off before another analgesic regime has been established. Before considering PCA remember that most women prefer to be free of all drips and catheters as soon as possible so that they can care for their babies.

Do not add anti-emetics to PCA infusions as these drugs enter the breast milk and affect the baby. NSAIDs also enter the milk and some units prefer to avoid them in breastfeeding mothers.

Further reading

Briggs *et al.* (2002) *Drugs in pregnancy and lactation*, 6th edn.
Hale (2004) *Medications and mothers' milk*, 11th edition.

12

Paediatrics

Children and babies frequently have operations and come to the recovery room. In the recovery room cardiac arrest and emergencies are three times more common in children than in adults. Children's anatomy and physiology is not similar to that of a scaled-down adult; they pose special problems.

Most complications are caused by laryngospasm following difficult intubation, or an overdose of anaesthetic drugs. Infants under the age of one month are at greatest risk because they are more likely to have major surgery, and tend to be sicker than older children.

Prematurity

The age of premature babies is calculated in postconceptual weeks. A baby born at 28 weeks and now 4 weeks old, is 32 weeks postconception.

Premature babies are less able to maintain their body temperature, swallow, suck or even breathe properly. Asphyxia during birth predisposes them to brain damage. If they are given 100% oxygen they are at risk of developing retinopathy of prematurity (ROP). They are also at risk of intraventricular haemorrhage, respiratory distress syndrome, bronchopulmonary dysplasia, anaemia, and apnoeic episodes. They may have a patent ductus arteriosis and are at risk of necrotizing colitis.

Premature babies normally consume oxygen at about 8 ml/Kg/min (compared with a full term baby's 7 ml and an adult's 3.5 ml). Their respiratory rate can be as high as 60 breaths/min with tidal volumes of 110–160 ml/Kg/min.

Compared with full-term babies, premature babies are more sensitive to anaesthetic agents. The volatile anaesthetics prevent their heart rate from increasing and their baroreceptors and chemoreceptors do not trigger responses, so they do not compensate for hypoxia or failing perfusion. They are also particularly intolerant to hypothermia.

For the purposes of this book:

- premature babies are those born before the 37th week from conception;
- neonates are babies those within 44 weeks from the date of conception;
- infants are under the age of one year;
- babies include neonates and infants;
- children are aged 1 year to 12 years;
- adolescents are between the age of 13 and 16 years.

Respiratory system

Neonates and infants

Neonates have a high metabolic rate; their oxygen consumption is about 7 ml/Kg/min, which is twice that of an adult's 3.5 ml/Kg/min and is the reason they desaturate more rapidly than an adult.

The dead space volume of the neonatal airways is proportionally the same as an adult's, so they must breathe twice as quickly to meet their high oxygen demands. Children become hypoxic and cyanosed rapidly.

Neonates cannot alter their volumes so they alter their rates instead.

Although neonates, and to a lesser degree infants, have pliant chest walls, their lungs are stiffer than an adult's. The alveoli are thicker walled, and events such as pneumonia or neonatal respiratory distress syndrome make their lungs even stiffer. They only use their diaphragms to draw air into their lungs. They compensate for this by having a high respiratory rate (about 32 breaths/min).

When neonates breathe in, instead of their lungs filling fully with air, their little chest walls tend to cave in. This results in a reduced amount of air entering their lungs. Furthermore at the end of expiration there is proportionately less air left in their lungs than in an adult. This means that neonates do not have a big reservoir of air (*functional residual capacity*) left in their lungs at the end of expiration, and without this store they become hypoxic quickly. After an anaesthetic, babies' muscles are sometimes too fatigued to breathe. Babies should be completely awake before the anaesthetist leaves them.

While the hearts of babies and children are relatively resistant to hypoxia, their brains are not.

Airway obstruction

Neonates breathe through their noses, and their narrow nasal passages are easily blocked by nasal secretions.

Factors contributing to an obstructed airway in neonates and infants are:

- large heads, short necks and prominent occiputs;
- big floppy tongues;
- large tonsils and adenoids;
- a large stiff epiglottis;
- a high larynx, with a small opening which is prone to oedema if it is traumatized or the infant is over-hydrated; the narrowest part of a child's airway is at the cricoid cartilage;
- the ribs are flexible making forceful coughing difficult;
- neonates and infants less 2–3 months old cannot breathe through their mouths.

Airway problems seen in the first postoperative hour include:

- airway obstruction caused by the tongue obstructing the nasal pharynx;
- laryngeal spasm;
- croup following extubation;
- respiratory depression;
- aspiration;
- apnoea.

Signs of an obstructed airway in an infant or child are:

- supracostal, intercostal and subcostal retraction;
- inspiratory stridor or crowing;
- nasal flaring;
- decreased or absent breath sounds.

Since neonates and younger babies cannot increase their tidal volume to increase their minute volume they need to increase their respiratory rate.

If a spontaneously breathing baby cannot sustain a PaO_2 greater than 60 mmHg (7.89 kPa) or a $PaCO_2$ less than 60 mmHg (7.89 kPa) it should be re-intubated. Intubation in babies is not difficult. An emergency tracheostomy is almost never required.

Foreign body aspiration

Foreign body aspiration (FBA) presents with an abrupt onset of coughing or respiratory distress, using every available muscle to breathe. It occurs if a child has inhaled something through the larynx into the lower airway. Give oxygen and call for help.

If the aspiration is severe the child is unable to make much sound, unable to breathe, becomes cyanosed quickly and loses consciousness. Establish an airway and start *basic life support* (BLS).[1]

Apnoea in the newborn

Neonates commonly stop breathing after having a general anaesthetic. This *apnoea* becomes serious if it lasts longer than 15 seconds, severe if the pulse oximeter reveals desaturation, and critical if associated with bradycardia, cyanosis or pallor.

Infants born prematurely, or those babies with a history of respiratory distress syndrome or bronchopulmonary dysplasia, are susceptible to apnoea following even short general anaesthetics. Their susceptibility to apnoea persists for the first 6 months of life, and can occur up to 12 hours after surgery. It is more common if muscle relaxants were used. For this reason, all infants who have been premature babies and all infants who are less than three months (52 post-conceptual weeks) are unsuitable for day case surgery. They need hospital admission and respiratory monitoring for the first 24 hours. Monitor infants of less than 45 conceptual weeks for 18 hours post anaesthesia. Monitor all infants under 6 months of age (64 post-conceptual weeks) with a pulse oximeter, and if possible a respiratory monitor for at least two hours postoperatively.

Factors contributing to episodes of apnoea in the recovery room are:

- immaturity of the central nervous respiratory control centres;
- depression of the chemoreceptor response to hypoxia by residual anaesthetic agents; and
- residual effects of muscle relaxants.

Pneumothorax in infants

Pneumothorax, where air escapes from the lungs into the pleural cavity, is not uncommon. It occurs if their little lungs are over-inflated, and can easily happen if the baby coughs during intubation or extubation. Physical signs, such as an absence of breath sounds, are difficult to detect, but the heart's apex beat may be displaced as the mediastinum shifts. Shine a light through the chest wall from behind and you may see the outline of the collapsed lung. Cyanosis and bradycardia are late signs. If a baby's oxygen saturation suddenly deteriorates, or their respiratory rate rises, think of pneumothorax. Always keep the necessary equipment to drain a pneumothorax sterilized and ready.

Children

Prevent airway obstruction, caused by the tongue falling back into the pharynx, by routinely nursing children in the recovery position. If this fails gently extend the head to relieve the obstruction. Call for help now. If the obstruction is still not relieved then insert a nasal airway. Nasal airways are better than oral airways in children because they are less likely to stimulate gagging, vomiting or laryngospasm. Give 100% oxygen until the airway is completely clear. Use gentle suction, and if this is not successful have a proper look at the pharynx with a laryngoscope.

Keep nasal airways available when recovering children.

Laryngeal spasm

Stimulation of the pharynx causes a *reflex* contraction of the intrinsic muscles of the larynx. This *laryngeal spasm* tightly closes the glottis. Often no air can pass, but occasionally you will hear stridor.

Laryngeal spasm is the body's emergency response to prevent foreign material entering the lower respiratory tract. Spasm can be triggered by mucus, blood or other material in the pharynx and sometimes merely by suction of the upper airway. Be gentle when using a sucker.

The incidence of laryngeal spasm is higher in children under the age of 9 years and reaches a maximum between the ages of 1–3 months. Patients with Down's syndrome are particularly susceptible to laryngeal spasm. The problem is more likely to occur if the child has a respiratory tract infection. Laryngeal spasm is a frightening event. It may not resolve spontaneously until the child has become deeply and dangerously hypoxic. Seek help early.

Initial management of laryngospasm

- Give oxygen by mask.
- Call for help.
- Fetch the emergency paediatric trolley.
- Attach a pulse oximeter.
- Attach an ECG monitor.

Then attempt to relieve the spasm by firm pressing behind the angles of the jaw to lift it forward. Try ventilating the child using firm *positive pressure* from a mask. This may fail. Attempts to strenuously ventilate the patient by forcing air into the pharynx will worsen the obstruction.

Further management of laryngospasm

If the above measures fail to relieve the obstruction within 30 seconds a dose of 1% lidocaine 1.5 mg/Kg intravenously usually resolves the spasm. If lidocaine is unsuccessful the anaesthetist should give succinyl choline 0.5 mg/Kg intravenously together with atropine 20 μg/Kg and then '*bag and mask'* the patient until the situation is assessed. The patient may need intubation for a short spell.

Acute *pulmonary oedema* is an uncommon complication of laryngospasm. It is probably caused by the violent swings in intrathoracic pressure generated as the child struggles to breathe sufficiently to overcome the obstruction.

Croup

A hoarse voice, or a barking cough are signs of developing croup. These signs tend to resolve spontaneously. Croup usually occurs because the delicate mucosal lining of the trachea is irritated by the endotracheal tube and become oedematous. Croup is caused by oedema partially closing the airway just below the larynx. It occurs in about four per cent of children who have been intubated. Oedema fluid easily accumulates in the loose submucosal tissue, where the cricoid cartilage forms a complete ring around the trachea.

Infants are more susceptible than older children, because they have a smaller larynx (4 mm in diameter compared with 8 mm in an adult) so that an equivalent amount of oedema reduces the diameter of the trachea by a proportionally greater amount. Rarely the cough progresses to stridor, a far more serious problem, heralding complete airway obstruction and respiratory arrest. The signs of croup or stridor usually occur within the first hour after extubation but it can be much later.

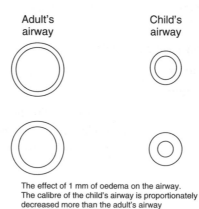

Adult's airway   Child's airway

The effect of 1 mm of oedema on the airway.
The calibre of the child's airway is proportionately
decreased more than the adult's airway

Figure 12.1 The effect of one millimetre of oedema on the cross-sectional area of a child's and an infant's bronchus

When to get help

Get help immediately if there is stridor or you can see signs of increased work of breathing with rib and subcostal retraction, or if the child is unsettled, worried or restless.

Anaphylaxis may also present with stridor, wheeze and an urticarial rash. Later the face and tongue swell.

How to manage stridor

Sit the child up, summon help, give oxygen, and get ready to give humidified oxygen and nebulized adrenaline.

To prepare the adrenaline for the nebulizer, take 2 ml of 1:1000 solution of adrenaline and make it up to a total of 5 ml in 0.9% saline. Put it into the nebulizer's reservoir and give it using a flow rate of oxygen of 5 L/min.

Adrenaline reduces the oedema by causing vasoconstriction in the inflamed mucosa. The effects are short-lived, lasting about 2 hours. If affected children are undergoing day case surgery, then they should be admitted as an inpatient overnight for observation.

Always get an expert to assess the child. A child with severe airway obstruction may look reassuringly pink on supplemental oxygen with satisfactory pulse oximeter readings, but be gravely hypoventilating and danger of totally obstructing their airway.

Stridor means airway obstruction; treat it immediately. It is a dangerous waste of time to confirm the obstruction with lateral cervical X-rays.

The anaesthetist may need to reintubate the child. Prepare a range of endotracheal tube sizes because children with stridor need a smaller tube diameter than they normally would.

Respiratory depression

$$\text{The normal respiratory rate in children} = 24 - \frac{\text{age}}{2}$$

As a rough guide the normal respiratory rate in children. If the child's respiratory rate is less than this, or their breathing is weak and shallow then they have respiratory depression.

Children recover quickly and predictably from muscle relaxants so look for other reasons for the respiratory depression. Infants pulling their legs up when they cry are unlikely to have residual muscle relaxation causing their respiratory depression; similarly older children should be able to lift their heads from the pillow.

When to worry

Get help immediately if the child:

- is anxious, unsettled or restless;
- has an oximeter reading < 95%;
- is fatigued, listless or their conscious state is deteriorating;
- appears to be working hard to breathe.

Other reasons for residual muscle paralysis following relaxant anaesthesia are hypothermia, hypocalcaemia or acidosis. Under these circumstances the anaesthetist should not hesitate to re-intubate the infant and transfer him to intensive care for observation and monitoring.

Opioids also contribute to respiratory depression. They may need naloxone 4 µg/Kg to reverse the effects of the opioids. Naloxone only lasts for 30–40 minutes and when it wears off the respiratory depression may recur.

Fentanyl is very slowly metabolized in babies and should not be used in the recovery room.

Aspiration

Suspect aspiration if a child suddenly develops a wheeze or a cough. Infants are susceptible to aspiration because they have a short oesophagus, their cough *reflex* is not well developed and their laryngeal competence is decreased for 6–8 hours following extubation.

Table 12.1 Endotracheal tube sizes

Age	Weight (Kg)	Tube size (mm)	Length to tip (cm)
Neonate	3.5	3.0	8.5
2 months	5	3.5	9
6 months	8	4.0	10
1 year	10	4.0	11

Endotracheal tube specifications

For children older than one year:

$$\text{Tube size} = \frac{\text{age (yr)} + 4}{4}$$

$$\text{Tube length} = \frac{\text{age (yr)} + 12}{2}$$

Assisted ventilation in infants < 10 Kg

Aim for:

- respiratory rate 30–40 per minute;
- inflation pressure of up to 25 cm H_2O;
- fresh gas flows of 4 L/min;
- positive end expiratory pressures of 5 cm H_2O.

Salivary gland enlargement

Sometimes acute engorgement of the parotid, submaxillary or sublingual glands occurs during anaesthesia and persists in the recovery room. Their face appears to be bloated, as if the child has mumps, and the glands are felt as firm masses. The problem usually subsides with an hour and is not dangerous unless it causes airway obstruction.

Cardiovascular physiology

Pulse rates

A neonate's cardiac muscles contract less forcibly than older children; and they are also stiffer. This means that if neonates need to raise their cardiac output, the only way they can do so is by increasing their heart rate.

As soon as babies are settled check their notes to find out their preoperative baseline pulse rate, because pulse rates vary widely from baby to baby. The pulse rate is an excellent guide to their physical progress in recovery room. A return to the preoperative pulse rate is a happy sign that all is well.

Table 12.2 Normal paediatric heart rates and blood volumes

Age	Heart rate (beats/min)	Blood volume (ml/Kg)
1 day	95–150	100
1 week	90–160	90
1 month	120–180	85
6 months	110–170	80
12 months	90–150	75
6 years	70–135	70

Bradycardias

The cardiac output in children is rate-dependent, and as a result a bradycardia causes hypotension. The sympathetic innervation of the heart is not as well developed as the parasympathetic, making babies prone to bradycardia. They do not tolerate bradycardia well; for instance apnoea and bradycardia may follow suctioning the pharynx and this can quickly cause severe hypoxaemia.

A child's heart is relatively resistant to hypoxia, so that by the time hypoxia is severe enough to cause a bradycardia cardiac arrest is near and brain damage has already occurred.

Bradycardia causing hypoxia in children is a grave sign.

Ensure a clear airway and oxygenate the child while preparing to give atropine. Notify the anaesthetist. Atropine alone without oxygenation is not effective. If bradycardia does not respond quickly then commence the advanced life support protocol with cardiac massage and prepare to give adrenaline.

Tachycardia

Children often have a high resting pulse rate. Look in the notes to find the preoperative rate and use this as a guide. A child in the recovery room with a tachycardia may be either in pain or hypovolaemic. Attach an ECG. Suspect hypovolamia if the child has cool hands and poor capillary return in the fingernail beds.

Tachyarrhythmias are uncommon in children, but if they do occur it is usually a narrow complex *supraventricular tachycardia* (SVT). The anaesthetist may choose to treat this with either vagal stimulation, or if that fails with intravenous adenosine 0.05 mg/Kg up to 0.25 mg/Kg.

Transient viral myocarditis in the first few weeks following a respiratory infection occurs occasionally in children. Usually the irregular pulse is not noticed by the parents and resolves without incident, but if the child has an operation during this period they may develop a supraventricular tachycardia in the recovery room. An ECG with looping ST segments in all leads adds weight to the diagnosis.

Hypertension

Acute hypertension in a child is unusual. It may reflect over-enthusiastic fluid replacement, and is more common in children with pre-existing kidney disease.

Fluids in children

By the age of 3 years the volume of body water has decreased from 80% of body weight at birth to the adult value of about 60%. Of this, a third of the volume is in the extracellular space and two-thirds is in the intracellular compartment.

The extracellular compartment is further divided into interstitial fluid (lying between the cells), and intravascular fluid (*plasma*). When fluid is lost from the body it initially comes from the smallest of the compartments – the plasma.

Why give fluids?

Intravenous fluids are given for four reasons: maintenance, replacement of losses (including catch-up for fasting), resuscitation, and as a vehicle for intravenous drugs.

When to give fluids

Most well children undergoing minor surgery do not need intravenous fluids when they return to the ward. Conversely, those having major or prolonged surgery where continuing losses are anticipated, or where the child is unable to take oral fluids for some time, need intravenous replacement and maintenance fluids.

Hypovolaemic children, or those that are shocked will be resuscitated either before surgery, or while they are in the operating theatre. Sometimes resuscitation needs to be continued in the recovery room.

What sorts of fluid are available?

Isotonic crystalloid solutions contain the same concentration of ions as blood, and so they exert the same osmotic pressure. Examples of isotonic fluids include: 0.9% normal saline, Hartmann's solution (Ringer's lactate) and Plasmalyte®. *Third space fluid* in the gut is an isotonic fluid with small variations in potassium and other ions.

Hypotonic fluids contain fewer ions than are present in the blood, and so exert a lower osmotic pressure. This means that when you give a hypotonic fluid, water floods into cells everywhere, until the osmotic balance is re-established. Examples of hypotonic fluids are 5% dextrose in water, and 4.5% dextrose and 1/5 normal saline. These fluids are used to replace water lost in dehydration.

What fluids to give

The choice of intravenous fluid depends on the cause of the problem, and usually replaces what was lost.

Heavily bleeding patients need blood. Gastrointestinal loss is replaced with isotonic crystalloid solutions, preferably Hartmann's solution or Plasmalyte®. Most paediatric anaesthetists no longer routinely use 4% dextrose and 1/5 normal saline as fluid replacement during surgery.

For simple dehydration, where a child has been fasting and has not been drinking water, then 4.5% dextrose and 1/5 normal saline is still used.

On admitting the child to recovery room

As soon as practical after the child has been admitted to the recovery room check what fluids were given in theatre. A baby of up to 15 Kg should have received approximately 20 ml/Kg. Children weighing from 15–30 Kg need approximately 15 ml/Kg and older children 10 ml/Kg.

Hypovolaemia

Acute reduction in plasma volume is called hypovolaemia, and unless treated rapidly progresses to shock. Bleeding and loss of fluid into the gut are the commonest causes of postoperative hypovolaemia.

Hypovolaemia is a grave threat to neonates and infants. An adult can lose of their blood volume without noticeable effect, in a neonate a 10% loss of blood volume is life-threatening. A 2.5 Kg neonate, with a normal blood volume of about 250 ml is severely shocked by a blood loss of only 20–25 ml, which is the amount of blood absorbed on one small well-soaked gauze square.

A loss of surprisingly little fluid from *plasma* activates physiological compensatory mechanisms. These include neuroendocrine responses that cause the kidney to retain sodium and water, and vasoconstriction and a tachycardia. In effect children go white or mottled, have a fast heart rate, cool hands, and low urine output. Hypotension is a late and serious sign of hypovolaemia. For most purposes you can estimate a child's normal blood pressure to be 80 + (age in years × 2) mmHg.

Young infants may not develop a tachycardia. If the fluid loss has been slow the baby may also have a sunken fontanelle.

Do not be afraid to give fluids to neonates,
hypovolaemia is a greater threat than fluid overload.

Capillary refill time

Capillary refill time is a useful and easy test to determine whether the child is mounting a neuroendocrine response to hypovolaemia. Press on the child's sternum or finger for 5 seconds, remove the pressure and then time how long it takes for the white blanche mark to fade. In normally hydrated children this should be less than 3 seconds. If it takes longer than that then assume the child is hypovolaemic and prepare to give intravenous fluids.

If hypovolaemia is suspected check the drains and catheters for continuing loss. Check the haemoglobin (or haematocrit) and prepare to cross-match blood.

How much fluid to treat hypovolaemia?

First give 20 ml/Kg of Plasmalyte® or Hartmann's solution, and repeat it as necessary if the capillary refill time is more than three seconds. If you need to repeat it more than once then seek advice from the anaesthetist.

How to calculate fluid deficit

A child's fluid deficit is calculated from an estimation of their fluid deficit expressed as a percentage of body weight (not their body water). For example a child weighing 10 Kg who is estimated to be 5 per cent dehydrated has an isotonic fluid deficit of 500 ml.

Ongoing losses from drains are measured and then replaced with a similar fluid. For instance blood is replaced with blood, and gastrointestinal losses with Plasmalyte® or Hartmann's solution.

4.5% dextrose and 1/5 normal saline is NOT an appropriate fluid for unwell children.

Shock

Shock is a clinical diagnosis based on a set of symptoms and signs that occur when the circulation is insufficient to meet the metabolic demands of the tissues and to remove their waste products. The pathological marker of shock is lactic acid produced by hypoxic tissues.

Delivering oxygen to the tissues depends on a chain of events: the heart pumps oxygen and nutrients dissolved in the blood through a series of vessels to the tissues when they are used. The type of shock depends on where this chain of events is disrupted. Cardiogenic shock occurs when the pump fails. Haemorrhagic or hypovolaemic shock occurs when there is not enough blood or body fluids. If the normal vascular tone is lost, the *resistance* vessels (arterioles) dilate causing the blood pressure to fall. This loss of peripheral resistance can be caused by tissue factors (anaphylaxis or toxins). Septic shock disrupts all three links in the chain: the heart, body fluids, and the vessels.

Diagnose shock early, and treat it vigorously.

Shock is a progressive phenomenon, but roughly falls into three phases: compensated, uncompensated, and irreversible. Compensated shock presents with oliguria, tachycardia and poor capillary return time, uncompensated shock occurs when the blood pressure falls and the pulse rate drops, and irreversible shock is a post-mortem diagnosis where the organ damage is so severe that recovery is impossible.

Haemorrhagic shock

Diagnosis

If possible check the urine output. The volume should be greater than 2 ml/Kg/hr. Hypotension in older children is a disastrously late sign of hypovolaemia. If it does occur then it begins with a falling systolic pressure, rising diastolic pressure and a muffled apex beat when you listen with a stethoscope.

If the child looks pale check the pulse rate and the blood presure. The pulse rate should return to the preoperative rate, and if not: worry.

Management

- Give high flows of oxygen with a face mask.
- Lay the child flat and lift the legs on to a pillow. Do not tip the child head down.
- Call for help.
- Prepare to give fluids rapidly. Ideally, this requires two short wide-bore cannulae, one in each cubital fossa.
- Prepare to take blood for full blood count, electrolytes and urea, glucose, and cross-matching.
- Give blood; use either cross-matched or rhesus negative type specific blood.
- Look for a source of bleeding.
- If sepsis is thought to be a possibility then collect blood for culture.

Give a fluid bolus of 20 ml/Kg through a blood warmer of isotonic crystalloid and then recheck the capillary refill, pulse rate, and blood pressure. Suitable crystalloids are Plasmalyte®, Hartmann's solution or 0.9% saline. Do not give dextrose-containing solutions.

Then check the capillary return time. If it is longer than 3 seconds then repeat the dose of 20 ml/Kg of isotonic crystalloid.

If further boluses are required, then use blood: either low antibody-titre O negative, or type-specific blood, or if there is time fully cross-matched blood.

Transfusion in infants

Blood volume is higher in the neonate, 90–100 ml/Kg compared with the 70–80 ml/Kg in the adult. When replacing blood give it to the nearest 10 ml above the estimated loss. For example, if the estimated blood loss is 35 ml, then give 40 ml. It is safer to slightly overload neonates and infants than to have them plasma volume deplete.

Crystalloid versus colloid debate

Over the past decade there has been much controversy about which is the best type of fluid to give to resuscitated shocked patients. In the early stages of shock, it probably does not matter whether you use a crystalloid, or a colloid such as 4.5% human albumin or Gelofusin®. If you use crystalloid, you need to give three times the volume to have the same effect as a given volume of colloid.

Intraosseus injection

Finding a vein can sometimes be a problem in shocked children. Rather than attempting saphenous vein cut downs, the anaesthetist may site an intraosseous needle. This approach is life-saving and under used. It has two advantages: bone marrow can be collected for haemoglobin and electrolytes (but not glucose concentrations), and it is possible to run fluids in rapidly. If children are conscious they will need a local anaesthetic. It is a strictly sterile procedure. The infusion should be discontinued once intravenous access has been established.

Figure 12.2 Tibial site for intraosseous injection

Problems with dextrose solutions

Do not use 5% dextrose for replacement or maintenance fluids. Even a small rise in blood glucose to 8 mmol/L can cause an osmotic diuresis leading to excessive extracellular fluid loss. If you use 5% dextrose to replace isotonic fluid lost during surgery the infant's serum sodium concentration will fall, and water will move into the cells. This shift may cause cerebral oedema in which case the infant develops signs of irritability, restlessness, a mew-like cry, drowsiness, vomiting and in severe cases, convulsions.

Routine fluid replacement

Normal maintenance fluids are fluids given to otherwise well children who are not taking any fluids by mouth. Normal fluid maintenance replacement should not exceed 2400 ml per day

The volume of maintenance fluid replaces the normal urine output and insensible losses (sweat, loss through the lungs and in the stools). As children grow older, they require proportionately less fluid.

Weights in Kg	ml per day	ml per hour
3–10	100 × weight (Kg)	4 × weight (Kg)
10–20	100 + (50 × (wt – 10))	40 + (2 × (wt – 10))
> 20	1000 + (20 × (wt – 10))	40 × (1 × (wt – 10))

For instance:
An 8 Kg baby needs:

$$8 \times 100 = 800 \text{ ml per day}$$
$$4 \times 8 = 32 \text{ ml per hour}$$

An 18 Kg baby needs:

$$1000 + (50 \times (18\text{–}10)) = 1400 \text{ ml per day}$$
$$40 + (2 \times (18\text{–}10)) = 56 \text{ ml per hour}$$

A 30 Kg child needs:

$$1500 + (20 \times (30\text{–}20)) = 1900 \text{ ml per day}$$
$$40 + (1 \times (30\text{–}10)) = 60 \text{ ml per hour}$$

Which fluid to use

For otherwise well children use 0.45% sodium chloride with 5% glucose and add 20 mmol/L of potassium chloride (KCl).

Do not use the above solution if the:

- serum potassium is elevated beyond 4.5 mmol/L;
- serum sodium is less than 136 mmol/L;
- child is hypovolaemic or shocked;
- child is dehydrated.

Kidneys

For the first two years of life blood flow through the kidneys, and consequently the glomerular filtration rate are proportionally lower than in an older child. Until about the age of 8 months, the kidney tubules are unable to excrete a large sodium or water load, which is the reason that in infants the maintenance fluid of choice is 4.5% dextrose and 1/5 normal saline.

In children oliguria is considered to be a urine output of less than 1 ml/Kg/hr. Once fluids are replaced the oliguria that accompanies hypovolaemia usually resolves. If oliguria persists the paediatrician or anaesthetist may use a diuretic and support the circulation with an ionotrope.

Central nervous system

Intracranial haemorrhage

The cerebral vessels in the premature baby are fragile and thin-walled. If neonates are circumcised or intubated without adequate anaesthesia their blood pressure will surge abruptly. This may rupture intracranial, especially intraventricular, vessels. If a neonate's conscious state deteriorates for no obvious reason in the recovery room consider this possibility.

Blood–brain barrier

In neonates the blood–brain barrier is not yet fully functional. This means that drugs such as antibiotics and opioids cross the blood–brain barrier more readily, which prolongs their action. Bilirubin too can cross the blood–brain barrier and cause kernicterus in babies with blood group ABO or rhesus incompatibility with their mother.

Emergence phenomena

Otherwise healthy children are often restless after anaesthesia, especially children who have had their entire anaesthetic with sevoflurane.

Never turn your back on a child.
They get into trouble quickly.

Liver

In neonates and young infants the liver enzymes are not fully functional and cannot easily breakdown many drugs. Opioids, for example, have a longer action. Consequently they should be used in small doses, and the dosing interval should be longer.

Metabolism

Glucose

Babies' immature livers do not store much glycogen. Glycogen can be quickly mobilized into glucose that is essential for the brain's *metabolism*, and without it brain damage occurs quickly.

Hypoglycaemia is common in the stressed neonate, especially if it has had a period of prolonged fasting, or becomes stressed by hypovolaemia, pain or hypothermia. Children most at risk are those weighing less than 15 Kg.

Hypoglycaemia is defined as a blood glucose of less than 2.2 mmol/L, at a level of 1.7 mmol/L permanent brain damage is imminent. It is difficult to diagnose as signs and symptoms vary. It usually presents as muscle twitching, an *obtunded mental state*, convulsions or just a reluctance to breathe.

It is far better to predict and then prevent hypoglycaemia than to wait until signs appear with the risk of brain damage. Accordingly measure the blood sugar concentrations of stressed babies as soon as they are admitted to the recovery room.

Use an infusion of 10% glucose to prevent hypoglycaemia.

An increasingly drowsy infant may be hypothermic

Thermoregulation

Hypothermia

Babies and infants have a large surface area when compared to their volume. This means that heat is lost proportionately more quickly than in adult. Under about the age of 6 months infants do not sweat, neither do they shiver nor vasoconstrict in response to cold. Neonates lose heat even more rapidly because they have little subcutaneous fat to insulate them.

During anaesthesia heat is lost predominately by radiation, but also by conduction, convection and evaporation. Considerable amounts of heat can be conducted to cold mattresses and blankets.

Hypothermia causes respiratory depression, decreased cardiac output, tissue hypoperfusion and lactic acidosis, increases the risk of infection, decreases the breakdown of drugs and decreases platelet function. Hypothermia is the most common reason for blood failing to clot.

Special brown fat is located between the scapulae, in the mediastinum and around the kidneys. It comprises about 4% of a neonate's body weight. As a once-only response, babies can metabolize brown fat to provide heat energy should they become cold, but this requires a plentiful supply of oxygen. Brown fat can, at the best, only provide energy for a few hours. Once the brown fat is metabolized it is not replaced.

The optimal ambient temperature (neutral thermal environment) to prevent heat loss is 35°C for premature infants, 32°C for neonates, 30°C for infants and children, 28°C for adolescents and adults.

Hypothermia causes profound problems for babies. Unless they were well wrapped or under special lights in theatre nearly all have cooled to a certain extent by the time they come to the recovery room. Compared to an adult, infants have a much bigger surface area in relation to their body weight.

Measure the temperature of a baby
as soon as possible after arrival in recovery room.

Babies are often cool when they come to the recovery room. Keep small infants warm. Cover their heads with a woollen or gamgee hat, infants lose heat through their bald heads quickly. Ideally they should go straight into an incubator after surgery. Their oxygen requirement is high; so make sure that 28% oxygen flows into the incubator.

Anaesthesia makes small infants drowsy postoperatively. If the infant becomes lethargic and floppy and its respiration and pulse rate are slow, assist his breathing with a Cardiff™ or small Ambu Bag™ and summon someone to help you. Warm the baby and check his blood sugar.

Hyperthermia

Hyperthermia can occur. Babies do not sweat, instead they simply vasodilate and go red. Consider the following causes:

- an overdose of atropine – the baby will have a rapid pulse > 150 beats/min;
- an infection;
- CO_2 retention;
- malignant hyperthermia.

Pharmacology

Children under 12 years do not respond to drugs in the same way as small adults; this particularly applies to neonates. Children's doses may be calculated from adult doses by body weight, or more reliably, by body surface area. The upper outer lateral aspect of the thigh is the only safe intramuscular injection site in children.

Ideal body weight in children

A well-nourished child's approximate ideal weight

Age less than 9 years: weight in Kg = $(2 \times age) + 9$

Age more than 9 years: weight in Kg = $age \times 3$

$$\text{Approximate dose for a child} = \frac{\text{Surface area of child } (m^2) \times \text{adult dose}}{1.8}$$

Keep a weight-for-age nomogram available in case you do not know the child's weight. Having determined the correct dose of a drug you may need to convert this into millilitres of drug as supplied by the maker. Under a stressful situation it is easy to make mistakes. So make up charts to convert directly from body weight to millilitres of solution and tie the charts to your paediatric resuscitation trolley.

Calculate drug doses from an ideal weight based on height and age. If you need to calculate doses on weight alone, never give more than you would to a 50 Kg patient. Be careful of sedatives, which may cause hallucinations; also anti-emetics, which can cause dystonic reactions.

It is better to use a table such as Table 12.3 to calculate approximate drug doses. Even using this table does not ensure safety because some drugs, such as aminophylline, have a small margin between the therapeutic dose and the toxic dose. If you have any doubts about the safety of a drug, or how to use it in children, consult the literature or a paediatric specialist. Be especially cautious and give drugs slowly to babies in their first 30 days of life.

Table 12.3 Paediatric drug doses

Age	Average body weight (Kg)	Percentge of adult dose
Neonate*	3.5	12.5
1 month*	4.2	14.5
3 months*	6	8
6 months	8	22
1 year	10	25
2 years	13	28
3 years	14	33
4 years	16	35
5 years	18	40
6 years	20	45
7 years	22	50
8 years	25	54
9 years	28	60
10 years	30	66
11 years	35	70
12 years	40	75
13 years	43	80
14 years	50	100

*Applies to full term but not to premature infants.

Pain relief

How to assess pain

Children waking from anaesthesia are often distressed, frightened, disoriented and in pain. Small children quickly respond to the warmth of a cuddle. It may not be possible to pick the child up but touch is very reassuring. A toddler out of his routine is anxious and upset; but a toddler out of his routine, and in pain, is inconsolable and very, very angry.

Ideally pain relief should be established in theatre or even preoperatively. Depending on the site of the surgery a combination of regional techniques such as caudals; with opioids and/or paracetamol (Panadol®) suppositories can be used to suit most circumstances. Never let a baby or child cry in pain. Incremental small doses of opioids, especially pethidine are ideal for quickly settling small patients. Paracetamol suppositories are less reliable. Intravenous paracetamol can be given; the dose is 15 mg/Kg.

> *Do not use aspirin in children,*
> *because it may cause Reye's syndrome.*

Babies

Postoperatively it is sometimes difficult to tell whether babies are crying because they are in pain, or simply because they are hungry. As soon as possible allow babies feed. Milk has a calming effect because it releases endogenous opioids, and is unlikely to cause any harm.

Diazepam suppositories 0.1 mg/Kg are sometimes used to relax the painful adductor spasms that occur when babies have plaster splints applied.

Reye's syndrome

Reye's syndrome is a very rare fulminating encephalopathy associated with liver failure that occurs in children. It follows after an acute virtal illness, and is thought to be aggravated by aspirin. The child becomes drowsy, confused, ataxic and starts to vomit, and may bleed. It has a high mortality. Do not use aspirin in children or adolescents.

Morphine and pethidine are effective analgesics for children, but the onset of action of pethidine is quicker than morphine. Titrate the initial doses of these drugs to achieve the desired effect.

Opioids are metabolized in the liver. Pethidine has pharmacologically active metabolites and occasionally these cause twitching and even seizures; especially if doses are repeated.

All the side-effects of opioids seen in adults also occur in children. Up to the age of 3 months the duration of action of opioids is unpredictable. Fentanyl in neonates or babies is metabolized slowly and unpredictably giving it a long action. It can readily cause respiratory depression and excessive sedation. Avoid all opioids in babies after neurosurgery.

Providing the child can be monitored closely in a special care unit, continuous morphine infusions are useful after major surgery. The loading dose is 0.1 mg/Kg before the end of surgery then 0.5 mg/Kg added to 500 ml of Hartmann's solution and given via an infusion pump or burette at 10–40 ml/hr.

Continuous epidural, with or without opioids, can be used successfully if the child is going to a supervised area, such as intensive care. Use 0.5 ml/Kg of 0.25% bupivacaine and infuse at a rate of 0.1–0.15 ml/Kg/hr.

Vomiting

Although children frequently vomit after anaesthesia they are not usually distressed. Clean the mouth and pharynx carefully and allow the child to sit up. Since most children only vomit once, use anti-emetics cautiously because they can cause severe dystonic reactions. Severe or intractable vomiting occurs in about two per cent of children postoperatively.

Using intraoperative NSAIDS instead of opioids for analgesia reduces the incidence of postoperative vomiting. If children are vomiting do not remove the intravenous line. Use either 0.9% saline or Hartmann's solution while children are vomiting; never use 5% dextrose.

Children who are older than 18 months and have uncontrolled postoperative vomiting may need rescue therapy. Use a combination of granisetron 40 µg/Kg and droperidol 50 µg/Kg.[2]

Dystonia

Anti-emetics can cause dystonic reactions in children. Dystonia causes the child to become stiff, with their arms held rigidly at their sides, their neck extended and their teeth clenched. Extra-orbital muscle spasm causes upward and outward deviation of the eyes.[3]

Another name for the side-effect of dystonia is the extrapyramidal syndrome. Although alarming and uncomfortable the effect is reversed with benztropine (Cogentin®) as a 0.02 mg/Kg bolus given intravenously.

Psychological aspects

Infants

Infants under the age of 6 months of age are not usually upset when separated from their mother, and readily accept comfort from a stranger.

Figure 12.3 Cuddle crying children

Younger children

Children up to the ages of 4 or 5 years are upset when separated from their mother and disturbed by unfamiliar faces and surroundings. It is difficult to comfort or reason with children of this age, especially when they are crying or distressed. Children are comforted by seeing their mothers as they emerge from their anaesthetic and staff are more accepting of the mother's presence. Children are extremely perceptive and readily detect anxiety in their parents. Thoroughly brief the mother on what to expect beforehand so that she does not convey her anxiety to the child. It is wise to keep other visitors and relatives away from patients who are recovering from anaesthesia. They may become upset to see someone vomiting or in pain.

Older children

School-aged children are more frightened of the prospect of being disfigured by the surgery than the possibility of pain. They are more easily reassured by strangers, and not so disoriented by unfamiliar places.

Adolescents

Adolescents are shy about their bodies, keep them well covered and do not embarrass them. They tend to fear going to sleep for their surgery, or dying during the procedure. They are not so worried by pain, but do fear losing control of themselves or their surroundings.

Teenagers and young adult patients can become restless while waking up. They roll about and may try to climb off the trolley before they can be reasoned with. Make sure the trolley sides are raised and there is a strong person to help restrain the patient. Secure the intravenous lines, nasogastric tubes and other drains, otherwise they may be pulled out during this restless phase.

When emerging from any of the volatile agents, younger patients sometimes develop muscle rigidity and experience violent shaking. This muscle activity uses a lot of energy, and consequently a lot of oxygen, so try and keep their oxygen masks on and cover them with warm blankets.

From their early teenage years through young adulthood, many patients seem surprisingly resistant to sedative and analgesic drugs. An alarmed young person diverts most of his blood supply to his muscles (a part of the flight response). When drugs are given intravenously they are more likely to be pumped to their muscles rather than their brain.

Cardiac arrest

Cardiac arrest in children is usually caused by lack of oxygen to the heart. The principal causes of cardiac arrest in children in the recovery room are hypoxia caused by respiratory obstruction and haemorrhage.

Children under the age of 1 year are most at risk. There is less time to respond to apnoea in children because they become hypoxic so quickly. Children nearly always have asystole or bradycardia as the initial rhythm.

Cardiac arrest is usually preceded by:

- respiratory distress with tachypnoea, cyanosis, distress and decreased breath sounds;
- tachycardia, bradycardia;
- hypotension or reduced pulse volume;
- poor perfusion with tachycardia, poor capillary return, cool or mottled peripheries;
- deterioration in conscious state;
- flaccidity.

The presence of any one of these signs needs urgent resuscitation. Summon help immediately.

The most common arrhythmias are severe bradycardia, pulseless electrical activity or asystole; all of which have a bad outcome. Ventricular arrhythmias such as ventricular fibrillation and ventricular tachycardias usually only occur in children with pre-existing cardiac disease.

How to recognize cardiac arrest

You cannot feel either the brachial pulse or the apex beat;
    or
    The pulse rate is less than 60 beats/min;
    or
    You are not sure.

Then immediately:

- Call for help.
- Stimulate the child and assess the result.
- Then start the ABC of resuscitation.

A = Airway

Position the head in a neutral position (for children aged less than one year), or the *sniffing position* (for older children).

Open the airway with head tilt, chin lift and a jaw thrust.

Insert an oropharyngeal airway.

B = Breathing

If the child is not breathing immediately start assisted ventilation. Use the right-sized resuscitating bag: for an infant under 2 years use a 500 ml bag; for older children use an adult 1500 ml bag. Use an appropriate-sized mask which should not overlap the chin and gives a good airtight seal. Use an oxygen flow rate of 15 L/min and attach a reservoir bag to give 100% oxygen. If necessary, clear the mouth and pharynx with a Yankeur sucker. Ventilate to produce a normal rise and fall of the chest. The recommended ventilation rate is rate is 10 breaths/min. Do not over-inflate the chest, because there is a risk of causing a pneumothorax. The anaesthetist may decide to intubate the child. Once circulation is restored, ventilate the child at a range of 12–20 breaths/min to achieve a normal PCO_2, and monitor expired CO_2.

C = Circulation

If there are no signs of circulation, or if the pulse is less than 60/min or you are not sure then commence external cardiac compression. Attach an ECG to determine the cardiac rhythm.

Cardiac massage

When performing cardiac massage remember the heart is positioned under the lower third of the sternum in children. Place the index finger of the lower hand just under the line between the nipples. The area of compression is at the junction between the middle and ring finger. Compress the heart with either two fingers or the heel of your hand depending on the size of the child use about 100 compressions per minute. You get the number about right by singing (silently) to the beat of 'Happy birthday to you' at normal speed (but don't pause at the end of each line).

Figure 12.4 Position of thumbs on baby's chest for cardiac massage

Important points:

- Do not stop cardiac compression except for defibrillation.
- Compress the sternum to about one-third the depth of the chest.
- For infants use two fingers.
- For neonates, the best technique is the two-hand hold. Grasp the baby with both hands to encircle its thorax and with your thumbs pointing to the baby's head. Now compress the lower third of the sternum.
- During cardiac massage do not stop to check the pulse unless the ECG is showing an organized rhythm.
- After DC shock, continue cardiopulmonary resuscitation (CPR) for two minutes before stopping to check the pulse.

The brachial pulse is easier to feel in chubby children than the carotid. Neonates, infants and small children have short necks. Do not hyperextend the neck, just lift the head forward a little into a neutral position. Insert a Guedal airway, use an appropriate sized mask, and ventilate at a rate of 40–60 per minute with puffs of 100% oxygen.

Recent changes

Cardioversion

Unlike adults, cardioversion is rarely needed in children. The most common tachyarrhythmia in children is paroxysmal supraventricular tachycardia. This comes on abruptly with a rate exceeding 220 beats/min. Other reasons for cardioversion are pulseless electrical activity (PEA), *ventricular fibrillation* (VF) and *ventricular tachycardia* (VT). Adult defibrillators can be used in patients aged 8 years or older.

Cardioversion should be done with a single 4 joule/Kg shock. Repeated shocks damage the myocardium. Use appropriate-sized paediatric paddles. This is 4.5 cm for infants weighing less than 10Kg and 8cm for older children. If necessary, you can use the larger 8cm paddles by placing them on the chest and back. The entire surface of the paddle must contact the chest wall over its entire surface area.

Most modern defibrillators have a preset maximum dose of 80 joule when the paediatric paddles are connected. Remember that small babies who have been stressed or starved are at risk from hypoglycaemia and need their blood glucose levels assessed following cardioversion.

Drugs

The dose of adrenaline is 10 µg/Kg for each dose. Drugs should be given intravenously or by the intraosseous route, and only as a last resort down the endotracheal tube.

When to stop?

The outcome of paediatric cardiac arrest is poor. Failure to achieve a return to spontaneous respiration after 15 minutes has dismal outcome. The exceptions for this are arrests associated with hypothermia, hyperkalaemia, and bupivacaine toxicity. If in doubt consult a paediatrician for advice.

Notes

1. Resuscitation Council (UK) (2005) *Guidelines.*
2. Campbell D (2001) *Australian Prescriber* 24:19–20.
3. Fujii Y, Toyooka H, Tanaka H (1998) *Anesthesia and Analgesia* 8:761–5.

13

The elderly patient

As we grow older, our bodies change. They adapt to the physiological needs of that time in our lives. We need to take into account each patient's physical fitness, intercurrent medical problems, psychological state, and the medication they are taking as well as the type of surgery and anaesthetic they have undergone.

Old age

Old age is a process; not a disease

In industrialized countries the population is ageing and about 12 per cent are over the age of 65 years. Half of those over the age of 65 will come to surgery before they die.

Elderly people are defined as those over the age of 65 years, while the *aged* is a subgroup of those over 85 years. Old age in itself is not a disease, but old people inherit the residual effects of past and continuing illnesses while undergoing a progressive decline of organ function.

Not everyone ages at the same rate. Physiological age varies enormously with chronological age. Some individuals are decrepit in their early 60s, while others are sprightly and active into their late 80s. It can be difficult to assess the physical condition of elderly patients, because their mobility is limited by the pain and stiffness of arthritis.

Often chronic illness, undiagnosed disease, malnutrition, multiple pathology and particularly *polypharmacy* are unwelcome companions to the elderly. Older patients coming to surgery should write down a problem list of every symptom, both major and trivial, that troubles them. In the recovery room this problem list will enable you to see patterns emerging so that you can separate the effects of the ageing process from disease. For instance elderly patients who cannot cough effectively may have chronic airway disease, in which case they might benefit from humidification or a BiPAP mask, or they may simply be physically weak, in which case gentle physiotherapy could help them cough up retained secretions. If they have low muscle mass they may still be affected by the residual effects of muscle relaxants.

It is helpful to have a list of all the patient's problems, even the ones that seem trivial. It is difficult to make sensible decisions if you do not have access to all the facts.

How to predict problems in the elderly

Three factors predict problems likely to occur in the recovery room:

1. surgery lasting longer than 45 minutes;
2. obesity;
3. poor cardiopulmonary function.

How function alters with age

We do not die quickly; we slowly degenerate over many years. As nerve cells and muscle cells everywhere inevitably die, they are not replaced with more muscle and nerve cells, but with collagen, amyloid and fat.

Collagen and elastin

The scar tissue of ageing is *collagen*. *Elastin* is the elastic springy connective tissue found almost everywhere, especially in the walls of arteries and arterioles, the heart, lungs, joints, tendons. Its job is to return things to their original shape. A young person's skin is tight, but with ageing it becomes loose and saggy. As we age, elastin unravels, loses its springiness and converts to stiff unyielding *collagen*. Elastin allows young blood vessels to spring back if they are stretched. However, as elastin turns into collagen it loses its elasticity and becomes stiffer. If blood vessels do distend in the elderly they stay dilated to eventually form aneurysms.

Age causes floppy lungs

All other things being equal, the elderly are as fit as the combined capacity of their heart and lung function allows them to be. The heart and lungs work together as a single *cardiopulmonary unit* supplying oxygen to the tissues and removing their metabolic waste.

Lungs in elderly people are less elastic, their chest walls are stiff, their respiratory muscles are weak, the airways are floppy and collapse more easily, and the alveolar surface area is reduced. All this means that gas exchange is less efficient.

The elderly become hypoxic more rapidly, are slower to respond to oxygen therapy, and cannot cough efficiently making sputum retention more likely.

Oxygen levels fall in the elderly

While breathing air the arterial PaO_2 falls with age from about 100 mmHg (13.3 kPa) in a fit young person, to about 80 mmHg (10.5 kPa) in an 80-year-old.

Oxygen demands are highest as the patient first emerges from anaesthesia. For this reason some anaesthetists prefer to extubate their patients in the recovery room, rather than transporting an unstable patient on the short trip from the operating theatre. Pain, coughing, hypertension or a tachycardia aggravates any hypoxia. Shivering or shaking can increase oxygen requirements sevenfold.

Diffusion hypoxia is a special problem unique to the recovery room. For about 10 minutes after the end of a general anaesthetic nitrous oxide seeps out of the blood into the lungs, displacing oxygen. You may see the patient's oxygen saturations decrease. Treat this with high flows of supplemental oxygen. Notify the anaesthetist if the patient's saturations fall to 90%.

Spinal and epidural anaesthesia may cause problems too because the vasodilatation caused by the regional block diverts blood to the lower limbs. With less peripheral *resistance* to push against, the heart needs to increase its force and rate of contraction to maintain the blood pressure. This increased work requires an increase in oxygen supply. If the heart does not receive enough oxygen, it becomes ischaemic and begins to fail.

How the heart ages

All forms of cardiac disease are more prevalent in the elderly. Circulation time is slower, and the vascular system more rigid. As the myofibrils in the heart die they are mostly replaced by collagen tissue. With fewer myofibrils and more collagen the heart becomes stiffer (less compliant), and it cannot contract so forcibly. Consequently, it is no longer able to compensate quickly for sudden changes in blood pressure or blood volume.

Why joints are stiff

Old joints are stiff. Joints and tendons lose their ability to flex and absorb shocks as springy elastin converts to stiffer collagen. Older people cannot run and jump easily because their tendons and ligaments no longer stretch to absorb the shock of impact. Be careful how you move and position them so that you do not injure their backs, hips, shoulders and knees. Be especially careful of moving patients who have had regional blocks, without warning pain ligaments and tendons are easily overstretched and torn. This is a potent cause of the backache which is so often reported after spinal, and epidural anaesthesia, where the lumbar arch has not been supported properly in the operating theatre or afterwards in the recovery room.

Why skin is fragile

Old peoples' skin is thin and easily torn by simple things such as turning them over, or removing adhesive dressings. Be particularly careful if they have bruises or brown staining on their arms or legs – this is a sure sign of atrophied skin. The elderly are very susceptible to pressure sores and need cushioning under bony protuberances such as their sacrum and heels.

Age and malnutrition

Many elderly patients suffer from malnutrition, especially the lack of dietary protein and vitamins. Vitamin and mineral deficiency places them at risk of poor wound healing and low resistance to *nosocomial infection*.

The *aged* (people older than 85 years) are usually thin, and have little subcutaneous fat. Because of their wasted muscles they are weak and cannot cough effectively, or move quickly. They need help to sit up or roll on to their side.

The elderly lose heat quickly

Elderly people cannot rapidly increase their metabolic rate to compensate for heat loss, so that their temperature is likely to fall further on the operating table than younger people. Additionally, the aged have less insulating subcutaneous fat to prevent heat loss. Hypothermia delays the enzymatic degradation of drugs, prolonging their action.

How the kidneys decline

With ageing, kidney function declines. We lose about one per cent of our *nephrons* each year after we turn 30. By the age of 70 years less than 70 per cent of the nephrons are still working. This delays the excretion of many drugs.

The liver is robust

As the years pass the liver loses little function, and provided the blood supply to the liver is good, and the patient is not hypoxic, septic or hypothermic the elderly liver metabolizes drugs just as efficiently as a younger person. However, if the blood supply to the liver is reduced, or the liver is affected by disease, such as cardiac failure, or the patient has a high alcohol intake then drugs are not cleared as efficiently, which prolongs their effect.

The liver is sensitive to the amount of circulating endotoxins from bacteria in the bloodstream, and is particularly likely to be affected after bowel surgery. This effect is aggravated during abdominal surgery when blood flow to the liver decreases by about half. To prevent problems occurring later in the ward it is particularly important that these patients are kept well oxygenated, well perfused, and have no pain in the recovery room.

How drugs affect the elderly

The elderly are usually taking multiple medications, and frequently a few pharmacologically active herbal remedies as well. More than half those admitted to our hospitals are taking inappropriate drugs, have drug conflicts, or are not taking their medication consistently, or at the correct interval. This is a major cause of morbidity, and unless detected before surgery can cause problems in the recovery room. For example NSAIDs are a common cause for acute postoperative oliguria, and garlic pills can cause bleeding.

A slow circulation time delays the onset of even fast-acting drugs such as naloxone. Naloxone may take 3 minutes or more to produce an effect in an older person, where in the younger patient it works within 90 seconds.

In general most drugs used during anaesthesia, and in the recovery room, initially have a more pronounced effect and last longer in the elderly than in the young. Most of the differences occur because an old person's physiology differs to that of a younger person.

Much of the body mass in a younger person is muscle with its high water content. In the elderly the bulk of their body mass is fat with its low water content. This means that the elderly have proportionately less water in which water-soluble drugs can dissolve, and proportionally more fat in which fat-soluble drugs can eventually disperse. In the elderly water-soluble drugs, such as the muscle relaxants, have less water in which to dissolve, and are therefore more concentrated.

Muscle relaxants

Although older people seem to need the same dose of muscle relaxant as younger people, the drugs take longer to act, and wear off more slowly. This can cause a problem in short procedures, because residual paralysis may persist into the recovery phase. Residual paralysis causes jerky movements, and patients are unable to lift their head clear of the pillow for 5-seconds. Notify the anaesthetist if you encounter this problem.

Midazolam

Midazolam is a safer drug for the elderly than diazepam. In older people midazolam is dispersed more widely, and its plasma concentrations decrease more slowly, particularly if it has been infused rather than given in a single dose. The reason why equivalent plasma levels cause more sedation in the elderly is unclear.

In their rush to get people out of the recovery room, some units use flumazenil (a benzodiazepine receptor antagonist) to reverse the effects of midazolam. This practice is unwise, because flumazenil wears off after about 45 minutes, leaving any residual midazolam to re-exert its effects. There are occasional reports of sudden deaths, because recovery room staff did not realize that midazolam may cause cardiorespiratory depression later in the ward.[1] This disaster is more likely if opioids have been used during or after the procedure.

Diazepam

Diazepam is sometimes used for uncomfortable day case procedures such as angiography. Diazepam slowly soaks into fat and slowly leaches out causing a prolonged effect. A standard 10 mg dose of diazepam may cause psychomotor retardation in the elderly for duration of the number of hours equivalent to their age in years. An 80-year-old person is still measurably slower to react to a red traffic stop light 80 hours after their last dose. Consider this effect when discharging elderly patients, who have received diazepam, after day procedures.

Morphine

Opioids are well tolerated in the elderly, however the effective dose may vary widely; a small dose of morphine can profoundly sedate one 80-year-old, while another similar 80-year-old may require a much higher dose to get adequate pain relief. The older brain is more susceptible to opioid-induced respiratory depression. As a general rule elderly patients need small doses, and longer intervals between doses.

Fentanyl

The opioid fentanyl causes problems in the elderly. A proportion of an injected dose of fentanyl binds to skeletal muscle cell membranes. While the patient is not moving it stays there, but once the patient starts to move around, the muscle blood flow increases and the fentanyl is washed back into the circulation. This rush of fentanyl is probably the cause of the delayed respiratory depression sometimes seen many hours after the last dose.

In summary

Two useful questions to ask about the elderly, but particularly about the aged, are:

- Should I use half the normal dose and give it twice as slowly?
- Is this drug really necessary?

Confusion and postoperative delirium are common

Postoperative confusion is common. Although hypoxia is the principal culprit, sometimes it is simply poor eyesight or hearing problems that disorientate the patient. Despite their confusion elderly people have an accurate perception of pain, and discourtesy. Respect for their dignity helps reduce the feelings alienation.

> *In the agitated and confused patient you must eliminate two killers: hypoxia and hypoglycaemia.*

Hypoxia is common. Acute hypoglycaemia is rare, however if it is not diagnosed and treated promptly it causes permanent brain damage. Those at risk include diabetics, especially those who are taking insulin, and alcoholics who, under certain circumstances, cannot manufacture glucose in their livers to maintain their blood glucose levels.

How to predict problems

Often there are signs of a developing acute brain syndrome in the recovery room that predict a full-blown *delirium* later in the ward. About 50 per cent of patients who fracture their femurs become confused postoperatively. As always hypoxia, in one of its many guises, is the prime suspect. Even though cardiopulmonary function may be adequate, if the patient has bled during the operation, the resulting anaemia will contribute to hypoxia. A blood transfusion does not necessarily prevent the problem. Stored blood picks up oxygen readily, but does not so easily download it to the tissues. It takes about 12–18 hours for the body to fully restore the oxygen-carrying ability of transfused blood. Merely because the oxygen saturation meter is reading 98% does not mean that the tissues are taking up oxygen.

An older person, who has been hypoxic even for a minute or two, will suffer brain damage. They may take hours or days to recover, and they may never recover completely. It is far better to prevent confusion than to have to manage it.

Other contributors to postoperative confusion include:

- pre-existing dementia;
- hypotension during the anaesthetic;
- anti-cholinergic medication such as atropine, and the phenothiazines;
- previous stroke or transient ischaemic attack;
- vascular disease including cerebrovascular or ischaemic heart disease;
- paradoxically, benzodiazepines occasionally aggravate confusion.

How to manage acute agitation and confusion

It is difficult to treat and manage confusion, restlessness, agitation and aggression. Agitation is harmful. The accompanying surge of noradrenaline and adrenaline raises the heart rate and blood pressure, putting the patient at risk of myocardial ischaemia.

> *You cannot drug a patient into mental competence.*

Start by giving high concentrations of oxygen by mask. Orient your patient by telling them where they are, and why they are there. Attach an ECG. Check the patient's blood pressure, pulse rate and perfusion status. All this is far easier said than done. An agitated fearful patient is not likely to be cooperative. They will not tolerate a mask; they can rip out their lines and become aggressive. Notify the anaesthetist; and prepare to sedate the patient. Every anaesthetist has a recipe for such occasions, but a useful one contains a mixture of haloperidol and midazolam. Once order has been restored, you will have a patient with a clouded conscious state whose airway needs protection. Check their blood gases, and blood glucose levels. Make a plan for their ongoing management. This may require the help of the intensive care unit.

How to communicate with the elderly

Deafness isolates older people from those around them. If a patient has a hearing aid, put it back as soon as they are conscious. Some recovery rooms have background music playing. Older patients with hearing aids find background noise distracting because it distorts how they hear voices. Turn the music off. Look at their faces when you speak to them. Speak slowly and clearly.

> *Sensory impairment leads to frustration.*
> *Frustration leads to withdrawal or anger.*

If older patients are in pain it is difficult for them to process new information. They are likely to forget what you have just said to them. A patient in pain will find it difficult to concentrate on what you are saying.

Age does not mean loss of intelligence, and older patients deeply resent being treated as child-like. Older patients find it easier to deal with one piece of information at a time. If you need to give instructions then present each point separately and make sure it is understood before moving on to the next point.

Respect cultural differences. Ethnicity, cultural beliefs and social norms affect patients' expectations. Remember that older people, even if born in the country, were raised in a different generation. They have different attitudes to privacy, modesty and communication. Many dislike being called by their first names, they have been taught to 'grin and bear' pain, not to 'worry other people', and the hospital staff 'know best'.

The disorientation of coming to hospital, the pain and discomfort the time without food or fluids all contribute to disorientate elderly people. Sedatives have a serious affect on their memory. The effect can be insidious. For many hours, and even days after an anaesthetic the patient's ability to process and remember information is blunted. They may appear to have understood what you have just told them, but a few minutes later the whole conversation has become a hazy blur in their memory, or has disappeared completely. If there are important points that the patient should know then make this clear to the nurses from the ward so that they can write instructions down for the patient or to alert the patient's relatives.

Note

1. National Confidential Enquiry into Patient Outcome and Death (2004) *Scoping our practice*, published 13 October.

14

Respiratory physiology

Terminology

Clinicians use special jargon when talking about respiratory medicine. The terms are not difficult to understand, but used carelessly they can be confusing.

Symbols

- O_2 = oxygen
- CO_2 = carbon dioxide
- H_2O = water
- PO_2 = partial pressure of oxygen
- PaO_2 = partial pressure of oxygen in arterial blood
- $PaCO_2$ = partial pressure of carbon dioxide in arterial blood
- FIO_2 = fractional inspired content of oxygen
- H+ = hydrogen ion
- [H+] = hydrogen ion concentration
- pH = a logarithmic scale for measuring hydrogen activity
- FRC = functional residual capacity

Units

- cm H_2O = centimetres of water pressure
- mmHg = millimetres of mercury pressure
- kPa = kilopascals of pressure
- For example: 7.60 mmHg = 1 kPa
- 1.32 mmHg = 10 cm H_2O

In the UK and parts of Europe the kilopascal (kPa) is the preferred unit for measuring pressure, whereas in Australasia and the US they use mmHg.

There are two principal gases: oxygen (O_2) and carbon dioxide (CO_2). Cells use oxygen to burn carbohydrate, fats and amino acids to produce energy, which cells use for doing things. This process is called *oxidative metabolism*.

The three terms *concentration, tension,* and *partial pressure*, all mean roughly the same thing. They are used to express how much of a particular gas is present in each litre of a mixture of gases.

Gases exert pressure, even when they are dissolved in fluids (for example the bubbles in beer). PCO_2 is the shorthand for pressure of carbon dioxide; similarly PO_2 is the pressure exerted by oxygen. By convention we use the Pappenheimer notation to describe the physical state of gases and fluids in biology (see the box below).

The term *fractional inspired concentration of oxygen* (FIO_2) is used to describe the concentration of oxygen in inspired air. Room air contains 21% oxygen, and therefore the FIO_2 is 0.21. Using the FIO_2 we can calculate the pressure exerted by oxygen in a mixture of gases such as air. This is discussed in the box describing Dalton's law of partial pressures.

Most oxygen face masks used in the recovery room deliver an arterial FIO_2 of 0.36 (36% oxygen) at a flow rate of 6 L/min.

For a healthy person breathing air ($FIO_2 = 0.21$) the normal arterial PaO_2 is about 100 mmHg (13.3 kPa). The PaO_2 declines with age and at 80 years is about 80 mmHg (10.5 kPa).

Giving patients supplemental oxygen raises their FIO_2. In a person with normal lungs as you increase their FIO_2, their PaO_2 rises roughly in proportion. If their FIO_2 doubles so will their PaO_2. However, in a patient with diseased lungs this does not occur.

Pappenheimer notation

Respiratory physiologists use the Pappenheimer notation as a shorthand for describing gases in various situations.

1. Upper case 'P' applies to pressures, e.g. PO_2 = partial pressure of oxygen.

2. Upper case 'A' applies to gases, e.g. PAO_2 = partial pressure of oxygen in alveolar gas.

3. Upper case 'I' applies to inspired gas, e.g. FIO_2 = fractional inspired concentration of oxygen.

4. Lower case 'a' applies to gases dissolved in arterial blood, e.g. $PaCO_2$ = partial pressure of carbon dioxide in arterial blood.

Oxygen transport

Four steps ensure oxygen from the outside air reaches the mitochondria in the cells.

1. Breathing.
2. Gas transfer between the lungs and the blood.
3. Transport of oxygen in the blood to the tissues.
4. Oxygen diffuses to mitochondria.

Breathing

Breathing is a process where air containing oxygen is inspired into the lungs, and carbon dioxide laden air is expired. The thorax behaves like a closed box that alters in size and shape with each breath. On inspiration, the cavity of the thorax enlarges, and the elastic lungs expand to fill the space. On expiration, the thorax returns to its former size and air is expelled. Then there is a short pause before the process starts over again.

In forced, or deep, inspiration the accessory respiratory muscles of the neck and shoulder girdle are recruited to assist. Laboured breathing occurs when the patient is using their accessory muscle to assist each breath.

Never ignore laboured breathing. Find the cause.

In contrast, *expiration* relies on the springiness of the lungs to drive the air out again. It is a passive process. If patients use the accessory muscles in their neck or abdomen to breathe they probably have some form of airway obstruction.

Humidification stops the airway drying out

As air is sucked through the upper airway, it is warmed and humidified. It then passes through a bottleneck in the larynx, and flows down either the left or right bronchi, and on through another 20 branches of airways, to reach the alveoli. Here oxygen diffuses into the blood, and carbon dioxide diffuses into the lungs.

Normal respiratory rate

The normal respiratory rate is 12–14 breaths/min. Each breath contains about 400 ml (*tidal volume*). About half the tidal volume reaches the alveoli where gas exchange occurs; but the other half remains in the airways as *dead space volume* where no gas exchange is possible. If the tidal volume is less than the dead space volume carbon dioxide banks up in the alveoli and blood causing the $PaCO_2$ to rise.

A rising respiratory rate is a useful sign, warning that the patient is becoming physiologically unstable. Once the rate reaches 18 breaths/min you should start looking for a cause.

A rising respiratory rate? Find the cause.

Functional residual capacity acts as an oxygen store

At the end of a quiet expiration about 3 litres of residual air remain in the lungs. This volume is called *the functional residual capacity (FRC)*. The FRC acts as a small oxygen store that we draw on when we breathe out, talk, or hold our breath. If it were not for this residual air we would turn blue every time we breathed out, and pink when we breathed in. As we grow older our lungs lose their elasticity and become floppy and the FRC becomes larger. Neonates and infants have proportionally the same FRC as an adult, but because they use oxygen twice as fast as an adult they become hypoxic quickly once they stop breathing.

Less air is stored in the FRC during, and directly after general anaesthesia. When a person lies down their abdominal contents push their diaphragm up into the thorax. This partly collapses the bases of the lung. This is the physiological reason pregnant or very obese patients become breathless when lying on their backs.

Respiratory centres drive breathing

Respiratory centres in the brainstem regulate breathing. They act like a biological computer, which receiving input messages from the lungs and elsewhere, then processes the signals and organizes an appropriate output response. This sequence is an example of a feedback control loop maintaining *homeostasis*.

Chemoreceptors sense oxygen and carbon dioxide tensions

Some of the inputs come from *chemoreceptors* in the aorta, carotid arteries and brainstem. When brainstem chemoreceptors detect a tiny increase in $PaCO_2$ levels, they stimulate the respiratory centres to make the patient *breathe-up* deeply and quickly. This causes the person to 'blow-off' the carbon dioxide to restore a homeostatic equilibrium. We are all familiar with becoming short of breath when we run up a flight of stairs. All that extra muscular activity produces a lot of CO_2, which accumulates in our blood, and is sensed by brainstem chemoreceptors. To restore homeostasis the chemoreceptors stimulate our breathing to get rid of the excess CO_2.

In contrast, the chemoreceptors' sensitivity to a falling PO_2 is not good. In most people the arterial PaO_2 has to fall to at least 55 mmHg (7.24 kPa) before the carotid chemoreceptors make us breathe-up. In 10 per cent of people the chemoreceptors do not work at all.

Drugs depress chemoreceptors

Anaesthetic drugs depress chemoreceptors. Why is this important in the recovery room? If a patient has a general anaesthetic with volatile agents or receives an opioid we cannot depend on their normal reflexes to stimulate breathing. The reasons are: first, that opioids depress the brainstem chemoreceptor response to a rising $PaCO_2$ and so the respiratory rate slows, and the tidal volume decreases. Second, the carotid body chemoreceptor response to hypoxaemia is abolished by even a tiny amount of residual volatile anaesthetic agent. These effects last for 6 hours or more after the end of anaesthesia.

Dyspnoea is a subjective feeling

Patient are said to be *dyspnoeic* when they feel short of breath. Dyspnoea is a sign that the patient is working hard to breathe. If your patient becomes dyspnoeic find the reason their work of breathing has increased. Anything impeding breathing (for example asthma, a pneumothorax, or bronchospasm); or increasing the stiffness of the lung (for example fibrotic lung disease, pneumonia, *pulmonary oedema*; or gas, fat, or air embolism) causes dyspnoea.

Reflexes guard the airway

Epithelial receptors guard the airway to stop foreign material becoming inhaled into the lungs. When stimulated these receptors cause sneezing, coughing, gagging, breath-holding or laryngospasm. Spraying the throat or airway with local anaesthetic abolishes the protective reflexes, consequently increasing the risk that the patient might aspirate material into their lower airway.

Gas transfer in the lungs

The surface area of the lung is about 70 square metres; about the size of a tennis court. Oxygen does not diffuse easily and needs this large surface area to move across the membranes separating the alveolus from the bloodstream. In contrast carbon dioxide diffuses easily, and only needs about a fifth of the area that oxygen requires. This is the reason that the arterial PaO_2 decreases in proportion to the area of damaged lung, while $PaCO_2$ does not start to rise until 75 per cent or more of the lung's membranes are severely damaged.

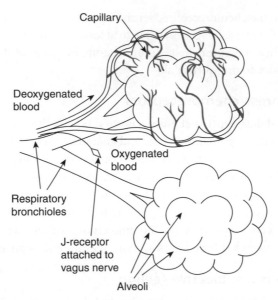

Figure 14.1 Two terminal respiratory units. Gas exchange takes place in the *terminal respiratory unit* (TRU). Ironed out flat they would cover an area of about 70 m². Each TRU is composed of a collection of 20–30 alveoli fed by an arteriole, encased by a capillary network and drained by small veins. Each TRU is polygonal in shape and about the size of a match-head. During surgery and anaesthesia TRU collapse and turn from pink to grey. If the fragile capillary network is damaged then the capillaries leak fluid into the spaces between the TRUs accumulating there to cause *interstitial oedema*. If fluid then leaks into the alveoli themselves it produces *alveolar oedema*. Near the junction of the TRUs and the bronchioles there are little strands of smooth muscle that act as stretch receptors called *J-receptors*. Fluid collecting in the lung's interstitial spaces stretches the J-receptors. They send an impulse up the vagus nerve to the brainstem respiratory centres, which in turn increase the rate and depth of breathing making the person feel breathless

How shunting causes hypoxia

In a normal lung less than five per cent of the blood bypasses oxygenated alveoli. In contrast, in patients with pulmonary disease larger proportions of blood are *shunted* through the diseased lung so that blue deoxygenated blood emerges still blue at the venous end. The blue deoxygenated blood then mixes with red oxygenated blood in the pulmonary vein. The result is a *venous admixture*, which causes the overall PaO$_2$ to fall.

Why giving oxygen may not be effective

Paradoxically, the more severe the patients' lung disease, the less effective is supplemental oxygen in raising their PaO$_2$.

Consider the case of a person with a totally blocked right main bronchus but a normally aerated left lung. In this case, blood flowing through the right lung will not be oxygenated, while the blood flowing through the left lung is fully oxygenated. This creates a 50 per cent shunt and the arterial PaO_2 will be about 40 mmHg. Such a patient is severely hypoxaemic, so that even if you give them 100% oxygen the PaO_2 will not increase by more than about 10 mmHg.

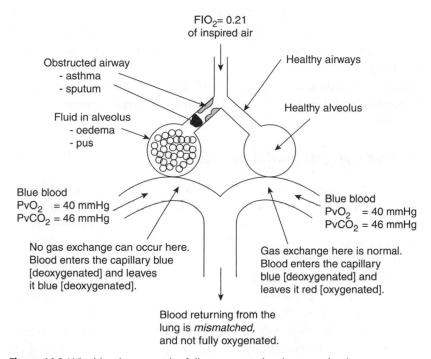

Figure 14.2 Why blood may not be fully oxygenated – shunt mechanisms

How atelectasis causes hypoxia

Surface tension tends to stick alveolar walls together. Normally, the alveoli secrete a natural detergent (*surfactant*) to overcome surface tension. During long anaesthetics the alveolar cells stop producing surfactant, and many alveoli collapse (*micro-atelectasis*). Blood now shunts past the collapsed alveoli causing PaO_2 to fall. In the recovery room once patients deep breathe and cough effectively they blast open collapsed alveoli.

How hypoventilation causes hypoxia

Measuring blood gases gives a good estimation of the carbon dioxide concentration in the alveoli. If a patient does not exchange enough tidal air into and out of their lungs then the concentration of CO_2 builds up in the alveoli, displacing oxygen to cause hypoxaemia. This is the reason patients who *hypoventilate* become hypoxic.

Carbon dioxide diffuses so easily across the alveolar capillary membrane that a patient's arterial $PaCO_2$ is almost the same as their $PACO_2$ in their aveolar gas. The alveolar gas approximates to the end-tidal CO_2 measured with the carbon dioxide monitor.

According to *Dalton's Law of Partial Pressures* the more carbon dioxide in the lungs, the less room there is for oxygen (and vice versa). Roughly, for every 10 mmHg rise in arterial $PaCO_2$, the PAO_2 in the lungs decreases by 10 mmHg.

Unlike carbon dioxide, oxygen is a poorly diffusible gas, so its concentration in arterial blood does not give a useful estimate of oxygen concentrations in the lungs.

Dalton's law of partial pressures

The concentration of gas in either air or a solution is measured by its *partial pressure.* The partial pressure is measured in millimetres of mercury (mmHg), or kilopascals (kPa). In a mixture of gases the partial pressure of a particular gas is the pressure that the gas would exert if it alone occupied the space available to it.

Nearly 200 years, *Dalton's law of partial pressures* effectively said; "if you add up the partial pressures of all the gases in a mixture, you will get the total pressure they exert".

At sea level the total pressure of the dry gases in the atmosphere is 760 mmHg (100 kPa), but only 21 per cent of this is oxygen so that the pressure oxygen exerts is $21/100 \times 760 = 160$ mmHg, while almost all the remaining gas is nitrogen so that the pressure it exerts is $79/100 \times 760 = 600$ mmHg. In room air there is also some water vapour. The pressure it exerts depends on the *humidity* in the room, but even in a steamy bathroom the pressure of water vapour in the air would be about 37 mmHg. The amount of CO_2 is a physiologically trivial 380 parts per million.

Gases also dissolve in fluids, and they can exert considerable pressure there. You will appreciate this if you have prompted them to escape from solution by shaking up a can of fizzy drink. The normal pressure exerted by dissolved oxygen in arterial blood could support a column of mercury 100 mm high or a column of water 1.36 metres high. This is what we imply when say the PaO_2 of arterial blood is 100 mmHg (13.3 kPa).

Diffusion hypoxia

For about 5 to 10 minutes after the end of a general anaesthetic nitrous oxide diffuses from the circulation back into the lung, displacing oxygen. This *diffusion hypoxia* is common and especially hazardous in elderly people who have floppy lungs, and an increased functional residual capacity. It is also a hazard in neonates and infants who have higher oxygen consumption. This is another reason to give high concentrations of oxygen to all patients recovering from general anaesthesia.

Oxygen transport to the tissues

Once in the alveoli oxygen diffuses across the alveolar–capillary membrane into the red cells where it loosely binds to haemoglobin. The blood flow then carries oxygen to the tissues where it diffuses into the cells.

Enormous amounts of oxygen are carried by haemoglobin inside the red cells. For example; 140 gm/L of haemoglobin carries 195 ml of oxygen; in contrast only 3 ml of oxygen is dissolved the *plasma*.

At the arterial end of a capillary the PaO_2 is about 100 mmHg. As the red cell moves along the capillary it unloads oxygen and picks up carbon dioxide. On its journey the PaO_2 progressively falls so that by the time it reaches the venous end of the capillary the $P\bar{v}O_2$ is only 40 mmHg.

There are four interlinked processes involved in supplying oxygen to the tissues:

1. Healthy lungs to ensure good gas exchange.
2. Good cardiac output to pump blood to the tissues.
3. Sufficient haemoglobin to carry the oxygen.
4. Metabolic factors affecting the shape of haemoglobin.

The ability of haemoglobin to carry oxygen to the tissues and then release it is reduced by metabolic factors such as hypothermia, disordered electrolytes in the blood, and particularly alkalosis.

Table 14.1 Causes of tissue hypoxia

Disease	Hypoxia
Anaemia	Possible
Anaemia + cardiac failure	Probable
Anaemia + cardiac failure + lung disease	Certain
Anaemia + cardiac failure + lung disease + fever	May be lethal

Massive blood transfusions produce a *functional anaemia* that may cause hypoxia. Stored red cells, near their expiry date, pick up oxygen easily enough, but are reluctant to release it to the tissues. In effect the blood enters the tissues pink, and emerges pink at the other end.

Patients dying from septicaemia or severe shock have cells that are so deranged they cannot use oxygen even if it is delivered to them.

Oxygen diffuses in mitochondria

Once in the tissues oxygen diffuses into the mitochondria. Cells use about 80 per cent of the oxygen to generate energy (oxidative metabolism), and the remaining 20 per cent to mop up the hydrogen ions they produce as a waste product.

How oxygen makes energy

Oxidative metabolism is a process where oxygen reacts (burns) with carbon in sugars, fats and proteins to form carbon dioxide and energy. Enzymes neatly confine this process to tiny harmless graded steps that allow the energy to be harvested and stored in high-energy compounds, principally as adenosine triphosphate (ATP), and yet not allow the heat produced to get out of control and cook the cell.

ATP and other similar compounds act like little rechargeable batteries. Cells use these to provide thermodynamic and electrochemical energy to kick-start and maintain biochemical reactions.

How oxygen mops up hydrogen ion

Oxidative metabolism releases large numbers of highly reactive hydrogen ions (H^+). Unless these are removed as soon as they appear they accumulate to disrupt cell metabolism and eventually kill the cell.

The moment hydrogen ions (H^+) are released a chain of mitochondrial enzymes immediately attach two of them to oxygen (O) to form harmless water (H_2O). Any stray ones that escape are mopped up by, and stored in *buffers* until they can be dealt with.

To form water, cells need an adequate supply of oxygen, but oxygen has to be delivered at a high enough pressure to push it into the cells, and at a sufficient volume to meet cellular needs. If oxygen supply fails then the hypoxic cells, for a short time, will shift into anaerobic metabolism, to produce lactic acid and a small amount of energy. The cells are now running on emergency power, but this cannot go on for long. Unless oxygen supply is restored lactic acid accumulates, enzymes fail, and if metabolism grinds to a halt the patient dies.

Clinically, a patient is said to be *hypoxic* when excess lactic acid collects in their blood. If the patient's oxygen supply is restored before too much damage is done, the liver's massive enzyme reserves turn lactic acid back into energy which is dissipated as heat.

Too much oxygen is toxic

Premature babies and neonates (weighing less than 1500 gm) who are exposed to prolonged periods of high concentrations of oxygen, which is then abruptly ceased are at particular risk of *retinopathy of prematurity* (ROP). ROP was formerly known as retrolental fibroplasia. It occurs where abnormal retinal vessels grow into an area where normal vessels have not yet developed. It can lead to lifelong visual impairment or blindness. If detected early it can be treated with laser surgery. In addition to low birth weight and prematurity, other factors contributing to the risk of ROP include anaemia, blood transfusions, respiratory distress, and breathing difficulties.

Older patients receiving 100% oxygen for more than 4–6 hours, or 50% oxygen for more than 16 hours, progressively stop secreting surfactant and risk developing lung damage called *bronchopulmonary dysplasia* which may be irreversible.

Oxygen supports combustion

Although oxygen itself does not burn, flammable material burns extremely vigorously in oxygen. Keep naked flames and sources of electrical sparks at least 2 metres away from an oxygen source.

Some patients are resistant to carbon dioxide

In a normal person a small rise in $PaCO_2$ vigorously stimulates breathing. Some patients with severe long-standing chronic obstructive airways disease have chronically raised $PaCO_2$. Their central chemoreceptors are no longer sensitive to changes in carbon dioxide tension. Instead their carotid chemoreceptors responding to a PaO_2 less than 60 mmHg (7.89 kPa), and drive their respiration. These *blue bloaters* may stop breathing if given more than an FIO_2 of 0.28 (28% oxygen). Blue bloaters are easy to recognize because they have *cor pulmonale*. They are plethoric, cyanosed and blue-faced, with oedematous (bloated) ankles, and they are breathless with minimal exercise. Using opioids in such a patient is a recipe for disaster, because they will have a respiratory arrest.

Never deprive blue bloaters of supplemental oxygen 'just in case they might stop breathing'. Watch them closely. If their respiratory effort fails, their $PaCO_2$ will rise even further. They will become drowsy, hypertensive and may sweat. Assist their breathing with a bag and mask. Treating persistent hypoventilation in blue bloaters is difficult. If you put them on a ventilator, they are difficult to wean. Many can be helped though an acute episode of *respiratory failure* with an intravenous infusion of the non-specific stimulant, doxapram, but this is not always successful.

15

The respiratory system

More than a third of the patients coming to surgery have respiratory disease that is severe enough to limit their day-to-day activities, or requires treatment. The pre-admission clinic should have identified and optimized these problems before the patient comes to surgery.

The events leading to hypoxia can start at any point between the patient's lips and their mitochondria. On inspiration, oxygen-rich air flows along a series of airways into the lungs, where the oxygen enters the bloodstream. Here it is loaded on to haemoglobin in the red cells and pumped through the circulation to the tissues, to finally diffuse into the cells where it is used. Weak points in this sequence are: the patency of the airways, the health of lungs, the quantity and quality of the haemoglobin, the adequacy of cardiac output, and various metabolic factors.

Hypoxia

Above all you must make sure patients under your care do not become hypoxic. The onset of hypoxia is subtle. Frequently, it is neither obvious nor predictable, but quickly maims or kills. If you thoroughly understand how and why hypoxia occurs, and how to recognize it, then you are better equipped to prevent it.

The terms *hypoxia* and *hypoxaemia* mean different things. Hypoxia occurs when the tissues do not receive enough oxygen to meet their metabolic needs. The cells respond by temporarily switching to anaerobic metabolism, but the accumulating lactic acid soon poisons them. Brain tissue is irreversibly and quickly damaged by lack of oxygen.

Hypoxaemia occurs when the arterial PaO_2 falls to 60 mmHg (7.89 kPa) or less.

Lactic acidosis is a sign of tissue hypoxia.

Common causes of hypoxaemia

In the recovery room the most common reason for hypoxaemia is a mismatch of perfusion to under-aerated parts of the lung caused by small airway collapse during the anaesthetic. Risk factors include older age, obstructive lung disease, obesity, raised intra-abdominal pressures (such as following laparoscopy) and immobility. Suspect hypoventilation if the patient is drowsy, has received intra-operative opioids, has pinpoint pupils, or cannot sustain a 5-second head lift.

Therapeutic targets

The pulse oximeter is the guardian of safety in the recovery room.

Aim for:

- oxygen saturations above 95% (equivalent to a $PaO_2 > 80$ mmHg 10.53 kPa);
- the ability to sit up, deep breath and cough effectively;
- respiratory rate between 12–14 breaths/min;
- tidal volume of 7 ml/Kg or more;
- clear airways with no wheeze.

Clinical signs

Hypoxia presents with a progression of symptoms.

Early signs include:

- difficulty in concentrating;
- confusion, restlessness, and agitation;
- signs of adrenergic discharge: cool hands and feet, tachycardia;
- oxygen saturation falls below 90%;
- cyanosis.

Later signs include:

- pallor;
- ischaemic chest pain;
- loin pain is possible;
- ST segment depression on ECG;
- hypotension;
- sinus bradycardia;
- convulsions;
- nodal bradycardia;
- coma;
- death with an asystolic arrest.

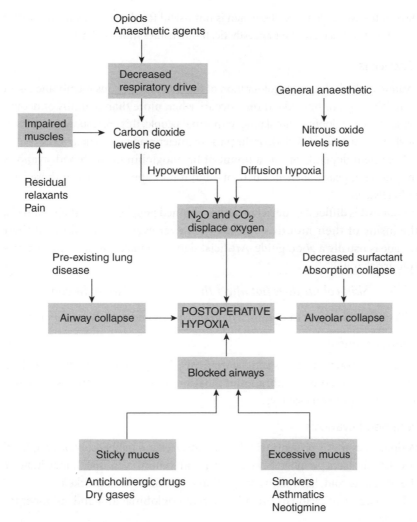

Figure 15.1 Causes of postoperative hypoxia

Since there are many reasons for the earlier signs of hypoxia, it is easy to be misled, and to miss the diagnosis.

*Hypoxia is difficult to assess, at first it may give no signs,
and the absence of cyanosis does not exclude it.*

The best sign of early hypoxia is the inability of the patient to concentrate. Even mild hypoxia makes it difficult to recite backwards the months of the year (or the days of the week). This excellent sign is not useful for the first few minutes after the patient wakes from their anaesthetic, but becomes more so later.

Cyanosis

Cyanosis, with its bluish discolouration of the skin and mucous membranes, is an unreliable sign of hypoxia. It only occurs when more than 3 grams of deoxygenated haemoglobin is circulating. In normal people, this corresponds to a PaO_2 of about 50 mmHg (6.6 kPa), or the pulse oximeter reading less than 85%.

Because it depends on the amount of haemoglobin in the blood, cyanosis may never appear in *anaemic* patients, and it may appear earlier in those with *polycythaemia*.

Cyanosis is difficult to detect in darker-skinned people. Check their nailbeds, the inside of their mouth, or inside the lower eyelid. The colour of their tongue is usually a good guide. Artificial light also makes it difficult to assess colour accurately.

Skin colour does not affect the accuracy of an oximeter.

There are two types of cyanosis: *central cyanosis* and *peripheral cyanosis*.

Central cyanosis

Severe hypoxaemia causes central cyanosis. The patient will have blue lips, tongue and mucous membranes. If a patient has central cyanosis, they will also have peripheral cyanosis.

Peripheral cyanosis

Peripheral cyanosis presents with blue hands, feet and nailbeds. Poor peripheral circulation causes peripheral cyanosis (without central cyanosis). It may indicate the patient is cold, has venous congestion in the limb, or is shocked.

Rare causes of cyanosis include methaemoglobinaemia and sulphaemoglobinaemia.

How to prevent hypoxia

- Give oxygen to patients during their transport from the operating theatre to the recovery room.
- As a minimum precaution give oxygen by mask at 6 L/min for at least 10 minutes after their anaesthetic.
- Nasal prongs do not give enough oxygen, and are useless in the recovery room as patients tend to breathe through their mouths.
- Once they are conscious sit patients up.
- Encourage them to deep breathe and cough.

How to manage hypoxia

Initially:

- Give 100% oxygen with a bag and mask.
- Call for help and summon the anaesthetist.
- Check the airway is clear, the patient is breathing, and air is going in and out of the chest.
- Attach standard monitoring: ECG, pulse oximeter, blood pressure cuff.
- Use a stethoscope to check that air entry is distributed to both lungs.
- Are patients breathing normally? If you are uncertain then use a respirometer to check their tidal and minute volumes. Their tidal volume should be greater than 5 ml/Kg. If it is less than this, then support their breathing with a bag and mask and find a reason.

Later:

- Take arterial blood gases, check the haemoglobin levels, and order a chest X-ray.
- Further therapy could include intubation and the application of *positive end expiratory pressure* (PEEP) and the use of nitric oxide.

Hints

- Treat hypoxaemia (oxygen saturations less than 92%) with high concentrations of oxygen.
- Treat hypoventilation (raised end-expired CO_2) by improving breathing.
- Monitor all patients with a pulse oximeter, but know its limitations.
- Assume that your patients are severely hypoxic if they are restless, agitated, confused or have a clouded conscious state.
- Eliminate the more serious causes of hypoxia: pneumothorax, cardiac tamponade, gas embolism, and anaphylaxis.
- Opioids may cause respiratory depression, which in the elderly may last for many hours.
- Send elderly patients to the ward on oxygen.
- Naloxone (Narcan®), an opioid antagonist, works for about 30–40 minutes, and may wear off before the effects of the opioid. You can prolong naloxone's action by 10–15 minutes if you give it intramuscularly.
- It is difficult to give oxygen to active children, because they may not tolerate a mask over their face. Studies show that, in the recovery room, up to 30 per cent of children have moderate to severe hypoxia at some stage.

Table 15.1 Signs of hypoventilation and hypoxia

Signs of hypoventilation	Signs of hypoxia
High $PaCO_2$	Low PaO_2
Drowsiness	Inability to concentrate and anxiety
Coma	Restlessness
Bounding pulse	Vasoconstriction cyanosis
Vasodilation	Hypertension and tachycardia
	Breathlessness
	Bradycardia
	Asystolic cardiac arrest
Treat by improving ventilation	Treat with oxygen

Hypoventilation

Hypercarbia occurs once the arterial $PaCO_2$ rises above 45 mmHg (5.92 kPa). Someone with hypercarbia is, by definition, hypoventilating. Clinicians prefer to use the term hypoventilation instead of hypercarbia. Hypoventilation may be acute or chronic.

Chronic hypoventilation occurs with severe chronic obstructive airways disease. Over time, as the patient's PCO_2 creeps up, the kidneys retain bicarbonate to balance it; in this way the plasma pH remains normal.

Acute hypoventilation occurs commonly in the recovery room because patients' breathing is frequently depressed by opioids, or the incomplete reversal of muscle relaxants. This prevents carbon dioxide being washed out of their lungs. As their minute volume decreases, they develop a progressive respiratory acidosis and eventually become hypoxaemic. For this reason patients who have received an opioid need supplemental oxygen

Hypoxia causes agitation and anxiety.
Hypercarbia causes drowsiness, and lethargy.

Clinical signs

Hypoventilation presents with a progression of signs:

- initially breathlessness (but not if the patient has received an opioid);
- tachycardia;
- hypertension;
- drowsiness;
- ventricular extrasystoles;
- flushing and cutaneous dilatation;
- coma.

In an otherwise healthy person hypercarbia causes hypoxaemia once the $PaCO_2$ exceeds 80 mmHg (10.53 kPa). If the patient is receiving supplemental oxygen hypercarbia is not lethal in itself until the $PaCO_2$ exceeds 120 mmHg (15.79 kPa).

How to manage hypoventilation

If a patient is not breathing deeply enough, or has respiratory rate of less than 8 breaths a minute, then give oxygen while you assess the problem.

Is the respiratory centre depressed?

All opioids depress the rate and depth of breathing. Babies and the elderly can remain affected by the short-acting ones such as fentanyl after admission to the recovery room. Look for the signs of opioid intoxication: pinpoint pupils, shallow breathing and pallor. Patients affected by excessive opioids will take deep breaths and cough actively when you ask them to, but then resume their shallow breathing.

Are the respiratory muscles weak?

Residual paralysis from muscle relaxants may persist after the patient is admitted to the recovery room, but more insidiously it may return when the anti-cholinergic drug used to reverse the muscle relaxant in the operating theatre wears off. This takes about 30–40 minutes. Patients with residual paralysis move jerkily like a floppy rag doll. They are unable to lift their heads from the pillow and maintain this for 5 seconds. You can test peripheral muscle strength by asking patients to squeeze your fingers. Offer your forefinger and middle finger and ask them to squeeze them as hard as they can.

Airways obstruction

Airway obstruction can be total or partial. It can occur at any point between the lips or nose and the alveoli. The commonest points are in the oropharynx, or at the airway's narrowest point between the vocal cords in the larynx.

Anatomy of the airway

Figure 15.2 illustrates the anatomy of an airway. Simply placing the head on a pillow and extending the neck usually opens up an obstructed airway.

Neonates are obligate nose breathers. They cannot breathe through their mouths, so if their nose becomes blocked they will struggle for breath. Their whole chest may be drawn in by the respiratory effort.

The main cause of airway obstruction is due to the tongue falling back into the pharynx to block the airway. This is more likely to occur if the patient is lying on their back.

Tongue has fallen back
to obstruct airway

Figure 15.2 How to maintain an airway

Total airway obstruction

Total airway obstruction is silent and lethal. Simply because you can see the chest move up and down does not mean any air is going in or out. See-saw breathing is a sign of a totally obstructed airway. While trying to breathe the patient's chest falls away as their abdomen rises, and vice versa. However, with ordinary breathing, both the abdomen and the chest wall rise and fall together.

Obstruction of an artificial airway

Patients awakening from anaesthesia often clench their jaws tightly shut (trismus). If their endotracheal tube or laryngeal mask happens to be between their teeth, they will bite down and occlude the lumen. Prevent this by inserting a Guedel airway alongside their endotracheal tube. If the patient does clench their teeth you can sometimes provoke them to open their mouth momentarily. To do this gently poke a flexible sucker straight back along the floor of their nose to stimulate a gag reflex. The lumens of endotracheal tubes can be obstructed by mucus plugs, kinks in the tube, or a cuff that has herniated over the distal end of the tube. If the endotracheal tube is obstructed, then remove it.

Stridor

Stridor is the crowing noise made by turbulent airflow as it is forced through a narrowing in the larynx or upper airway. Stridor trumpets disaster. Once the airflow through the larynx is narrow enough to cause stridor complete airway obstruction is not far off. Get help quickly.

Stridor means death is near.

Snoring is a form of stridor caused by soft tissues collapsing around the upper airway. Relieve it by extending the patient's head.

In the recovery no one should be allowed to snore.

Laryngospasm

Laryngospasm is another cause of stridor. You will hear a harsh crowing noisy as the patient tries to breathe in. A conscious patient who is struggling to breathe will panic.

Laryngospasm is a common and dangerous sign that something is irritating the larynx or pharynx, and causing the true and false vocal cords to clamp shut. Normally this reflex prevents food or fluid entering the lungs when we eat or drink. However, in the recovery room it becomes rapidly life-threatening if not relieved.

Extubation sometimes triggers laryngospasm particularly in children, and is more likely if intubation has been difficult or traumatic. About 20 per cent of children get stridor after tonsillectomy. Laryngospasm is also common after bronchoscopy, or surgery on the upper airway and thyroid surgery.

Initial management

- Give 100% oxygen by mask – even a few breaths helps.
- Send someone to fetch the anaesthetist.
- You will need two assistants. The first assistant to attach your standard monitors: ECG, oximeter, and measure the pulse rate and prepares to measure blood pressure. The second assistant to fetch the emergency trolley (cart) and prepares to draw up drugs for intubation.
- Meanwhile inspect the patient's airway with a laryngoscope and suck out the pharynx.
- Firmly thrust the patients jaw forward with your fingers behind the angle of the mandible and pull firmly upwards. (Ask an anaesthetist to teach you this very useful manoeuvre.)
- Once you are sure the airway is clear, use a bag and mask to apply firm continuous *positive pressure* to relieve the spasm.

If this is unsuccessful:

- An intravenous bolus of 1.5 mg/Kg lidocaine often resolves the problem;
- If this fails then the only option is urgent intubation.

Other problems:

- Attempts to inflate the patient may cause the stomach to distend with gas. A nasogastric tube may be needed to deflate the stomach;
- *Pulmonary oedema* occasionally occurs in young people who try vigorously to inspire against a close glottis.

Laryngeal oedema

Laryngeal function is disturbed for at least 4 hours after tracheal extubation. Keep patients who have been intubated under observation for this period. This precaution is especially important in children who have been intubated for day case surgery. Oedema in the upper airways occasionally follows extubation in children, and more frequently in neonates and infants. A small amount of reactive oedema will intrude on the narrow lumen rapidly occluding it.

Mild cases respond to warmed and humidified oxygen. However, it may be necessary to use nebulized adrenaline to shrink the mucosa. Take two 1 ml ampoules of 1:1000 adrenaline and make them up to 5 ml in 0.9% saline. Give this by oxygen-driven nebulizer at a 5 L/min flow through a face mask. The effect lasts about 2 hours. Although this seems to be a big dose for a small child, it is most effective.

Other causes of *laryngeal oedema* occur with:

- thyroidectomy, carotid endarterectomy, or other operations on the neck;
- airway burns;
- trauma to the neck;
- subcutaneous surgical emphysema.

Vocal cord damage

Vocal cord paralysis or damage is a rare complication of surgery, it is easily diagnosed, because the patient is unable to say "Eeeee" in a high-pitched whine like a mosquito.

Vocal cord paralysis occurs if the laryngeal nerves are damaged during thyroid or major neck surgery. Unilateral vocal cord paresis presents as hoarseness in the recovery room but usually resolves over several weeks.

Bilateral vocal cord paralysis is serious. It presents with upper airway obstruction as soon as the patient is extubated but it does not respond to standard measures to control stridor. Applying firm continuous positive airway *pressure* with a bag and mask may temporarily overcome the obstruction. Laryngoscopy reveals motionless vocal cords lying slightly apart (adducted) and a narrow V-shaped aperture. The patient will need a tracheostomy.

Patients with rheumatoid arthritis or other connective tissue diseases have tenuous attachments where their laryngeal muscles insert into cartilage. The muscles easily tear off their insertions during intubation, or if the patient coughs on the endotracheal tube.

Cough

Coughing signals irritation in the larynx or lower airway. This protective reflex so explosively expels material in the airway that the velocity of the ejected air exceeds the speed of sound. With paroxysms of coughing, patients may be unable to get their breath; they become distressed and turn purple in the face. The venous congestion aggravates bleeding in head and neck surgery, and can cause catastrophic bleeding following eye, ear or neurosurgery. The raised vascular pressures can cause retinal detachment. Coughing may contribute to cardiac arrhythmias and disrupt abdominal sutures; or in the elderly break their ribs (cough fractures).

A cough progressing to stridor is life-threatening.

Frequently, coughing is a problem after rigid bronchoscopy or laryngeal surgery. Patients may not be able to get their breath between paroxysms and become cyanosed, hypoxic and distressed. Sit them up, and give high doses of humidified oxygen. Attach a pulse oximeter. Summon the anaesthetist. Listen to the chest with a stethoscope. A localized wheeze may suggest aspirated foreign material, usually into the right lower lobe posteriorly.

Nebulized lidocaine 1.5 mg/Kg in 5 ml of saline will settle almost any cough. If not, then sedation and intubation allows time to appraise the situation.

Morphine is an effective cough suppressant, but pethidine or tramadol are not. With excessive sputum production, it is unwise to suppress cough, because any accumulating sputum will block airways causing partial lung collapse.

Dyspnoea

Dyspnoea is a subjective feeling of breathlessness. In the recovery room dyspnoea is always a warning sign of something serious. Causes include: pneumothorax, cardiac failure myocardial ischaemia, anaphylaxis, aspiration and late in haemorrhagic shock. Patients with cardiac failure become uncomfortable if they attempt to lie flat; conversely shocked patients feel worse sitting up.

Sputum retention

Sputum retention is common in smokers and those with chronic bronchitis. Some people, especially those with severe emphysema, are unable to cough effectively enough to eject their sputum. Sputum sticking in their larynx may cause stridor. Humidified oxygen helps keep the sputum liquid enough to cough up.

Some elderly patients (especially those with brainstem ischaemia) lie there oblivious of the gurgle they make every time they breathe. Most of these patients have such poor laryngeal and pharyngeal protective reflexes that you can simply open their mouth, and with the aid of a laryngoscope and Magill forceps pass a soft plastic sucker down their trachea. Thoroughly pre-oxygenate them first. Do not distress them by persisting with suction if they do not cough.

Wheeze

Wheezing indicates irritation, inflammation or oedema of the bronchioles. As air passes along narrowed tubes it causes their walls to vibrate producing an audible sound like the reed vibrating in a clarinet. You will hear wheeze best if you listen near patients' mouths as they breathe out forcibly with their mouth wide open.

> *In the recovery room a developing wheeze*
> *is always potentially serious.*

Causes of wheeze include aspiration, anaphylaxis, developing pulmonary oedema, and pulmonary embolism; but almost never asthma.

Aspiration

By far the most common cause of wheeze starting in the recovery room is aspiration of a small amount material from the pharynx into the lower airway. This usually occurs shortly after extubation, especially if the patient is lying on their back. Immediately after the patient has aspirated the wheeze will be confined to one lung.

> *Consider any wheeze occurring within an hour*
> *of an offending stimulus to be anaphylaxis.*

Anaphylaxis

Anaphylaxis may present with a generalized wheeze, as may acute cardiac failure. Anaphylaxis usually presents immediately, or a few minutes after some offending substance is given intravenously. In this case wheezing frequently precedes profound cardiovascular collapse. Occasionally the reaction may take an hour or more to develop. Offending substances include blood, or its products, penicillin, morphine, muscle relaxants and NSAIDs or a plasma expander or anything else to which the patient is allergic.

Cardiac failure

Acute left ventricular failure with pulmonary oedema is often a result of fluid overload during or after the anaesthetic. Check the fluid balance sheet. If the patient has received more than 2 litres of fluid during their procedure then suspect pulmonary oedema. Other causes of acute pulmonary oedema include heart failure caused by acute myocardial infarction or ischaemia.

Gas embolism

Air or gas embolism is a worrying cause of wheeze. If a patient starts to wheeze abruptly, immediately check that the central venous catheter connection has not come apart.

A chest X-ray helps diagnosis

A chest X-ray can help with the diagnosis of wheeze. At first, cardiac failure shows up as a generalized haziness on the film. Later this may coalesce into the classic bat's wing picture stretching out from the hilum of the lung. Aspiration shows nothing at first, and it may take several hours or more to develop a picture of localized haziness, especially in the right lower lobe. The chest X-ray after air or gas embolism may never show anything at all.

Cardiac failure or asthma

Because wheeze is common to both conditions acute left ventricular failure is often confused with an acute asthmatic attack. It is extremely unlikely elderly patients will have their first acute asthma attack in the recovery room. To help with the diagnosis, eliminate the possibility of fluid overload with a chest X-ray; or consider the possibility of an acute allergic reaction to a drug, blood or plasma expander.

All wheezes are not asthma.

Difficult airways

Anticipate that you may have difficultly in maintaining an airway in patients with:

- short or fat bull necks;
- stiff necks;
- prominent upper teeth;
- underslung jaws;

- Down's syndrome;
- Turner's syndrome;
- patients who cannot open their mouths widely;
- previous cervical spine surgery.

Cervical spine disease

X-rays studies in patients with rheumatoid arthritis show 20 per cent have cervical spine instability. It is possible to cause *subluxation* of the atlanto-occipital joint when you extend the neck. This may sever the spinal cord, or damage their vertebral arteries; be gentle. Patients with rheumatoid arthritis often have temporomandibular joint (TMJ) stiffness and are unable to open their mouths widely.

Other causes of airway obstruction include a forgotten throat pack after surgery on the upper airway, laryngeal oedema after neck surgery, tracheomalacia occurring after long-standing tracheal compression, and a foreign body at any point in the airway.

Aspiration of foreign material

Aspiration of stomach contents into lungs is every anaesthetist's nightmare. Aspiration occurs if the laryngeal reflexes fail to prevent foreign material entering the trachea and lower airways. A flood of blood or gastric acid may kill the patient. Lesser degrees of aspiration cause a progression of stridor, wheeze, respiratory distress and partial or complete collapse of the lungs.

The foreign material can be:

- vomitus, gastric secretions, blood, pharyngeal secretions;
- a piece of tooth, a forgotten throat pack, a fragment of adenoid tissue or the top your sucker.

If there is any evidence of aspiration the patient needs to be re-anaesthetized and the situation assessed with a rigid bronchoscope. Every recovery room needs the provision to do an urgent adult or paediatric bronchoscopy.

Aspiration pneumonitis

Depending on the amount and nature of the aspirated material, acute chemical aspiration pneumonitis may be fatal. This event is particularly fulminant and deadly in pregnant patients where it is termed Mendleson's syndrome (although the term is now used for all aspiration pneumonitis).

Many patients aspirate small quantities of fluid from their pharynx soon after they emerge from anaesthesia. The immediate consequences are few, but these small amounts probably contribute to postoperative chest infections in the elderly that surface a day or so later. To prevent aspiration nurse your patients in the recovery position.

Any sedated patient is at risk of aspiration.

Suspect aspiration if the patent has vomited or regurgitated and then becomes wheezy, tachypnoeic, and coughs vigorously. They may desaturate as the wheeze develops. Usually, these initial symptoms resolve with humidification and bronchodilation, but the real trouble starts several hours later as the patient becomes progressively hypoxaemic, tachypnoeic and develops respiratory failure.

It is difficult to predict which patients are going to develop severe aspiration pneumonitis and respiratory failure. The published advice is not helpful, and the evidence quoted is based on limited animal research. What is clear is that aspiration of large volumes (> 25 ml) is more serious than small volumes, that particulate matter (such as milk curds) causes more problems than clear fluid, and that acid aspiration is the most devastating event of all.

How to manage massive aspiration

Massive aspiration is an emergency. As with all emergencies, you will need three additional staff to help you. One person to monitor the vital signs, the second to prepare drips, drugs and fetch trolleys, and the third to summon the anaesthetist and be ready to run errands. Your job is to keep the patient alive by preserving their airway and ensuring oxygenation.

If an unconscious patient vomits or regurgitates then:

- immediately place the patient in the left lateral position with a 30° head-down tilt;
- suck out the pharynx including the nose;
- ventilate with 100% oxygen;
- get help to attach oximeter, and ECG;
- send for the anaesthetist;
- prepare to re-intubate the patient for bronchoscopy;
- expect bronchospasm, and prepare to treat it.

Later treatment may include:

- fibreoptic bronchoscopy to unblock airways and assess the damage. A rigid bronchoscopy may make the problem worse because the air injector used to ventilate the patient blasts aspirated material deeper into the lungs;
- give salbutamol by aerosol, or intravenously if necessary;
- bronchial lavage is not recommended. It tends to spread the aspirated to unaffected parts of the lungs;

- steroids are contraindicated because they impair the immune response, and prevent localization of the inevitable infection;
- prophylactic antibiotics are not recommended at this early stage, because they select out the resistant bacteria;
- transfer to intensive care, but avoid ventilation if possible. Ventilation abolishes the vital ability to deep breathe and cough;
- antibiotic therapy when the principal (usually anaerobic) bacteria have declared themselves and the patient has developed a fever.

How to prevent aspiration pneumonitis

- Where possible, nurse each patient in the recovery position until they are fully conscious.
- Identify those at risk; they are people who are likely to have full stomachs, or have gastro-oesophageal reflux, or any disease that would prevent them guarding their airways should they vomit or regurgitate.
- Treat all pregnant women as high-risk patients.
- Proper but not prolonged fasting preoperatively. Water usefully dilutes gastric acid and should be freely available until 2 hours before induction.
- Use prophylactic ranitidine and antacids 2–3 hours before surgery, and then give them 0.3 molar sodium citrate 30 ml just before induction, and then roll them over to spread it around.

Pneumothorax

When air, which is normally confined to the lung, escapes into the pleural space and is trapped there it causes a *pneumothorax*. Pneumothorax is usually accompanied by pleuritic pain that is so sharp and severe that the patient dare only to breathe in short shallow pants, and stops abruptly with a grunt when he feels pain. Other signs include an unexplained tachycardia, hypotension, wheeze, short sharp inspiratory movements, cyanosis and sometimes *surgical emphysema*.

A pneumothorax may occur:

- during the insertion of intercostal, cervical, or supraclavicular brachial plexus blocks;
- during the insertion of a central venous line or pulmonary venous catheter;
- in patients with bullae in the lung (congenital or acquired with emphysema); Marfan's syndrome, chest trauma or rib fracture, and barotrauma;

Surgical emphysema

Surgical emphysema occurs when air or gas escapes into the tissues. There is a peculiar crackling feeling to the skin and subcutaneous tissues. The most likely cause is a breach in the pleura and a hole in the lung during operations on the neck, rib resection, kidney operations, trauma to the rib cage; and following external cardiac massage where ribs are fractured. It also occurs with distension and rupture of alveoli if the expiratory limb of the anaesthetic circuit or ventilator becomes obstructed. The gas tracks along the sheaths of the blood vessels to the hilum of the lung, from where it spreads to the neck and chest wall. Sometimes the crackling crepitations can be felt in the suprasternal notch. This is diagnostic of air in the mediastinum and may follow a ruptured bronchi, or mid-line trauma such as a stab wound.

- after thoracic surgery if the tubing on a chest drain becomes kinked or occluded in some way. If the drain tube stops bubbling exclude this cause first;
- following nephrectomy, where the pleura has been accidentally breached or a rib resected for easier surgical access;
- as a complication of laparoscopic surgery.

If the escaped air or gas collects under pressure it causes a tension pneumothorax. The collection of air progressively grows in size to squash the lungs, heart and major blood vessels. Blood vessels get kinked and the cardiac output falls. In the recovery room the patient may suddenly panic, collapse, go blue in the face and struggle to breathe, with almost undetectable pulses. Sometimes the neck veins will be grossly distended. The displaced heart and lungs push the trachea to the opposite side. No breath sounds can be heard on the affected side, and if you percuss the chest the note will be booming (similar to what you hear if you percuss a pillow). Listening with the stethescope at the same time as the percussion improves your ability to diagnose a pneumothorax.

In neonates sometimes simply holding a bright light behind the chest will reveal the pneumothorax.

A tension pneumothorax is a medical emergency.

Cricothyroid puncture

There are a number of commercially available tracheostomy sets which are designed for quick and easy insertion. However, in an emergency situation, where the patient is becoming cyanosed, or his conscious state is deteriorating, you may not have time to organize this. You may have to perform an acute cricothyroid puncture.

Figure 15.3 Improvised cricothyroid puncture set

Take the largest bore intravenous cannula you have, (preferably 10 G or bigger) and insert it through the cricothyroid membrane into the trachea. Attach the barrel of a 2 ml syringe into the needle and then jam a No. 8 endotracheal 15 mm adaptor into the barrel of the syringe. It will now be possible to attach the cannula to a self-inflating bag or T-piece to support the patient's oxygenation until a tracheostomy or other means of establishing an airway can be achieved.

Figure 15.4 Location of cricothyroid puncture

Initial management

- call for help;
- sit patient up;
- give high concentrations of oxygen;
- attach pulse oximeter and ECG.

Further management

If the patient has collapsed with a suspected pneumothorax, and you are unsure what side is affected, then aspirate each side with 23 G needle through the second intercostal space in the mid-clavicular line on either side. If you freely aspirate air on one side then you will need to insert an intercostal catheter on that side. While preparing to insert the catheter push a 14 G cannula through the same spot you found free air when you aspirated. This will relieve the pneumothorax quickly.

Ventilators

Ventilators support the breathing of patients who are not able to breath for themselves. They are used on paralysed patients under anaesthesia, and in the intensive care unit to manage acute respiratory failure for whatever the cause. They are occasionally used in the recovery room where a patient does not reverse properly from their muscle relaxants.

About normal breathing

The normal respiratory rate is about 12 to 15 breaths/min. The active inspiratory phase takes about one second, the passive expiratory phase, takes about 2 seconds where air and the pause lasts for just under two seconds. The ebb and flow of air give a tidal volume of about 400 ml with each breath so that the normal minute volume is about 5 litres. Depending on the health of the lungs, it takes an intrathoracic negative pressure of minus 3 to minus 7 cm H_2O to suck the tidal volume into the lungs.

How a positive pressure ventilator works

Breathing in is easy

Ventilators impose intermittent positive pressure ventilation (IPPV) on the lungs; they blow them up like a balloon, and then pause to allow them to passively deflate. In normal lungs the pressure needed to inflate them is 7–15 ml H_2O.

Breathing out may be a problem

Air is forced out of the lungs by the springiness of this elastic tissue. This works well in young people with healthy lungs, but ageing causes the lung elastin to degenerate into collagen. The young have compliant lungs, which when stretched behave like an elastic band. In contrast the elderly have non-compliant lungs that behave more like chewing gum. The result is that, in the elderly, more air remains in the lungs at the end of the expiration and their functional residual capacity is higher.

How ventilators work

Ventilators inflate the patient's lungs, and then allow time for expiration. They generate a *positive pressure*, then cycle from the inspiratory phase to the expiratory phase and back again. Most ventilators deliver a fixed volume of gas before cycling to the expiratory phase, and have controls to alter the volume, the timing or the pressure of gas delivered.

On top of this basic design are added safety features including alarms to warn if the preset conditions are not achieved, and safety release valves to prevent barotrauma.

Other features include provision to: nebulize and humidify the gas; apply a sigh; adjust the inspiratory waveform; provide intermittent mandatory ventilation; allow the patient to trigger the switching mechanism; control of oxygen concentration and applying positive end-expiratory pressures.

Figure 15.5 The respiratory cycle

Ideal ventilators should be:

- simple to operate;
- easy to maintain;
- compact;

- robust;
- portable;
- economical to run.

 Ventilators should be able to generate:

- an inspiratory flow rate of 100 litres/min;
- tidal volume between 50 and 1500 ml;
- rates between 5 and 50 per minute;
- variable inspiratory and expiratory ratios.

How ventilation affects pulse pressure

The outcome of this pumping effect on the veins in the thorax is that the blood pressure rises on inspiration and falls on expiration. You can often see this if the patient has an arterial line. The reverse happens if the patient is breathing spontaneously; the pulse pressure falls on inspiration and rises on expiration.

Pulse pressure rises on inspiration and falls
as pressure in the great veins decreases.

Figure 15.6 Pulse pressure rises on inspiration and falls as pressure in the great veins decreases

 This effect is more obvious if the patient's vascular volume is under-filled. So if you see this arterial wave pattern developing on the monitor suspect the patient vascular volume is depleted. You can confirm this by looking for the *postural drop* in their systolic blood pressure.

 Maintain a normal $PaCO_2$ in a ventilated patient in the recovery room.

Typical ventilator settings

For an unconscious adult patient with normal lungs the usual settings are:

1. Respiratory rate = 14 breaths/min.
2. Inspiratory pressure = + 5 cm H20.

3. Inspiratory time = 1.2 seconds.
4. Expiratory time = 3.5 seconds.
5. Tidal volume = 8 ml/Kg.
6. The sigh mechanism = 40 sighs an hour.

Adverse effects of IPPV

The lungs are designed to suck air in to them, but not to be blown up under positive pressure like a balloon. Blood flow through the alveolar capillary units depends on the mean pulmonary pressure imposed by the ventilator rather than the peaks and troughs.

Adverse effects of positive pressure ventilation include:

- depression of the myocardial contractility so that cardiac output falls;
- activation of the sympathetic nervous system;
- disturbance of the blood flow through the lungs, kidneys, and brain.

Positive end expiratory pressure

Positive end expiratory pressure (PEEP) improves oxygenation by recruiting alveoli that would otherwise not be aerated. This increases the surface area of the alveoli available for gas exchange and prevents *terminal respiratory units* collapsing at the end of expiration. PEEP keeps the intrathoracic pressure continually elevated. Typical pressures are between 2.5 and 15 cmH$_2$O.

Advantage

PEEP keeps small airways open, especially the non-axial airways, which otherwise would be closed. It therefore reduces the lungs' dead space. PEEP increases the total available surface area of the respiratory units by opening up airways in the apex and mid-zones of the lung.

Disadvantage

PEEP increases the risk of barotrauma to lungs, and it causes cardiac output to fall and lowers the blood pressure.

BiPAP

Bi-level positive pressure airway pressure (BiPAP) is used to restore the functional residual capacity in patients who have have difficulty in emptying the air out of their lungs.

BiPAP is also used to treat high-pressure pulmonary oedema, and pneumonia. The patient wears a tight fitting mask strapped over their mouth and nose. When the patient starts to breathe in, the device delivers an inspiratory positive airway pressure (IPAP) to help the patient achieve a larger tidal breath. When the patient finishes inspiration, the machine allows the patient to exhale passively with a little bit of back pressure support (PS) to splint the floppy airways open to the expiratory positive airway pressure (EPAP).

$$PS = PAP - IPAP$$

Most machines allow the patient to take a spontaneous breath in (assist mode), or they can be set to cycle in (control mode).

Normal settings are:

IPAP 5–10 cm H_2O

EPAP 3–5 cm H_2O

If the patient's oxygen saturations fail to improve then the settings are adjusted in 3–5 cm H_2O increments.

BiPAP is not easy to use. It requires persistence to make BiPAP work effectively. If the patient's respiratory rate rises to 20 breaths/min or they start to use their accessory muscles to help them breathe, then it is time for the anaesthetist to reassess the situation.

Lung diseases

Asthma

Asthma is a chronic lung disease with reversible airway obstruction. It occurs when a usually trivial stimuli causes the bronchioles to become inflamed and oedematous. In some countries asthma affects up to 10 per cent of the population, and is particularly common in children. For most surgery the patient's peak flow rate (PFR) should not be less than 150 L/sec, but for abdominal or thoracic surgery the PFR needs to be at least 220 L/sec.

In the recovery room, asthma usually does not cause problems, because volatile anaesthetic gases are superb bronchodilators. If a non-asthmatic patient starts to wheeze then suspect aspiration, anaphylaxis or cardiac failure.

Asthma never presents for the first time in the recovery room.

Because morphine can release histamine it may theoretically cause bronchoconstriction in asthmatics, but this does not seem to happen. On the other hand NSAIDs often aggravate bronchoconstriction and should not be used in asthmatics unless they tell you they have had them in the past without problems.

Chronic obstructive airways disease

Smoking is the main reason for chronic obstructive airways disease (COAD). In older people the usual reason is cigarettes and, in those under the age of 40 years, marijuana remains a suspect.

COAD ranges between two extremes. At one extreme is *emphysema*, where the lung's *parenchyma* is extensively damaged. The walls between the terminal respiratory units are destroyed forming large blebs in the lung where air gets trapped. In severe cases these patients are more comfortable breathing in short shallow breaths – the so-called pink *puffers*.

At the other end of the range is *chronic bronchitis* where years of inflammation have destroyed the cartilage rings holding the bronchi open. Consequently airways become floppy and collapse. Moreover mucosal goblet cells proliferate producing large amounts of sputum.

With COAD and asthma the patient has no trouble breathing in, but because small airways collapse, getting the air out again is a problem. These patients (called *blue bloaters*) are more comfortable taking deep gulping breaths, and then blowing out through pursed lips which creates back pressure on the airways. The back pressure splints their floppy airways open allowing them to expire more fully. Sometimes anaesthetists add expiratory retard valves to their circuits to achieve the same effect.

The closer the surgical incision is to the diaphragm, the greater the respiratory problems in the recovery room. Pain from upper abdominal or thoracic incision severely limits respiratory effort. Epidural analgesia gives optimal pain relief. In contrast, morphine depresses ventilation, and pethidine dries secretions making sputum more difficult to cough up.

Patients with COAD are more comfortable, and have better gas exchange if they sit up in the recovery room. Give 35% oxygen by mask and where possible humidify the inspired air. Encourage deep breathing and coughing. If patients find it difficult to breathe, become distressed or hypoxaemic then consider short-term respiratory support with continuous positive airway pressure (CPAP) or BiPAP masks. Arterial blood gases help decide about ongoing management. Anaesthetists are reluctant to re-intubate patients with COAD, because they are difficult to wean from artificial ventilation.

Embolism to the lungs

Various materials can be carried in the blood stream to lodge in the lungs. This event can obstruct blood flow and cause an inflammatory response. The most common emboli are air, blood clots, fat and amniotic fluid.

Air embolism

Air embolism occurs when air, or some other gas, enters the circulation, usually through a vein. Air embolism causes the patient to collapse abruptly. In the recovery room, it usually occurs during the insertion, or accidental disconnection of a central venous line. About 100–200 ml of gas abruptly entering a vein is enough to cause a cardiac arrest. About 100 ml of air can be sucked through a 14-gauge needle in one second with a negative gradient of 5 cm H_2O. Despite these alarming facts, most air emboli are minor, and their effects transient.

Once a large bolus of air enters the right ventricle, it makes the blood froth. The churning mass of bubbles blocks blood flow to the lungs. Unable to achieve a cardiac output the patient suddenly becomes hypoxic, cyanosed, hypotensive, with a feeble pulse, tachycardia and engorged neck veins and has a cardiac arrest. You may hear the characteristic *mill-wheel murmur* if you listen over the posterior chest wall. The murmur sounds as if water is squelching around inside a Wellington boot.

Signs of less severe embolism are a strident dry cough, wheeze, chest pain and breathlessness.

Detectable air embolism occurs during 11 per cent of Caesarean sections. Air enters the circulation when the surgeon is handling the uterus. If the patient is awake, she usually becomes breathless, alarmed, hypotensive and her oxygen saturations decline. The anaesthetist will notify the surgeon, and then manage the problem appropriately depending on its severity. However, the patient may still be alarmed and fearful when she returns to the recovery room. Her chest may still feel painful, if necessary a small dose of morphine usually helps her. Comforting reassurance from the nursing staff that her distress will pass quickly is a better option.

Gas embolism occurs quite frequently in the operating theatre. During laparoscopy carbon dioxide under pressure is used to inflate the peritoneum. Sometimes some of the gas enters the venous circulation and is carried to the right heart.

Occasionally bubbles of gas pass through a patent foramen ovale or ventricular septal defect to enter the left ventricle and embolize to some distal vascular bed. Since 18 per cent of the cardiac output goes to the brain there is an 18 per cent chance of the gas bubble causing a stroke.

What to do first

In the recovery room most gas embolism occurs during the insertion of a central venous line, or if the line is accidentally disconnected allowing air to enter. Immediately stop further air entering the vein; if necessary put your finger over the hole where air is going in. Call for help. Give high concentrations of oxygen. Tip the patient into a 15° head-down position so that the hole is below the heart level. Do not put them in a steep head-down tilt, because you will jeopardise gas exchange in their lung.

Turn the patient on to their left side (*Durrant's manoeuvre*). This manoeuvre may possibly lessen the amount of air entering the pulmonary arteries. Attempt to aspirate air from the central venous line (this is not usually fruitful). If you cannot feel the carotid pulse then treat the patient as a cardiac arrest. Some clinicians feel cardiac massage may help break up the froth. There are reports of extreme cases of air embolism being treated successfully with direct large bore needle aspiration of the right ventricle, cardiopulmonary bypass, or thoracotomy.

What to do next

The patient needs high flow oxygen for at least 6 hours to help wash the nitrogen out of their blood, and absorb the air from the bloodstream. Hyperbaric oxygen rapidly speeds this process, but it is not always available.

Fat embolism

Fat embolism syndrome (FES) is a major hazard affecting 10 per cent of patients who have had major bone trauma. FES occurs 12–72 hours after bones are broken either from trauma or with orthopaedic surgery. Broken or cut bone releases fat globules from the marrow into the circulation. Almost instantly, plasma lipases degrade the fat into fatty acids that are toxic to the cells lining the lung's capillaries. The damaged alveolar capillary membrane allows fluid to leak into the lung's interstitium and alveoli causing pulmonary oedema. To add to the disaster, the fat can trigger disseminated intravascular coagulation.

Fat emboli syndrome may present in the recovery room, especially in trauma cases admitted the previous day or after surgery such as on the tibia. As pulmonary oedema develops the patient becomes progressively breathless, and their oxygen saturation begins to fall. Damage to the capillaries in the brain allows fluid to leak out to cause cerebral oedema resulting in headache, confusion and eventually a deteriorating conscious state. Although not always present a good clinical sign are tiny pricks of purple petechia on the patient's trunk, under their fingernails, and even in their retina.

Early stabilization of fractures and good resuscitation helps prevent this disaster. There is no specific treatment apart from preserving oxygenation. Mortality can reach 45 per cent in florid cases. Occasionally, FES also occurs after bone marrow transplantation and liposuction.

Venothromboembolism

Thromboembolism

It is unlikely you will encounter pulmonary embolism (PE) in the recovery room, but it is the number-one killer on the ward and in the weeks following discharge from hospital. If blood clots (thrombi) form in the great veins of the legs and pelvis, they can break off and lodge in the lung, plugging blood vessels like a cork. The effect may be catastrophic. Within a few seconds the patient collapses, becomes desperately short of breath, frightened and panics. They can have a cardiac arrest and die. A chest X-ray or ECG may reveal little or nothing at this early stage. If you listen over the affected area with a stethoscope, you will hear a transient wheeze. Treatment involves giving oxygen, treating bronchospasm and anticoagulation with heparin.

Deep vein thrombosis

Deep vein thrombosis (DVT) is the ninja of the post operative period; stealthy, concealed and deadly. Deep vein thrombosis occurs when blood clots form in the large veins in the legs, or pelvis.[1] Deep vein thrombosis is one part of a syndrome called *venothromboembolic disease* (VTE). Other components to the syndrome include pulmonary embolism and post-thrombotic venous disease. DVT is particularly common after orthopaedic surgery, pelvic surgery and in patients with heart failure, cancer, or those who have had previous clots. It becomes more common as people age, and it may occur spontaneously. Patients over the age of 60 years are at particular risk. The incidence of DVT ranges from 36–84 per cent in patients who did not receive anticoagulants after total hip replacement or hip fracture surgery.[2] After major hip surgery, where patients have not received DVT prophylaxis, the risk of fatal pulmonary embolism is as high as 13 per cent. Even with DVT prophylaxis the rate of VTE is still 18–20 per cent although few of these progress to pulmonary emboli.

Why DVT occurs

Over one hundred years ago Professor Gustav Virchow described a triad of risk factors for deep vein thrombosis. They were changes in blood flow, changes in the vessel wall, and altered blood coagulability.

All surgery changes the volume of blood supplying the legs. Bandages or plasters impede flow. Spinal and epidural anaesthesia allow blood to gush through the lower limbs so fast that clots do not get a chance to form.

Changes in the vessel wall can occur in diabetics who become hyperglycaemic while in the recovery room. Blood glucose levels greater than 12 mmol/L cause vascular endothelial cells to shrivel up and pull away from their neighbours, exposing basement membrane where clots readily form.

Finally, physiological stress such as pain, or hypovolaemia, or even fear increases blood's tendency to clot.

Women who are pregnant, or taking oral contraceptives, or hormone replacement therapy are at risk of venothromboembolism. If they have surgery they require DVT prophylaxis, but if women are not having surgery, the risk of VTE is very small indeed.

Who needs prophylaxis?

Measures to prevent venothromboembolism start in the recovery room. Any patient over the age of 40 years who is having major surgery lasting longer than 30 minutes needs prophylaxis.

How to prevent DVT

Measures include:

- adequate hydration, leg exercises, and good analgesia to prevent hypercoagulopathy;
- maintaining the blood glucose in diabetics to be in the range 7–10 mmol/L;
- check bandages and prevent any restriction to blood flow;
- order suitable DVT prophylaxis before the patient is discharged from the recovery room:
- graduated elastic compression stockings;
- intermittent pneumatic leg compression;
- anti-coagulation.

While in the recovery room get the patient to flap their feet up and down, and flex their knees at least 20 times every 15 minutes.

Recovery room staff have a major role in preventing VTE.

A uniform enforced hospital policy on measures to prevent DVT gives the best results. However, even with the best regimes the relative risk reduction is probably only 60–80 per cent. Prophylaxis is no guarantee that thrombosis will not occur. Although PE is uncommon in the recovery room, deep vein thrombosis often starts here.

Anticoagulants

Unfractionated heparin

Unfractionated heparin (UH) is a fast-acting anti-coagulant with a short half-life of about 90 minutes. The dose is 5000 units subcutaneously (s/c) twice daily.

Its effect can be monitored with an activated partial thromboplastin time (*aPTT*). It can be reversed with protamine.

Low molecular-weight heparins

Low molecular-weight heparins (LMWH) are selective anti-coagulants causing less systemic effects than UH. There are number of LMWH, but the two most commonly used are enoxaparin and dalteparin, while fondinaparinux is reserved for high-risk cases.

Enoxaparin (Clexane®) is given once a day. The standard adult dose is enoxaparin 40 mg s/c. In patients weighing less than 50 Kg, or those with renal failure use half of this dose.

Dalteparin (Fragmin®) is given twice a day. The standard adult dose is 5000 units s/c 1–2 hours preoperatively and repeated 12 hourly in high-risk patients. In patients weighing less than 50 Kg, or those with renal failure use half of this dose.

Fondinaparinux is a synthetic pentasaccharide derived from unfractionated heparin. It has a long half-life of 21 hours. It is more efficacious than warfarin, but not as safe. It is best reserved for patients with an extreme risk of DVT. The dose is 2.5 mg s/c injection for 5–9 days. Give the first dose 6 hours after surgery. It is unsafe to use in patients who have an epidural catheter in place.

Table 15.2 How to use the heparins

Risk of DVT	Type of surgery	Best practice
Extreme risk	Major orthopaedic surgery with risk factors*	Fondinaparinux
High risk	Major surgery in patients > 60 yrs Major surgery in patients with one or more risk factors* All joint replacements All multiple trauma Thrombophilia	Daltaparin
Moderate risk	Major surgery in patients < 60 yrs Minor surgery with risk factors*	Heparin
Low risk	Minor surgery and no risk factors Diagnostic laparoscopy Transurethral resection at prostate Endoscopic surgery e.g. TURP	Early mobilization

* Risk factors include previous DVT or pulmonary embolism, active cancer, pregnancy, postpartum < 1 month, inflammatory bowel disease, body mass index > 30, hormone replacement therapy, or oral contraceptive pills, thrombophilia, and varicose veins.

Mechanical devices

If heparins are contraindicated use intermittent pneumatic compression (IPC), and graduated compression stockings. Do not use IPC in patients with severe peripheral vascular disease, severe peripheral neuropathy, lower limb oedema, or if the leg has a breach in the skin such as ulcers or eczema.

Intermittent calf compression

Devices that apply intermittent calf compression are useful where a LMWH is contraindicated, for instance after intracranial, inner ear, or some forms of plastic procedures.

Graduated stockings

Properly fitted graduated stockings are clearly effective in reducing the incidence of deep vein thrombosis.[3] Graduated pressure stockings apply graded degrees of pressure to the lower limb. The greatest pressure is at the ankle, and the pressure exerted by the stocking progressively decreases further up the leg. Graduated stockings prevent venous stasis increasing the rate of blood flow, protect from vessel injury and improving venous valve function. It is not known whether full thigh-length stockings are more effective than the shorter knee-length stockings. They are, however, not without risk, and must not be used on patients who have vascular disease affecting blood flow to the lower limb because they may cause limb ischaemia.

Notes

1. The National Working Party on the Management and Prevention of Venous Thromboembolism (2001) *Best Practice Guidelines for Australia and New Zealand*, 2nd edn, HEMI.
2. Greets WH, Heit JA, Clagett GP et al. (2001) *Chest* 119 (supp)132–175.
3. Ammarigini SV, Lees TA (2000) Cochrane Review, The Cochrane Library Issue 3.

16

Cardiovascular physiology

The heart, circulatory system and the lungs work together as an integrated *cardiopulmonary unit*. The lungs transfer oxygen to the blood, and evict the waste carbon dioxide, while the heart pumps enough blood, at enough pressure, through the circulation to deliver enough oxygen and nutrients to the tissues and organs, and to remove their metabolic waste products.

The heart is a sturdy little *volume pump*, but it is not a *pressure pump*. Being a volume pump it supplies blood to the organs at low pressures. However, if the heart is forced to pump blood at high pressures it will, sooner or later, fail.

Blood pressure oscillates. When the ventricles contract (*systole*) the blood pressure in the arteries rises, and as they relax (*diastole*) the pressure falls. The pressure at peak of the pulse wave is the *systolic blood pressure*, and the trough is the *diastolic pressure*. The difference between the two pressures is called the *pulse pressure*.

In the recovery room adequate blood flow with good tissue perfusion, a clear conscious state and a good urine output, is more important than a high blood pressure.

The heart consists of two *demand* pumps set in *series*. The right side of the heart is a low-pressure pump; it supplies the lungs. Simultaneously the left side of the heart working as a high-pressure pump feeds blood to the organs and muscles. Because they are set in series each pump feeds the other, and being demand pumps they adjust their output to the metabolic needs of the tissues. Sometimes the heart cannot keep up with the demands of the tissue for oxygen and nutrient. This does not necessarily mean the heart is diseased. When you get puffed running up stairs, your heart is failing to meet the demands of your muscles: this is not heart disease. If you get puffed doing normal day-to-day activities then some sort of cardiopulmonary dysfunction is probable.

What is cardiac output?

Cardiac output is the volume of blood the heart pumps out every minute. In a resting individual the normal heart rate is about 72 beats a minutes. It ejects 70 ml of blood (*stroke-volume*) with each beat.

Cardiac output = heart rate × stroke-volume

Thus the cardiac output = $72 \times 70 \approx 5000$ ml/min

Role of heart rate

One might suspect that the faster the heart beats the more blood it pumps out. This is partly true, but it depends on the age of the person. With exercise or increased demand an older person's stroke volume does not increase, consequently they compensate by increasing their heart rate instead. Similarly, neonates depend on their high heart rate to maintain cardiac output. In most adults, the heart becomes increasingly inefficient at rates more than 130 beats per minute. In the recovery room, worry about an adult's heart rate if it exceeds 100 beats per minute. Always look for a cause of tachycardia.

Role of stroke volume

Healthy hearts can double their stroke-volume with ease. In young people, this pump, a little larger than the size of your clenched fist, can increase its output to 20 L/min or more, however this ability declines with age and deteriorating physical fitness. Athletes often have stroke-volumes exceeding 130 ml per beat (and so do severely obese people).

Three factors determine stroke-volume:

1. preload;
2. myocardial contractility;
3. afterload.

So that we can compare the cardiac output in people of different sizes it is standardized to a *cardiac index*; this is the cardiac output per square metre of body surface area, which at rest, is about 3 L/metre^2.

Table 16.1 Where the cardiac output goes

Organ	Proportion of cardiac output
Heart	4%
Brain	15%
Kidneys	25%
Muscle	5–20% depending on demands
Liver	15–25% depending on proximity to a meal
The rest	15%

Every time the ventricle contracts it ejects about half the blood it contains (*ejection fraction* of 50%). Those with *systolic heart failure* have ejection fractions of 40% or less. Ejection fractions are measured with transthoracic echocardiography.

Starling's law describes contractility

Over a hundred years ago two physiologists, Frank and Starling, noted that like an elastic band: "The more the myocardial fibres are stretched during diastole, the more they will contract during subsequent systole, and therefore the more blood will be expelled." This initial stretching is now called *preload*.

Cardiac preload

Within limits, the more cardiac myocytes are stretched (preload) the harder they contract. The myocytes, however, are damaged if they are overstretched. The preload on the ventricles is determined by how hard the atria needs to contract to fill (prime) the ventricles with blood.

Ventricular pump priming by atrial contraction contributes to 25 per cent of the cardiac output in a normal person, and over 50 per cent in patients with diastolic dysfunction. If a patient with diastolic failure develops atrial fibrillation, then their cardiac output may drop disastrously.

Cardiac contractility

Healthy muscles contract more forcibly than unhealthy ones. Many factors reduce the ability of ventricular muscle to contract forcibly; they include old age, hypertension, ischaemic heart disease, the long-term effects of chronic alcoholism, and there are many others.

Cardiac afterload

Blood pressure is a result of the balance between the volume of blood ejected with each beat (*stroke-volume*), and the *resistance* the arterioles (*afterload*) impose on blood flowing through the systemic vascular bed.

If the arterioles dilate reducing afterload, then the blood pressure falls, and if they constrict, increasing the afterload, the blood pressure rises.

Diseases of cardiac muscle

Without resting, the human heart beats about 100 000 times each day, and has an all-up lifetime budget of about 2.5 billion beats. After 2 billion contractions it is not surprising that cardiac myocytes start to simply wear out and degenerate.

Apart from old age many other insults affecting the ability of cardiac myocytes to fulfil their destiny. Myocytes degenerate faster and die if they have to pump at high pressures as occurs with hypertension or aortic stenosis.

Diastolic failure

Overworked cardiac myocytes wear out prematurely, and as they die they are replaced by collagen and amyloid scar tissue, making the heart muscle stiff (*incompliant*). Eventually this causes *diastolic cardiac failure*.

The ventricles cannot stretch enough in order to increase their stroke volume. In the recovery room, the only effective way to treat this frustrating problem is to increase the preload by giving additional fluids to forcibly fill the atria. The stretched atria may then respond by contracting harder forcing blood through the mitral valve to stretch the stiff left ventricle, and in turn the ventricle contracts more forcibly. There is a risk in giving extra fluids because it increases the pressure in the pulmonary veins, which can cause pulmonary oedema. It is possible to indirectly measure the pulmonary venous pressure as a pulmonary artery wedge pressure. Exceeding a pulmonary wedge pressure greater than 22 mmHg is unsafe.

Systolic failure

Systolic heart failure occurs where a process, such as inflammation or a chronically poor oxygen supply, directly damages heart muscle causing the ventricles to become dilated and flabby. A flabby dilated heart contracts weakly and cannot eject its stroke volume in a normal way. This condition is called a *dilated cardiomyopathy*.

The lipid-based cell membranes of cardiac myocytes slowly degenerate if continually exposed to a fat dissolving toxin: alcohol. Alcoholic cardiomyopathy is responsible for one-third of dilated cardiomyopathies.

Systolic failure is treated with *ionotropes*, which stimulate the heart to contract more forcibly; and vasodilators, which reduce afterload making it easier for the flabby heart muscle to eject its stroke volume.

Arrythmias

In the recovery room, arrythmias usually occur if the heart muscle receives an inadequate oxygen supply to meet its demands. Although suboptimal oxygenation is responsible for most arrhythmias, there are other causes including thyrotoxicosis, exogenous or endogenous catecholamines, and diseases directly affecting heart muscle itself.

Diseases of heart muscle

Diseases directly affecting heart muscle include structural abnormalities (septal defects and abnormal valves), haemochromatosis, infections (particularly viruses), AIDS, and amyloidosis.

How blood pressure is controlled

A normal blood pressure in an adult is considered to range between 110–130 mmHg systolic, and 65–80 mmHg diastolic. It is kept within this range by a number of homeostatic feedback mechanisms. Patients coming to surgery with poorly controlled blood pressure are at a higher risk of adverse cardiac events in the recovery room. It is often stated that people with blood pressures up to 180/110 are unlikely to run into problems perioperatively. We feel that this is a flawed assumption. If a hypertensive patient gets a tachycardia in the recovery room, they often develop ECG changes, such as ST depression and ventricular extrasystoles, which herald myocardial ischaemia.

Homeostasis

Interlinked feedback control mechanisms stabilize the circulation. These include:

- baroreceptors to sense pressure changes;
- chemoreceptors to sense changes in the composition of the blood;
- sensory nerves to carry the information to central processors;
- processors in the central nervous system to coordinate these mechanisms;
- effector nerve to instantly make adjustments;
- hormones to maintain the changes over a long period.

Baroreceptors

Baroreceptors are special stretch receptors located in the walls of the veins, and arteries near the heart. There are two types of stretch receptors: *high-pressure baroreceptors* located in the arch of the aorta, and the carotid arteries; and *low-pressure baroreceptors* in the great veins and right atrium.

Baroceptors sense changes in mean blood pressure, and instruct the autonomic nervous system to restore the blood pressure to an optimal level. General anaesthetics blunt baroreceptor function, particularly if the patient is also taking long-term vasodilator anti-hypertensive drugs. If a patient is taking ACE inhibitors or angiotensin receptor blockers, do not suddenly sit them because their blood pressure will fall, and with it their cerebral perfusion. Should this occur they will feel nauseated, faint and may lose consciousness, and even have a seizure.

Neural regulation

If the arterial blood pressure falls, the fast-acting sympathetic nervous system, backed up by several slower-acting hormones, attempt to increase cardiac output and decrease the arteriolar calibre to restore the blood pressure.

Feedback in response to a fall in blood pressure

Sequence
1. Blood pressure falls.
2. Arterial baroreceptors detect fall in blood pressure.
3. Message sent to vasomotor centre.
4. Vasomotor centres trigger sympathetic nerves to fire.
5. Sympathetic nerves release noradrenaline:
   – arterioles constrict impeding blood flow
   – heart muscle contracts more forcibly
6. Blood pressure rises.
7. Baroreceptors detect rise in blood pressure and stop sending signals to the vasomotor centre.

Figure 16.1 Negative feedback control of blood pressure

Chemoreceptors

Chemoreceptors respond to chemical changes in the blood. One type of chemoreceptor located in the arch of the aorta and carotid bodies, responds to hypoxia. Their job is to stimulate breathing should blood oxygen levels fall. They start firing vigorously once the PaO_2 falls below 60 mmHg (kPa = 7.89) or where the oxygen saturation is less than 90%. Even tiny amounts of volatile anaesthetics blunt this response, and so for several hours after a general anaesthetic, the rate and depth of breathing may not increase if the patient becomes hypoxaemic.

The MET score

The heart must be able to attain and sustain the demands placed on it during the postoperative period. Instead of reporting a patient's cardiac function as 'poor', or 'good', or 'excellent' we now calibrate this with the MET (Metabolic Exercise Tolerance) score.

One MET is the amount of oxygen used each minute by a 70 Kg man at rest (3.5 ml/Kg/min): 2 MET is the amount of oxygen used when walking at 2 kilometres per hour, while 10 MET is roughly equivalent to jogging at 10 kilometres per hour.

METs can be measured by exercising the patient on a static bicycle or a treadmill, but an estimate can be gleaned simply from the scale shown in Table 16.2.

Table 16.2 MET score

MET	Equivalent physical activity
1 MET	Watching TV, writing at a desk, eating a meal, washing dishes.
2 MET	Walking from room to room, showering, walking around a supermarket, hanging out the washing, making a bed, playing lawn bowls.
3 MET	Carrying bags of groceries from car, pushing full supermarket trolley, vacuuming floors, and walking up one flight of stairs without becoming short of breath. Playing golf (but not carrying their golf bag).
4 MET	Sweeping yard, raking up leaves, walking up 2 flights of stairs carrying 7 Kg load. Walking 4 km in one hour.
5 MET	Walking briskly, climbing four flights of stairs without breathlessness, mowing lawn with power mower.
35 MET	Olympic athlete running the 400 metres.

Following major surgery, such as a hip replacement where the operation is long and tissue damage considerable, we can expect a large postoperative inflammatory response. To perfuse the inflamed tissue the patient must be able to attain, and maintain, a MET score equivalent to 3 to 4 or more. If the MET score is less than 4, then a postoperative adverse cardiac event is likely to occur, either in the recovery room, or later in the ward. For minor surgery, where the operation is short and there is little tissue damage, then a MET score of 2 to 3 is sufficient.

Perioperative adverse cardiac event

If the patient has clinically silent or apparently stable heart disease postoperative physiological stresses may either reveal, or destabilize it.

What is a postoperative adverse cardiac event?

In the recovery room acute cardiac problems include one or more of cardiac ischaemia, arrhythmias, hypotension, cardiac failure, acute pulmonary oedema, cardiogenic shock or even death. For convenience these events are lumped together as *postoperative adverse cardiac events* (PACE).

Typically, PACE surfaces at two distinct times. The first is the *avoidable stress response* that occurs in the recovery room. The second *obligatory stress response* peaks on the second and third postoperative day.

Avoidable response

During the induced coma of a general anaesthetic the patient is protected from the pain and undesirable reflex responses caused by surgery. On emerging from their protective coma, patients are confronted by a barrage of one or more physiological insults including fright, pain, hypothermia, hypoxia, abrupt blood pressure changes, acid-base disturbance, the effects of circulating biochemical cytokines released from injured tissue, the persisting effects of anaesthetic drugs; and possibly the immunosuppression from homologous blood transfusion. This may well be the most severe physiological onslaught the person has ever experienced. Skilled care in the recovery room can avoid, or at least modify these responses.

Obligatory responses

On the second and third postoperative day the cardiac output has to rise to the task of perfusing inflamed tissue. The normal resting cardiac output for an average adult is about 5 litres a minute. On the second day after a total hip replacement, or major vascular surgery this increases to 8.5 L/min or even more. This 70 per cent increase in cardiac output must be sustained until at first the inflammatory response, and later the tissue repair process have resolved. Prostate, and thyroid operations and cataract extractions cause less tissue damage, and therefore less relative risk of PACE.

Leaving other factors aside, the risk of PACE is directly proportional to the mass of tissue damaged by the surgery. You can give a haircut to a patient with severe heart disease, but a total hip replacement, where kilograms of tissue are damaged, is likely to be fatal. Unless your patient can increase their cardiac output during and after surgery to adequately perfuse their tissues then they will die.

The first signs of problems appear in the recovery room as the patient experiences the stress of emerging from their anaesthetic. If they develop signs of ST-depression on their ECG, or a tachycardia with hypotension despite having a normal vascular volume, or their oxygen saturations dip below 95% while they are receiving oxygen, then you can confidently predict perioperative adverse cardiac events two days later in the ward.

Electrophysiology

The essentials

The heart runs on tiny electrical currents. Unless every cardiac myocyte contracts at exactly the right moment the heart would pump chaotically.

To organize and coordinate this activity, the heart uses tiny electrical currents called *action potentials* to kick-start the myocytes.

The sino-atrial (SA) node ticks away like a clock, normally generating about 70 electrical impulses a minute. Each electrical impulse then starts on a journey through the heart as a wave of *depolarization*.

The firing rate of the SA nodes is sped up by sympathetic nerves, circulating adrenaline and certain drugs (such as atropine). It is slowed by the *parasympathetic nervous system* and certain drugs (such as neostigmine and β-blockers).

Each impulse then plays follow-the-leader through the heart down the same well-beaten path. From the SA node the impulses wash through atrial muscle like a wave, stimulating (*depolarizing*) each myocyte to contract as they pass. As the atrial muscle contracts it pushes blood through the mitral and tricuspid valves into the left and right ventricle respectively. When the wave of depolarization hits the atrioventricular (AV) node it is delayed momentarily to allow time for the ventricles to fill with blood. In less than 120 milliseconds it fizzes, like a lighted fuse, down specialized Purkinje fibres in the bundle of His. Then the depolarizing wave fans out through special conducting tissue along the branches of the right and left bundles to the ventricles to sweep up from the heart's apex jolting each cell into action. All this happens in an orderly sequence, like a cascade of falling dominoes, each activating the one next to it. In this way ventricular contraction squeezes blood, in a twisting anti-clockwise vortex, upwards and out through the aortic and pulmonary valves into the aorta and pulmonary arteries.

It takes about 120 milliseconds to eject the stroke-volume from the ventricles during systole, and it takes about another 200 milliseconds for the cardiac myocytes to recover enough to contract again. During this *refractory period* the exhausted ventricles relax, receive their oxygen and nutrient supply through the coronary arteries, and fill with blood to be ready to start pumping over again.

At the beginning of diastole, the heart muscles begin to relax, and the backward pressure of blood in the arteries snaps the pulmonary and aortic valves shut. This stops blood refluxing back into the heart. Then the whole cycle starts again.

Electrocardiograph (ECG)

We routinely monitor the electrocardiograph (ECG) on most patients in the recovery room. The trace is displayed on the monitor's screen. Built into the monitors are alarms for cardiac rate, rhythm, and many have facilities for arrhythmia and ST analysis. Although monitors are mostly reliable, you still need to observe your patients carefully.

P-Wave
– disappears in AF
– saw-tooth in atrial flutter
– inverted in junctional rhythm

PR interval
– prolonged in heart block
– shortened in WPW syndrome

QRS
– abnormal shape indicated conduction abnormalities

ST segment
– raised, depressed or sloping indicates serious ventricular problems eg. ischaemia

QT interval
– prolonged in ↓ mg^{++} and ↓ Ca^{++}
– shortened in ↑ K^+

T-wave
– peaked = ↑ K^+
– flat   = ↓ K^+
– inverted = irritation (ischaemia or inflammation)

U-wave
– if prominent = ↑ Ca^{++}

PR interval	0.12–0.20s
QRS complex	0.08–0.12s
QT interval	0.35–0.42s

Figure 16.2 The normal ECG complex.

An ECG uses electrodes stuck on the skin to measure the sum of the electrical action potentials on the body surface. Impulses passing towards an electrode record a positive deflection on the trace while those passing away from the electrode cause a negative deflection. Each electrode samples the sequence, direction and magnitude of the impulse as it travels from its origin in the atria to its extinction in the ventricles.

At any instant an ECG trace reveals the overall direction the electrical impulses are going. If the electrical currents are aberrant, or going in the wrong direction, they appear as an abnormal waveform on the ECG trace.

Monitors can deceive you. Sometimes false alarms occur or alarms fail to go off when they should. ECG leads can fall off the patient simulating asystole, or electrical interference may simulate ventricular fibrillation. Never silence the monitor alarm without checking the patients pulse, and blood pressure manually.

Do not ignore the monitor, and never ignore the patient.

Describing ECGs

Learn to recognize and describe ECG traces. Sooner or later you will have to tell someone what is happening over the telephone. This takes practice.

1. If the patient is hypotensive – call for help immediately.

2. What is the heart rate?
   - a bradycardia is less than 60 bpm;
   - a relative tachycardia is greater than 80 bpm;
   - a tachycardia is greater than 100 bpm.

3. Is the rhythm regular? Look at lead II.

4. Is the QRS complex wide or narrow?

5. Is there a P wave in lead II and are they all the same shape?

6. Are there signs of ischaemia? The best lead to detect ischaemia is CM5. Is the ST segment raised above, or depressed below the isoelectric line? Is the ST segment sloping?

7. Is the pulse oximeter showing a decreasing saturation?

Since it takes a lot of experience to read an ECG competently, we can only cover the barest rudiments of this skill. Let us be pragmatic; for those who are not competent at reading an ECG it is better to use the information provided by the monitor to help with the diagnosis rather than analysing every little bit of the trace yourself. Or consult a colleague who can read an ECG.

If you do not understand something, or what you are doing, or what is wrong with your patient, then consult someone who does.

Pacemakers

Implanted electronic pacemakers are used to maintain cardiac output in patients who are having symptoms caused by *sick sinus syndrome*, bradycardias, heart blocks, or recurring or uncontrollable atrial tachyarrhythmias.

Permanent pacemakers

Types of pacemakers

There are two types of implanted pacemakers: anti-tachycardia pacemakers, which terminate arrhythmias, and anti-bradycardia pacemakers that simulate normal pacemaker function. There are also implantable defibrillators.

Pacemakers are described by an internationally accepted code. Most patients carry a card describing the make of the pacemaker, when it was inserted, when the battery was last checked and a 5-letter code on specifying what the pacemaker does.

1st letter chamber paced	2nd letter chamber sensed	3rd letter response to sensed event	4th letter (optional) programmability	5th letter (for implanted devices)
A = atria	A = atria	I = device inhibited	O = not programmable	O = none
V = ventricles	V = ventricles	T = device triggered	P = rate + output	P = anti-tachycardia pacing
D = dual (both atria and ventricles)	D = dual	D = ventricular sensed event with device triggered Atrial sensed even with device inhibited O = off – device unresponsive	M = multiple C = telemetric R = rate responsive	S = shock delivery D = both

For example DDD = both chambers paced, both chambers sensed. This pacemaker generates an atrial impulse inhibiting the patient's atrium from generating a normal impulse. The pacemaker then senses whether the impulse it generated has arrived at the ventricle. If not, then it generates an impulse to stimulate the ventricle.

Reasons for pacemaker malfunction during surgery include:

- threshold changes where the heart muscle becomes more or less sensitive to the pacemaker's pulse;
- the pacemaker failed to generate an impulse;
- or a lead or electrode has become displaced.

VVI pacemakers can be disrupted by tiny electrical currents even those generated when muscles contract; for instance fasciculation caused by succinyl choline. Many anaesthetists prefer that VVI mode be switched to VVO mode with a special magnet before they start the anaesthetic.

Temporary pacemakers

Temporary pacemakers are inserted as a stop-gap measure where symptomatic bradycardia, atrioventricular blocks, or sinus arrest cause the cardiac output and blood pressure to fall. The leads are inserted into a large vein, in the same way as a central venous catheter, and fed into the right ventricle to depolarize it. The usual reason for using a temporary pacemaker in a surgical patient is as a precautionary measure, where the patient has a high-grade trifasicular block.

What to check

As soon as the patient with a pacemaker is admitted to recovery room put on an ECG monitor and do a full 12-lead ECG. If the ECG rhythm strip (lead II), does not show regular pacemaker spikes, the pacemaker may either be faulty, or set in demand mode. Check each pacemaker spike is followed by a widened QRS (similar to an extrasystole).

Sometimes pacemakers are turned off during surgery. Before the patient returns to the ward they should be turned on again using a special magnet, which is placed over the pacemaker.

Pacemakers need normal serum potassium levels to function properly. Check the serum potassium concentrations if arrhythmias occur, or the pacemaker misbehaves.

The electromagnetic fields generated by diathermy or electrosurgery does not upset modern pacemakers, but older models can be damaged by current surges. Cardioversion can damage pacemakers. If possible consult a cardiologist before performing cardioversion on a patient with a pacemaker in place.

Do not insert central lines or pulmonary flotation catheters into patients with pacemakers because the catheter may dislodge the pacemaker wire from the right ventricle.

17

Cardiovascular disease

Cardiovascular disease is common. The principle problems, in order of prevalence, are hypertension, cardiac failure, ischaemic heart disease, and valvular heart disease.

About 40 per cent of patients over the age of 40 attending a hospital for surgery have some form of cardiovascular disease such as hypertension, vascular disease, or ischaemic heart disease. If these problems are optimized before surgery it reduces the risk of them surfacing in the recovery room.

Proper preoperative management alleviates many
problems in the recovery room.

Hypertension

Hypertension is due to either, or both, an elevated cardiac output, or an increase in peripheral resistance. Increased levels of circulating *catecholamines* cause most hypertension in the recovery room. Adrenaline and noradrenaline are released as the sympathetic nervous system is activated in response to actual or perceived stress. The elevated blood pressure increases cardiac work, which in turn increases the heart's need for oxygen and nutriment.

The heart is only perfused during *diastole*. Because tachycardias shorten diastolic time they reduce coronary blood flow and cardiac oxygen supply. If a tachycardia (which reduces coronary perfusion) accompanies hypertension (which increases cardiac oxygen demand), the combination becomes a potent cause of cardiac ischaemia.

Tachycardia + hypertension → cardiac ischaemia.

Acute hypertension

Check the patients' medical records to elicit their preoperative blood pressure. Normal blood pressure ranges from 110/65 to 130/85. In the recovery room the patients' blood pressures should ideally remain within 15 per cent of their preoperative blood pressures.

Risks associated with hypertension include:

- arrhythmias;
- myocardial ischaemia, myocardial infarction;

- cardiac failure;
- strokes – subarachnoid, or cerebral haemorrhages;
- bleeding from the operative site.

Causes of acute hypertension include:

- pain;
- hypoxia;
- CO_2 retention;
- full bladder;
- over-transfusion;
- vasopressors;
- obstructed airways;
- shivering;
- hypoglycaemia;
- phaeochromocytoma;
- carcinoid.

Hypertension should be treated if it is associated with:

- a systolic pressure above 180 mmHg;
- a diastolic over 105 mmHg;
- ventricular premature beats;
- ST changes on the ECG;
- a deteriorating conscious state.

The elderly, or those with pre-existing heart disease, are at risk of cardiac ischaemia and arrhythmias, especially if they also develop a tachycardia. If you see ventricular extrasystoles on the monitor then suspect myocardial ischaemia. Controlling the hypertension usually resolves the extrasystoles.

Chronic hypertension

Chronic hypertension is endemic in the community affecting about half the population over the age of 65 years. In patients with chronic hypertension, haemorrhage or a rapid infusion of intravenous fluids can cause unexpectedly large swings in their blood pressure. These swings are hazardous for the same reasons as that of acute hypertension.

Patients should have taken all their cardiac medication on the day of surgery. Check in their medical record that they have done so. Many patients are already taking a β-blocker such as atenolol, metoprolol, or bisoprolol. If their β-blockers are withdrawn abruptly then patients may experience rebound hypertension, tachycardia, sweating, ventricular arrhythmias, and possibly sudden death.

Malignant hypertension

Fulminating (malignant) hypertension can cause cerebral oedema if the blood pressure rises acutely beyond 220/120 mmHg. Control the blood pressure urgently if the patient shows signs of:

- headache;
- deterioration in mental state;
- an up-going plantar (Babinski) response;
- drowsiness;
- disorientation;
- nystagmus;
- muscle weakness.

Malignant hypertension may cause cardiac ischaemia and cardiac failure with a gallop rhythm, rales in the lung bases, and retrosternal chest pain. If fulminating hypertension occurs unexpectedly consider undiagnosed phaeochromocytoma, tetanus, carcinoid syndrome, or spinal cord damage.

Principles of management of hypertension

Give oxygen, attach a pulse oximeter and an automated blood pressure device.

- Sit the patient up: it sometimes helps.
- Attach an ECG.
- If the patient has new ST segment changes then give sublingual glyceryl trinitrate.
- Eliminate hypoxia and hypoglycaemia as a cause.
- Check that the patient has taken their morning antihypertensive therapy before coming to the operating theatre.
- If patients are in pain then:
  - control it with intravenous analgesia;
  - they may need a regional anaesthetic block.
- Check the intraoperative fluid chart to see if it balances.
- Notify the anaesthetist.

Depending on the cause of the hypertension the anaesthetist may:

- use a vasodilator such as nitroglycerine, hydralazine or nitroprusside;

- reduce the force of the myocardial contraction and the heart rate with a β-blocker, or decrease central sympathetic drive with clonidine.

Be prepared because the anaesthetist may want to:

- give an infusion of antihypertensive drugs with a syringe pump;
- give each drug infusion though a separate intravenous line;
- use intra-arterial continuous blood pressure monitoring.

Hypertension in a healthy patient?
Consider pain or fluid overload.

Antihypertensive drugs

Nitroglycerine

Glyceryl trinitrate (GTN) is a short-acting drug that relaxes vascular smooth muscle and improves myocardial oxygenation. It is suitable for those with ischaemic heart disease, or where you wish to improve pulmonary blood flow. Its effect wears off in 5–8 minutes. *Tachyphylaxis* may become a problem.

Hypertension with myocardial ischaemia

If the patient is showing signs of myocardial ischaemia, with either chest pain or ST changes on the ECG, give sublingual glyceryl trinitrate, and send for the anaesthetist.

If a reflex tachycardia occurs, then the anaesthetist may give a β-blocker such as metoprolol 5–20 mg intravenously over 2 minutes to control the rate.

If the patient is hypertensive but does not have a tachycardia, then give a sublingual or an oral spray of glyceryl trinitrate (Anginine®). Since GTN works for about 10 minutes, it will give you time to get help and to set up a glyceryl trinitrate infusion to control the blood pressure. The initial rate for a GTN infusion is 10 μg/min, increasing in increments up to 200 μg/min. GTN infusions take 3–4 minutes to stabilize blood pressure and the effects wear off in about 8–10 minutes. It may cause a headache.

Hydralazine

Hydralazine is a direct-acting peripheral arteriolar vasodilator. It causes a reflex tachycardia, with increased cardiac contractility, so it may cause cardiac ischaemia. The diastolic blood pressure responds to a greater extent than the systolic pressure.

Hydralazine for moderate hypertension

If the patient is not showing signs of myocardial ischaemia the anaesthetist will probably use hydralazine 5–20 mg slowly intravenously to reduce blood pressure.

Hydralazine takes about 15–20 minutes to reach maximum effect, and works for about 3–4 hours. A second dose may be given within 4–5 hours, using about two-thirds of the original loading dose. As hydralazine's effects are unpredictable, dilute it and give in 5 mg increments every 5 minutes. Any reflex tachycardia can be controlled with a small dose of metoprolol 5–10 mg intravenously.

β-blockers

Do not use β-blockers as a first line therapy for hypertension in the recovery room. Both α- and β-receptor stimulation causes hypertension. β-blockers only block β-receptors, leaving unmodified α-stimulation to cause peripheral vasoconstriction. Using β-blockers to reduce the heart's ability to contract, while simultaneously requiring it to pump blood through vasoconstricted vessels, decreases tissue blood flow and may precipitate heart failure.

Labetalol

Labetalol is a selective α_1 blocker and a non-selective β-blocker. Bradycardia may become a problem where larger doses are used. It reduces blood pressure by reducing cardiac output and heart rate, and decreasing the peripheral vascular resistance. It has a long half-life of between 3.5 and 6.5 hours depending on the dose given.

Clonidine

Clonidine is a centrally acting α_2-agonist that reduces blood pressure by damping down the activity of the sympathetic nervous system. Clonidine is not a first line agent. It may cause the blood pressure to rise transiently before it falls.

Phentolamine

Only used occasionally, phentolamine is a short-acting α_1-blocker arteriolar vasodilator. Its effects wear off after 6–10 minutes.

Nitroprusside

Sodium nitroprusside (SNP) (Nipride®), a potent ultra-short-acting vasodilator, is the best drug to control of malignant hypertension. It causes a reflex tachycardia, and vasodilates cerebral arterioles.

As SNP is metabolized cyanide is released, which in turn is metabolized to thiocyanate inside red cells. Thiocyanate toxicity causes hypoxia, disorientation, muscle spasms, and tinnitus. Cyanide toxicity is possible if the patient has had a long operation, such as inserting Harrington's rods, where large doses of SNP were used to induce hypotension.

Nitroprusside for malignant hypertension

In severe or fulminating hypertension, where the blood pressure is greater than 220/120 mmHg, the anaesthetist may buy time with a nitroprusside infusion while organizing alternative measures. The blood pressure will fall within 30 seconds, and will bounce back about 2–4 minutes after turning off the SNP.

Warning about vasodilators

If vasodilating drugs are used in patients who are unable to increase their cardiac output, they will become profoundly hypotensive.

Antihypertensive medication? Was it given preoperatively?

Do not use vasodilating drugs in patients with:

- aortic or mitral stenosis;
- hypertrophic obstructive cardiomyopathies;
- cardiac tamponade;
- restrictive pericarditis;
- head trauma;
- hypovolaemia;
- epidural or spinal anaesthesia;
- closed angle glaucoma.

Hypotension

Hypotension is common in the recovery room. It quickly causes renal damage, myocardial ischaemia or strokes, and especially so in those who suffer from chronic hypertension.

In the recovery room patients become hypotensive once their mean blood pressure falls below 20 per cent of its preoperative values. A patient with a preoperative mean blood of 100 mmHg, is hypotensive if it falls to 80 mmHg. Prepare to correct hypotension once mean blood pressure falls by 15 per cent of its preoperative values, and to treat it when it falls by 20 per cent.

When to worry about hypotension

Send for the anaesthetist if your patient:

- is restless, anxious or agitated;
- has chest discomfort, angina or finds it difficult to get their breath;
- complains of nausea, fading vision or their conscious state deteriorates;
- oxygen saturation falls below 93%.

Do not worry if the patient's:

- mean blood pressure is within 15% of the baseline reading;
- **and** they are resting comfortably;
- **and** have a good perfusion status;
- **and** their pulse rate is less than 80 beats/min and greater than 55 beats/min. Elderly people and infants drop their cardiac output if their pulse is less than 55 beats/min.

Physiology of hypotension

All the causes of hypotension fall into two groups; those caused by:

- decreased cardiac output, and
- decreased systemic vascular resistance.

The blood pumped by the heart needs to push against a peripheral resistance to maintain the blood pressure.

$$\text{Blood pressure} = \text{cardiac output} \times \text{peripheral resistance.}$$

To maintain cardiac output the heart needs three things:

1. Enough blood returning to it from the great veins (*preload*).
2. To be able to contract forcibly enough (*myocardial contractility*).
3. To have a resistance to push against (*afterload*).

As arterioles dilate the heart must increase its output to maintain the blood pressure. If the heart fails to achieve this, then blood pressure falls.

From this we can see that hypotension could be caused by:

- Not enough preload: hypovolaemia, blood loss, tension pneumothorax, and supine hypotensive syndrome in the grossly obese or pregnant patient where the gravid uterus or pressure from fat impedes venous return to the heart;
- impaired myocardial cardiac contractility; ischaemia; arrhythmia; drugs used;
- during the anaesthetic: cardiac tamponade;
- reduced afterload: spinal or epidural blocks, residual effects of antihypertensive therapy, adrenocortical insufficiency and anaphylaxis or anaphylactoid reactions.

Often there is a combination of these factors causing hypotension: for instance hypovolaemia in a patient who is on antihypertensive therapy; or epidural or spinal anaesthesia in patients with cardiac failure.

Why it is bad to tip hypotensive patients head down

If a patient becomes hypotensive, it is common practice for staff to tip the trolley head down, presumably because they erroneously believe it increases venous return and improves blood pressure. Tipping a person head down seriously disrupts oxygen transfer from the lungs to the blood, makes breathing difficult because the diaphragm has to lift the abdominal contents to move, slows cerebral blood flow, risks regurgitating stomach contents, and is most unpleasant.

The best way to demonstrate this is for you to put a pulse oximeter on your finger, climb on to a trolley and get someone to tip you 35° head down. Most people's oxygen saturation fall by 2–3%. You will find it more difficult to breathe and most uncomfortable.

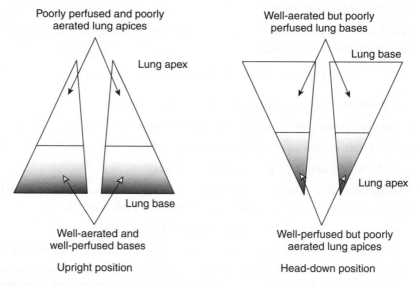

Figure 17.1 Effect of head down tilt

Why is this so?

The human lungs are designed to operate best when their owner is either upright, or lying flat. They are shaped a bit like tall narrow pyramids. In the upright position the bases of the lungs are better perfused, and better ventilated. Air travels almost in a straight line along axial airways to reach the lower lobes, and blood does not have to be pumped uphill to get there. The bases of the lungs have a much larger surface area available for gas exchange than the apices. When people lie on their back, air passes almost straight to the dependent lungs, which lie in gutter-shaped depressions on either side of their spinal columns.

However, when people are tipped into the head-down position, most of the air is directed to the bases of their lungs, but most of the blood is diverted toward the tip of the pyramid where there is not so much surface area for gas exchange. Consequently there is a mismatch of ventilation (V) to perfusion (Q). In jargon clinicians sometimes call this *V/Q imbalance*.

Management

Immediately

- Lift the patients' legs above their *isophlebotic point*, blood runs downhill into their central circulation. The veins in the legs hold about 400 ml of blood: this neither disturbs lung function, nor engorges their brains.
- Increase the inspired oxygen concentration.
- Check the ECG trace for asystole, ventricular fibrillation or pulseless ventricular tachycardia. These are treated as a cardiac arrest.

Validate the blood pressure

Confirm the blood pressure with your sphygmomanometer. Ensure the non-invasive blood pressure monitor is working properly. Is the blood pressure cuff the correct size? Measure the blood pressure on the other arm. If you are using an arterial line then flush the line, open the three-way tap to air to check the *transducer* is properly zeroed. Check that the waveform is pulsatile and not damped. Check that the oximeter reading is greater than 95%.

Is hypotension expected?

Expect hypotension:

- Immediately following spinal or epidural anaesthesia.
- Following cardioactive drugs: vasodilators, β-blockers, or pethidine.
- In patients who take long-acting vasodilating drugs for hypertension:
  - angiotensin-converting enzyme (ACE) inhibitor drugs with names ending in '-pril'; such as enalapril, and ramipril;
  - or angiotensin receptor blockers (ARB) with names ending in '-sartan'; such as irbesartan or candesartan.

What to do:

- Put the legs on a pillow (but do not tip the patient head down), while replacing vascular volume.

- Notify the anaesthetist who may use a vasopressor, such as metaraminol or phenylephrine, if the blood pressure does not respond to a volume load.

Volume resuscitation is the first priority,
especially after neuraxial blocks.

Is hypotension unexpected?

Consider:

- tachyarrhythmia: supraventricular tachycardia, atrial fibrillation or ventricular tachycardia;
- bradycardia < 45 beats/min;
- anaphylaxis;
- blood loss;
- impaired venous return for example pneumothorax, cardiac tamponade;
- air embolism – has the central line come apart?;
- CO_2 retention (especially after laparoscopy);
- trash emboli (orthopaedic or major trauma surgery);
- amniotic fluid (obstetric surgery);
- water (urological surgery and hysteroscopy);
- myocardial ischaemia;
- transfusion incompatibility;
- septic shock;
- acute adrenal insufficiency;
- rupture of the mitral valve.

Is hypotension unresponsive?

- Get help.
- Check airway, breathing.
- Prepare for chest X-ray, blood gases, 12-lead ECG.
- Prepare to insert central venous lines, or pulmonary artery catheters.
- In the intubated patient, transoesophageal echocardiography can provide useful information about myocardial function, and how adequately the ventricles are filling.

Drugs used to manage hypotension

Vasopressors are drugs that contract the smooth muscle in the walls of arterioles causing them to constrict. These drugs increase the systemic blood pressure in septic shock and during cardiopulmonary resuscitation. Some, but not all, vasopressors are *catecholamines*.

Catecholamines include naturally occurring substances such as noradrenaline, adrenaline and dopamine. Non-catecholamine vasoconstricting drugs include ephedrine, metaraminol, phenylephrine and methoxamine.

Adrenaline

Adrenaline is a hormone produced by the adrenal gland. It is the 'hormone of exercise'. It increases heart rate and cardiac output, and in physiological amounts increases blood flow to skeletal muscle and the heart, while decreasing blood flow to the gut and kidneys.

Noradrenaline

Noradrenaline is the neurotransmitter for the sympathetic nervous system. It is potent and causes generalized arteriolar constriction everywhere except the brain. It is also produced in the adrenal gland where it is a precursor for adrenaline.

Dobutamine

Dobutamine is a synthetic drug resembling dopamine, and causing less tachycardia. It does not maintain the blood pressure as effectively as dopamine, but increases cardiac output without a parallel increase in heart rate. As the heart rate is slower, and the blood pressure is slightly higher, myocardial perfusion is better than with drugs that increase the heart rate. This is a valuable asset for the ischaemic, failing heart.

Dopexamine

Dopexamine is a synthetic β_2 agonist that dilates blood vessels in muscle and gut. It simultaneously increases the force of cardiac contraction, and decreases peripheral resistance; this improves tissue blood flow. It also improves renal blood flow.

Ephedrine

Ephedrine is a synthetic vasoconstrictor. Its effects are similar to adrenaline although it lasts longer. It is often used to counteract the hypotension caused by vasodilation after the insertion of an epidural or spinal anaesthetic. It is the best vasopressor to use during pregnancy because it does not greatly affect uterine blood flow.

Phenylephrine

Phenylephrine is a synthetic vasoconstrictor similar to noradrenaline. It produces profound vasoconstriction and as the blood pressure rises, it triggers a baroreceptor response that causes the heart rate to fall. It lasts about

15–20 minutes. Some anaesthetists use it to counteract the hypotension produced by spinal anaesthesia.

Metaraminol

Metaraminol is a synthetic vasopressor with actions similar to phenylephrine. If it is given by infusion then *tachyphylaxis* becomes a problem where more and more drug has to be infused to achieve an effect. A single dose lasts for 20–60 minutes.

Methoxamine

Methoxamine is a long-acting (1–2 hours) potent synthetic vasopressor similar to phenylephrine.

Vasopressin

Arginine vasopressin (AVP) is simply another name for naturally occurring *antidiuretic hormone* (ADH). Infused at higher than physiological concentrations it causes profound vasoconstriction in all vascular beds. It acts in an entirely different way to other vasopressors and is increasingly being used *off-label* to support the blood pressure in septicaemic shock and increasingly during cardiac arrest in the place of adrenaline.

Acute coronary syndrome

Emerging from an anaesthetic after major surgery is physiologically stressful. In susceptible patients this may cause *acute coronary syndrome* (ACS) to appear for the first time in recovery room. If staff fail to recognize ACS, the patient will return to the ward at risk of having a myocardial infarct in the next few days.

The acute coronary syndrome consists of a collection of ischaemic events with the shared underlying pathology of rupture of a coronary artery plaque, endothelial inflammation, and thrombosis. Clinically the syndrome includes unstable angina, acute ischaemia and evolving myocardial infarction.

Physiology

Cardiac ischaemia occurs when the heart's oxygen demands exceed its oxygen supply. When a person is at rest, their heart uses about 8 ml/100 mg/min, however with heavy exercise this may rise to 60 ml/100 mg/min. The hearts of people with hypertension have to work much harder than normal.

Oxygen demands

Oxygen demands depend on how much energy the heart muscle needs to function properly. The harder the cardiac myocytes *work*, the more oxygen they consume. The heart demands a lot more oxygen to sustain a high cardiac output, or a high blood pressure. Unless the oxygen is delivered properly to the heart muscle either the muscle becomes irritable and contracts incoordinately (usually seen as ventricular ectopics on the ECG monitor) or it fails to maintain its output and the patient becomes hypotensive.

Oxygen supply

Oxygen supply depends on the amount of oxygen carried in the blood, and how fast the coronary blood flow can deliver it. The amount of oxygen carried to the tissues by the blood depends on the oxygen content of the blood and the partial pressure at which it is delivered.

How fast the coronary blood flow can deliver oxygen depends on the mean blood pressure, the patency of the vessels, and the viscosity of the blood.

Blood can only flow through cardiac muscle when it is not contracting. Consequently almost all the ventricles' coronary perfusion occurs during diastole. With tachycardia the time taken for diastole gets shorter, and consequently the blood supply to both ventricles decreases.

Tachycardia decreases coronary blood flow.

Cardiac ischaemia in the recovery room

What is known:

- Postoperative myocardial infarction is the most common cause of death in patients undergoing non-cardiac surgery.
- If patients develop any indication of myocardial ischaemia during the operation or in the recovery room they are at increased risk of arrhythmias, ischaemic episodes, or cardiac failure in the first postoperative week, which probably extends through the following weeks.
- Most postoperative infarcts occur on the second or third postoperative day when the inflammatory response peaks.
- About half of postoperative infarcts are clinically silent with no chest pain; and of those patients who do infarct about half will die.
- Proper preoperative management of *ischaemic heart disease* (IHD) with aspirin, a statin, an ACE inhibitor, and possibly a β-blocker reduces cardiac complications postoperatively.
- Anxiety, fright, or pain is a potent cause of ischaemic chest pain.
- In patients with known ischaemic heart disease prophylactic GTN infusions do not help prevent ischaemia in the recovery room. This is because GTN has a brief action, and a tendency to cause *tachyphylaxis*. For these

reasons, it is better to withhold GTN in the recovery room until signs of ischaemia develop.

Who is at risk of ischaemic heart disease (IHD)?

The 40% rule

40% of patients

with IHD have few or no risk factors;
with IHD don't get classical angina;
with IHD have normal looking ECGs;
with vascular disease have severe IHD;
with diabetes > 10 years have IHD;
Smokers > 40 years have IHD;
with eGFR = 50 ml/min/1.73m2 have IHD.

In the recovery room be alert for the possibility of myocardial ischaemia in younger people with major risk factors.

Preoperatively:

- men aged > 50, and women aged > 60 years;
- those who have smoked for > 10 years;
- history of dyslipidaemia;
- hypertension;
- diabetes;
- myocardial infarction in a first-degree relative age <55 years;
- *android obesity*.

Postoperatively:

- major vascular surgery;
- emergency surgery;
- prolonged surgery > 3 hours;
- intraoperative arrhythmias, hypertension or hypotension;
- painful surgery in those aged > 45 years.

PACE

PACE is useful shorthand for *perioperative adverse cardiac events*. It includes such events as cardiac ischaemia, arrhythmias hypotension, shock, cardiac failure, acute pulmonary oedema, cardiogenic shock and death.

For elective surgery the risks of PACE are unacceptably high in those with:

- a myocardial infarct in the past 6 months, but especially within the past 3 months;
- a coronary artery stent inserted in the past 3 months, and probably within the last 6 months;
- unstable angina preoperatively; congestive cardiac failure at the time of surgery.

Such patients should not come to theatre for elective surgery. If they present for emergency surgery you can expect problems to arise in the recovery room.

How to recognize myocardial ischaemia

Diagnosing myocardial ischaemia depends on two features:

- chest pain;
- ECG changes.

Chest pain

Patients describe ischaemic chest pain (*angina*) as a heavy crushing pain behind their sternum and often as a tight band around their chest. Cardiac pain may be accompanied by pain radiating down the arm or up into the jaw or neck. In the recovery room these symptoms warn of impending myocardial infarction.

Any pain above the umbilicus relieved by rest or GTN, is angina until proven otherwise.

More than 40 per cent of postoperative patients with myocardial ischaemia get no warning signs, because they feel no pain. The nerve fibres carrying pain sensation from their hearts are already dead, because their blood supply has ceased. This is especially likely in patients with microvascular disease such as smokers, and diabetics.

As the oxygen supply fails the heart begins to fail. The patient may look grey, sweat, become hypotensive, develop a tachycardia, develop an irregular pulse (ventricular extrasystoles), have poor perfusion status, feel anxious, complain of breathlessness, and faintness or collapse.

Angina does not have to be chest pain. It may present with an aching pain anywhere above the umbilicus. It can radiate to neck, or jaw, or either arm (or both) and even to the top of the head. Occasionally angina is misdiagnosed as pain arising from the gallbladder.

ECG changes

The ECG monitor helps diagnose ischaemia. At first myocardial ischaemia presents with a tachycardia, and a few ventricular ectopic beats. As ischaemia worsens, the ST segment sinks below the isoelectric line. After an infarct the ST segment rises above this point.

Automated computerized ST analysis in leads II and V5 detects about 80 per cent of myocardial ischaemic episodes. Set the monitor to diagnostic ECG filtering mode.

ST analysis may mislead you if the patient is taking digoxin, has a bundle branch block, has a pacemaker, or is a fit young athlete. Isoelectric J-point depression developing for the first time in the recovery room is diagnostic of an ischaemic heart.

How to diagnose acute coronary syndrome

In the recovery room be particularly alert for ischaemia in patients who have:

- previously had coronary artery bypass surgery;
- diabetes;
- chronic kidney disease with an eGFR < 60 ml/min/1.73 m^2;
- or a coronary artery stent inserted within the past year.

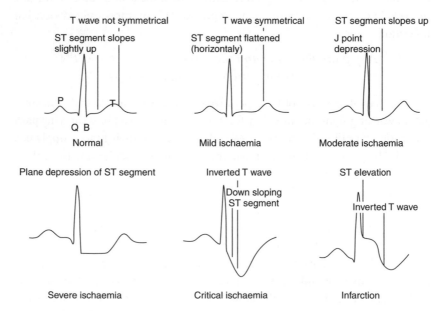

Figure 17.2 ECG stages in ischaemia

Signs to look for:

- transient hyperacute tall T-waves;
- flattening of the ST segment;
- down-sloping ST depression is serious;
- new onset left bundle branch block.

Consult the anaesthetist immediately if[1]:

- The patient has repeated chest pain or discomfort, or if the symptoms last more than 5 minutes.
- There are persistent ECG changes of ST depression = 0.5 mm, or new T-wave inversion > 2 mm.
- Transient ST-segment elevation (= 0.5 mm) in more than two contiguous leads on the ECG printout.

Prepare to resuscitate patients if:

- their systolic blood pressure < 90 mmHg, cool peripheries, sweating, or develops a mitral regurgitation murmur;
- their pulse rate > 120 beats/min or worse develops a supraventricular tachycardia;
- they feel faint, anxious and feel as though they are 'going to die';
- they collapse.

ST changes may not occur in a patient with acute coronary syndrome.

Hints

- Elderly patients, diabetics, long-term smokers, and women may present with atypical symptoms such as neck, jaw, back or epigastric discomfort, sweating, nausea or vomiting.
- Age is an important factor. The older the patient the more likely they are to have ischaemic heart disease. They do not need to have any of the classic risk factors, although younger patients with acute coronary syndrome generally have one or more risk factors.
- ST changes on the ECG may not occur in patients with acute coronary syndrome.

What to do if the patient develops cardiac ischaemia

Call for help. At least two trained staff should be attending the patient. Bring the cardiac 'crash cart' to the bedside. Make sure everything is ready in case you need to defibrillate the patient.

Improve oxygen supply:

- Give oxygen by mask, and continue it in the ward for the first 2–3 days;
- Give sublingual glyceryl trinitrate (GTN) 300 μgm;
- Improve coronary blood flow by treating diastolic hypotension.

Patients with ischaemic heart disease who become anaemic are at higher risk. Perioperatively their haemoglobin should be maintained above 100 gm/L.

Reduce oxygen demands:

- Treat tachycardia with a β-blocker such as metoprolol.
- Prevent hypertension and tachycardia by treating pain, controlling fluid balance, and treating anxiety.
- Keep blood pressure within 20% of baseline preoperative levels.
- Reduce afterload with GTN.
- Prevent or correct hypothermia to prevent shivering.
- The anaesthetists may use GTN to reduce preload and improve coronary blood flow. Start GTN at 10 μg/min, and then increase the dose by 10 μg/min until the symptoms resolve, or the mean blood pressure falls below 90 mmHg.

What to do next

Give aspirin as soon as possible. Give the patient 300 mg of soluble aspirin tablet dissolved in a glass of water. First discuss this with the surgeon, especially where bleeding may be a disaster such as after neurosurgery, open eye or middle ear surgery.

Persistently raised or lowered ST segments greater than 0.5 mm or new T-wave inversion greater than 2 mm suggest severe ischaemia. This means that one or more of the patient's coronary arteries is partly or completely obstructed. The sooner the artery is unblocked, the better the outcome for the patient. Involve a cardiologist immediately. It may be necessary to transfer the patient to a tertiary institution. Although patients who have just had surgery are not suitable for fibrinolysis they may have *percutaneous intervention* (PCI) such as a coronary stent or balloon angioplasty. Ideally balloon angioplasty needs to be done within 60 minutes of the onset of signs or symptoms, because longer delays result in poorer outcomes. By the time 12 hours have elapsed and where the patient is haemodynamically stable there is little point in performing an angioplasty.

What investigations to order

In the mean time investigations should include 12-lead ECG; full blood examination (FBE); serum electrolytes and creatinine; and blood glucose. Take blood for troponin T levels. If troponins are not done in your hospital then order serum creatine kinase also known as CK-MB levels, but raised levels may be misleading because CK-MB is released from bowel smooth muscle during abdominal surgery.

Acute coronary syndrome? Involve a cardiologist immediately.

How long to monitor patients

Even if a patient develops only transient postoperative myocardial ischaemia in the recovery room, they should be transferred to a special unit where they can be continuously monitored with an ECG until the stress phase of surgery is over. If continuous monitoring is unavailable then patients require serial ECGs at least every 8 hours. After uncomplicated major surgery the stress phase usually lasts 4–6 days.

Heart failure

Cardiac failure not only affects the heart; it is a multisystem disorder with abnormalities in cardiac and skeletal muscle; alterations in renal function; chronic stimulation of the adrenergic nervous system, and a complex pattern of neurohormonal changes.

What is heart failure?

Pragmatically, *heart failure* occurs when a person's heart cannot pump enough blood to their tissues for them to go about their daily business. If you are not anaemic, do not have lung disease but you get puffed shopping, or making the bed you probably have heart failure. As we grow older our capacity to exercise declines. There may be nothing much wrong with our hearts but we are unlikely to be able to run up steep hills against gale force winds carrying a 60 Kg pack like an elite soldier.

Exactly what constitutes heart failure is not well defined, and clinicians use many different terms to describe it. *Left-sided failure* and *right-sided failure* are the most commonly used terms. Left-sided failure clinically presents with one or more symptoms of exertional dyspnoea, a large heart and crackles in the lung bases. In contrast right-sided failure is characterized by oedema in the legs or over the sacrum, raised jugular venous pressure and possibly liver congestion. The term *congestive cardiac failure* is reserved for left-sided cardiac failure that is severe enough to produce right-sided failure. The clinical signs vary in severity from patient to patient.

The clinical findings and treatment of heart failure are best understood by reviewing normal cardiac function, and the effects of disease. Despite all the different descriptions of heart disease there are only three ways the heart can fail. It can have problems with:

1. rate and rhythm;
2. contractility;
3. excessively high output.

Rate and rhythm problems

Heart rate is too slow:

- sinus bradycardia;
- heart blocks;
- drugs, such as neostigmine, and β-blockers.

Heart rate is too fast:

- sinus tachycardia;
- uncontrolled atrial flutter or fibrillation;
- paroxysmal supraventricular tachycardia;
- drugs, such as atropine and adrenaline.

Contractility problems

Cardiac contractility problems occur with:

- ischaemic heart disease;
- various forms of *cardiomyopathy*;
- high-output failure when a normal heart has to output higher than normal volumes because of an intercurrent medical illness.

Systolic heart failure

Systolic failure is usually caused by ischaemic heart disease or cardiomyopathy. Of the many causes of cardiomyopathy, alcoholism is the most frequent culprit.

With systolic failure the heart muscle becomes stretched and flabby. It has lost its ability to contract forcibly enough to eject the normal amount of half of its blood volume during systole. If the patient has chronic systolic failure then the preoperative chest X-ray (CXR) shows a large heart, an echocardiogram will show an ejection fraction less than 40%, and the patient will have a MET score less than 3.

Only two things cause acute systolic failure in a previously well patient: acute myocardial infarction or ischaemia, or gross iatrogenic fluid overload.

Pulmonary oedema

Cardiogenic pulmonary oedema

In the recovery room acute left ventricular systolic failure presents with *pulmonary oedema*. These patients feel breathless, and are wheezy; if you listen near their mouth you can hear crackles when they breathe. A stethoscope reveals showers of crackles all over their lungs. The patients panic if they are lying flat and struggle to sit up. They usually have a tachycardia. They cannot lie flat (*orthopnoea*) and may be cyanosed or even coughing up frothy pink sputum. Their urine output is low, and they may be sweaty, and cyanosed with cold hands.

These symptoms are easy to recognize, although the early stages may be mistaken for asthma or aspiration. A chest X-ray confirms the diagnosis revealing a snowstorm appearance in both lungs, and pulmonary vascular congestion. Blood gases show signs of tissue hypoxia; typically a metabolic acidosis, and a low PO_2 less than 60 mmHg (7.89 kPa) and a low PCO_2 less than 30 mmHg (3.95 kPa).

Non-cardiogenic pulmonary oedema

Acute pulmonary oedema can also occur without systolic failure.

Naloxone not only reverses all the effects of opioids, but also the patient's *endogenous* pain-killing endorphins, and may suddenly catapult the patient into agonizing pain. In younger people the shock may causing such an abrupt rise in pulmonary vascular pressures that intravascular fluid is forced through the alveolar capillary membrane into the airspaces of the lung, causing pulmonary oedema.

Young patients who forcefully inspire against a closed airway can so badly damage their alveolar–capillary membrane that fluids transudate from their blood stream into their alveoli. You sometimes see this after an episode of severe laryngospasm or coughing.

With septicaemia, bacteria release endotoxins, which damages vascular endothelial membranes in all tissues. This event allows fluid to leak out of the capillaries and collect in the interstitium of the lungs causing interstitial pulmonary oedema. This phenomenon is occasionally seen in the recovery room in patients who have had urological surgery, or where abscesses were drained.

How to manage pulmonary oedema

To treat acute pulmonary oedema, first keep your patient alive, then identify the problem, find the cause, and treat it.

First

- Sit the patient up as much as possible.
- Give high oxygen concentrations by mask.
- Inform the anaesthetist.
- Do a full 12-lead ECG to identify ischaemia and arrhythmias.
- Give furosemide 0.5 mg/Kg slowly IV and repeat in 20 minutes if the urine output is < 100 ml/hr.
- Give morphine 0.1 mg/Kg IV slowly to relieve distress, slow their breathing, and lower pulmonary vascular pressures. Use morphine and no other opioid.
- Give GTN 600 µg sublingually while preparing an infusion.

Later

The anaesthetist may consider additional measures:

- Invasive blood pressure monitoring: arterial, central venous, and possible pulmonary artery catheters.
- GTN infusion to lower vascular pressures.
- Dobutamine infusion to increase cardiac contractility.
- Positive pressure ventilation.
- Intra-aortic balloon pump to assist the circulation.
- Transfer to intensive care unit.
- Urgent cardiology consultation.

Monitor

ECG, pulse oximetry, non-invasive blood pressure, urine output, blood gases, serum electrolytes, urea, troponin T levels, and a chest X-ray.

Diastolic heart failure

As each cardiac muscle degenerates and dies, it is replaced by stiff (*incompliant*) collagen tissue and the heart slowly becomes fibrotic. Unable to stretch enough to increase its stroke-volume, the only way the heart can increase its output is to beat faster. Usually patients with diastolic failure have preoperative resting pulse rates of 80 beats/min or more.

The commonest reason for chronic diastolic failure is sustained or poorly treated hypertension. The myocytes simply wear out and die from overwork. Once hypertensive patients have established ECG evidence of left ventricular hypertrophy they are destined to get diastolic dysfunction.

Unable to increase their stroke volume patients with diastolic dysfunction are susceptible to hypotension if they vasodilate. Vasodilation can be caused by epidural or spinal anaesthesia, and some drugs. Then the only way the heart can increase its output to maintain the blood pressure is to increase its rate.

You may encounter other conditions simulating diastolic failure where the stroke-volume of the heart is limited by:

- gas embolism, which is occasionally seen after laparoscopy or hysteroscopy;
- acute pulmonary embolism;
- tension pneumothorax;
- pericardial tamponade after thoracic surgery;
- aortic or mitral stenosis.

Features of acute diastolic failure may not be as obvious as those of acute systolic failure, but they include tachycardia, hypotension, nausea, vomiting, and faintness or syncope on sitting up. Peripheral perfusion is poor and urine output is low.

A useful warning is to look at patient's preoperative heart rate and resting blood pressure. If they have hypertension and a resting heart rate higher than their diastolic blood pressure then suspect chronic diastolic heart failure.

Management

First

- Give high concentrations of oxygen by mask.
- Inform the anaesthetist.
- Exclude a pneumothorax. Patients with a pneumothorax are more comfortable sitting up.

Monitor:

ECG, pulse oximetry, non-invasive blood pressure, central venous pressures, urine output, blood gases, serum electrolytes, urea, troponin T levels, and a chest X-ray. Continuing management depends on the cause of the failure.

High-output heart failure

High-output cardiac failure occurs, not because there is anything wrong with the heart, but rather that some other disease is making the heart work too hard.

If the demands are too great the heart eventually fails. In addition if the patient also has heart disease, then the heart fails sooner, rather than later.

What causes high output failure?

Anaemia

Anaemic patients have less haemoglobin to carry oxygen so their hearts have to pump blood around faster to maintain tissue oxygen supply.

Obesity

With each 10 Kg of extra weight the resting cardiac output increases by a 1000 ml a minute. A normal person's resting cardiac output is about 5 litres a minute. In contrast, a person who is 40 Kg overweight (say weighing 110 Kg) has a resting cardiac output of 9 litres a minute. Following a total hip replacement, their cardiac output must increase by an additional 40 per cent. Consequently, on the second and third day following surgery their heart must sustain a resting cardiac output of about 14 litres a minute. This is one reason that obese people are at higher risk of cardiac failure after major surgery.

Thyrotoxicosis

Thyrotoxicosis speeds up tissue metabolism so that their oxygen needs increase hugely.

Paget's disease of the bone

With Paget's disease large blood vessels in the bone allow blood to flow from the arteries into the veins with little resistance. To prevent hypotension the cardiac output has to rise.

Incompetent cardiac valves allow blood to reflux

The ventricles of patients with incompetent heart valves have to cope with a backward reflux of blood in addition to ejecting their stroke volumes. This is analogous to a heart with each beat having to pump two stroke-volumes forward into the aorta only to have one stroke-volume to reflux back into the ventricle.

Severe intra-abdominal sepsis

Intraperitoneal sepsis may result in up to half the cardiac output being shunted through inflamed peritoneum, thus depriving other organs and tissues of their oxygen supply. This huge afterload reduction causes hypotension, tachycardia and a high cardiac output. Additionally bacterial endotoxins released from the septic source accompanied by circulating shock factors often cause the heart to contract more weakly, resulting in catastrophic septic shock.

Cardiogenic shock

Postoperative cardiogenic shock is usually caused by a massive myocardial infarction, or occurs in a patient with pre-existing severe systolic heart failure. Patients are hypotensive, cyanosed, cold to touch, sweating with almost no urine output. They may have altered conscious state, with dilating pupils. Their blood gases show a severe metabolic acidosis and hypoxia. Perfusion of gut, kidneys, liver and pancreas fails, and skin and muscle circulation almost cease. Once the left ventricular output falls by about 35 per cent the consequent noradrenergically induced vasoconstriction is so intense the patient will not survive.

Cardiogenic shock is managed the same way as severe acute systolic dysfunction. In desperation clinicians sometimes use adrenaline or even noradrenaline infusions to improve cardiac function, but usually to no avail.

Pericardial tamponade

Cardiac *tamponade* occurs when more than 150–300 ml of fluid acutely collects in the pericardial sac. The collecting fluid squashes the heart, preventing it filling enough to eject an adequate stroke volume.

Bleeding into the pericardial sac can occur with chest trauma, a dissecting aneurysm, or after thoracic or upper abdominal surgery (especially hiatus hernia repair, or oesophagectomy). Diagnosing tamponade is not easy; but clinically hypotension, tachycardia, dyspnoea, and especially distended neck veins and facial suffusion give a clue.

On the ECG monitor you might see *electrical alternans* (alternating big and small QRS complexes) and low voltages. When patients inspire their systolic pressure may fall by more than 20 mmHg, and their peripheral pulse may even disappear altogether. This *pulsus paradoxus* also occurs with hypovolaemia. Usually patients need to return to theatre to have the fluid drained, but occasionally the surgeon may aspirate the fluid (*pericardiocentesis*) with a wide bore needle.

Valvular heart disease

Aortic valve sclerosis is common in people older than 65 years, and about 3 per cent of those older than 75 years have severe aortic stenosis. Preadmission clinics usually assess symptomatic valvular heart disease with echocardiography before surgery. This test assesses both the function of the valves and the ventricular ejection fraction. Those with a reduced ejection fraction (EF) of less than 40% are particularly at risk.

People with valvular heart disease such as aortic or mitral stenosis or incompetence have *fixed cardiac outputs* so that they cannot increase their cardiac outputs to meet tissue demand.

Mitral valve disease is more common in younger people who have had rheumatic fever, while it accompanies aortic stenosis in older people who have atherosclerosis.

To withstand major surgery patients with mitral valve regurgitation need an *ejection fraction* above normal (EF > 50%).

Patients with stenotic valvular heart disease become abruptly hypotensive if their cardiac output falls, or if they vasodilate. Bradycardias may cause hypotension, and tachycardias do not allow enough between each beat time to squeeze blood though the narrow valve openings.

If the patient has aortic or mitral stenosis they may develop pulmonary oedema if given enough fluid to raise their preload; or severe hypotension if they incur peripheral vasodilation with spinal or epidural anaesthetics.

People with incompetent valves have ejection fractions greater than 50% and may consequently progress to develop a form of high output cardiac failure.

How to manage valvular heart disease

In the recovery room prevent your patient developing a tachycardia, or abrupt changes in blood pressure. Do not allow your patient to suffer pain, hypoxia, or hypovolaemia; or have any other reason to develop a tachycardia. Do not discharge patients to the ward unless they are pain-free, have stable circulations, a good urine output and warm dry hands.

Those with valve disease or septal defects are susceptible bacterial endocarditis and need antibiotic prophylaxis for dirty surgery, or if they have been intubated. Dirty surgery includes bowel, dental or urological surgery including endoscopy. Check your hospital's protocols for using prophylactic antibiotics, and check that they have either been given in theatre; or give them now.

Arrhythmias

Arrhythmias are irregularities in the heartbeat. There are two pathological mechanisms that alter the heart's rate or rhythm: abnormal impulse generation and abnormal impulse propagation.

Arrhythmias are best seen in lead II on the ECG.

Abnormal impulse generation

Although the cardiac impulse usually originates in the SA node and follows an orderly path through the heart, irritable cells can disrupt the sequence by imposing their own rhythm. Myocardial cells irritated by ischaemia, electrolyte imbalance, or inflammation depolarize spontaneously generating stray *ectopic cardiac beats*.

Abnormal impulse propagation

Arrhythmias can arise at any point on the cardiac impulse's journey from the SA node to its final extinction in the ventricles. Impulses are diverted from their usual path when a group of myocardial cells become hypoxic or die. The abnormal diversion causes the heart to either beat irregularly, or in an uncoordinated way. Impulses blocked or delayed while passing through the AV node cause *heart blocks*. Impulses blocked in one of the major branches of the bundle of His cause right or left bundle branch blocks. Damage to the component branches of the left bundle cause anterior or posterior hemiblocks.

Clinical aspects

Minor arrhythmias are common in patients recovering from anaesthesia. If you notice a slow, fast irregular or absent pulse attach an ECG monitor. It is not always easy to immediately identify the type of arrhythmia on a monitor screen. If the arrhythmia persists do a formal 12-lead ECG to establish its nature.

Patients may complain of one or more of the following: palpitations, chest pain, nausea, faintness, or breathlessness. All these are signs of hypotension or myocardial ischaemia.

Causes of arrhythmias

Patient factors

Factors specific to the patient may cause arrhythmias including pain, hypoxia, myocardial ischaemia, hypercarbia, hypertension, hypotension, electrolyte imbalance particularly potassium, and magnesium; and drugs such as tricyclic antidepressants and digoxin.

Surgical factors

Factors caused by the surgery include thoracic operations (especially if the pericardium is damaged), unrelieved pain (particularly from upper abdominal surgery), operations on eyes, ears and upper jaws stimulate the vagus nerve (causing bradycardia), and drugs such as cocaine or adrenaline used to reduce bleeding.

Anaesthetic factors

Anaesthetic drugs can contribute to arrhythmias. These include residual effects of drugs such as fentanyl or neostigmine causing bradycardia, or atropine causing tachycardia. Adrenaline used with local anaesthetics may cause tachyarrhythmias.

A new wide QRS complex rhythm needs urgent attention.

When to worry about arrhythmias

Innocent arrhythmias usually have rates between 60 and 120 beats/min; the ECG shows narrow QRS complexes, the blood pressure remains within 20% of preoperative levels, and the oxygen saturation greater than 95%.

Notify the anaesthetist if the patient's heart rate is greater than 200 minus the patient's age. Also notify the anaesthetist if the:

- pulse rate is < 50 beats/min;
- oxygen saturations fall below 93%;
- QRS complexes become widened;
- regular heart rhythm suddenly becomes irregular;
- ST segments rise above or fall below the isoelectric line;
- patient feels: faint, becomes hypotensive, complains of chest pain, is nauseated, or their conscious state deteriorates;
- perfusion status deteriorates.

Figure 17.3 The principle causes of arrhythmias in the recovery room

Arrhythmia with hypotension? Call for help!

Tachycardia

Tachycardia is defined as a pulse rate exceeding 100 beats per minutes, or in children a rate 20 per cent greater than their preoperative baseline rate. Once the pulse rate exceeds 150 beats/min it is either a *supraventricular (SVT) or ventricular tachycardia* (VT). An SVT may show P-waves on the ECG trace (although they may be difficult to detect), and ventricular tachycardias do not.

In adults, look for a reason for a pulse rate exceeding 80 beats/min. Tachycardia is a response to an activated sympathetic nervous system, and something must be activating it.

If the heart rate is greater than 80 beats/min then find the cause.

At heart rates above 130 beats/min the ventricles do not have time to fill properly and so their stroke-volume progressively declines. Older patients tolerate tachycardia poorly; they readily become hypotensive or develop myocardial ischaemia.

Sinus tachycardia

With a sinus tachycardia the P-waves are present; the QRS width is normal (less than 120 ms); and the rhythm regular.

Lead II

Figure 17.4 Sinus tachycardia

Sinus tachycardia is an excellent early warning sign of developing disaster: hypoxia in the early stages, bleeding, hypovolaemia, dilutional anaemia, cardiac failure, early cardiac ischaemia, hypoglycaemia, hypercarbia, malignant hyperthermia and sepsis. Other causes are agitation, developing thyroid storm after a thyroidectomy, pneumothorax, and drugs used to control local bleeding during surgery such as adrenaline or cocaine.

To treat sinus tachycardia you need to treat the cause. Unrelieved sinus tachycardia may progress to supraventricular tachycardia.

Sinus tachycardia warns of impending problems.

A β-blocker is often used to slow the heart rate if tachycardia is causing signs of myocardial ischaemia. The anaesthetist may start with the short acting β-blocker, esmolol as an infusion of 50–200 μg/Kg/min. If this is effective therapy is converted to a long-acting β-blocker, metoprolol or atenolol, once the situation is controlled.

Atrial fibrillation

In *atrial fibrillation* (AF) the P-waves are absent, and the rhythm is irregular, but the QRS width remains normal. The usual cause of AF in the recovery room is acute myocardial ischaemia. AF also may occur if the pericardium is disturbed during surgery. Other uncommon causes of AF include acute pulmonary embolism and thyroid storm. If your patient becomes hypotensive then prepare for cardioversion with a synchronised direct-current defibrillator. Seek skilled help.

Lead II

Figure 17.5 Atrial fibrillation

Atrial ectopic beats

Atrial ectopic (AE) beats are common and nearly always benign.

Normal P wave

Abnormal P wave
distorts T wave

Figure 17.6 Atrial ectopic beats

Multifocal atrial tachycardia

Multifocal atrial tachycardia (MAT) is uncommon. Its irregular rhythm is easy to confuse with AF, but MAT has three or more P-wave morphologies. Look at lead II. It is usually seen in the elderly where it indicates hypoxia or myocardial ischaemia.

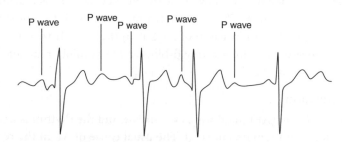

P wave   P wave   P wave   P wave   P wave

Figure 17.7 Multifocal atrial tachycardia

Hazardous tachycardias

More serious tachycardias are:

1. Narrow complex tachycardias (QRS complex < 120 ms, that is less than 3 little squares on the ECG paper).

2. Broad complex tachycardias (QRS complex < 120 ms, that is more than 3 little squares on the ECG paper).

Narrow complex tachycardias

Narrow complex tachycardias have a rate exceeding 150 beats/min. Their QRS duration is less than three little squares on standard ECG paper.

Atrioventricular node re-entry tachycardia

With AV nodal re-entry tachycardia the pulse rate may exceed 160 beats/min, but the QRS complex is not widened. It usually starts and stops abruptly. The commonest cause is *Wolf–Parkinson–White syndrome* (WPW), a congenital abnormality of the conducting system. The ECG shows PR intervals less than 0.12 seconds, with a slurred upstroke on the R wave. Use DC reversion if the patient is hypotensive. Do not use adenosine, verapamil, or digoxin to try to slow the rate, because these drugs may, paradoxically, divert the cardiac impulse down the aberrant pathway and cause the heart rate to increase.

Figure 17.8 Atrioventricular node re-entry tachycardia

Atrial flutter with block

With *atrial flutter* with block can present usually has a fixed number of flutter waves before a QRS complex. With atrial flutter with 2:1 block the rate is almost exactly 150 beats/min. Look for saw-toothed flutter waves in lead II. This arrhythmia indicates myocardial ischaemia, or digoxin toxicity. Often, it will respond to a cold wet towel placed on the patient's face. If that fails, prepare to give adenosine 6 mg by rapid IV injection, followed by a saline flush. If necessary another 12 mg dose can be given 3 minutes later. Adenosine often causes bronchospasm in asthmatics.

Flutter waves

Flutter waves

Lead II

Figure 17.9 Atrial flutter with 3:1 block

Broad complex tachycardias

Broad complex tachycardias have a rate greater than 150 beats/min, and QRS greater than 120 ms (more than 3 little squares on the ECG paper). They are invariably serious and, apart from torsade de pointes, are almost always due to acute cardiac ischaemia. You will find it difficult to identify the underlying rhythm. Prepare for urgent resuscitation. Give high flow oxygen by face mask. Call for help. If you cannot feel a pulse then it is a *pulseless arrhythmia*: start the *advanced cardiac life support algorithm*.

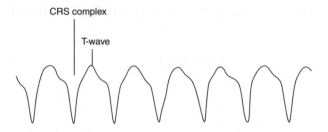

CRS complex

T-wave

Figure 17.10 Ventricular tachycardia

Ventricular tachycardia

With *ventricular tachycardia* (VT) and the patient is hypotensive then use DC cardioversion; otherwise give amiodarone 150 mg IV over 10 minutes, followed by 300 mg infusion in 1 hour. When patients are stable they will be transferred to the intensive care unit.

Ventricular fibrillation

With *ventricular fibrillation* (VF) there are no clearly identifiable QRS complexes, and the pulses are absent or weak. This is a *cardiac arrest*. Start the *advanced cardiac life support algorithm*. Use asynchronized DC cardioversion. When the patient is stable, organize to transfer them to the intensive care unit.

Figure 17.11 Ventricular fibrillation

Torsades de points

Torsades de points is a vicious polymorphic ventricular tachycardia. The QRS complexes appear to twist about the baseline on the ECG trace. The patient's preoperative ECG may show a prolonged rate corrected QT interval (*QTc* greater than 400 ms), and possibly U-waves in leads V2, and V3. Most patients have a congenital abnormality of their calcium channels called the long QT syndrome (LQT), but others are taking drugs that prolong the QT interval such as lithium, haloperidol, erythromycin, terbinafine; or cardiac drugs such as amiodarone, sotalol or disopyramide.

Note "Spiral Pattern"

Figure 17.12 Torsades de points

Hypokalaemia and hypomagnesaemia aggravate the problem. In the recovery room torsades sometimes occurs if a susceptible patient has received isoflurane during the anaesthetic. It is usually treated with magnesium sulphate 2 gm IV (4 ml of the 50% solution) infused over 10 minutes. Organize to transfer the patient to ICU for ongoing infusion and observation.

Bradycardia

Bradycardia is defined as a pulse rate less 60 beats/min. However bradycardia rarely causes problems until the rate is 45 beats/min or less.

Bradycardia causing hypotension is an emergency.

Sinus bradycardia

With sinus bradycardia the ECG complexes are normal in form, and the rhythm is regular.

Many athletes have slow pulse rates; other causes include intraoperative fentanyl especially if propofol was used, calcium channel and beta-blockers (even timolol eyedrops), residual effects of neostigmine used to reverse muscle relaxation, and after carotid surgery.

Lead II

Figure 17.13 Sinus bradycardia

Do not treat bradycardia unless your patient is hypotensive. Then give oxygen, and a small dose of atropine 0.4 mg IV over one minute.

Serious causes of bradycardia include heart blocks, near-death hypoxia, myocardial ischaemia (especially after anterior infarction), critically raised intracranial pressure hypothermia, high spinal cord injury, and myxoedema.

Trifascicular block

Trifascicular block is misnamed, because the block only involves two fascicles. When two fascicles are blocked simultaneously (such as the right bundle branch and the left anterior hemi fascicle) it is called a bifasicular block. A delay in transmitting the impulse from the sino-atrial node through the atrioventricular node is called an *AV conduction block* (or first degree heart block). The combination of all three (LAHB + RBBB + AV conduction block) is called a *trifascicular block*. It is caused by ischaemic heart disease, hypertension or other degenerative heart diseases.

At one time, many patients with trifasicular block were electively paced with a pacemaker for major surgery, but unless the patient is having faints or dizzy turns this is not longer necessary. Trifasicular block can progress to complete heart block in the recovery room. If it does, the pulse rate will drop to 40 beats/min or less and the patient may require a temporary pacemaker.

Complete heart block

Complete heart block (third degree heart block) is a life-threatening arrhythmia. The pulse is less than 40 beats/min, and the rhythm irregular. Look for it in lead II. With complete heart block a QRS complex does not necessarily follow each P-wave, because the atria and ventricles are contracting independently from one another.

Figure 17.14 Complete heart block

In the recovery room, the onset of complete heart block strongly suggests acute myocardial ischaemia. Give oxygen. Notify the anaesthetist. The patient may become hypotensive, and feel nauseated. The anaesthetist may try in order: atropine 0.4–1.2 mg IV slowly. If that fails, then an isoprenaline infusion (0.5–20 μg/Kg/min), or less optimally an adrenaline infusion (2–10 μg/Kg/min) is used to maintain the pulse rate and blood pressure. This will give you time to organize the insertion of a cardiac pacemaker. Some recovery rooms keep a transcutaneous pacemaker to use as a stop gap measure.

Other important arrhythmias

Ventricular ectopic beats

Ventricular ectopics (VES) are also called ventricular premature beats (VPBs) or ventricular extrasystoles. These premature contractions arise from an irritable ectopic focus where impulses arrive earlier than expected in the cardiac cycle.

Figure 17.15 Ventricular ectopic beats

About half the population have occasional ectopic beats, especially if they have recently indulged in caffeine, alcohol, or nicotine. Less than 3 ectopic beats a minute are not a worry. If there are more than 5 ectopic beats, or if the beats have different morphology, then they warn of impending problems. Important causes of VEs include; hypoxia; hypercarbia; myocardial ischaemia; hypertension; pain, anxiety or fear; hypomagnesemia and hypokalaemia.

Bigeminy

Bigeminy occurs when a normal beat is followed by a ventricular ectopic to be followed by a pause. During this compensatory pause the myocytes recover before the next cycle begins.

Figure 17.16 Bigeminy

Bigeminy indicates more serious problems than the occasional VE such as myocardial ischaemia, hypertension, digoxin toxicity; high sympathetic drive; hypokalaemia or hypomagnesemia. In the recovery room it usually resolves when the cause is corrected, or progresses to ventricular tachycardia. Principles of management are to give oxygen, treat pain, treat hypertension, consider a giving a GTN sublingually or intravenously, and cautiously slow the pulse rate with intravenous metoprolol.

A patient with ventricular ectopics, who has myocardial ischaemia or poor peripheral perfusion, is likely to die suddenly.

Anti-arrhythmic drugs

Atrioventricular conduction blockers

Adenosine

Adenosine, an endogenous purine nucleoside, is a potent atrioventricular blocking drug. This drug is used to treat both wide complex and narrow complex supraventricular tachycardias arising in the SA or AV node, but not for atrial flutter. Its therapeutic effect lasts for 20–30 seconds. The dose is titrated starting with 50 µg/Kg IV, and then give incremental doses of 50 µg/Kg IV every two minutes. The mean dose required to revert AV nodal re-entry arrhythmias ranges from 100–250 µg/Kg. Side effects of dyspnoea, chest pain, hypotension, nausea and flushing and headache are common, but they only last for about 30 seconds. If used in a patient taking dipyridamole it may cause heart block.

Beta-blocking drugs (β-blockers)

β-blockers block the effects of catecholamines, such as, noradrenaline and adrenaline. They slow the heart rate and make the heart contract less powerfully. This effect is useful in hypertension, and angina. Principally they are used to control supraventricular tachycardias. They may cause bronchoconstriction, make asthma worse, and mask the signs of hypoglycaemia, hypovolaemia and hypercarbia. All β-blockers are about equally efficacious. The two most widely available are metoprolol and atenolol. Cardioselective β-blockers have fewer vascular, respiratory and metabolic side-effects, and are less likely to cause bronchoconstriction.

Metoprolol

Metoprolol is a cardioselective β-blocker. The dose is 0.1–0.15 mg/Kg IV. Give it over 1 minute. It has a half-life of 3–4 hours, and is metabolized by the liver. It aggravates asthma and cardiac failure, and may cause AV block in patients taking verapamil.

Esmolol

Esmolol is a short-acting, cardioselective β-blocker used to control the heart rate in patients with supraventricular tachycardias. It works in less than 5 minutes, and has an elimination half-life of 9 minutes. It is used as a 10 mg/ml solution, with a loading dose of 500 μg/Kg over one minute. This is followed with a 4-minute maintenance infusion of 50 μg/Kg/min. The dose is varied to get the desired effect. If the ventricular rate does not fall and the blood pressure remains stable, then repeat the loading dose, and increase the maintenance dose in steps of 50 μg/Kg/min to a maximum of 200 μg/Kg/min. Once the heart rate is under control it can be maintained with another agent, such as digoxin, propanolol, or metoprolol. It aggravates asthma and cardiac failure, and will cause AV block in patients taking verapamil.

Drugs prolonging the refractory phase

Once a myocardial cell contracts, it takes a short time to recover before it can contract again. This is called the *refractory phase*. Amiodarone and sotalol are drugs that prolong the refractory phase. They are useful for suppressing abnormal *depolarization* in irritable myocardial cells.

Sotalol

Sotalol is useful for treating atrial fibrillation and flutter, arrhythmias in Wolff–Parkinson–White syndrome, ventricular tachycardia, and ventricular premature beats. Unlike other β-blockers it only slightly depresses the heart's contractility, but may cause sinus bradycardia. The dose is 0.5–1.5 mg/Kg IV over

10 minutes. The kidney excretes it, and its effect lasts about 6 hours. Atropine 0.6–2.4 mg IV is used if there is excessive bradycardia causing symptoms, such as hypotension, dyspnoea, or mental state changes. Bradycardia and heart block are more likely if the patient is hypokalaemic.

Amiodarone

Amiodarone is the most effective drug for acute arrhythmias. It is unlikely to reduce cardiac output. Vasodilation causes troublesome hypotension occurs if amiodarone is given too rapidly to patients in heart failure. Make up 300 mg in 50 ml of 5% dextrose. (It is not compatible with 0.9% saline). The oily vehicle causes thrombophlebitis, so infuse it into a central vein.

The initial loading dose is 4–5 mg/Kg (about 0.7–0.8 ml/Kg) given over 20 minutes. The maintenance dose is 0.3–0.4 mg/Kg/hr for the next 24 hours. If the rate control remains poor an extra 1 mg/Kg may be given over one hour, and repeated if needed. As amiodarone is a non-competitive adrenoceptor antagonist, it potentiates the effects of β-blockers or calcium channel blockers increasing the risk of hypotension and bradyarrhythmias.

Cardiac glycosides

Digoxin

Digoxin usually slows the ventricular rate in atrial fibrillation, but does not revert the heart to sinus rhythm. It is sometimes used in atrial fibrillation to increase myocardial contraction, and slow the rate of impulse transmission through the AV node. The loading dose is up to 10–15 µg/Kg IV, given over 20 minutes and a further 5 µg/Kg after 6 hours. The lower dosing range is used in the elderly. Never give digoxin intramuscularly, because it causes massive muscle necrosis.

New onset atrial fibrillation with hypotension?
Use DC reversion.

Calcium blockers

Verapamil

Verapamil slows AV node conduction. It is useful to control atrial fibrillation and flutter, but vasodilation may cause the blood pressure to fall. It does not revert the heart to sinus rhythm. It is likely to cause severe bradycardia, heart block, or even asystole if used with β-blockers. The dose is 0.1–0.2 mg/Kg IV given over 10 minutes. If an infusion is needed, then give verapamil at a rate of 5 µg/Kg/min. If the patient is taking a β-blocker do not use verapamil.

Magnesium

Magnesium is an essential co-factor for the production of *ATP* in biochemical reactions. It is a physiological calcium antagonist. Magnesium deficiency is associated with cardiac arrhythmias, cardiac failure and sudden cardiac death. It can precipitate refractory ventricular fibrillation. Magnesium supplementation may decrease the incidence of post-ischaemic arrhythmias. Suspect magnesium deficiency in patients who have been on diuretics, have had large intestinal fluid losses, or who are hypokalaemic. Since magnesium spreads evenly through out the extracellular fluid, it needs a large loading dose. The kidneys rapidly excrete magnesium, so to maintain blood levels, the loading dose is followed with a constant intravenous infusion. It works mainly by presynaptic inhibition of neuro-transmitter release in peripheral nerves, or by direct inhibition of cardiac muscle, or by vascular smooth muscle dilation. Magnesium also blocks the vagus nerve causing a tachycardia. Apart from its anti-arrhythmic activity it is a bronchodilator, a tocolytic, and has renal vasodilator activity. Calcium is an effective antagonist of magnesium's effects.

Note

1. Aroney CN, Aylward P, Kelly A-M (2006) *Medical Journal of Australia* 184:S1–S32.

18

Cardiopulmonary resuscitation

Cardiac arrest is best managed by following the published guidelines and recommendations of the International Liaison Committee on Resuscitation. These guidelines use current best medical evidence, and cover basic, advanced and paediatric life support. Every health care worker must be competent in performing cardiopulmonary resuscitation (CPR) to the level of basic life support (BLS). Competence depends on three things: early detection of cardiac arrest, maintenance of coronary and cerebral oxygenation, and the time to defibrillation. In the recovery room nurses witness most of the cardiac arrests. They must be able to commence resuscitation, and be confident about applying defibrillation without a doctor present.

New terminology (current up until 2007)

- *CPR* = cardiopulmonary resuscitation. This includes external cardiac massage and respiratory support, which may be either bag and mask ventilation, or intubation and ventilation.
- *DCR* = direct current cardioversion with a defibrillator.
- *Lidocaine* is the new accepted rNNi nomenclature for lignocaine.
- *Pulseless VT* = pulseless ventricular tachycardia.
- *Pulseless electrical activity* (PEA) has replaced the term *electromechanical dissociation* (EMD).
- *Rescue breathing* has replaced the term expired air ventilation (mouth-to-mouth resuscitation), because it includes skilled workers using bag-and-mask techniques.
- *Rescuer* is a term that includes anyone trained in the CPR, whether or not they are a trained health care worker (a nurse or doctor).
- *Two-rescuer* CPR means that while one person is maintain the airway and ensuring adequate tidal air exchange, the other is performing external cardiac massage.
- *VF* = ventricular fibrillation.

Recent changes

An international consensus on resuscitation

In 2002 The American Heart Association in collaboration with the International Liaison Committee on Resuscitation (ILCOR) published a consensus statement, *Guidelines 2000 for Cardiopulmonary Resuscitation and Emergency Cardiovascular Care*.[1] These guidelines are accepted in most countries including Australasia, and those of the European Economic Union. The guidelines were further revised in 2005.[2]

Since the publication of *Guidelines 2000* there have been many changes in techniques and terminology.

Fundamentals

The aim of CPR is to supply enough oxygen to the myocardium and brain to prevent irreversible damage. Success depends on being able to maintain a clear airway, give high concentrations of oxygen, institute efficient cardiac massage, and early defibrillation. The resuscitation technique is based on basic cycles, each of 2 minutes duration.

There is no firm published data on the success of witnessed arrests in the recovery room, but a number of facts are evident.

A hypoxic heart will not respond to resuscitation.

- The outcome improves if staff practice CPR regularly on a mannequin.
- Most cardiac arrests are caused by the profound physiological stresses occurring as the patient emerges from anaesthesia. The effects of these stresses are magnified by any underlying ischaemic heart disease.
- Irritable myocardium responds by developing ventricular extrasystoles, this progresses to ventricular tachycardia, and finally ventricular fibrillation.
- Progressive untreated hypoxia ends in an asystolic arrest.
- Pulseless electrical activity is usually caused by unrecognized bleeding.
- Some cardiac arrests in the recovery room have reversible causes. Detect them early.
- Successful cardiac massage depends on pushing fast enough (100 beats per minutes) and hard enough. In the elderly this sometimes means fracturing ribs. Ribs heal: brains do not.
- Shock advisory external defibrillators (SAEDs) are useful for inexperienced staff.

Basic life support

Basic life support (BLS) consists of life saving-techniques, which can be used by trained (but not necessarily medical) responders with only the basic skills to maintain an airway, perform *rescue breathing*, and external cardiac massage.

Table 18.1 The steps in basic life support are:

D	Danger	look for hazards.
R	Response	look for signs of life (talk to the patient, shake the patients shoulder). Send for help.
A	Airway	tilt the head slightly down, open the mouth and allow material to drain out. Suck out the mouth if you have a sucker.
B	Breathing	look, listen, feel – if ineffective breathing give 2 rescue breaths.
C	Compression	If the patient does not show signs of life do not delay by feeling for a pulse. Commence compressions immediately: ratio of 30 compressions to 2 breaths; compressions are over the lower half of the sternum; press hard and fast at 100 compressions a minute with 5 cycles (30 compressions and 2 rescue breaths completed over 2 minutes; do not stop – minimize any interruptions to CPR.
D	Defibrillate	Attach an automated external defibrillator (AED) as soon as possible and attach the three leads to the patient.

In contrast to advanced cardiac life support (ACLS) it does not include using drugs or invasive techniques. Effective basic life support buys time until trained medical responders arrive to provide ACLS. The best outcome is achieved if CPR is started immediately, and if the arrhythmia is VF or pulseless VT.

Advanced cardiac life support

Compression:ventilation ratio

- Press the centre of the chest, at a rate of 100 per minute with minimal interruptions.
- Push hard, push fast.
- Universal ratio of 30 compressions to 2 breaths for all two-rescuer CPR for adults.
- Universal ratio of 15 compressions to 2 breaths for all two-rescuer CPR for children.
- Attempts to intubate the patient must not interrupt CPR for more than 20 seconds.

Paddle placed just to right of sternum under clavicle

Paddle placed just to left of nipple with centre of paddle in mid clavicula line

Figure 18.1 Defibrillator paddle positions

Defibrillation

There are three types of defibrillators:

1. *Monophasic defibrillators* sent a direct current in one direction only.

2. *Biphasic defibrillators* send the current first one way, and then back again, and deliver the same success rate with lower energy levels, and less myocardial injury.[3] These are better defibrillators.

3. *Automated external defibrillators* (AEDs) are able to detect the type of rhythm and automatically give an appropriate shock.

How to defibrillate

Two breaths first and then shock for VF arrests.

- Use shock first for ventricular fibrillation (VF) and pulseless ventricular tachycardia (VT).
- It is probably best to use direct current reversion (DCR) first, and then commence CPR.
- All nurses must be trained to use DCR and give it before a doctor arrives.
- Time to defibrillation is the key to survival.
- Use three shocks on the first cycle, and thereafter only use one shock.
- When using manual biphasic defibrillators use energy levels of 150 joule.
- When using monophasic defibrillators give 300 joules.
- In children use biphasic energy levels of 1–2 joule/Kg for defibrillating ventricular fibrillation and pulseless ventricular tachycardia.

Table 18.2 Detect and correct the 5Hs and 5Ts

Hypoxia	Thrombosis–coronary
Hypovolaemia	Tension pneumothorax
Hypothermia	Tamponade–cardiac
Hyperkalaemia	Toxins and drugs
Hypokalaemia	Thromboembolism to the lungs

About the drugs

The best way to give these drugs is via a central venous catheter, and failing that a large bore catheter in a big vein in the arm (not in the back of the hand!). However, if the only vein available is in the arm, then after injecting the drugs lift the arm so that they run into the central veins.

Do not inject drugs in leg veins because of the risk of thrombosis. Many drugs used in ACLS, including adrenaline, calcium chloride, sodium bicarbonate, and potassium chloride, are toxic if they get outside the vein and can cause horrendous tissue damage if the patient survives. There is no place for injecting drugs directly into the heart. In desperation a double dose of lidocaine, adrenaline and atropine (but not other drugs) can be instilled down the endotracheal tube.

The following notes are a summary of the consensus of the effectiveness of drugs in cardiopulmonary resuscitation.

Adrenaline

- Adrenaline is considered to be the best vasopressor to use in cardiac arrest.
- Adrenaline is cheap, and readily available.
- Give 1 ml of adrenaline 1:1000 every 3 minutes during CPR. If you are injecting it into a peripheral vein make it up to 10 ml in saline first. Long-term prognosis is not improved by higher doses.

Vasopressin

- There is no significant difference in the outcome of cardiac arrest whether adrenaline or vasopressin is used to support blood pressure.
- "At this stage there is insufficient evidence to support or refute the use of vasopressin as an alternative to, or in combination with, adrenaline in any cardiac arrest rhythm" (Australian Resuscitation Council Guidelines 2006).

Amiodarone

- Use amiodarone for pulseless VT and VF.
- Amiodarone is the only anti-arrhythmic drug that improves short-term outcome. Give amiodarone 300 mg after the second 2-minute cycle.
- If DCR fails to revert the rhythm then consider giving another 150 mg.
- Follow this with an infusion of amiodarone 15 mg/Kg over the next 24 hours.

Lidocaine

- Although lidocaine has been traditionally used its efficacy is equivocal. It may have a place in pulseless VT or VF that fails to convert with DCR.
- The initial bolus dose is lidocaine 1 mg/Kg with an additional 0.5 mg/Kg if you are desperate.
- There is no place for lidocaine infusions while you are still performing CPR.

Atropine

- Atropine has a place in severe bradycardia.
- Use atropine 1.2 mg intravenously, to a total dose of 3 mg.
- It is worth a try in asystolic arrest although there is no consistent evidence it helps. No matter what the treatment the outcome is poor anyway.

Calcium

- No proven place during CPR.
- Has a place in the treatment of hypocalcaemia, hyperkalaemia and over-dose of calcium channel-blocking drugs.
- Dose is calcium gluconate 10 ml of 10% solution.

Magnesium

- No proven place during CPR.
- May be useful in treating *torsade de points*, digoxin toxicity, documented hypokalaemia and documented hypomagnesaemia.
- May have a use when adrenaline and DCR fail to revert pulseless VT or VF.
- Give 5 mmol bolus of magnesium sulfate, which may be repeated once and followed by an infusion of 20 mmol over four hours.

Potassium

- Use for persistent VF for known or suspected hypokalaemia.
- Give well diluted potassium chloride 5 mmol slowly over 5 minutes intra-venously.
- Bolus potassium may stop the heart.

Sodium bicarbonate

- Use for known or suspected severe acidosis, hyperkalaemia or after 15 minutes of CPR.
- The trigger for using bicarbonate occurs when blood gases show the pH is less than 7.10.
- Dose is 1 mmol/Kg intravenously very slowly over 3–5 minutes.
- Do not mix in line with calcium because it will clog the giving set with chalk.

Pulseless electrical activity

Pulseless electrical activity occurs where the heart is generating coordinated electrical activity but there is no discernable cardiac output. Prognosis with this arrhythmia is dismal (as it is with asystole). There is no point in performing DCR. Look for causes for this arrhythmia. In the recovery room particularly look for exsanguinating haemorrhage and tension pneumothorax.

Asystole

Asystole occurs when the heart is not contracting, there is no discernible ECG rhythm – there is a flat line on the monitor. Asystole is often associated with end-stage hypoxia. Unrelieved hypoxia produces a progression of sinus tachycardia to sinus bradycardia to nodal bradycardia to slow wide QRS complexes and finally a flat line on the ECG – asystole.

Asystole has a poor prognosis, few patients are successfully resuscitated, and almost none leave hospital.

Other measures

Fluids

It is life saving to give fluids if you suspect the patient is *hypovolaemic*, but otherwise they will not affect the outcome.

About therapeutic hypothermia

Therapeutic *hypothermia* with cooling to 33°C reduces subsequent neurological damage and deficit by 2.5-fold and results in a good outcome.[4]

Notes

1. *Circulation* (2000) 102:1–371.
2. *Circulation* (2005) 112:1–211.
3. Tang W, Weil MH, Sun S *et al.* (1999) *Journal American College of Cardiologists* 34:815–22.
4. Bernard SA, Gray TA, Buist MD *et al.* (2002) *New England Journal of Medicine* 346:557–63.

19

Shock

Shock is a clinical diagnosis based on a series of clinical events that occur when the circulation is neither sufficient to meet the metabolic demands of the tissues and organs, nor adequate to remove their metabolic wastes.

Clinically established severe shock is easy to recognize. The patient has a low or unrecordable blood pressure, no urine output, and is pale and sweaty, with gasping respiration and a deteriorating conscious state. Unfortunately, by the time all these features are present the patient is moribund and unlikely to survive. Consequently, it is important to detect and treat shock vigorously long before this irreversible stage.

By the time you diagnose shock, you should have already recognized the symptoms and be treating them. Get help as soon as you notice your patient's perfusion status is deteriorating. The aim of resuscitation is first to restore tissue oxygen supply, and then find and treat the cause of the shock.

By the time you diagnose shock, you should already be treating it.

Types of shock

Maintaining satisfactory blood flow to the tissues requires a pump (the heart) and a distribution system (the blood vessels). If either of these components fail, then shock follows.

The type of shock depends on which component fails, and in the manner they do so. Shock has many causes, but those most commonly encountered after surgery are acute haemorrhage, acute heart failure, sepsis, and anaphylaxis.

Hypovolaemic shock

Hypovolaemic shock occurs when the blood vessels do not contain sufficient blood to fill them. Bleeding is the most common cause, but hypovolaemic shock also occurs where tissue fluid is lost from the circulation with burns, bowel obstruction, or vomiting and diarrhoea.

Normovolaemic shock

Normovolaemic shock occurs when patients' blood pressure falls even though their blood volume is normal.

- *Cardiogenic shock* occurs if the heart fails to pump sufficiently to maintain blood pressure.

- *Septic shock* occurs when bacterial toxins so severely damage the blood vessels that capillaries leak fluid into the tissues, and the smooth muscle in arterioles cannot contract enough to sustain the blood pressure.

- *Anaphylaxis* occurs when an immunological response releases large amounts of inflammatory mediators into the circulation. These biochemicals injure arterioles and capillary membranes allowing intravascular fluid to leak into the tissues.

- *Endocrine shock* occurs if there is insufficient cortisol available for vascular smooth muscle to contract properly to a sympathetic nerve stimulus. Another form of endocrine shock occurs with myxoedema where not enough thyroxine is available for normal tissue metabolism.

Stages of shock

If impending shock is recognized and treated promptly, in most cases its progression through the stages of *compensated* shock, *uncompensated* shock, and *irreversible* shock can be thwarted.

Compensated shock

In the stage of compensated shock the blood flow to the brain and heart are preserved at the expense of the so-called *non-essential organs*: the kidneys, gut, skin and muscles. In this stage of shock the patient usually has a tachycardia, cool skin, and a urine output less than 0.5 ml/Kg per hour. Compensated shock generally responds well to treatment, but if not then it progresses to decompensated shock.

> *The blood pressure does not necessarily fall in compensated haemorrhagic shock.*

Decompensated shock

In the stage of decompensated shock the body's compensatory mechanisms begin to fail, and organ perfusion is severely reduced. Oxygen starved tissues produces lactic acid as they switch to from *aerobic* to *anaerobic metabolism* in an attempt to maintain their function.

Hypoxic tissue releases inflammatory mediators. These depress myocardial contractility and damage capillaries allowing intravascular fluid to leak away into the tissues. Damaged or dead tissues release factors that can trigger *disseminated intravascular coagulation* (DIC).

It is only in the later stages of shock there is profound hypotension. Do not rely on hypotension to diagnose haemorrhagic shock, especially in young people. Their blood pressure may not fall in the stage of compensated shock, and by the time it does fall they may be near death.

It is safer to regard any patient who has cool hands and a tachycardia greater than 100 beats/min as becoming shocked, until some other cause is found to exclude the diagnosis.

Irreversible shock

As shock progresses the tissues are so starved of oxygen that organs fails and die. Irreversible shock is a post-mortem diagnosis.

Signs of shock

Signs of shock include:

- rising pulse rate;
- rapid breathing becoming shallow;
- low urine output;
- anxiety;
- pallor and later sweating;
- confusion.

Bleeding is the most likely cause of shock in the recovery room. Two excellent signs that your patient may be bleeding are that their blood pressure falls by more than 20 mmHg as you cautiously sit them up at 45°, and it takes more than 2 seconds for blood to return when you squeeze a fingernail bed.

Treatment of haemorrhagic shock

Managing shock involves restoring the oxygen supply to the organs, controlling bleeding, and only then finding the cause.

Call for help when you detect deteriorating tissue perfusion. Lay the patient in the position they feel most comfortable, but never head down. If the patient is bleeding they will feel more comfortable lying flat; but if they are developing cardiogenic shock with pulmonary oedema, they may prefer to sit up a little.

Give high flows of oxygen Hudson® mask. They should have wide bore intravenous cannula. If you suspect a patient is bleeding then they need a drip in both arms. To ensure that intravenous infusions run quickly, remove any three-way taps and other plastic paraphernalia because they impede flow.

Read more about the bleeding patient in chapter 25.

What happens in the tissues

During the hypoperfusional stage of shock, cells do not receive enough oxygen to allow the mitochondria to make their little packets of chemical energy called adenosine triphosphate (ATP). Cells use ATP to kick start biochemical reactions. As the oxygen supply fails, at first the cells produce a limited emergency supply of ATP using a process called anaerobic metabolism. However, once this limited back-up supply of ATP is exhausted, the cells' membrane pumps fail and fluid leaks through the membranes causing the cells to swell and die. In the meantime anaerobic metabolism releases lactic acid into the blood causing a metabolic acidosis. Metabolic acidosis is a biochemical marker of cellular hypoxia.

Meanwhile the body attempts to compensate for the acidosis. The patient starts to hyperventilate. Hyperventilation removes carbon dioxide from the body, which temporarily restores the blood's pH to more normal levels.

If the crisis is successfully treated, then shock does not progress. If not then, as the body's compensatory mechanisms fail, cells start to disintegrate. The surviving cells stagger along on their emergency energy supply producing more and more lactic acid. Protein-rich fluid leaks from the blood, through damaged capillary walls to collect in the tissues. The remaining blood becomes more concentrated and syrupy impeding flow in the microcirculation. The sluggish blood flow further deprives tissues of their oxygen supply, and delays toxic waste removal. Eventually the process becomes irreversible. Brain damage and death follow.

Steroids

Little is known about the physiological role of cortisol. The body seems to use this hormone to respond to stress, such as trauma, bleeding, starvation, infection or emotional stress. Cortisol helps cells make certain enzymes and structural proteins, while suppressing the activity of others. In large amounts, cortisol suppresses the body's immune response to foreign antigens.

On average, the adrenal glands produce about 30 mg of cortisol each day, but the adrenal glands in a super-stressed surgical patient who has infection, pain which is possibly aggravated by hypoxia and fluid imbalance, may put out 300 mg or more of cortisol a day.

Many patients take steroids, such as prednisolone, to treat chronic inflammatory disease, for example asthma or rheumatoid arthritis. Prednisolone, in doses exceeding 10 mg daily, suppresses the adrenal gland's ability to make cortisol. This means that when a crisis arrives the adrenal glands simply cannot make enough cortisol to meet the extra demands.

In the recovery room, hypotension may occur after surgery unless the anaesthetist has given supplemental hydrocortisone during their surgery. The patient's blood pressure may steadily decrease. Typically, about 10 to 20 minutes after arriving in the recovery room, the patient's blood pressure starts to fall. The low blood pressure neither responds to an intravenous fluid load, nor even doses of noradrenaline. Once you give 50–100 mg of hydrocortisone intravenously, their blood pressure bounces back within minutes as new receptors are made.

Consequently, patients who take higher doses of steroids need supplemental hydrocortisone for several days after surgery. Make sure they have hydrocortisone ordered before they leave the recovery room. Typical doses are for major surgery are hydrocortisone 50 mg intravenously 4 times a day for 4 days; and for minor surgery 50 mg for the first day.

Equivalent steroid doses

Cortisol 100 mg = 80 mg hydrocortisone

= 20 mg prednisolone

= 16 mg triamcinolone

= 4 mg dexamethasone

= 2 mg betamethasone

Shock in children

Children who are becoming shocked, present differently to adults. Hypotension in children signals the onset of irreversible shock. This problem is discussed more comprehensively in the chapter on paediatrics.

Crisis Management

Where to look

Be prepared

Emergencies happen. Be prepared. Before the start of each day check all your trolleys and equipment, including your defibrillator, and make sure all new staff know where everything is kept.

Crisis protocol

A *crisis protocol* is an organized approach to manage the patient whose life is in danger. It is often difficult to diagnose what has happened to the collapsed patient, but the fundamentals of basic life support are the same for all emergencies.

Prepare a set of flow charts (*algorithms*) on 5 × 8 inch filing cards setting out how to diagnose and treat emergencies. These cards are your *crisis protocols*. Put them in a box on the desk where everyone can refer to them. Practice simulated disaster management monthly.

How to practice

In an emergency you must keep your patients alive while you find out what has gone wrong. There are three aspects to resuscitation: first, keeping your patient alive; second, finding out what is wrong; and third is the organization of the resuscitation. Practice resuscitation techniques regularly. It is a bit like a ballet; everyone must know their part, and keep out of each other's way.

Successful resuscitation depends on practice, practice, practice.

As you practice your crisis protocols consider:

- What are the problems?
- What is the worst thing that can happen?
- What is the normal response?
- How do I assess the problem?
- What is the immediate management?
- What is the follow-up?

When patients suddenly deteriorate, for instance their blood pressure falls, or seizures occur, or they cannot breathe properly, then follow your crisis protocol. Because you will have to act quickly, both diagnosis and treatment must be performed at the same time, even when the cause of the problem is far from clear.

During a crisis make a presumptive diagnosis, consider the differential diagnosis, and plan management. To do this, answer the following questions:

- What is the problem?
- What else could it be?
- What are we going to do about it?

Keep your patient alive

Use the alphabet of resuscitation

Use the A, B, C, D, E, F plan – but first check the patient's conscious state and their carotid pulse. If you cannot feel the carotid pulse or the patient is unconscious then start advanced cardiac life support protocol.

Check the carotid pulse
then
A, B, C, D, E, F

A = Airway:

Check the patency of the patient's airway. Gently suck out mucus, blood and other debris with Yankeur sucker. Use a bag and mask giving 100% oxygen to ventilate your patient.

Oxygen saves lives.

B = Breathing:

Check that air is moving in and out of the lungs. If you hold the chin up you can feel this in the palm of your hand. Insert an airway. Check the oxygen saturation. If you are having difficulty in getting oxygen into and out of the patient's lungs then consider upper and lower airway obstruction. Check from outside the airway, to the airway wall, is there a foreign body in the lumen?

C = Circulation:

Feel for a carotid pulse. If it is absent start *advanced cardiac life support (ACLS) protocol*. Check blood pressure, pulse rate and rhythm, re-evaluate perfusion status, attach ECG.

What's gone wrong?

D = Drugs

Review drugs for effects or side-effects. If blood, drugs, or plasma expanders are being infused, then consider some form of reaction; turn off the drip. Consider: Wrong drug, Wrong rate, Wrong route.

E = Endocrine

Consider the three Hs:

1. Hypoglycaemia. Check blood glucose with a glucose meter.

2. Hypothyroidism as a cause of delayed emergence.

3. Hypoadrenalism as a cause of refractory hypotension.

F = Fitting?

Consider:

- Hypoxia;
- Hypoglycaemia;
- Hypocalcaemia;
- Hyperpyrexia;

- Hypocarbia;
- Water intoxication;
- Epilepsy, eclampsia;
- Drugs.

Work out what is wrong

The cause is often obvious such as a cardiac arrhythmia, or laryngospasm, but you will still need to

LOOK × 5

LISTEN × 4

FEEL × 4

Look

1. Wound sites and drains.
2. Appearance: Pallor? Cyanosis? Flushing? Sweating? Agitation?
3. Respiration: rates, depth, rhythm.
4. Neck: Jugular vein distension? Swelling of tissues? Tracheal deviation?
5. Strip to expose whole body to ensure you aren't overlooking something.

Blood loss is usually obvious, but it can be hidden beneath the sheets. Blocked chest drains can cause respiratory difficulty. Difficulty in breathing can indicate airway obstruction, inadequate reversal of muscle relaxants, cardiac failure, or allergy. Bleeding into the neck can cause airway obstruction and cause the face to become suffused. Distended neck veins may indicate tension pneumothorax, cardiac tamponade, *TURP syndrome*, or gross fluid overload or pulmonary embolism by clot or air. A tension pneumothorax may push the trachea to the opposite side. Strip the patient to reveal abdominal swelling, and many other problems.

Listen

1. Patient's complaints.
2. Air entry: wheezes with mouth open?
3. Stridor and other breathing noises.
4. Heart sounds: muffled? murmur gallop rhythm?

If patients say something is wrong, never pass it off as anxiety or attention-seeking. If they cannot breathe properly or are feeling breathless, then something is wrong. Listen to the breath sounds with a stethoscope. Assess adequacy, pattern, and distribution of ventilation. Possible problems include bronchospasm, pulmonary oedema, lobe collapse, pneumothorax, haemothorax, and cardiac tamponade.

Stridor is a sign of impending total airway obstruction. It is an medical emergency – get help immediately. Wheeze suggest: anaphylaxis, aspiration, asthma, acute pulmonary oedema, allergy to drugs or infusions, or embolism. Heart sounds may be muffled if there is a pneumothorax or pericardial effusion – this is a difficult sign to interpret.

Feel

1. Heart and pulse: rate? intensity? rhythm?
2. Head: sweaty? fever?
3. Hands: perfusion? grip strength, and leg movement on both sides?
4. Head lift to check residual muscle relaxation.

Take both wrists and check that the pulse in each is equivalent. Check the carotid pulse and the femoral pulses. Look for differences in volume and rhythm. A 12-lead ECG may reveal arrhythmias. Cold hands are an excellent sign of noradrenergic discharge, warning of problems such as haemorrhage, hypoxia, hypoglycaemia, and pain. Warm hands and a bounding pulse suggests hypercarbia, thyrotoxicosis. Sweating or fever suggests reaction to blood or drugs, malignant hyperthermia, serotonergic syndrome, thyrotoxic crisis, and neuroleptic malignant syndrome. Loss of grip, strength, or weakness in the legs only on one side of the body suggests stroke, or if on both sides consider the effects of residual muscle relaxants, neostigmine overdose, myasthenia or other neuropathies and myopathies, or massive stroke.

How to monitor resuscitation's progress

Write everything that could possibly be relevant on a special chart, or in the patient's notes. Once you have an established problem list it is much easier to set priorities and follow what is going on.

Organization of a resuscitation

All trained staff in the recovery room should be adept at managing advanced cardiac life support. Everyone taking part in resuscitating a patient must know their role, but teaching how to organize resuscitation is often overlooked. At the beginning of each shift each member of the recovery room staff should know what their role would be if an emergency occurs.

Start with the three Cs

1. Call for help, summon the anaesthetist or surgeon, emergency trolley and the defibrillator.

2. Check pulse, colour, oximeter and ECG;

3. Check the clock, and note the time.

Monitor: ECG, blood pressure, pulse rate and rhythm, respiratory rate, oximetery.

Get HELP:

H Help – it takes four staff to manage a crisis:

> Person 1. To manage the airway.
>
> Person 2. To monitor the blood pressure, pulse, and perfusion, and perform external cardiac massage if needed.
>
> Person 3. To get drugs, equipment, and take blood tests.
>
> Person 4. To supervise the resuscitation, liaise with other staff and write the problems and treatment on a whiteboard where everyone can see it. This person should help the others too.

E Emergency trolley and other equipment as needed.

L Look in the patients notes for clues: such as allergies, cardiac disease, previous pneumothorax, problems with previous anaesthetics and so on.

P Prepare to take blood for laboratory analysis. Phone the laboratory and warn them of the problem.

Monitoring

Patients who have been involved in multiple trauma, or undergone prolonged major surgery with extensive blood loss should be monitored with the following when they arrive in the recovery room:

- ECG;
- nasogastric tube;
- 14 G cannula in their right internal jugular vein to give fluids and measure their central venous pressure;
- 14 G cannula attached to a blood warmer in their right forearm;
- 14 G cannula in their left forearm;
- 20 G cannula in their left radial artery to measure their arterial blood pressure and to collect samples for blood gases estimation;
- urinary catheter attached to 100 ml burette;
- warming mattress or convection heater at 37°C;
- sometimes a pulmonary artery flotation catheter to measure wedge pressures.

Anaphylaxis

Anaphylaxis is an acute, life threatening allergic reaction to a foreign substance (*antigen*). Examples of antigens include penicillins, blood, or its products, muscle relaxants, and latex,

Anaphylaxis is easy to diagnosis if the patient suddenly collapses with wheeze and hypotension immediately after being given an offending antigen. However, it may not be so easily recognized if the signs and symptoms creep up slowly over many minutes or even an hour or more. Anaphylaxis is often fatal if it is not recognized and treated.

Early signs include:

- sensation of warmth or itching, especially in the groin or axilla;
- flushing or mottled rash over the upper part of the body;
- restlessness, acute anxiety, or panic;
- nausea and vomiting;
- feelings of tightness in the chest.

Later:

- erythematous or urticarial rash similar to hives;
- developing oedema of face, eyelids, and neck;
- crampy abdominal pain.

Progressing to:

- hypotension sometimes severe enough to cause coma;
- bronchospasm, cough, dyspnoea, wheeze;
- laryngeal oedema with dyspnoea, stridor, drooling, and hoarse voice;
- tissue hypoxia with cyanosis; arrhythmias and cardiac arrest.

Laryngeal oedema or developing facial oedema is life-threatening. The onset of stridor warns that total airway obstruction is only moments away. If patients are conscious they may panic. At this stage intubation is often difficult, because the normal anatomical landmarks will be obscured. Airway management in the patient needs a skilled anaesthetist. Prepare equipment for intubation, and if that fails, an emergency cricothyroid puncture, or to insert a mini-tracheostomy. In some cases a surgeon may perform a formal open tracheostomy.

Principles

- Suspect any unexpected reaction to a drug as an anaphylactoid reaction.
- Almost every type of drug that can be injected (except ketamine and the benzodiazepines) has been reported to cause anaphylaxis.

- Usually the patient deteriorates rapidly.
- Use adrenaline at the first suspicion of anaphylaxis: it is safe and effective.
- The combination of adrenaline and plasma volume replacement will return cardiac output to acceptable levels. Do not use polygelines, such as Gelofusin® because they occasionally cause allergic responses.
- Although steroids and histamines are used as follow-up therapy, they take many hours to act.

Immediate management

1. Call for help.
2. Stop any potentially offending substance.
3. Maintain the ABC – airway, breathing and circulation. Give 100% oxygen. You may need to start advanced cardiac life support.
4. Attach an ECG, pulse oximeter, and automated blood pressure monitor.
5. Get the emergency trolley, and prepare for a rapid infusion of fluids.
6. Lay the patient flat, and raise the limbs. Do not tilt them head down.
7. Insert a large wide bore drip to infuse large volumes of 0.9% saline.
8. Give adrenaline. (Patients taking β-blockers may need much larger doses than recommended below.)

Adults

For adults open an ampoule of adrenaline 1:1000 (1 mg in 1 ml).

If the patient weighs

- less than 50 Kg then give 0.25 ml of adrenaline,
- between 50 and 100 Kg then give 0.5 ml of adrenaline,
- more than 100 Kg give 0.75 ml of adrenaline.

Use intramuscular adrenaline initially, If either there is no response to the intramuscular adrenaline, or the blood pressure or pulse is unrecordable then give adrenaline 5 ml of 1:10 000 slowly intravenously over 5 minutes.

Children

For children dilute an ampoule of 1 ml of 1:1000 adrenaline and make it up to 10 ml in saline. The syringe now contains adrenaline 1:10 000. Use this diluted adrenaline and give 0.25 ml per year of age slowly (over 5 measured minutes) into a drip running in a large vein.

Later management

Once your patient's blood pressure is restored:

- Give hydrocortisone 5 mg/Kg intravenously.
- Give promethazine 0.5 mg/Kg (maximum dose 50 mg) intravenously slowly over 10 measured minutes.
- Treat wheeze with 2 ml of 0.5% salbutamol through a nebulizer and face mask.
- If the wheeze remains unrelieved then give salbutamol 1.5 µg/Kg intravenously.
- Prepare to transfer the patient to ICU for further treatment. It may be necessary to give an adrenaline infusion for several hours.
- Take 10 ml of blood in a plain tube for serum tryptase concentrations, but wait one hour after the event.

Anaphylaxis and anaphylactoid reactions

Anaphylaxis

Anaphylaxis occurs when the immune system reacts in a cataclysmic way to a trivial stimulus. The reaction requires that the person has previously encountered the antigen and built up a partial immunity to it. When the person re-encounters a similar antigen an explosive allergic reaction occurs.

When an antigen binds to IgE on the surface of mast cells or basophils these cells instantly release a flood of inflammatory biochemicals into the surrounding tissues. Some of these biochemicals cause the smooth muscles in arterioles to relax, while others damage basement membranes in capillary beds all over the body to soon allow fluid to escape from the circulation into the tissues.

In the most extreme case within seconds to minutes every arteriole in the body dilates, so that the blood pressure falls catastrophically and can cause cardiac arrest. However the reaction may take an hour or more to run its course. If the patient survives the first insult, capillary beds all over the body, especially in the lungs, gut and skin, leak a flood of fluid into the tissues causing oedema. The face puffs up, the lungs fill with fluid, and the airways narrow causing wheeze. It is rare for anaphylaxis to take much more than an hour to develop.

To be safe, treat either anaphylactic, or anaphylactoid reactions with adrenaline.

Anaphylactoid response

Anaphylactoid responses occur when some drug or chemical causes the mast cells to release histamine, either locally or throughout the whole body.

The reaction is not immune-mediated, does not require previous exposure to an antigen, does not involve IgE, but is related to the dose and the speed of the injection.

Since it is almost impossible clinically to tell the difference between an anaphylactic response and an anaphylactoid response, treat all these types of reactions with adrenaline.

Seizures

A fitting patient? Exclude hypoxia and hypoglycaemia.

Causes of seizures:

- Hypoxia;
- Hypoglycaemia;
- An epileptic patient who has not taken their medication;
- Water overload, including the TURP syndrome;
- Eclampsia;
- Malignant hypertension;
- Hypocalcaemia, hypomagnesemia;
- Drugs.

Seizures and fits are both terms for the same thing. Drugs that may cause seizures are local anaesthetics, pethidine, rarely propofol and occasionally acute withdrawal of benzodiazepine or antiparkinson drugs.

There are reports that propofol may rarely cause seizures in the recovery room from minutes to hours after the last dose. Be cautious about early discharge of a patient if any abnormal muscle movement occurs such as twitching or jerking. If this occurs admit the patient for overnight observation.

Pethidine can cause a seizure. Its toxic metabolite 6-norpethidine is excreted only by the kidney. Do not use pethidine in patients with renal failure.

Immediate management

Seizures usually start with the patient losing consciousness and becoming rigid (tonic phase); this is followed shortly by generalized jerking movements (clonic phase), which may persist for some time. Seizures cause cerebral hypoxia and if not quickly treated can cause permanent brain damage.

- Call for help. It takes two competent staff to manage seizures.
- Turn the patient into the recovery position and gently restrain them so they do not fall off their trolley.

- Start the ABC: clear the airway, assist breathing, and give 100% oxygen by mask. Do not try to force anything between their teeth.
- Attach an ECG, pulse oximeter and automated blood pressure machine.
- Do not leave the patient.
- Check that the blood sugar concentration is > 3.5 mmol/L. If they are hypoglycaemic give 50 ml of 50% glucose into a large vein in a free-flowing drip.
- If the patient is even possibly an alcoholic give thiamine 100 mg intravenously to prevent Wernicke's encephalopathy.

Further management

- Thiopental 2–7.5 mg/Kg IV is the best option. Usually this immediately terminates the seizure, but you will now have a comatose patient to manage. Continuing seizures are best controlled with a thiopentone infusion of 1–5 mg/Kg per hour.
- Diazepam 0.15 mg/Kg IV (maximum adult dose 20 mg). This is a second line drug.
- To prevent further seizures give phenytoin 7.5 mg/Kg intravenously into a saline infusion. If the patients are not already taking phenytoin then load them with a further 1000 mg over the next 30 minutes.
- Send bloods for measurement of blood glucose, calcium, magnesium, phosphate, and if relevant, anticonvulsant drug levels.
- If the patient remains comatose, they will need to be intubated, have urinary catheter inserted, and transferred to ICU for further management.

Endocrine emergencies

Consider the three Hs.

1. Hypoglycaemia as a cause of agitation and sweating.
2. Hypothyroidism as a cause of delayed emergence.
3. Hypoadrenalism as a cause of refractory hypotension.

Major disasters

Most hospitals have a detailed Major Disaster Plan designated (Code Brown), with nominated key staff responsible for specific prearranged duties. The operating theatres should already have their own plans in place, with portable packs containing equipment, and drugs prepared for this eventuality.

Because of their expertise, the recovery room staff may be asked to form a mobile team to go to the site of the disaster, or allocated to a primary receiving hospital near the site. However it is more likely you will stay put to form a back-up support hospital taking the overflow of casualties.

Apart from the overwhelming number of casualties in a major disaster, most of the problems are logistic, and of these the biggest problem is communication. Your recovery room will work closely with the emergency department (now called a receiving station), the operating theatres, and the intensive care unit.

Do not be surprised if the hospital switchboard is totally overwhelmed and jammed, and the receiving station staff too busy to answer the phones. They will be constantly engaged, and you will not get through. Do not rely on the mobile phone network, because with major disasters, such as 9/11 and the Madrid bombings, the phone networks became so clogged they were unusable.

Allocate the three most experienced senior staff to establish a command centre at the recovery room desk, set up lines of communication, assess priorities, gauge capability and gather information so available resources are used most efficiently. The best way to do this is for each of the commanders to personally visit the ICU, the receiving station and the operating theatres at regular intervals. Our experience shows first-hand reconnaissance by visiting these areas saves a lot of time and makes everything work more efficiently.

21

The kidney

Renal failure after major surgery carries 60 per cent mortality, and if systemic sepsis develops then mortality approaches 90 per cent. If the kidneys fail the patient is more likely to develop gastrointestinal bleeding, respiratory infections, cardiac failure, poor wound healing and generalized sepsis. If we can anticipate and recognize developing renal failure, then we have a chance to ameliorate these calamities.

Physiology

Homeostasis

The kidneys help maintain body *homeostasis* by controlling the volume and composition of the extracellular fluid, and by excreting water-soluble wastes. The kidneys regulate the balance of water, sodium, potassium, hydrogen ion and other water-soluble substances in the body. They also produce hormones, erythropoietin, activated vitamin D, renin and *prostaglandins* and excrete water-soluble drugs.

Each kidney is a collection of 1 200 000 nephrons forming a high pressure blood ultrafiltration system. A *nephron* is a long tube lined with epithelial cells. At the proximal entrance of the nephron is a sieve (*glomerulus*) and the other end of the tube opens into the renal pelvis. Fluid passing through the sieve is called the *filtrate*. As filtrate moves along the nephron useful substances pass back into the bloodstream, while metabolic wastes stay in the nephron to be excreted. Normally the glomerulus will not allow red blood cells, or larger proteins, such as albumin, into the filtrate. If the glomerulus is damaged then albumin or even blood appears in the *urine*.

Glomerular filtration rate

The *glomerular filtration rate (GFR)* is the volume of urine entering the glomerular end of the renal tubule each minute. In a healthy young adult, this is about 125 ml/min or 180 litres per day, but only 2 litres is passed as urine. To reabsorb the remaining 178 litres of filtrate, and to concentrate the urine in the tubules, the kidney needs a good oxygen supply to generate energy for the ion pumps. The kidneys fail to concentrate *urine* if deprived of sufficient blood flow or oxygen supply.

Measuring actual GFR is cumbersome. In the recovery room the best we can do is to measure the urine output. The blood electrolyte results measure the concentrations of a biochemical called *creatinine*.

Creatinine is produced as muscle protein, and is broken down. The amount building up in the blood, the serum *creatinine concentration*, is used as a surrogate marker of renal function. Serum creatinine levels can be misleading in the elderly, obese or those on unusual diets. As a rule, if patients have a raised serum urea level and a normal creatinine then they have kidney disease.

Normal serum creatinine and raised urea?
Then consider chronic kidney disease.

Chronic kidney disease

The two principal markers of the kidneys' health are the volume of urine they form and how effectively they concentrate sodium in the urine. Complications of chronic renal disease increase as the GFR falls. For this reason GFR is the best indicator of the severity of kidney disease.

How to stage chronic kidney disease

The year 2000 saw the introduction of a five-stage classification of *chronic kidney disease* (CKD) based mostly on a formula that estimated glomerular filtration rate (eGFR). Most pathology laboratories now report an eGFR with the electrolyte results.[1]

A normal eGFR is greater than 60 ml/min/1.73m^2 but this does not automatically mean the kidneys are healthy. We need to look for other markers of kidney damage such as albuminuria, proteinuria, hypertension, and haematuria.

Since 2002 the stages of chronic kidney disease have been modified several times and are continually being reviewed. Here is the latest version.

Table 21.1 Stages of chronic kidney disease

Stage	eGFR	Description
1	≥ 60	No kidney damage
2	≥ 60	Mild kidney disease if: Proteinuria Hypertension Diabetes Age over 50 years Family history
3	30–59	Moderate decrease in kidney function
4	15–29	Severe decrease in kidney function
5	<15	End-stage kidney disease

Limitations of the eGFR

The formula needs to be modified for:

- Asian: Japanese, Chinese, Vietnamese;
- Maori or Pacific Islanders;
- Australian aboriginals;
- African Americans.

How the tubules modify urine

Once fluid passes through the glomerulus' sieve it enters the *renal tubule*. Each tubule has three parts: the *proximal tubule* reabsorbs almost everything that is useful, and excretes most of the unwanted waste; the *loop of Henle* works with the collecting tubule to concentrate the urine, and the *distal convoluted tubule* and *collecting ducts* fine tunes the composition of the filtrate.

Fig. 21.1 How the kidney concentrates urine

Most of the waste is urea, a breakdown product from food and cellular metabolism. Importantly, the kidney excretes many drugs.

Kidney blood flow

Each kidney is about the size of your clenched fist. Compared with their size their blood supply is enormous. About 25 per cent of the 5-litre cardiac output passes through them. This blood supply of 1250 ml/min is far more blood than they need for their metabolic requirements. Their high blood flow gives them the agility to rapidly adjust the composition or volume of body fluids to meet the physiological circumstances. They quickly filter out, and excrete the water-soluble noxious wastes in the body. Every hour, the kidneys process about 60 litres of fluid; this is equivalent to the entire volume of the body's water.

How the kidney conserves sodium

Every day the kidneys filter 25 000 mmol of sodium ions, but excrete less than 0.5 per cent of it. The kidneys defend the volume of the *extracellular fluid* (ECF), and if necessary do this at the expense of every other priority. They protect the ECF volume and composition by reabsorbing sodium and other substances and water in varying quantities. Where necessary the kidneys can retain all the sodium in the filtrate, and with it most of the water.

How the kidneys maintain their blood flow

The flow through the glomerular capillaries is *autoregulated*. As blood pressure rises and falls the intrarenal arterioles constrict and dilate to keep the blood flowing at a constant rate. This enables urine to form at an almost constant rate. If the mean arteriolar pressure falls below 80 mmHg autoregulation is lost, and urine output starts to fall.

Once the mean blood pressure falls below 80 mmHg the kidneys' health is at risk.

How kidneys maintain their GFR

To produce urine the kidneys need sufficient perfusion pressure to *force* fluid from the blood through the glomerular membrane to form the *filtrate*. It is a bit like turning a hose on a bed sheet stretched out on a washing line. When the water pressure is low not much water passes through the sheet and most of it runs off. However, if you now turn up the water pressure more will pass through the bed sheet. Likewise with higher pressure more fluid will pass through the glomerulus into the tubules.

Even if the blood flow through the kidney decreases, it can temporarily compensate for this. The kidney maintains the pressure across the glomerular sieve by leaving the inflow (*afferent*) arteriole wide open, while constricting the outflow (*efferent*) arteriole. This causes blood to dam up in the glomerulus. A hormone, angiotensin II, and the noradrenergic nervous system mediate this outflow shutdown.

If the patient has been taking *angiotensin-converting enzyme* (ACE) inhibitors, or *angiotensin receptor blocking* (ARB) drugs then the efferent arteriole cannot constrict effectively. Despite blood flowing freely through the glomerular tuft, there is not enough pressure to form urine.

The kidneys' ability to keep forming urine despite being deprived of their blood supply does not mean that they are well oxygenated, or healthy.

Simply because the kidneys are making urine does not mean they are healthy.

In a healthy person glomerular filtration stops and urine output ceases once the mean blood pressure falls to 60 mmHg. This pressure corresponds to a driving pressure in the glomerular tuft of about 30 mmHg. In patients with vascular disease (such as diabetics or long-term smokers) glomerular filtration ceases at mean blood pressures higher than 60 mmHg because the kidneys blood vessels are too clogged to maintain enough blood pressure in the glomerular tuft to form urine.

How anaesthesia affects the kidney

Even patients with normal kidneys experience transient renal impairment after anaesthesia. During general anaesthesia, organ perfusion slows because volatile agents depress myocardial contraction, and dilate arterioles everywhere. Blood tends to flow along paths of least resistance; consequently some blood flow is diverted away from the kidneys.

How surgery affects the kidney

The body interprets surgery as a life-threatening physical injury. Evolutionary pressures have finely honed a sequence of survival responses. In anticipation of losing blood or tissue fluid a number of hormones are released; *antidiuretic hormone* (ADH), the *glucocorticoids*, and *aldosterone*. These hormones prevent the kidney from wasting precious body fluids and help it get rid of excessive potassium released from dead and dying cells The sympathetic nerves release noradrenaline causing vasoconstriction that slows intrarenal blood flow,

Surgery disrupts renal function and body fluid balance.[1] By far the most common cause of kidney damage is the combination of hypotension and hypovolaemia. Surgery involving an infected field, releases showers of Gram-negative bacterial *endotoxins* into the bloodstream. These can damage the glomerular filter, and the capillaries serving the tubules.

If, during aortic surgery, the surgeon clamps the aorta above the renal arteries the kidneys progressively become hypoxic. More than 30 minutes of clamp-time causes substantial ischaemic damage.

Surgery also damages tissues and causes pain, and the more major the surgery, the greater the mass of injured tissue. *Cytokines* released by damaged cells flood into the circulation to damage *basement membranes* everywhere.

Unfortunately the kidneys and lungs, with their high blood flows, bear the brunt of this assault.

Hepato-renal syndrome

Jaundiced patients are at particular risk of kidney damage because of the high levels of bilirubin in their blood.[3] The combination of hypoxia, low renal blood flows, bacterial endotoxins and bilirubin contribute to a form of polyuric renal damage called the *hepato-renal syndrome*. Once established, it is almost invariably progressive and often fatal. In jaundiced patients, ensure adequate hydration by giving at least one extra litre of crystalloid overnight, and another in the morning.[2] Good pain control also improves renal perfusion. Using either mannitol or furosemide to prompt a *diuresis* does not improve the prognosis.

Hypovolaemia

Unless a hypovolaemic or bleeding patient rapidly receives fluids to restore their vascular volume the kidney blood supply may fall from 1250 ml/min to

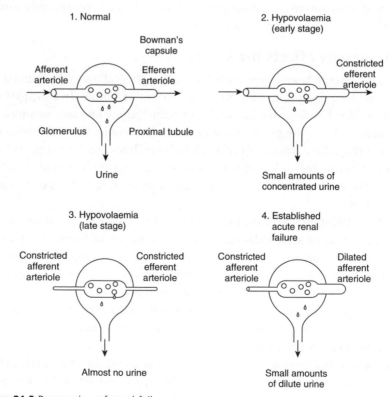

Fig. 21.2 Progression of renal failure

250 ml/min or less. The kidneys can survive for 30–60 minutes on as little as one-tenth of their normal blood supply (125 ml/min). Despite deprivation of their blood supply, at first the kidneys are able to maintain a urine output; but they can no longer efficiently concentrate urine. As a priority, the kidneys tend to protect their GFR, rather than supply their tubules with oxygen.

A well-oxygenated healthy kidney responds to hypovolaemia by concentrating the urine, reabsorbing almost all the sodium and most of the water. The urine entering the bladder now has high osmolarity, but a low sodium concentration.

If the blood supply fails and the kidney becomes hypoxic, then the ion pumps in the tubules fail. Without enough oxygen they are unable to pump sodium back into the blood so it stays in the filtrate and is excreted in the urine. Now the urine has a high sodium content.

We can measure sodium concentration in the urine with flame photometry. This is a simple procedure for most laboratories. In the recovery room, a urinary sodium concentration greater than 40 mmol/L suggests renal impairment.

Postoperative hypovolaemia can occur because of:

- bleeding;
- bowel obstruction;
- peritonitis;
- prolonged vomiting.

During surgery the anaesthetist will start to resuscitate the patient but often it is necessary to continue this process in the recovery room.

Bleeding

As a patient bleeds there is an ordered progression of responses. These involve the sympathetic nervous system (adrenaline and noradrenaline), and hormones (ADH, angiotensin II, and aldosterone). Initially the urine output is maintained, but as the kidneys become hypoxic they start to fail to concentrate urine and the sodium content of the urine rises; then urine production falls and finally stops altogether.

As blood is lost the kidneys progressively shut down their circulation. In doing so, they divert up to a 1000 ml/min of their 1250 ml/min blood supply to boost the volume of the central circulation. At the same time *aldosterone* primes the pumps in the tubules to retain sodium and water; and the urine output slows and may stop. ADH prevents the kidney from excreting water, while angiotensin II helps raise the systemic blood pressure, and prompts the adrenal glands to release aldosterone to stop sodium loss in the urine.

Bowel surgery

Following abdominal surgery extracellular fluid is lost in a number of ways. Fluid transudates into the bowel, or collects as effusions in the peritoneum (this retained fluid is called *third space loss*); or it escapes through drains, or with bleeding. During major abdominal surgery up to 10 ml/Kg/hr of water is lost simply by evaporation from the open peritoneum. Dry anaesthetic gases remove water from the lungs. Unless these losses are replaced, the patient will develop *hypovolemia*, and the kidneys will attempt to compensate by retaining fluid.

Peritonitis

With an inflamed peritoneum large amounts of fluid can accumulate as third space loss in the peritoneum.

How kidneys guard their blood supply

Once the kidneys' blood supply decreases they respond by secreting an enzyme called renin. Renin cleaves a prohormone, *angiotensinogen* into angiotensin-I. Angiotensin-I is converted in the lung by *angiotensin-converting enzyme* (ACE) to angiotensin-II. Angiotensin-II is a potent vasoconstrictor. As it circulates it causes vascular smooth muscle everywhere to spasm including the kidneys' own arterioles. As arterioles shut down, the systemic blood pressure rises. With haemorrhage, the combined effect of angiotensin-II and noradrenaline on the skin's arterioles makes people go white. The shutdown of the blood supply to the gut, skeletal muscle, kidney and skin, diverts valuable blood to the heart, lungs and brain.

The kidneys are selfish organs. As blood loss progresses they ensure (temporarily) that their own blood flow is not affected by producing a prostaglandin that overrides the vasoconstriction. However if the patient has been taking an NSAID, the kidneys cannot make the prostaglandin, and the kidneys fate is sealed.

Most anaesthetists prefer that patients stop taking their NSAID at least 4 days before major surgery, especially if they are elderly, as NSAIDs are a major risk factor for postoperative renal dysfunction.

Avoid using NSAIDs in patients who have bled during surgery.

ACE inhibitors increase the risk of postoperative renal dysfunction because the renin-angiotensin system can no longer compensate if renal perfusion falls.[4] In patients taking ACE inhibitors it is important to maintain *normovolaemia* so that they do not become hypotensive.

Acute tubular necrosis

Unless blood volume and oxygen supply are rapidly restored the kidneys' tubular cells degenerate and die. Damage to the capillaries slows intra-renal blood flow by 40–50 per cent. This process of both endothelial and tubular damage is termed *acute tubular necrosis* (ATN).

At this stage, even if the cardiac output and blood flow is restored, the damaged intra-renal blood vessels prevent blood from circulating properly within the kidney. The patient becomes anuric. Given ideal conditions the dead tubular cells and damaged endothelium will eventually be replaced, and with dialysis, normal renal function usually returns in about 3–6 weeks.

Renal vascular disease, diuretics and nephrotoxins such as gentamicin accelerate the progression of these events.

Who is at risk from renal damage?

The following are at risk of renal damage during, or after, surgery:

- patients over the age of 65 years;
- people with severe arterial disease ('vasculopaths');
- diabetics;
- surgery where the aorta is cross-clamped;
- patients with pre-existing renal disease;
- those undergoing major vascular surgery, especially if they require blood transfusion;
- patients taking NSAIDs;
- patients with systemic sepsis;
- those having bowel surgery;
- pre-eclampsia;
- trauma and crush injury.

How kidneys age

Renal blood flow decreases by about one per cent a year after the age of 30 years, and by the age of 90 years has halved. Estimated renal plasma flow falls from about 650 ml/min in 30–40 year olds to about 290 ml/min in the 80s.

Any disease affecting nephrons, affects the GFR.

As we age our kidneys' nephrons progressively die, and are replaced by fibrous tissue. Because the elderly have fewer nephrons, a small insult such as a brief fall in blood pressure, may have a large effect.

Drugs and the kidney

How kidney disease affects drugs

With chronic kidney disease the glomerular filtration rate (GFR) falls, and the incidence of adverse drug reactions rises. Once the GFR falls below 30 ml/min the kidney fails to efficiently excrete water-soluble drugs. Adverse drug reactions may occur because kidney disease prolongs the half-life of some drugs and their metabolites.

Reduce the doses of drugs, and increase the dosing interval in patients with an estimated glomerular filtration rate (eGFR) less than 30 ml/min 1.73m^2.

How drugs affect the kidney

Drugs may decrease renal perfusion

Drugs can damage kidneys by decreasing their perfusion, impairing intrarenal blood distribution, being toxic to tubules, or causing interstitial nephritis.

Drugs decreasing renal perfusion include diuretics, angiotensin converting enzyme inhibitors (the 'prils' eg. enalapril), and angiotensin receptor blockers (the 'sartans' e.g. irbesartan), and vasodilators. In critically ill patients, especially those with sepsis, these drugs may aggravate hypotension, and impair the kidney's defences that normally preserve glomerular filtration and medullary blood flow.

Drugs can be toxic to the tubules

Because the kidneys have an enormous blood supply, and the renal tubules concentrate the fluid flowing through them, any toxins present in the tubules are also concentrated. Many drugs are concentrated to toxic levels including gentamicin, high dose furosemide, and amphotericin.

Drugs can cause interstitial nephritis

Some drugs can cause interstitial (allergic) nephritis. These include β-lactams (penicillins and cephalosporins) and non-steroidal anti-inflammatory drugs.

NSAIDs cause kidney ischaemia

Non-steroidal anti-inflammatory drugs (NSAIDs) disrupt intra-renal blood flow, especially in the elderly. They can disrupt the blood supply to the renal tubules. NSAIDs should be stopped four days before surgery, and preferably not used in patients over the age of 65 years, or those with chronic kidney disease.

Morphine

Because morphine is partly metabolized by the kidneys its action may be prolonged in patients with diseased kidneys. Morphine's metabolite morphine-6-glucoronide is a more potent analgesic and respiratory depressant than morphine itself. Although a single loading dose of morphine is well tolerated in patients with kidney disease, increase the intervals between subsequent doses by 30 to 50 per cent.

Pethidine

Avoid pethidine in patients with chronic kidney disease, because its metabolite, 6-pethidinic acid, accumulates and may cause convulsions.

Avoid pethidine in patients with renal impairment.

Fentanyl

Although fentanyl is metabolized by the liver, and has no active metabolite, the drug's *clearance* is decreased in patients with an eGFR less than 15 ml/min. This will prolong its action.

Penicillins and gentamicin

Never combine gentamicin and penicillins in intravenous injections or infusions. Gentamicin splits open-lactam rings of penicillins chemically inactivating them both the gentamicin and the penicillin. The problem occurs especially in patients with stage 3 (or worse) chronic kidney disease, who retain higher levels of penicillin for longer than patients with normal renal function.

If patients with renal failure require both gentamicin and penicillin, then separate the doses by several hours.

Benzodiazepines

Because there is increased sensitivity to their effects in patients with kidney disease, reduce the dose of *benzodiazepines*, such as diazepam, oxazepam and midazolam, by 30 to 50 per cent.

Relaxants

Neuromuscular blocking drugs whose effects may be prolonged in patients with kidney disease include pancuronium, doxacurium, pipercuronium, and vecuronium.

Iodionated contrast media

Iodinated radio-contrast media used in angiography is hypertonic and concentrates in the blood disrupting intra-renal blood flow. To reduce the risk of radiocontrast nephropathy, give one litre of 0.45% saline before giving the contrast. Do not try to boost urine output with either mannitol or furosemide because these drugs further desiccate tubular endothelium making the outcome worse.

Diuretics

A *diuretic* is a drug promoting urine output. There are four types of diuretics.

1. *Loop diuretics* e.g. furosemide (previously called frusemide) inhibits chloride (and therefore sodium) reabsorption in the loop of Henle. Furosemide is a powerful drug.

2. *Osmotic diuretics* such as mannitol, which being hypertonic enter the filtrate and drags water along with it.

3. *Potassium-conserving diuretics*; such as spironolactone, an analogue of aldosterone, blocks the uptake of sodium ion.

4. *Thiazide* diuretics such as chlorothiazide and indapamide act at the proximal part of the distal tubule to prevent potassium reabsorption.

How to calculate drug dose

The doses of some drugs, such as gentamicin, are modified according to renal function. Check renal function before using any drug that is excreted by the kidney. After you have given a drug to patients with kidney disease, observe them assiduously for untoward effects.

The Crockoft–Gault Equation (1976) is used to estimate creatinine clearance from the plasma creatinine concentration. It is primarily used in the recovery room for determining the correct dose of gentamicin.

$$\text{Creatinine clearance} = \frac{(140 - \text{age in years} \times \text{lean body weight in Kg}}{815 \times \text{serum creatinine (mmol/L)}}$$

For women the value is 85 per cent of that estimated by the equation.

Although eGFR has supplanted creatinine clearance, appropriate drug doses in those with kidney disease are still calculated by the Crockoft–Gault equation.

End-stage renal disease

End-stage kidney disease (ESKD) occurs when the eGFR is greater than 15 ml/min, and dialysis is usually necessary when the eGFR is less than 10 ml/min.

There are two clinical types of end-stage kidney disease: *oliguric renal failure* with little or no urine produce, and *polyuric renal failure* where urine is formed but cannot be concentrated in the kidney tubules. Both types cause raised serum creatinine and urea concentrations, and are accompanied by the usual retinue of hypertension, anaemia, ischaemic heart disease, calcified heart valves, coagulopathies, chronic steroid dependence, poor wound healing and a susceptibility to infection.

Kidneys are precious and fragile.
Seek help from senior trained specialists.

If you have any doubt about the management of patients with end-stage kidney disease then consult a renal physician. Take care not to overload these patients with intravenous fluids. Most patients have been dialyzed before they come for elective surgery, and are relatively hypovolaemic so it is safe for them to receive up to a litre of Hartmann's solution during their operation. If they arrive with their second litre running then, in consultation with the anaesthetist, slow it to an 18-hourly rate.

Veins and arteries are precious

Veins in patients with end-stage renal failure are precious because they may be needed for haemodialysis. Never put drips in around the wrists or in the cubital fossa. Use the smallest possible cannula and a careful sterile technique to insert it (not just wipe with an alcohol swab). Never allow even a hint of thrombophlebitis to occur. If there is any sign of inflammation remove the cannula and re-site it in another place. Replace cannulas within 24 hours. Avoid taking blood gases from their precious radial arteries, use their femoral artery instead.

How to prevent postoperative renal failure

The recovery room has a major role in preventing postoperative renal failure, especially in patients who have risk factors. So:

- Give oxygen.
- Ensure that your patient is not *hypovolaemic*.
- Do not use NSAIDs in patients with an eGFR < 50 ml/min/1.73 m^2.
- Control pain. Pain activates a noradrenergic response, which reduces renal blood flow.
- Do not give nephrotoxic drugs to patients who are hypovolaemic.
- Avoid the so-called 'triple whammy' of furosemide, gentamicin and NSAID.

Classes of acute renal failure

There are three classes of acute renal failure:

1. *Prerenal acute renal failure* is caused by hypovolaemia, which diminishes renal blood flow. This is the most common cause of acute renal failure encountered in the recovery room.

2. *Intrinsic acute renal failure* occurs when there is damage to the renal parenchyma. This is more likely where radiocontrast dyes are used during surgery.

3. *Postrenal acute renal failure* occurs when the urinary tract becomes obstructed, usually with blood clots or stone fragments after urological surgery. However, occasionally the ureter is damaged during pelvic surgery.

What to do if urine output slows or stops

In the recovery room *oliguria* occurs when the urine output falls below 1 ml/Kg/hr. *Severe oliguria* occurs when it falls below 0.5 ml/Kg/hr, and *anuria* when no urine has been produced for the last 15 minutes.

Consider the likely possible causes for acute renal failure for example hypovolaemia (prerenal), toxic drugs (renal) and obstruction (postrenal).

Prerenal causes

Ensure that your patient is not hypovolaemic. Check their perfusion status; cold hands and a tachycardia suggest ischaemic kidneys. A hypovolaemic patient will drop their systolic blood pressure if you sit them up in Fowler's position at 45°.

Cold hands = cold kidneys.

Treat hypovolaemia

- Give oxygen and aim for saturations > 97%.
- Notify the anaesthetist.
- Treat hypovolaemia aggressively because it rapidly causes damage to the kidney.

If they are bleeding then give blood, or:

- Give 500 ml of a colloid first and follow this with Hartmann's solution.
- After each 500 ml of fluid check if they are still hypovolaemic by propping them up at 45°. If their blood pressure falls by > 20 mmHg then prepare to give another 500 ml of Hartmann's solution.

Suppress renovascular constriction

- Give oxygen and aim for saturations > 97%.

- Treat pain, because severe pain reduces renal blood flow. If possible use epidural anaesthesia.

- Be alert for a possible shower of bacteria especially after urological, or gastrointestinal surgery; or where the surgery has involved an infected site such as drainage of an abscess or fluid collection.

Renal causes

Check the patient has not been receiving nephrotoxic drugs leading up to or during their surgery. A common nephrotoxin is radiocontrast dye, especially if the patient is also taking metformin, or the patient is, or has been, hypovolaemic.

To prompt urine output

- Give oxygen and aim for saturations > 97%.

- If the patient's blood volume is normal you can prompt urine output with a small dose of furosemide and mannitol. Start with a combination of furosemide 0.5 mg/Kg and mannitol 1 gm/Kg.

- Use higher doses of furosemide if the patient has pigment associated *nephropathy* following haemolysis, *rhabdomyolysis* or massive crush injuries.

Postrenal causes

- Check the patency of the urinary catheter.

- Is an over-full bladder peeping over the pelvic brim?

When not to worry

If the patient has good perfusion with warm hands, is not in pain, has oxygen saturations > 95% and has neither received any nephrotoxic drugs, nor has been assaulted with a shower of bacteria, then the kidneys are probably not at risk.

Oliguria is not necessarily a sinister event, and in itself is not a reliable predictor of acute renal failure. This phenomenon of oliguria with well-perfused kidneys is more likely in a patient taking *angiotensin-converting enzyme inhibitors* (ACEIs).

Providing the patient has not been hypotensive or hypoxic at any time these drugs probably exert a protective effect on the kidney during major surgery. They certainly predispose to perioperative hypotension, especially in patients with cardiac failure.[5] In the case of warm kidneys, urine output will probably improve over the next hour or so. If there has been one or more kidney-damaging events during surgery it is worthwhile provoking an increase in urine output with a small volume load and a low dose of furosemide.

Drugs modifying renal function

0.9% saline

In patients with chronic kidney disease, *normal saline* contributes to hyper-chloraemia, and probably contributes to postoperative renal dysfunction.[6] If you need to give more than one litre of crystalloid fluid then use Ringer's lactate or Hartmann's solution.

Avoid large volumes of 0.9% saline in patients with renal disease.

Diuretics

Loop diuretics increase renal blood flow. Furosemide may shorten the oliguric period, but it has no clinical benefits when used to prevent or treat acute renal failure[7], and has no effect on mortality and may be harmful. High doses cause ototoxicity and damage a hypoperfused kidney.

Mannitol

Mannitol, is a complex polysaccharide. It acts an osmotic diuretic. Although it causes renal vasodilation, and has some theoretical advantages, in practice it can cause osmotic damage to proximal tubular cells. Mannitol is probably no better than a saline infusion. Its only proven place is to treat *rhabdomyolysis*.

Dopamine

Dopamine, a biochemical precursor of noradrenaline is used to treat acute cardiac failure and normovolaemic shock. In critically ill patients dopamine has a dark side. It may cause arrhythmias, and certainly jeopardises blood flow to the gut and liver. More obscurely it causes endocrine and immune dysfunction, and impairs surgical healing. To use dopamine is controversial. The consensus is that renal dose dopamine has no place in renal protection in the hypovolaemic, septic or hypothermic patient.

Dopexamine

Dopexamine is a synthetic β_2 agonist, it is useful after aortic surgery as it improves the cardiac output and therefore the blood supply to the kidneys.

Notes

1. Levey AS, Bosch J P, Lewis JB *et al.* (1999) *Annals of Internal Medicine* 130:461–70.
2. Sear JW (2005) *Br J Anaes* 95:20–32.
3. Wabash AM, El Heaney MO, Wafa EM *et al.* (2000) *Hepatogastroenerology* 47:1691–4.
4. Cittanova ML, Zubicki A, Savu C *et al.* (2001) *Anaesthesia and Analgesia* 93:1111–15.
5. Sear JW. (2005) *British Journal of Anaesthesia* 95:20–32.
6. Bennet-Guerrero E, Frumento RJ, Mets B *et al.* (2001) *Anesthesiology* 95:A147.
7. Kwok Mo, Sheridan DJ (2006) *BMJ* 333:420.

22

Fluid balance

Patients coming to the recovery room from theatre may have disturbed circulating and tissue fluid volumes for many reasons: they are fasted, they may have received intravenous fluids or lost fluid during their operation; or have ongoing losses from bleeding or bowel obstruction.

How surgery affects fluid balance

Postoperatively, sensors in brainstem and hypothalamus emerge from anaesthesia to encounter a whole host of neural and *cytokine* messages telling the brainstem and the *vital centres* that the body is injured. These inputs include pain, tissue trauma, hypothermia, hypovolaemia, sepsis, and hypoxia.

If we are injured, evolution has programmed us to hide, without food or water, for several days while recovering. The body uses a barrage of measures to preserve vital body fluids and maintain *homeostasis*. The sympathetic nervous system and several hormones regulate these measures. Hormones that are released include angiotensin, aldosterone, cortisol, and *antidiuretic hormone*. Their net effect is to stop the kidneys excreting precious extracellular fluids, and breaking down skeletal muscle (and some days later, fat) to provide an emergency food source. Some of these responses are potentially harmful, and most are no longer necessary, because we shelter, feed and give fluids to our patients.

Thrombophlebitis

Check established intravenous lines when you admit the patient to the recovery room. Thrombophlebitis is potentially lethal and can lead to septicaemia. If there is any sign of inflammation or pain along the course of the vein, then re-site the cannula and use a new giving set. Take the opportunity to replace cannulas if they have been there for 48 hours or more.

Intravenous cannula and their insertion

1. Assemble all the equipment you need and use standard precautions.

Thrombophlebitis *(continued)*

2. Choose the right cannula:

   Blood transfusion size 14 to 16 G

   Electrolyte solutions size 18 to 20 G

   Drug administration size 22 to 24 G.

3. It is easier to sit down to do difficult cannulations. Choose a vein on the forearm well away from the elbow or wrist, and preferably on the non-dominant arm. Insert the needle at the confluence of two veins. If there is no alternative other than to insert a drip near a joint, then splint the joint.

4. If you are inserting a cannula larger than size 22, then use a 30 G needle to raise a skin bleb with 1% lidocaine a few millimetres away from the vein. An alternative is to use an insulin syringe, with its a tiny needle that can barely be felt as it enters the skin.

5. Choose a vein on the forearm well away from the elbow.

6. Do not put cannulas in veins near flexures such as the elbow or wrist joint, because as the joint moves the cannula will abrade the inside of the vein causing inflammation. They are also likely to kink off. If you insert a drip near a joint, then use a splint.

7. Where possible avoid inserting drips in the back of the hand or foot. Cannulating veins in a lower limb carries a high risk of thrombophlebitis.

8. Use a sterile technique. Wear gloves, preferably sterile gloves on sick patients. Allow about 60 seconds for the skin prep to dry. Do not drag wet skin prep into the vein or it will cause thrombophlebitis.

9. Put on a transparent dressing to protect the insertion site. If these are not available, use a small adhesive dressing over the puncture wound, and fix the cannula with tape on top of this. Write the time and date on the plaster.

10. Use a transparent dressing to protect the insertion site. If these are not available, use a small adhesive dressing over the puncture wound and fix the cannula with tape on top of this.

11. Cannula should be replaced every 12 hours if blood is being infused, otherwise they should remain in place for no longer than 36 hours.

12. Fluids will flow faster if the cannula is short with a wide bore and the flask is hung on a high drip stand.

13. Chubby children who seem to have no peripheral veins will often have visible jugular veins.

14. In an emergency a valuable approach is to insert a large bore cannula into the femoral vein using a Seldinger wire technique and an 8.5 F sheath. In children who have no veins the anaesthetist may inset an intramedullary or intraosseous infusion. Use a large bore, short bevelled needle into marrow of the sternum or preferably the tibia taking care to avoid the epiphysial plates. Use an infusion pressure of up to 300 mmHg.

The body's fluid compartments

Functionally the body is divided into two compartments: the *intracellular fluid* (ICF) and the *extracellular fluid* (ECF). The two compartments are separated by a cell membrane. Only water can flow across cell membranes, and it does so to keep the ionic concentration (*tonicity*) of the fluid exactly equal on either side of the membrane. The *force* that drives water across the membrane is called *osmotic pressure*. Osmotic pressure is generated by the difference in the number of ions on each side of the cell membrane.

Facts

- The volume of the ECF is about 15 litres, of which 3 litres are *plasma*. The remaining 12 litres are in the interstitial space and bathe the cells in a warm swamp from which they derive their nutrients, and into which they jettison their wastes.

- The volume of the ICF is 30 litres, and about 2 litres of this volume are inside circulating red blood cells.

- Normal blood volume is about 5 litres or 70 ml/Kg.

- The capillary endothelium is freely permeable to water, *cations*, and *anions*, but not to larger proteins. Proteins such as albumin are principally confined to plasma.

- The principal cation in the ECF is sodium, but inside the cells it is potassium.

Fluids

Intravenous fluids can be *hypertonic, isotonic,* or *hypotonic.*

Most of the intravenous fluids we use in the recovery room are isotonic with plasma. This means they exert the same *osmotic pressure* as plasma. Isotonic fluids include *Ringer's solution*, 0.9% saline, and Hartmann's solution. When these solutions are given as an intravenous fluid into the

Fig 22.1 Fluid compartments

extracellular fluid, water neither enters nor leaves the cells. These fluids remain entirely in the ECF.

Some intravenous fluids are hypotonic. Water from these fluids will flow into cells causing them to swell. Although seldom used, 0.45% normal saline is a hypotonic solution; its osmotic pressure is half that of plasma.

Sometimes hypertonic solutions are used to correct serious problems with water balance. Examples of these solutions are 2N saline, 3N saline and 20% mannitol.

Table 22.1 Content of parenteral crystalloids in mmol/L

	Sodium	Potassium	Magnesium	Calcium	Chloride	Lactate	Acetate	Gluconate
0.9% saline	154	–	–	–	154	–	–	–
Hartmann's	131	5	–	–	111	29	–	–
Plasmalyte®	140	5	1.5	–	98	–	27	23
Ringer's lactate	137	4	–	3	142	–	–	–

Hypotonic solutions

Five per cent dextrose in water

Dextrose is simply another name for glucose: *5% dextrose in water* (D5W) contains 50 gm/L of glucose (278 mmol/L) dissolved in sterile water. As soon as it enters a vein it acts as an isotonic solution, exerting exactly the same osmotic pressure as plasma, but within a few minutes the cells take up the glucose, leaving the water behind. The water distributes itself evenly throughout the whole 45 litres of body fluid compartments. Two-thirds of the water enters the ECF, and one-third remains in the ECF.

If you give excess hypotonic fluid its water enters cells causing them to swell and disrupting their function. It may even cause red cells to burst (*haemolysis*) so releasing their haemoglobin into the plasma. Brain cells are confined inside a tight bony box the skull. If brain cells swell, the *intracranial pressure* (ICP) rises abruptly jeopardising the blood supply: this can be fatal.

Four per cent dextrose and 1/5 normal saline

'*4% and a fifth*' is a popular maintenance fluid in children. One litre is made up of 800 ml of 5% dextrose and 200 ml of 0.9% saline, but it is seldom used in the recovery room. Once a child weighs 10 Kg or is 7 months old, its kidneys are mature enough to cope with intravenous fluids used in adults.

Isotonic solutions

Colloids

Colloids exert enough oncotic pressure to balance the flow of fluid between the intravascular and the interstitial space. Colloids rapidly increase blood volume in hypovolaemic, shocked or bleeding patients, because they stay within the circulation much longer than crystalloids.

There are four principal types of colloids: human albumin, polygelines, dextrans, and starches.

Human albumin 5 per cent

Human albumin 5% (50 gm/L) is a purified, sterile, colloid derived from human plasma. It does not need to be cross-matched. Given intravenously it stays in the circulation, but within 18 hours it leaks away to distribute uniformly throughout the ECF. The metabolic half-life of albumin is 20 days, and the turnover in an adult is about 5 gm/day. As with all colloids it can cause circulatory overload, particularly in patients with cardiac failure or renal impairment. Occasionally, it can cause hypotension and rigors. Although never reported there is a theoretical risk of transmitting Creutzfield–Jakob disease (CJD), but not HIV or hepatitis viruses.

Polygelines

Polygelines are 3.5% colloid solutions prepared from gelatin. They do not carry diseases, they are cheap. They do not require refrigeration and are iso-osmotic with blood. Occasionally they cause allergic reactions, especially if the patient is hypovolaemic. Intravascular half-life is 4 to 6 hours in patients with normal renal function.

Other synthetic colloids

Hydroxethyl starch (pentastarch) in sodium chloride (Volvulen®) is a polysaccharide polymer derived from corn and similar to glycogen used to expand the intravascular volume. It has a plateau effect of 4–6 hours and is excreted by the kidneys more quickly than older solutions of polymers. It has little effect on haemostasis. The advised maximum dose is 15 ml/Kg. Pentastarch solutions are probably better than hetastarch solutions.

Dextrans are long-chained polysaccharides occasionally used as plasma expanders. The use of dextrans has declined because they sometimes cause kidney damage, allergic reactions and difficulty in cross-matching blood.

Crystalloids

Crystalloids are physiologically balanced salt solutions. They do not cause allergic reactions, they improve renal perfusion more effectively than colloids, and are cheap. However, they have a greater risk of causing pulmonary oedema, and they may aggravate acute respiratory distress syndrome more than colloids.

Normal saline

Normal (0.9% saline) is an isotonic solution containing 154 mmol of sodium chloride in a litre of distilled water. When you give 0.9% saline intravenously it rapidly distributes itself between the circulation and the interstitial fluid, but all of it remains in the ECF, and none of it crosses the cell membrane to enter the cells. Rapid infusions of 0.9% saline can cause a hyperchloraemic acidosis.[1] For most situations, particularly in shocked patients, Hartmann's solution is a better choice than 0.9% saline.

Hartmann's solution (Ringer's lactate)

Hartmann's solution is isotonic. When infused into a vein it all stays in the ECF. In addition to sodium ion, Hartmann's solution contains potassium, lactate, chloride and calcium ions. It is useful because it roughly approximates the ionic concentration of plasma, but does not contain any plasma proteins.

Ringer's solution

Ringer's solution is similar to Hartmann's solution, but contains no lactate ions.

Plasma-Lyte®

Plasma-Lyte 148® is a sterile isotonic solution for intravenous fluid therapy. It was introduced as a substitute for 0.9% saline. Rapid infusions of 0.9% saline can cause an acidosis, but Plasma-Lyte® consumes hydrogen ions as the acetate and gluconate are metabolized in the liver to carbon dioxide and water.

How the body controls fluids

The body has two systems for controlling fluid balance. One, the *low pressure baroreceptor system*, responds to the pressure of fluid in the great veins and right atria; in contrast the other entirely separate *osmoreceptor* system responds to changes in *tonicity* in the interstitial fluid. Grasp this point firmly: there are two separate fluid systems each with its own sensor.

Low-pressure baroreceptors respond to stretching the walls of the right atria. As they stretch they release *atrial-naturetic peptide* (ANP), a hormone that improves renal blood flow. Once they have a good blood supply the kidneys now excrete near-isotonic fluid.

Osmoreceptors in the *hypothalamus* detect changes in concentration of sodium ion in the ECF. This system controls the *tonicity* of the body water. As the tonicity of the ECF rises, the osmoreceptors release *antidiuretic hormone* (ADH). ADH forces the kidney to retain water to dilute the ECF. On the other hand if the concentration of sodium ion in the ECF decreases, the osmoreceptors stop producing ADH and the urine becomes more dilute. This system is a typical example of a physiological negative feedback loop.

What can go wrong

Either of these two systems can become disordered independently of each other. Conceptually, it is easier to regard each of them as separate 'tanks': one containing the 45 litres of *total body water*, and the other 15 litres of *isotonic fluid* in the ECF. The isotonic ECF is predominately a saline solution containing added electrolytes (potassium, chloride, bicarbonate, magnesium and trace elements).

Fluid out = fluid in

Fluid balance is achieved when the rate of fluid going in equals the rate of fluid being lost, and the patient is haemodynamically stable. If you work with this basic formula you will find postoperative fluid balance easier to manage.

$$Fluid\ requirements = continuing\ loss + catch\text{-}up\ fluid + maintenance$$

Disorders of fluid balance

It is best to estimate total body water and ECF volume separately. Replace blood loss with colloid. Replace isotonic fluid losses from the bowel (such as with vomiting or from fistulae) with Hartmann's solution. Assess and adjust potassium levels, magnesium and phosphate levels separately.

Maintenance fluid requirements

Postoperative fluid therapy is usually planned by agreement between the anaesthetist, surgeon and the recovery room nursing staff. Often the first 24 hours of fluid therapy are organized before the patient is discharged to the ward.

Adult maintenance

Adult maintenance fluids = 40 ml + 1 ml/Kg each hour.

A 70 Kg man will require 40 + (70 × 1) = 110 ml/hr. This is 2640 ml per day. Add 13.4 mmol of potassium per litre. For a routine adult patient who is expected to drink within a few hours' maintenance fluids would be 1 litre of saline and 2 litres of dextrose 5% daily. Give each litre over 8 hours.

Child maintenance

A solution of 1/5 normal saline and dextrose is a commonly used fluid for small children.

For the first 10 Kg give 4 ml/Kg/hr
Add a further 2 ml/Kg/hr for children weighing 10–20 Kg
Add a further 1 ml/Kg/hr for children over 20 Kg

Examples:

5 Kg infant would require 5 × 4 = 20 ml/hr or 480 ml/day

15 Kg child would require:
for the first 10 Kg give 4 ml/Kg/hr = 10 × 4 = 40 ml
add 2 ml/Kg/hr for the next 5 Kg = 5 × 2 = 10 ml
total requirements = 50 ml/hr or 1200 ml/day

28 Kg child would require:
for the first 10 Kg give 4 ml/Kg/hr = 10 × 4 = 40 ml
add 2 ml/Kg/hr for next 10 Kg = 10 × 2 = 20 ml
then add 1 ml/Kg/hr for next 8 Kg = 8 × 1 = 8 ml
total requirements = 68 ml/hr or 1632 ml/day

Consider putting these formulas on a wallchart in the recovery room.

Correct problems in the following order:

1. Correct the blood volume to protect and restore the perfusion of the patient's brain, heart and kidneys.

2. Estimate and adjust the ECF volume.

3. Calculate and adjust water balance.

4. Correct other electrolyte disturbances.

Restore the blood volume

In patients who are bleeding or who are saline depleted, the first thing to do is save their kidneys, by quickly restoring the blood volume. Preferably give bleeding patients blood, or failing that a colloid to restore their vascular volume rapidly as possible, and consequently preserve blood flow to their heart, brain, liver, and kidneys.

Correct the ECF volume

Because isotonic fluids cannot cross cell membranes they are confined to the ECF. Think of the ECF as tank of isotonic fluid (which is 98% saline) that can either can be too full (*saline overload*) or too empty (*saline deficit*).

ECF volume overload

Acute saline overload

In its most dramatic form acute *saline overload* presents with pulmonary oedema. Initially the patient has a tachypnoea (rate greater than 20 breaths/min) and cool hands. Fluid accumulating in the interstitium of their lungs triggers a rise in respiratory rate, and a noradrenergic response. The normal respiratory rate is 12–14 breaths/min. Measure the respiratory rate carefully by putting your hand on the patient's chest to feel it rise and fall.

As the saline overload progresses patients feel breathless, and then start to wheeze. They feel most uncomfortable lying down. At this early stage the chest X-ray shows peribronchial oedema (cuffing) and distended upper lobe veins. Later, the X-rays show a ground glass appearance of interstitial pulmonary oedema.

If you listen at the patient's mouth as they force out a deep breath, you can hear oedematous small airways softly, snap, crackle and pop open. As their oxygen saturation falls below 90% patients may feel panicky, and grope about the bed. You can now hear showers of crackles at the lung bases that do not go away with deep breaths. Now the chest X-ray shows the fluffy dense bat's wing appearance of alveolar pulmonary oedema.

How to manage acute pulmonary oedema

Sit the patient up, give high flow oxygen, and ensure their blood pressure is greater than 100 mmHg. If they are older then 60 years give furosemide 40 mg IV; in younger patients, give furosemide 10–20 mg IV. Wait 20 minutes. If the urine output remains less than 30 ml/hr, check their urinary catheter is not blocked, there is no chance of haemorrhage, and their systolic blood pressure is greater than100 mmHg. At this point the anaesthetist may double the dose of furosemide to 80 mg IV. If there is still no urine produced then further measures include seeking expert help, dobutamine infusions, active vasodilation with sodium nitroprusside, and if desperate the anaesthetist may venesect 500 ml of blood.

Chronic saline overload

Chronic saline overload is a feature of chronic congestive cardiac failure. If someone has demonstrable pitting oedema in their legs, they have at least 3 litres of excess fluid in their extracellular fluid space. Chronic saline overload is treated with furosemide, which forces the kidney to excrete near isotonic fluid.

ECF volume deficit

Saline deficit occurs with diarrhoea, protracted vomiting, and diabetic ketoacidosis, but in the recovery room it is most often seen in people who have had surgery to relieve a bowel obstruction, or have suffered severe burns.

The signs of saline deficit are the same as that of haemorrhage: poor peripheral perfusion, a urine output less than 0.5 ml/Kg/hr, and tachycardia greater than 100 beats/min. In young people the blood pressure does not fall until the situation is grave. People older than 50 years may become hypotensive, but this is an unreliable sign in a supine patient.

In people of all ages, hypovolaemia is always revealed by a *postural drop* in blood pressure. Take the patient's blood pressure, and then gently sit them up at 45°. If their systolic pressure falls by more than 20 mmHg then their vascular volume is low.

Postural drop in blood pressure is an excellent sign of low vascular volume.

Untreated saline deficit progresses to shock and metabolic acidosis. This metabolic acidosis is treated by replacing the fluid loss (deficit) with an isotonic fluid, such as Hartmann's solution or 0.9% saline. The patient's electrolyte results helps decide whether they need additional potassium, and possibly magnesium too.

Correct total body water

Unlike the saline, water readily crosses cell membranes, so its 'tank' has a volume of 45 litres and includes both the ECF and ICF compartments.

Water overload

The hallmark of water overload is a low serum sodium ion concentration. In the recovery room it is usually seen after endoscopic urological surgery or hysteroscopy where large amounts of water have been instilled, and then absorbed. Another common cause is the injudicious use of 5% dextrose, but it can also occur with severe chronic heart failure, and other more uncommon chronic conditions.

Acute water overload

With acute water overload patients complain of faintness, headache, tingling around the mouth, nausea, breathlessness, and a tight feeling in the chest. They may become progressively restless, confused, disoriented, start retching, develop muscle twitching and then wheeze (a sign of developing acute pulmonary oedema). The blood pressure rises, the pulse may slow, and *haemoglobinuria* causes the urine to turn brown. The ECG may show widening of the QRS complex and T-wave inversion. If not promptly treated the patient becomes cyanotic, hypotensive, and may have a cardiac arrest. All these signs are caused by the osmotic pressure of water entering cells, causing red cells to rupture, cerebral oedema; and disturbing cardiac myocyte function.

Management

Give high concentrations of oxygen by mask. Monitor blood pressure, pulse, respiratory rate, oxygen saturation and ECG. Send blood to laboratory for electrolytes, and haemoglobinaemia, and urine haemoglobin.

Use hypertonic saline as soon as water overload starts to cause symptoms. Give 1000 ml of 3N saline with the aim of increasing the serum sodium ion by 3 to 5 mmol/L over the first 2 hours. The principal risk of using hypertonic saline is saline overload. (Every 1000 ml of 3N saline will convert 2000 ml of the excess water into 2000 ml of isotonic saline; as well as infusing the equivalent of a further 1000 ml of N saline.) To overcome this, use furosemide 20–40 mg IV every 2–4 hours to get rid of the excess ECF volume.

A word of caution: if you find a premenopausal woman, or a child with a serum sodium ion concentration falling towards 130 mmol/L they are in grave danger of developing cerebral oedema with seizures. Postoperatively premenopausal women who develop hyponatraemic encephalopathy are 25 times more likely to die or have permanent brain damage than either men or postmenopausal women. Seek skilled help.

Chronic water overload

Don't attempt to correct long-standing compensated hyponatraemia with hypertonic saline, because you may cause a central pontine myelolysis resulting in the locked-in syndrome. This is a catastrophe. The patient is rendered quadriplegic, unable to move anything except their eyes, and is condemned to life on a ventilator. Patients with chronic hyponatremia and severe symptoms (e.g., severe confusion, coma, seizures) should receive hypertonic saline but only enough to raise the serum sodium by 3–5 mmol/L, which is enough to stop seizures.

Asymptomatic water overload

Asymptomatic acute water overload usually self-corrects over a number of days if the patient receives no further 5% dextrose or free water. A common error in such patients is to 'fluid restrict' them and give them furosemide, in which case they will probably become saline depleted too, and risk developing renal failure. Of course water overloaded patients can still have isotonic fluids if indicated because that fills a different tank. In men and postmenopausal females symptoms of confusion and renal failure occur progressively once the serum sodium ion acutely falls to less than 130 mmol/L.

Syndrome of inappropriate ADH secretion (SIADH)

SIADH is a rare cause of water overload. It usually only occurs in patients who were critically ill preoperatively. Consider the diagnosis if the serum Na^+ < 135 with corresponding plasma hypo-osmolality, but despite this the kidney continues to excrete sodium > 20 mmol/L and osmolality > 500 *mOsmol/Kg*), there is clinical evidence of *volume depletion* and the patient is not hypotensive.

Water deficit

It is uncommon to encounter an isolated water deficit in recovery room. Occasionally you may see water deficit in patients who have been febrile for some time. The hallmark of water deficit is an elevated serum sodium ion concentration (Na^+ > 142 mmol/L). It responds readily with 5 per cent dextrose. Each 1000 ml of 5% dextrose in an adult will decrease their serum sodium ion concentration by 3 mmol/L; conversely each 3 mmol/L rise in serum sodium ion concentrations indicates a deficit of 1000 ml of water.

Summary

Table 22.2 Water or saline?

Water status	Problem	Remedy
If Na$^+$ <135 mmol/L	= Water overload	Give no water
If Na$^+$ <130 mmol/L	= Severe water overload	Consider hypertonic saline
If Na$^+$ >143 mmol/L	= Water deficit	Give 5% dextrose
Saline status		
Postural drop >20 mmHg + Urine output <30 ml/hr + Tachycardia >100 bpm + Cool hands	= Saline deficit or Bleeding	Replace with 0.9% saline Ensure that there is no bleeding
Rising respiratory rate + Falling SaO$_2$ ± Wheeze ± Orthopnoea	= Saline overload	Stop IV infusion Give oxygen and furosemide Get a CXR

Correct other electrolytes

Hypokalaemia is easy to correct, but hyperkalaemia is dangerous and requires intensive care.

Hypokalaemia

Hypokalaemia is a serum potassium concentration of less than 3.5 mmol/L.

Hypokalaemia exacerbates residual paralysis from long-acting muscle relaxant drugs. Affected patients are unable to sustain a 5-second head lift. Suspect hypokalaemia if the patient had low serum potassium preoperatively or the ECG shows flattened or inverted T-waves. Hypokalemia is more likely to cause problems if the oxygen saturation is low, the PCO$_2$ high, or the patient has had anti-cholinergic drugs. Treat hypokalaemia by adding 26.8 mmol of potassium chloride to 1000 ml of dextrose or saline, and give it at a rate of not more than 13.4 mmol (one gram) an hour under ECG control. If extrasystoles occur, slow the infusion rate.

Never inject concentrated potassium chloride directly into the drip – it will kill your patient.

Hyperkalaemia

Hyperkalaemia is a serum potassium concentration exceeding 5.5 mmol/L.

Patients at risk include those with renal failure, burns, crush injuries, established muscle paralysis (whatever the cause), incompatible blood transfusions, or where haemolysis has occurred.

The ECG shows high-peaked T-waves especially in the precordial leads, but there should not be any prolongation of the QT interval as happens with other causes of peaked T-waves. As the hyperkalaemia worsens the PR interval becomes prolonged (> 200 ms), progressing to AV conduction defects, the QRS widens, and finally asystole occurs.

Treat arrhythmias with calcium gluconate 1 gram intravenously over two minutes into a fast-running drip into a big vein. If necessary repeat the dose once. If the serum potassium remains greater than 6.5 mmol/L, then treat it with a glucose and insulin infusion. Give one unit of insulin for every 4 grams of glucose. Measure the glucose and potassium levels every half an hour. Watch for signs of hypoglycaemia: sweating, anxiety, tachycardia and confusion. Alternatively you can use the ion exchange resin Resonium™ 15–30 gm as an enema. Persistent hyperkalaemia requires haemodialysis or peritoneal dialysis.

Fluids after surgery

Bowel surgery

For some days after bowel surgery, isotonic fluid transudates into the gut. Because this fluid is lost from the ECF, and is no longer accessible to the circulation, it is called *third space loss*. An atonic bowel can contain 6 litres or more of third space fluid. It may take up to 6 days for the bowel to recover its function, and for the fluid to be returned to the circulation. Following bowel surgery replace four-fifths of the fluid requirements with isotonic fluids such as saline or Hartmann's solution. The basic potassium requirement is 1 mmol/Kg/day. After bowel surgery requirements are usually double this amount. If you replace third space loss with 5% dextrose the patient will become hyponatraemic, and it is not uncommon for the serum sodium levels to be less than 132 mmol/L.

Neurosurgery

Many neurosurgeons prefer to keep their patients water depleted with higher than normal serum sodium levels. There is little evidence this reduces cerebral oedema. Indiscriminate fluid restriction causes saline depletion and jeopardises renal perfusion. Occasionally the surgeon may ask for an infusion of *mannitol* to reduce intracranial pressure.

Urological surgery

Following urological surgery, surgeons are anxious that blood clots do not form in the bladder or ureters where they may cause blockages. To prevent this and for the first few hours surgeons prefer the urine output to be at least 200 ml/hr. Such a high urine output may require a saline load of a litre or more with encouragement of a judicious dose of furosemide 10–40 mg intravenously.

Chronic renal failure

Patients with chronic renal failure are usually dialyzed before coming for major surgery and consequently may be relatively volume deplete. In addition to replacing the fluid lost during the surgery, they should not receive any more one litre of Hartmann's solution while in the recovery room. Most renal patients have many medical problems, such as diabetes, hypertension, ischaemic heart disease and anaemia. For this reason ask a renal physician to guide postoperative care. If you are in doubt about how to manage their fluid balance then measure the volume of their urine output. In addition to replacing any losses from drain tubes with Hartmann's solution, you can give them an additional 700 ml of 5% dextrose over the next 24 hours to cover *insensible fluid losses.*

Cardiac failure

If a patient has overt or stable cardiac failure you need to carefully balance the amount of intravenous fluid given against the volume of urine produced. Listen to their chests for developing fine moist sounds or wheeze suggesting saline overload. A respiratory rate rising beyond 14 breaths/min, or the reluctance to lie flat, are early warning sign of problems, in which case treat them for acute saline overload.

23

Metabolism

Homeostasis

At the core of the way we understand how the body controls its internal
environment, is the concept of *homeostasis*. This compound word is loosely
derived from the Greek meaning: '*to keep things still*'. Most of our work in
recovery room is to help the body maintain its homeostasis.

Homeostasis involves a collection of *feedback* mechanisms that keep our internal environment in a steady state despite fluctuations in our external environment.
For example, naked individuals can be exposed to temperatures as high as 42°C,
and as low as 28°C in dry air and still keep their core temperature constant.
Homeostasis is a three-step process. Sensors register the changes, sending a
message to a central processor, which coordinates mechanisms to compensate
for the change.

Feedback can either be positive reinforcement or negative inihibition

Figure 23.1 A feedback loop

For example, as we stand up blood pools in the great veins in our legs,
causing our mean blood pressure to fall transiently. Pressure sensors near the
heart detect the change in pressure, and send a message to a processor in the
midbrain. This signals the heart to increase its output, and the peripheral
vessels to constrict to compensate. This homeostatic feedback loop prevents us
from fainting every time we stand up.

What is stress?

A person at rest is in almost in equilibrium (homeostatic). In physiological
terms, a *stress* is something that moves the body away from its comfortable
resting state. Some stresses are minor, such as getting out of a warm bed in the

morning, while others are life-threatening, such as septicaemia following major bowel surgery. Other stresses include injury, infection, blood loss, dehydration, starvation, hypothermia, poisoning, and fear.

As a rule, stress response is proportional to the stress causing it and involves two sets of homeostatic mechanisms. The first is the autonomic nervous system (or *neural*) response, and the other is a hormonal (or *humoral*) response. The neural response works instantly; but the various hormonal responses take time to achieve their effect.

In response to a major stress, such as surgery, the body blends the neural responses to fit the immediate circumstances, and backs them up with lots of different hormones to maintain the initial response. Components of the response preserve body fluids, mobilize protein and fat stores to use as energy, prevent infection and heal the wounds.

Table 23.1 Some stresses encountered in the recovery room

Pain	Hypothermia
Fluid imbalance	Starvation
Haemorrhage	Infection
Hypoxia	Hypercarbia
Tissue injury	Anxiety/fear
Vomiting	Nausea

The autonomic nervous system

1. The sympathetic (noradrenergic) nervous system.
2. The parasympathetic (cholinergic) nervous system.

There is an intellectually appealing (but false) notion that these two systems work in opposition to each other. It is true they oppose each other in some aspects; for example the sympathetic system increases heart rate, while the parasympathetic nervous system slows it down. However, they evolved for two entirely different purposes and for the most part work independently of one another.

The sympathetic nervous system

The *sympathetic nervous system* (SNS) is part of the body's fight and flight response. Its control centre is in the hypothalamus; the nerve fibres leave the spinal cord in the thoracolumbar outflow to *synapse* in the sympathetic chain and then they accompany blood vessels to their target organs.

Fundamentally, an acute stress causes the body to respond either by preparing a person to run away (flight) or stay and face the consequences (fight).

Two separate *catecholamines* mediate the two separate responses.

The two catecholamines are:

1. *Noradrenaline* (a neurotransmitter), and

2. *Adrenaline* (a hormone) made by the adrenal medulla.

Following surgery the hypothalamus blends the effect of the two catecholamines to create an appropriate response that fits the circumstances.

Noradrenaline prepares the body for brief intense effort (to fight); and adrenaline dilates muscle vasculature, preparing the body for a sustained effort to run away (flight). In other words, noradrenaline is the neurotransmitter for inescapable life-threatening situations such as shock, sepsis, pain and hypoxia. In contrast, adrenaline is a hormone secreted predominantly for exercise.

There are two groups of catecholamine drugs: beta (β) agonists and alpha (α) agonists. Beta agonists increase the heart rate, and its force of contraction. Alpha agonists cause vasoconstriction in skin, muscle, kidney and gut.

Most catecholamine drugs have both alpha and beta effects. Noradrenaline has predominantly alpha effects causing peripheral vasoconstriction raising the blood pressure. Adrenaline has mixed alpha and beta effects increasing the heart rate and its force of contraction; also causing arterioles to constrict in the kidney, skin and gut, and vasodilation in muscle.

Hormonal back-up

Several hormones back up the stress response. A steroid, 'cortisol', enables the body to maintain a sustained adrenergic response to prolonged stress. Without cortisol the effects of noradrenaline would soon wear off, and the blood pressure falls. Another steroid, *aldosterone* slows the excretion of sodium ion, for example in a patient who is bleeding, or has lost some of their extracellular fluid.

Parasympathetic nervous system

The parasympathetic nervous system role is one of housekeeping: a 'rest and digest system'. It attends to the every day functions of digestion of food, stimulating salivary and other gastrointestinal glands, accelerating peristalsis.

Parasympathetic nerve fibres have their cell bodies in the central nervous system and their neurons run in the cranial nerves (CN III, VII, IX and X). The neurotransmitter of parasympathetic (cholinergic) nervous system is *acetylcholine*.

Simulating the parasympathetic nervous system slows the cardiac rate, constricts bronchi, and constricts the pupils. Drugs simulating the action of acetylcholine cause a bradycardia; they also stimulate bronchial secretions and salivation, and peristalsis. These drugs include neostigmine, physostigmine, and pyridostigmine. Conversely, atropine blocks the effects of acetylcholine on the heart, and causes tachycardia.

Temperature

The *core temperature* is the temperature of blood flowing through the thermo-regulatory centre in the anterior hypothalamus. This is not readily accessible so the benchmark is the temperature of blood in the pulmonary artery.

The centre for heat regulation lies in the hypothalamus, which tightly controls the body's core temperature around a *set point* that varies by less than 0.5°C. A normothermic patient has a *core temperature* between 36.5°C and 37.2°C. Outside this range, cellular metabolism is progressively disrupted.

Heat production and loss

Thermal balance occurs when heat production exactly equals heat loss. In hot environments we use less energy to maintain our body temperature, and in cold environments we use more. In humid atmospheres sweat cannot evaporate to lose heat.

In a *neutral thermal environment* a naked body neither loses nor gains heat. For adults this occurs at 28°C when the *relative humidity* is 60%. In premature babies the neutral thermal environment is 34°C, in neonates 32°C and in babies 30°C.

General anaesthetics abolish the body's ability to raise its metabolic rate, or vasoconstrict, to compensate for heat loss. In contrast, regional anaesthetics block the ability of blood vessels in the skin to vasoconstrict and preserve heat. Patients cool down during surgery because the operating theatre is maintained at 20°C, with a relative humidity of about 50%, which is well below the temperature of their neutral thermal environment.

How much patients cool down during surgery depends on the processes of conduction, convection, radiation and evaporation. For about the first 20 minutes on the operating table the patient's temperature stays stable. Then their core temperature falls rapidly over the following two hours, and more slowly after that.

The two main sources of heat loss during anaesthesia are evaporative heat loss from open abdomens, and radiant heat loss from exposed skin.

Hypothermia is a common after endoscopic urological procedures where large volumes of fluids are instilled and retrieved. This wash-in, wash-out of fluid is an example of convective heat loss. Giving two units of cold blood at 4°C will cause a fall in temperature of 0.5°C. This is an example of a conductive heat loss.

Table 23.2 Heat loss

Heat loss on the operating table	(%)
Convection	25–35
Conduction	< 10
Radiation	40–50
Evaporation	Varies
Heat loss in recovery room	
Radiation	50
Convection	30
Evaporation	10
Respiration	10
– humidifying air	8
– heating air	2

Cold patients

Waking up cold from an anaesthetic is a miserable experience, and long remembered by many patients: a warmed blanket is most welcome and comforting.

Shivering, particularly in older patients, puts unacceptable demands on the heart and lungs. If it is necessary use a convection air heater such as a BairHugger® or WarmTouch®. Cold patients do not metabolize opioid analgesics efficiently, and are at greater risk of hypoxia, hypoglycaemia, renal impairment, deep vein thrombosis and hypotension.

Air warming devices are not without risk. There have been reports of them contributing to cross-infection,[1] use a new blanket for each patient. It is possible to burn your patient if the blankets are not properly attached to the hose. Simply placing the hose under a sheet or blanket can cause a burn.

Hypothermia

All patients having surgery are at risk of hypothermia.

Occasionally active hypothermia is used to cool patients during cardiac and neurosurgery to protect the patient from brain damage where the blood supply to their brain heart needs to be temporarily interrupted. Induced hypothermia is being used increasingly to manage patients who have had a cardiac arrest and with those head injuries.

Hypothermia starts to cause clinical problems if the temperature falls below than 36°C, and once it falls below 35.8°C it has significant adverse outcomes.[2]

To delay the onset of hypothermia anaesthetists use warming blankets, and warm infused fluids, humidify inspired air, and try to reduce conductive and convective losses. Warming patients in the recovery room substantially reduces complications and the purchase of warming devices is cost-effective.[3]

What are the risk factors for hypothermia?

- Extremes of ages: thin elderly patients, neonates and infants.
- Long surgery (more than 3 hours) especially where the abdomen or thorax has been opened.
- Burns victims, especially those having skin grafts.
- Cachectic patients.
- Patients undergoing emergency surgery for major trauma.
- Those who are unable to shiver, such as paraplegics or quadriplegics (or those rendered temporarily so by spinal or epidural anaesthesia).

Neonates become hypothermic quickly. They have poorly developed heat regulatory mechanisms, a relatively high body surface area, no insulation from subcutaneous fat, and they do not shiver. They have a one-off mechanism for restoring their body heat by metabolizing stored brown fat, but once this is gone they are at grave risk of hypothermia.

The effects of hypothermia

Hypothermia slows down the body's metabolism by about 7 per cent per degree Celsius lost. The oxygen dissociation curve shifts to the left, indicating that haemoglobin hangs on to its oxygen more tightly. This means the oxygen pressures in the tissues have to fall further before the oxygen on the haemoglobin is released. Enzymes act sluggishly, or stop working altogether. Blood viscosity increases while the ability of blood to clot progressively fails.

After arriving in the recovery room a patient's core temperature continues to fall, before it begins to rise. This *after-drop* is caused by cold blood returning from the muscle beds and skin as the circulation to these areas is restored.

Hypothermia is now recognized as a major predictor of serious postoperative problems because it:

- promotes bleeding; this is a major problem;
- increases the chance of wound breakdown;
- increases the risk of pressure injuries;

- suppresses the immune system increasing the risk of infection (especially pneumonia);
- suppresses the cough reflex increasing the risk of aspiration;
- increases blood viscosity, which compromises the circulation to the surgical site. This may jeopardise the viability of skin flaps and patency of vascular grafts;
- may cause cardiac arrhythmias, and exacerbate cardiac failure;
- delays drug metabolism; especially of opioids, sedatives and muscle relaxants;
- delays discharge from hospital after surgery by an average of 2.6 days.

Shivering is not shaking

Shivering is a reflex response to cold. In contrast *shaking* is a complex neurometabolic side-effect of general anaesthesia. Both shivering and shaking produce vigorous muscle activity creating lots of heat, and using large amounts of oxygen. Oxygen consumption may rise to five- to sevenfold placing huge demands on the cardiopulmonary unit to supply it.

Shivering causes the blood vessels in muscle beds to vasodilate abruptly. Once shivering starts you may have to give additional fluid to prevent hypotension. Give warm fluids through an in-line blood warmer.

Epidural and spinal anaesthetics reduce shivering and delay warming. The reason for this is that the nerve fibres relaying information from the skin's temperature sensors to the patient's hypothalamus are anaesthetized. This prevents the hypothalamus from initiating shivering, causing the skin blood vessels to vasoconstrict. Consequently the patient remains vasodilated, radiates heat and only warms slowly.

Once the temperature falls below 34°C patients cease to shiver, and they become less and less conscious.

At temperatures below 28°C
the patient may appear dead.

How to detect hypothermia

Place the palm, but not the back, of your hand on the patient's chest. If they feel cold to touch, then measure their core temperature with either an infrared tympanic membrane sensor, or a skin thermistor placed over the temporal artery or an infrared temporal artery scanner. Core temperatures can also be measured by pulmonary artery catheter with a thermistor on its tip, or an oesophageal stethoscope with a thermistor embedded in it.

Table 23.3 Average temperatures

Site	Equivalent temperature °C
Core	37
Sublingual	36.2–36.8
Peripheral skin	26–35
Temporal artery	36.7–37
Axillary	34.5–36.2
Rectal	36.5–37.5

How to treat hypothermia

Monitor core temperature, blood pressures, pulse rate, ECG, blood glucose levels, and urine output.

Many patients remember feeling freezing cold when they wake. They are much comforted by a warm blanket. With mild hypothermia most patients are able to warm themselves if you protect them from further heat loss with socks, head covering, limiting skin exposure and forced-air convection heaters.

Do not discharge patients to the ward until their temperature is at least 36° C.

How to actively warm your patient

Forced-air convection heaters, such as a BairHugger™ or WarmTouch™, are the best way of warming a hypothermic patient. It can take 12 hours or more to rewarm severely hypothermic patients. Proceed slowly. Rewarming at a rate faster than 0.8°C per hour can cause arrhythmias. Give high concentrations of oxygen to cope with the increased oxygen requirements should the patient shiver.

How to passively warm your patient

Increase the ambient air temperature to at least 24°C.

The best way to protect patients from further heat loss is to cocoon them in insulating layers. Put a warm blanket next to their skin, cover this with silver metallic space-blanket and then cover that with another warm blanket. Space-blankets only reduce radiation loss, and are nearly useless if used on their own. The additional blankets prevent convective, conductive and evaporative losses.

If the patient's temperature is less than 34.5°C then keep them sedated and protect their airway until they are warmer. Following major surgery elderly, frail, and sick patients should remain intubated, paralysed and ventilated until their core temperature is at least 35.8°C. In intubated patients a heated humidifier usefully reduces further heat loss.

Hints

- If a patient is slow to warm then consider hypoglycaemia or hypothyroidism as cause.

- Avoid Hartmann's solution or Ringer's lactate because a cold liver is slow to metabolize lactic acid.

- The effects of drugs and anaesthetic agents are prolonged because they are metabolized and excreted more slowly.

- In patients with a temperature between 35.5–36.5°C use half the dose of opioid and wait twice as long for it to take effect.

> *Use small increments and small doses of drugs in hypothermic patients.*

Blood gases in hypothermic patients

Hypothermia increases the solubility of gases in body fluids and slows the thermodynamic activity of all chemical reactions in a proportionate way. If you need to measure the pH in a hypothermic patient measure the blood gases as you would for a normal patient at 37°C. This technique is called alpha-stat. There is no need to make corrections for temperature, which is called pH-stat.

Hyperthermia

Fever (pyrexia) refers to core temperatures of 37.8–40°C. *Hyperthermia* refers to a core temperature more than 40°C. At about 42°C brain enzymes are irreversibly damaged and muscle tissue breaks down (*rhabdomyolysis*) releasing myoglobin into the blood stream.

It is rare for a patient to become febrile in the recovery room, but it is always serious when it does happen. For each degree Celsius rise in temperature the body's oxygen consumption increases by about 15 per cent.

A patient's temperature rises if their body produces more heat than it loses. To produce heat the body needs food energy, and oxygen. While at rest the body produces about as much heat as an 80 watt light bulb. This heat keeps the core temperature at about 37°C.

Causes of a rise in heat production

Sepsis, especially following urological surgery or bowel surgery, or the draining of an abscess, or any surgery where Gram-negative bacteria escape into the circulation.

- Thyroid storm.
- Immunological reaction to blood or blood products.
- Shivering or shaking.
- Malignant hyperthermia.
- Drugs causing the serotonin syndrome.

Causes of failure to lose heat

- Atropine or other anti-cholinergic drugs prevent sweating.
- Core hyperthermia in the grossly obese.

Malignant hyperthermia

Malignant hyperthermia (MH) is a disorder of skeletal muscles. MH affects about 1:15 000 of the general population. It usually runs in families, as an inherited auto-somal dominant condition, although there are sporadic isolated cases. The skeletal muscles of affected individuals have abnormal calcium channels in their cell membranes. Certain triggering factors, such as *succinyl choline* and all the volatile anaesthetic agents, allow calcium to flood into muscle cells causing extreme and uncontrolled muscle contraction. This generates enormous amounts of heat, uses lots of oxygen and produces lots of carbon dioxide. Overheated and dying skeletal muscle cells release myoglobin, potassium and creatinine kinase into the blood-stream. The laboratory can detect these markers in the blood.

In the initial stages malignant hyperthermia may be difficult to diagnose. Sometimes it presents dramatically as a *metabolic storm* with high fevers, sweating, metabolic acidosis, tachycardia and masseter spasm causing tightly clenched jaws (trismus); but more usually it sneaks up insidiously with a tachycardia and a rising respiratory rate. Slow-onset MH usually presents a few hours later, after the patient has returned to the ward.

Drugs you can use safely in patients at risk of MH include benzodiazepines, droperidol, ketamine, all the opioids and the anti-emetics. Avoid controlling ventricular arrhythmias with calcium blockers such as verapamil and diltiazem, because they will cause hyperkalaemia if you use dantrolene.

Thyroid storm

Now rarely seen, a *thyroid storm* occurs where patients with suboptimally con-trolled thyrotoxicosis present for surgery. It may surface in the recovery room, but more usually 8–16 hours after surgery. It is triggered by preoperative stresses increasing circulating thyroid hormones. These include anxiety, apprehension, iodine withdrawal, pain, hypovolaemia, trauma or infection.

The consequent hypermetabolic state presents with hot flushed skin, tachycar-dia, atrial fibrillation, hypotension, and high blood pressures. The temperature rises to the range of 38 to 41°C. Treatment includes β-blockade, potassium iodide, and cortisol.

Acid base disorders

Our cells are bathed in an isotonic swamp (the extracellular fluid) kept at constant temperature (37°C) and require just the right amount of acidity to flourish. We constantly produce prodigious amounts of hydrogen ions as a product of metabolism. If we did not get rid of the excess hydrogen ions our cells would soon grind to a halt, overwhelmed by acidity.

Our bodies have many mechanisms to control the acidity (or hydrogen ion concentration) of the *body water*. The hydrogen ion concentration is kept at a constant level by the body diluting these ions, excreting them or *buffering* them.

Hydrogen ions

A *Hydrogen ion* (H^+) is a single proton; it carries a positive electrical charge. Hydrogen ion is present in very tiny amounts in the body, and too much or too little causes havoc to biochemical reactions. Normally homeostatic mechanisms control the hydrogen ion concentration in the extracellular fluid within a range of 38 – 45 nanomols per litre.

[H⁺] = hydrogen ion concentration in nanomol/L

Figure 23.2 Hydrogen ion and pH

What is an acid?

Acids are substances that *dissociate* in water to donate hydrogen ions to chemical reactions. *Bases* are substances that accept hydrogen ions.

Acids and bases are reciprocally related to each other. So, as the concentration of acid rises, the concentration of base falls by exactly the same amount. Every hydrogen ion accepted by a base (OH-) means that while there is one less hydrogen ion there is one more water molecule (H_2O).

How hydrogen ions affect biochemical reactions

Enzymes are complex proteins whose singular shape is necessary to catalyse biochemical reactions. Too much or too little hydrogen ion in the vicinity of the enzyme distorts an enzyme's shape so that it cannot work properly.

Acid-base disturbances become a life-threatening problem when the pH drops below 7.12 ([H^+] greater than 76 nmol/L) or rises beyond 7.55 ([H^+] less than 28 nmol/L). Outside this range important enzymes progressively fail, and the cardiovascular response to *catecholamines* declines.

How hydrogen ion affects haemoglobin

Excessive hydrogen ion, as occurs in the lactic acidosis of haemorrhagic shock, loosens haemoglobin's bond with oxygen so it is released more readily to the tissues. Conversely, an excess of base tightens haemoglobin's grip on oxygen so that it is not as readily released. In this way mild to moderate acidaemia protects tissues against hypoxia.

Where hydrogen ion comes from

Every day our cell's mitochondria produce staggering amounts of hydrogen ion as glucose is converted into energy. Fortunately more than 99.999999999% of the hydrogen ion (H^+) immediately combines with oxygen (O) to form harmless water (H_2O), which can be either used or excreted at leisure. This still leaves us with 0.000000001% of the hydrogen ion that must be dealt with promptly before it has a chance to upset body metabolism. Even in nanomol concentrations changes in the amount of hydrogen ion in body fluids disrupts the biochemistry of cells.

Excess hydrogen ion is buffered inside cells by phosphate compounds. Once outside the cell hydrogen ion is counterbalanced by bicarbonate ion (HCO_3^-). In this way hydrogen ion concentration is kept within the normal range. It is only when excessive hydrogen ion is being produced, or it cannot be excreted, that problems arise.

Acidosis and alkalosis

An *acidosis* occurs when too much hydrogen ion accumulates in the tissues. An *acidaemia* occurs when hydrogen ion concentrations in the blood rises beyond 45 nmol/L. Conversely, an alkalosis occurs when there is too much *base* in the tissues. An *alkalaemia* occurs when hydrogen ion concentration in the blood is less than 38 nanomol per litre.

The body can easily cope with a moderate acidosis, but is almost defence_ less against an alkalosis. Severe alkalosis may quickly maim or kill. Fortunately, alkalosis is rare, and usually is caused by some sort of medical intervention.

Acidosis and alkalosis are classified by whatever causes them. An excess or deficiency of carbon dioxide results in a respiratory acidosis, or alkalosis respectively; while an excess or deficiency of bicarbonate ion results in a metabolic acidosis or alkalosis. The lungs control carbon dioxide levels, while the kidneys control the absolute levels of bicarbonate.

Table 23.4 Normal values for blood gases

PH	7.35–7.42	[H+] 45–35nmol/L
PaO_2	85–100 mmHg	11.0–13.1 kPa breathing air
$PaCO_2$	37–42 mmHg	4.9–5.5 kPa
HCO_3	22–25 mmol/L	

Four steps to interpret blood gases

Step 1. What is the hydrogen ion concentration [H+]?

- If $[H^+] > 45$ nmol/L (pH < 7.35) the patient has an acidaemia.
- If $[H^+] < 35$ nmol/L (pH > 7.45) the patient has an alkalaemia.

Step 2. What is the arterial PaO_2?

- If $PaO_2 < 60$ mmHg (7.9 kPa) then the patient is hypoxaemic.
- If $PaO_2 < 35$ mmHg (4.6 kPa) then the patient is dying.

Step 3. What is the arterial $PaCO_2$?

- If $PaCO_2 > 45$ mmHg (5.5 kPa) then the patient is hypoventilating.
- If $PaCO_2 < 35$ mmHg (4.6 kPa) then the patient is hyperventilating.

Step 4. What is the actual bicarbonate?

- If it is nearly normal and the pH is abnormal then there is an acute respiratory component.
- If it is abnormal and the pH is abnormal then there is a metabolic component.

Tell the laboratory the inspired oxygen

When you send blood gases to the laboratory make a note on the request slip about the fractional *inspired oxygen concentration* (FIO_2). In a person with healthy lungs the FIO_2 and the PaO_2 rise in parallel. However, if there is something wrong with the lungs, for instance pneumonia or asthma, then this parallel rise does not happen.

The balance between acids and bases

Since too much or too little hydrogen ion concentration or activity in the body disrupts cell metabolism, the balance has to be just right for the enzymes and protein pumps in cells to function properly.

In the body several chemical reactions are involved in acid-base balance, but the principal extracellular reaction involves a balance between carbon dioxide, water on one side of the equation and hydrogen ion and bicarbonate ion on the other.

$$H_2O + CO_2 \rightleftharpoons HCO_3^- + H^+$$

Each component is in *dynamic equilibrium* with the others. They balance each other in much the same way that a weighing scale does.

If you add CO_2 to the one side of the balance the pointer will to swing towards a low pH (and higher hydrogen ion concentration). You can restore the balance to normal by either removing the CO_2, or adding HCO_3^- to the left side to counterbalance it. Similarly adding HCO_3^- to the left-hand pan will swing the pointer to a higher pH (and lower hydrogen ion concentration). You can restore the balance by either adding CO_2 to the right-hand pan, or removing HCO_3^- from the left hand pan.

Mathematically this balance can be represented as the *Henderson–Hasselbach equation*, which is often quoted, but because the calculations are difficult it is rarely used.

$$pH = 6.4 + \log_{10} \frac{[CO_2]}{[HCO_3^-]} \quad \text{at } 37°C$$

The *Henderson equation* is more practical because the sums are easy. The Henderson equation is exactly the same as the Henderson–Hasselbach equation, except that the logarithms have been taken out. What the equation says is that if you know two of the three variables, you can calculate the third.

If you want to know what the patient's PCO_2 was before they came to theatre, then use the Henderson equation.

Figure 23.3 Henderson equation

Now, if you know the PCO_2 and the HCO_3^- you can calculate the hydrogen ion concentration, and use the table to estimate the pH. In the Henderson formula you must use the actual bicarbonate levels from the electrolyte results; you cannot use the bicarbonate from the blood gas results, because the lab has already used the formula to calculate the bicarbonate from the measured pH and the PCO_2.

Respiratory causes of acid-base disorders

Carbon dioxide (CO_2) is produced in mitochondria as a waste product of oxidative metabolism. The pressure exerted by CO_2 in arterial blood is about 40 mmHg (5.3 kPa) and in venous blood about 46 mmHg (6.1 kPa). If a patient fails to breathe deeply enough to *blow off* carbon dioxide as fast as the tissues produce it then the excess CO_2 dissolves in body water releasing hydrogen ion (a strong acid) and bicarbonate ion (a weak base) to cause a *respiratory acidaemia*. Conversely, if patients blow off carbon dioxide faster than they produce it, the hydrogen ion levels falls in the blood and the patient will have a *respiratory alkalaemia*.

It is commonly believed that hydrogen ion is 'blown off' as carbon dioxide, but this is a mistake because there is no hydrogen ion (H^+) in carbon dioxide (CO_2). Instead, the mitochondrial enzymes shuffle the highly reactive hydrogen ion around to eventually link it to oxygen to make water (H_2O).

How hypoventilation causes respiratory acidosis

Hypoventilation is caused by:

- a side-effect of the opioids:
- residual effects of muscle relaxants;
- sedation caused by benzodiazepines such as midazolam or diazepam.

While at rest we produce about 200 ml of CO_2 every minute. Our total body stores of carbon dioxide are about one hundred times this amount (200 litres). If the patient has been *hyperventilated* during their anaesthetic, their body stores of CO_2 become depleted, and bicarbonate ions accumulate in the blood. This is revealed by a reluctance to breathe up in the recovery room, and blood gases will show a respiratory alkalosis. However, the CO_2 soon builds up to normal levels. During this time give high concentrations of oxygen to compensate for the patient's diminished *minute volume*.

An uncommon cause of an acute respiratory alkalosis, with low arterial $PaCO_2$ levels, (*hypocarbia*) is interstitial pulmonary oedema. Fluid accumulating in the lung's interstitial space triggers a reflex to make the patient hyperventilate to blow-off CO_2. The causes of interstitial pulmonary oedema include fluid overload, acute or chronic cardiac failure, septicaemia, fat or gas emboli, gastric aspiration or early acute respiratory distress syndrome.

Metabolic causes of acid-base disorders

A metabolic acidosis occurs if the liver fails to metabolize lactic acid, or the kidney fails to excrete acids.

The causes include:

- hypoxia, where the tissues produce lactic acid faster than it can be metabolized;
- unstable diabetics, where keto-acids accumulate;
- septicaemia, where bacterial endotoxins have damaged the liver so that it cannot deal with organic acids as fast as normal;
- renal failure, where the kidney can't excrete the acids.

Metabolic alkalosis is uncommon. Usually it is the result of severe potassium depletion, or injudicious use of sodium bicarbonate. Massive blood transfusion may cause a metabolic alkalosis, because the liver metabolizes sodium citrate (used as an anti-coagulant in the stored blood) to sodium bicarbonate. Metabolic alkalosis becomes a clinical problem once the pH exceeds 7.55.

Is the acid-base disorder an acute or chronic problem?

Disturbances that occur within minutes or hours are known as *acute disturbances*. Others creep up slowly over days or weeks, and are known as *chronic disturbances*. Patients with acute disturbances have an abnormal hydrogen ion concentration (pH) in their arterial blood. In patients with chronic disturbances, the kidneys or lungs have adjusted the balance of CO_2 and HCO_3^- to ensure the patient's pH is normal.

What to monitor in acid-base disorders

- Blood pressure, pulse rate, temperature.
- ECG.
- Respiratory rate, tidal volume and minute volume.
- Urine output.

Prepare to take:

- Arterial blood gases: pH, hydrogen ion concentration, PaO_2, $PaCO_2$, and bicarbonate.
- Blood samples for sodium, potassium, chloride, urea, creatinine, bicarbonate, anion gap, lactate, and glucose.

How to manage an acid-base disorder

Get help from someone who understands this complex problem. Never use sodium bicarbonate to treat respiratory acidosis, not only is it inappropriate, but it will make the problem worse.

Dangers with bicarbonate

Sodium bicarbonate corrects a metabolic acidosis, but it is tricky to use and best reserved for patients near death. In general bicarbonate is only used for patients with an arterial pH < 7.12 who are not responding to therapy, as is the case of a diabetic with ketoacidosis who is not responding to insulin; or when the patient is not responding to catecholamines during cardiac arrest.

Bad things about bicarbonate:

- In patients who have a metabolic acidosis bicarbonate slows their respiratory rate, causing excessive carbon dioxide to build up in body fluids.
- It alters the shape of haemoglobin molecules so that they do not release oxygen to the tissues as readily.
- It takes some days for the kidneys to excrete the excess in the urine.

Diabetes

In high-income nations more than 8 per cent of adults are now diabetic; while in some of the Pacific islands (such as Nauru) this approaches 100 per cent.

There are two principal forms of diabetes: Type 1 and Type 2 diabetes. These are two quite different diseases, with different causes, different natural histories, and requiring different management.

- *Type 1 diabetes*, formerly known as insulin-dependent diabetes mellitus (IDDM) is caused by insufficient insulin secretion; and occurs in about 10 per cent of diabetics.

- *Type 2 diabetes*, formerly known non-insulin-dependent diabetes mellitus (NIDDM) is caused by tissue resistance to the effects of insulin; and occurs in about 90 per cent of diabetics.

What is diabetes?

The World Health Organization (WHO) defines diabetes mellitus as 'a chronic disorder of carbohydrate, protein and fat metabolism caused by an absolute or relative insulin deficiency, fasting hyperglycaemia, glycosuria, and a striking tendency for atherosclerosis, microangiopathy, nephropathy and neuropathy'.

Table 23.5 Insulins

Class	Insulin	Onset (hr)	Duration (hr)
Ultra-short-acting	Lisipro	0.25	4–5
Short-acting	Neutral	0.5	6–8
Intermediate acting	Isophane	1–2.5	16–24
Long-acting	Ultralente	2–4	24–36

How surgery destabilizes diabetes

Surgical mortality rates are five times higher in diabetics than in non-diabetics. Properly functioning insulin promotes wound healing, white cell function, phagocytosis of bacteria, clotting, and prevents fat breakdown that causes ketone production. Postoperatively diabetics are at a higher risk of dying from primary infection, anastomotic breakdown, pneumonia, pulmonary emboli, and adverse cardiac and cerebrovascular events. All these problems can be traced back to insufficient insulin, excessive blood glucose concentrations, and tissue glycation. These processes cause endothelial dysfunction; most noticeably in small vessels.

Insulin

Insulin has two principal functions. First, it packs any glucose, fat and amino acids that are excess to immediate needs into storage as glycogen, triglyceride and cellular protein respectively. Second, and more importantly insulin prevents glycogen and protein stores being raided unnecessarily to provide energy. Without insulin, the liver frenetically mobilizes glycogen and cellular protein stores back to glucose. As glucose is released into the circulation blood glucose levels rise sharply.

The triglyceride in fat cells (lipocytes) is not converted back to glucose, but released as fatty acids, ketones and glycerol. All the tissues (except for brain) can use these compounds as a fast food energy source, but like fast food it may become indigestible in large quantities and then ketones appear in the blood.

The problem with type 1 diabetes is too much glucose production, rather than too little uptake by the cells. In contrast, the problem in type 2 diabetes is that the cells can neither use nor store the glucose delivered to them.

In both types of diabetes excess glucose slowly sticks to connective tissue and cell membranes. This process is called glycation, which essentially means the tissues are turning to caramel. The endothelial linings of small blood vessels take the brunt of glycation. The eventual result is atherosclerosis everywhere, but most importantly in the eyes, heart, brain and kidneys.

Diabetes in the recovery room

Postoperatively there are two big risks for diabetics: hyperglycaemia and hypoglycaemia. The normal range of blood glucose concentrations is 3.5 to 5.5 mmol/L. In the recovery room the blood glucose concentration of normal people, especially if they are in pain, may exceed 14 mmol/L. It is well known that untreated hypoglycaemia rapidly causes brain damage. However, it is less well known that if the blood sugar in a diabetic exceeds 12 mmol/L in the recovery room the risks of postoperative infection, strokes, myocardial infarction, ischaemia and deep vein thrombosis rise more than sevenfold.[4]

> *To prevent postoperative complications keep, the blood glucose levels within the normal range.*

Type 1 diabetes

Before coming to theatre for major surgery type 1 diabetics should be stabilized on a continuous infusion of insulin and glucose. They need a baseline infusion of 150 grams of glucose over 24 hours. To this baseline infusion is added a continuous infusion of regular insulin equivalent to their normal total daily requirements. For example, if a patient normally takes 20 units of prota-mine zinc insulin (Protophane®) in the morning, 12 units of regular insulin at lunch time, and 40 units of Protophane® at night, the total 24-hourly dose of insulin would be 20 + 12 + 40 = 72 units or 3 units per hour. This means the patient should come to theatre with an infusion of 50 grams of glucose running over 8 hours, and a regular insulin infusion of 3 units an hour.

Type 2 diabetes

Type 2 diabetics are controlled with oral hypoglycaemic drugs. Most type 2 diabetics use metformin, but sometimes they need an alternative drug, or a supplement with one of the sulfonylureas: gliclazide, glimepiride, or gliben-clamide; or one of the glitazones such as pioglitazone. These drugs are usually omitted on the day of surgery.

Problems with metformin

- Metformin decreases glucose absorption from the gut, increases glucose entry into cells and lowers the appetite. Lactic acid is produced by hypoxic tissue. Metformin prevents the liver metabolizing lactic acid efficiently. For this reason it is stopped 36 hours before surgery where tourniquets or vascular clamps are used (e.g. leg surgery), big operations where lots of tissue is damage (e.g. total hip replacements) or where large blood transfu-sions are necessary (e.g. abdominal aneurism repairs).

- Metformin induced lactic acidosis may present in the recovery room. The first sign will be a rapidly rising respiratory rate.

If a type 2 diabetic becomes acidotic, then suspect metformin as the cause.

- Metformin induced lactic acidosis is lethal in 50 per cent of cases and needs urgent and expert management.

- Metformin may cause acute renal failure if the patient receives X-ray radio-contrast media for angiography or intravenous pyelograms. To prevent this metformin is ceased 48 hours before the procedure and for 5 days after it.

- In patients taking metformin it is better to avoid large volumes of Hartmann's solution because it contains lactate.

How to manage diabetics

When managing diabetic in the recovery room aim to:

- keep the blood glucose concentrations within a range of 6–10 mmol/L;

- prevent, detect and treat hyperglycaemia and hypoglycaemia;
- prevent large swings in blood glucose concentrations;
- give enough insulin to prevent ketosis;
- detect and treat lactic acidosis;
- prevent and treat hypokalaemia, hypomagnesemia and hypophosphataemia.

Why hypoglycaemia is harmful

Hypoglycaemia occurs when blood glucose concentration less than 3.5 mmol/L.

Healthy people experience symptoms of an adrenergic alarm response once their blood glucose falls below 2.5 mmol/L. These include tachycardia, feeling alarmed and light-headed, pallor, palpitations, sweating and double vision. As it progresses patients can become confused, agitated or aggressive, with slurred or confused speech. They soon convulse and lapse into coma. If blood glucose concentrations fall below 2 mmol/L then hypoglycaemia causes irreversible brain damage and death.

Risk factors for hypoglycaemia include: type 1 diabetics, alcoholics, neonates, those with septicaemia, and severe liver disease.

In the recovery room the warning signs of hypoglycaemia may be camouflaged by β-blockers, residual anaesthesia or opioids. For this reason measure the blood glucose levels of all those at risk as soon as they are admitted to the recovery room, then every half hour thereafter, and just before discharge to the ward.

Every recovery room
needs a glucose meter.

How to manage hypoglycaemia

If the blood glucose is 3 mmol/L or less then give 30 grams of glucose intravenously into a big vein. You should see an improvement in the patient's conscious state within 2 to 3 minutes. Repeat the dose after 5 minutes. Start a 6-hourly litre of 5% dextrose. Check the blood glucose levels at 20 minute intervals until they stabilize at about 5 mmol/L. You may need to change the rate of the dextrose drip.

Hints

- Dextrose is the American name for glucose.
- Use 300 ml of 10% dextrose or 600 ml of 5% dextrose.
- One litre of 5% dextrose contains 50 grams of glucose.
- One litre of 10% glucose contains 100 grams of glucose.

- Keep a litre of 10% glucose with your emergency drugs.
- Glucose is cheaper and safer than glucagon.

Why hyperglycaemia is harmful

Hyperglycaemia occurs when the blood glucose concentration rises above 10 mmol/L. Normally blood glucose concentrations lie within the range of 3.5–5.5 mmol/L. With the physiological stresses of surgery, even in normal patients the glucose concentration may rise to 15 mmol/L or more. Generally the higher the stress levels (pain, hypovolaemia, or hypoxia) the higher the blood glucose concentrations.

Hyperglycaemia is a sign of a stressed patient.

In diabetics, within 20 minutes of their blood glucose concentration exceeding 12 mmol/L their vascular endothelium is damaged. Non-diabetics whose endothelium is healthy are not affected as much.

Keep the blood glucose of diabetics < 10 mmol/L.

Hyperglycaemia in a diabetic immediately after surgery is a disaster. The combination of high blood glucose, catecholamines, and *cytokines* released from injured tissue, wreak havoc on already diseased endothelial cells. Within 20 minutes they are so damaged there is an immediate risk of myocardial ischaemia or stroke.

Figure 23.4 Length of action of insulin

Hyperglycaemia in the immediate postoperative period carries over into the ward to cause a 15-fold increase in risk of vascular disasters such as stroke, myocardial infarction, deep vein thrombosis, and renal impairment in the first postoperative week. These effects are additional to the increased risks diabetics already have of infection, osmotic diuresis and poor wound healing.

How to manage hyperglycaemia

Measure the blood glucose concentration when the patient is admitted into the recovery room and check their urine for ketones. If their blood glucose is above 10 mmol/L then give one unit of regular insulin for every 10 Kg of lean body mass. Notify the patient's physician so that control can be continued in the ward.

Hints

- Insulin requirements usually rise in the recovery room.
- Usually, one unit of regular insulin (in a stable adult diabetic) lowers the blood glucose concentration by about 1.5 mmol/L, but after surgery one unit of insulin only decreases the blood glucose levels by about 1 mmol/L.
- Maintain the glucose infusion at a constant rate of 50 grams 8-hourly and vary the insulin dose. Not the other way around.
- 10 grams of intravenous glucose raises the blood glucose in an adult by about 1.5–2 mmol/L.
- Ketosis is a sign of insulin lack, and not excessive glucose. If your patient is ketotic then check the blood sugar levels and give more insulin.
- Monitor potassium levels because insulin causes potassium to enter cells, resulting in hypokalaemia.
- To convert mmol/L of glucose to mg/100 ml multiply the millimols/L by 18.
- Although insulin is adsorbed by glass and plastic, there is no need to initially prime the apparatus with glucose and insulin.
- Never use sliding scales to control insulin doses.

Why sliding scales are harmful

The *sliding scale* technique of controlling blood glucose levels relies on tailoring the dose of insulin or glucose to the amount of glucose in either plasma or urine.

Sliding scales are still recommended by some people to control blood glucose concentrations after surgery. This technique should be avoided. It allows dangerous swings in blood glucose. Following surgery it only takes a few minutes of high blood glucose levels to damage diabetic's endothelium. By the time you discover the hyperglycaemia, the damage may already be done.

*Check the blood glucose frequently when you have
a diabetic patient in the recovery room.*

Why endothelium suffers

Vascular endothelium is not merely a single plastic-like sheet of cells lining blood vessels. These sheets of lively cells move about on their basement membrane bed, retracting their edges to allow white cells to enter and leave the circulation, and then closing up the gap again. They busily release nitric oxide to dilate arterioles and improve blood flow, and if needed secrete endothelin to reduce blood flow. They also release other factors needed for blood to clot, and still others to stop it clotting in the wrong place.

In diabetics endothelial cells become glycated; their cell membranes are coated in sugary caramel-like goo (called advanced glycaemic end-products). The gummed-up endothelial cells tend to climb on top of one another, leaving behind patches of naked basement membrane where clots can form. Then curled up in a miserable heap, they stop releasing their factors, and partially obstruct blood flow particularly in the microcirculation.

Surgery damages tissues. The injured tissues release biochemicals into the circulation irritating endothelial cells. Now that the already sick endothelium in diabetics is further assaulted by circulating stress biochemicals, the additional osmotic effect of hyperglycaemia is too much to bear. The sick endothelial cells retreat to form scattered heaps on the walls of blood vessels. Clots form in places they should not, small arterioles become blocked, and atheromatous plaques rupture leaving raw surfaces for platelets to adhere to and form clots.

All these events give diabetics a much higher risk of suffering cardiac ischaemia, stroke (both haemorrhagic and embolic), venous thrombosis, renal dysfunction and disruption of blood flow to the surgical site.

Why nerves are damaged

If a patient has had diabetes for more than 5 years, especially if the diabetes is not well controlled, they are prone to developing peripheral and autonomic neuropathy. Patients with malfunctioning autonomic nerves respond unpredictably to fluid loads. They become hypotensive if you sit them up, and they may not feel chest pain (*angina*) if myocardial ischaemia occurs.

What is hyperosmolar plasma?

Patients with poorly controlled diabetes become much worse after surgery. This places them at risk of a hyperosmolar crisis.

A hyperosmolar crisis occurs when the blood glucose rises beyond 25 mmol. The concentrated glucose in the extracellular fluid osmotically sucks water out of cells. Middle-aged and elderly diabetics are at the highest risk. Initially the brain and kidney suffer most. Ketosis may or may not be present. The urine output rises, and as the brain cells shrivel the patient becomes confused, sleepy and may convulse. You can check the stability of the patient's diabetes over the previous 2–3 months by measuring their glycolysated haemoglobin levels (HbA/c). Normally the range is 5–7%; while levels exceeding 9% indicates increasingly poor control. As a rule elective surgery should be postponed in patients whose HbA1c exceeds 8%.

Obesity

Higher income nations have an epidemic of obesity; it now outranks tobacco as the biggest killer. More than 40 per cent of Australian adult men and 18 per cent of women are not just overweight, they are obese. The number has doubled since 1996 and most of this increase is in women between the ages of 40–59 years. Few morbidly obese men live to old age, but women fare better.

Many obese patients present for surgery either directly as a result of their obesity, or incidentally for other operations. Obese patients are now termed *bariatric patients*, and procedures used to treat obesity are *bariatric procedures*. Bariatric patients are more likely to have major joint replacement and back surgery. Procedures such as high gastric reduction, iliojejunal bypass, and laparoscopic stomach banding have become operations of last resort to treat life-threatening obesity.

Body mass index

Body mass index (BMI) is one way of classifying obesity. It is not ideal because it does not assess muscle mass. A super-fit body builder may well be classified as obese on the BMI scale.

$$BMI = \frac{\text{weight in Kg}}{\text{height in metres}^2}$$

Table 23.6 Body mass index

Status	BMI (Kg/m²)
Starving	< 17
Underweight	17–19
Normal	19–25
Overweight	25–30
Obese	30–35
Very obese	35–40
Morbidly obese	40–55
Super-morbidly obese	> 55

> *Problems arising in the recovery room increase progressively and steeply once a patient's BMI > 30.*

Life insurance companies have worked out the ideal body weight (IBW) that is associated with the lowest mortality rate for a given height and gender.

$$IBW (Kg) = height (cm) -100 (for men)$$
$$= height (cm) -105 (for women)$$

Most very obese people have life-threatening comorbid chronic diseases, such as hypertension, heart disease, diabetes, and *dyslipidaemias*.

How to manage obese patients

Obese patients weighing more than 150 Kg need special reinforced beds, trolleys and lifting apparatus. Organize to have these available before the patient comes to the recovery room.

Book an ICU bed for those patients with BMI greater than 50 or those with pre-existing cardiac or respiratory disease, CO_2 retention, or where the surgery is expected to last for more than 3 hours.

Following open abdominal and even laparoscopic procedures consider admitting morbidly obese patients (BMI > 40) overnight for continuing observation. Obese patients seem to tolerate laparoscopy quite well.

Respiratory problems

Preoperative respiratory function tests do not usefully predict postoperative problems. With their low *functional residual capacity*, obese patients are at high risk of postoperative hypoxia; so plan to give supplemental oxygen, particularly at night.

Morbidly obese patients have kilos of fat lying across their chests and bellies. If they lie on their back their fat sits on their chest like a sandbag, which makes breathing difficult. This becomes a problem especially after major abdominal or thoracic surgery. Once obese patients are fully awake, prop them up in Fowler's position (at about 45°) on their trolley. This move takes the weight off their chest and diaphragm and lets them deep breathe and cough more effectively. Sitting them up also reduces the risk of aspiration. On the other hand, if they have an *obtunded* mental state or are unconscious then lay them on their side in the recovery position.

Very obese patients have precarious airways that easily obstruct. Access to their pharynx is made difficult by a fat face, big breasts, short necks, limited cervical spine movement, high anterior larynx, and restricted mouth opening.[5] It is can be risky to use laryngeal masks in obese people, because should they regurgitate the laryngeal mask may divert stomach contents down the trachea.

Encourage obese patients to deep breathe, and cough. These manoeuvres blast open small airways increasing the functional residual capacity and improving oxygenation.

Never tip obese patients head down, because as their intra-abdominal fat pushes their diaphragm up it squashes the bases of their lung. They will almost immediately become hypoxaemic, and usually panic. Furthermore in a head-down position they are far more likely to regurgitate and aspirate stomach contents.

Does supplemental oxygen ever pose a risk?

Some super-morbidly obese patients with severe pulmonary hypertension (blue bloaters) may stop breathing if you give them more than 28% oxygen. The reason is that these patients need a hypoxic drive to breathe. Universally these blue bloaters have pitting oedema on the tops of their feet, plasma bicarbonate in excess of 34 mmol/L (reflecting a chronically elevated PCO_2), pulmonary hypertension, and right-side heart failure.

Beware of a blue bloater who becomes drowsy after surgery. There is a delicate balance between preventing hypoxia and preserving respiratory drive. Remember hypoxia kills – so you must treat it. If blue bloaters stop breathing support their ventilation with a bag and mask. Doxapram (Dopram®), a nonspecific respiratory stimulant, can help tide hypoventilating obese patients over this time to avoid them being intubated and ventilated.

Avoid respiratory depressant drugs, such as opioids and benzodiazepines, because they will probably cause a respiratory arrest.

Sleep apnoea

Snoring, with or without overt *sleep apnoea*, occurs in more than 80 per cent of morbidly obese people. During sleep they get a bradycardia when they stop breathing and a tachycardia when they start again. In the recovery room these patients need constant attention to maintain an unobstructed airway. If they start to snore then protect the patency of their airway. Sometimes you can use a nasopharyngeal airway to bypass their floppy soft palate. Many obese patients use CPAP mask at home, and in some cases they will bring them to recovery room.

Patients with sleep apnoea who receive opioids may simply stop breathing. These patients already have abnormal respiratory drives and they may not summon the respiratory effort to start breathing again. Propped up on pillows, sedated with morphine, and drowsy from a rising $PaCO_2$, their head lolls forward so that their chin rests on their chest, quietly obstructing their upper airway … a few feeble gasps … and it is all over. You find them dead on their trolley.

Deep vein thrombosis

The perioperative risk of venothromboembolism (VTE) in obese patients is more than twice that of normal patients. This particularly applies to those with *android obesity* ('beer bellies'). Start their leg exercises in the recovery room. Ensure they have received low molecular-weight heparin prophylaxis, and have their compression stockings properly fitted.

Predisposing factors include polycythaemia, prolonged immobilization leading to venous stasis, increased intra-abdominal pressure retarding venous flow from the legs, cardiac failure, and decreased fibrinolytic activity with increased concentrations of fibrinogen. VTE is the commonest complication of obesity surgery with an incidence of about 5 per cent. Arrange adequate prophylaxis.

Gastro-oesophageal reflux

Obese people often have as much as 75 per cent more fluid in their stomach than a normal patient. Even if they report no heartburn or reflux most obese patients have hiatus hernias, and this puts them at risk of regurgitation and pulmonary aspiration. The risk of aspiration is augmented by raised intra-abdominal pressure exerted by the mass of fat in their abdominal wall and cavity. A prudent approach would be to neutralize their stomach acids with oral ranitidine 2 hours before surgery, and 0.3 M sodium citrate 30 ml orally just before induction.

Aspiration of gastric contents into the lungs remains a danger well into the postoperative period after the patient returns to the wards.

Cardiac and circulatory problems

You will need especially large blood pressure cuffs. Normal-sized cuffs either will not fit, or if they do they overestimate the blood pressure.

Obese patients have a lower relative blood volume (50 ml/Kg) than a normal person (60 ml/Kg). Because their large capacitance veins are squashed by fat, and are less able to distend to hold additional fluids, they are at risk of pulmonary oedema if given injudicious intravenous fluids.

When very fat people lie down flat, the huge mass of fat in their abdominal cavity tissue falls back to tamponade their inferior vena cava. With the impeded venous return to the heart, their cardiac output plummets. Some super-morbidly obese patients cannot lie flat, and panic if they attempt to do so. They may even have a cardiac arrest. Have sturdy help at hand to help the patient sit up again if they begin to panic.

Core hyperthermia

Morbidly obese people may meltdown after surgery or trauma. Core hyperthermia occurs rarely, but can be lethal. Core hyperthermia occurs because obese patients have a thick layer of insulating fat surrounding them. Pain, hypovolaemia, or sepsis causes the circulation to the skin to shut down so that heat can no longer escape. After a few hours this bottled-up heat raises their core temperature to lethal levels.

Although cooking on the inside with a core temperature exceeding 41°C, the patient's skin is cold and clammy. They are in mortal danger. To save their life they need to be vasodilated to open up the blood supply to their skin so they can dissipate heat. The safest drug to use is a small dose of chlorpromazine 12.5 mg slowly IV. Chlorpromazine also helps reset the temperature-regulating centre in the hypothalamus. Rehydrate the patients with cold saline. Treat their pain with judicious intravenous morphine. In severe cases the treatment is similar to malignant hyperthermia, but they do not need dantrolene.

They require careful vasodilation, cooling and superb tissue oxygenation. Sometimes patients need to be intubated to help decrease their raised PCO_2. Additionally, you still need to consider the diagnosis malignant hyperthermia.

Nerve damage

Obese patients have a higher risk of intraoperative neural compression injury and pressure sores, so check pressure areas and movement and feeling in limbs. This applies particularly to hands. If the patient has been in the lithotomy position where there is risk of stretching the sciatic nerve then check that they can bend their knees and flap their feet up and down.

Numbness (*anaesthesia*) and tingling (*paraesthesia*) occur when a nerve is damaged. The nerve can be cut, stretched, compressed or made ischaemic, or damaged by an injection directly into a nerve. The incidence is about 1:800 operations.

There are anecdotal reports where automated blood pressure devices have been blamed for nerve damage in the upper limb, but these have not yet been substantiated.[6]

While patients are on the recovery room trolley, take care not to allow their elbow to rest on sharp edges, or extend their arms in such a way as to damage their brachial plexus.

Epidural anaesthesia

In obese people distended veins and substantial amounts of fat occupy the epidural space. This means that obese people require about 20% less volume of epidural drugs to achieve the same effect as thinner people.

Transport

Transport morbidly obese patients on their beds. Limit the number of transfers between beds, trolleys and tables to the minimum. Occasionally you may need to use special hydraulic lifting devices to manoeuvre super-morbidly obese patients around. Remember that many nurses have injured their backs while lifting patients. Do not attempt to move them on to hospital trolleys because it is possible the patient may accidentally slip out of control and on to the floor.

Drugs and doses

Calculate the drug dose in obese patients on their estimated *lean body weight* (LBW), not on their actual weight. Their lean body weight is approximately their height in centimetres minus their weight in kilograms.

Be especially careful with drugs with low therapeutic indices, because their toxic dose is a hair's breadth from the therapeutic dose; these drugs include digoxin, lithium, dipyridamole, and the aminoglycosides.

In some cases fatty changes in liver may not be reflected in routine liver function tests. Drugs such as opioids and others metabolized by the liver may be cleared slowly, requiring longer dosing intervals and smaller incremental doses.

In the recovery room it is best to give drugs intravenously. On the rare occasion it is necessary to give intramuscular drugs, use special long needles otherwise 'intramuscular injections' may never reach the muscle, and just stay in poorly perfused fat.

Benzodiazepines

It has been postulated the effects of *benzodiazepines* may persist for sometime, because large amounts can be soaked up by fat and dribble back once the drug is discontinued, causing prolonged sedation. This scenario is improbable.

Benzodiazepines do cause problems in the obese by exacerbating the effects of the *sleep apnoea syndromes*.

Opioids

Continuous intravenous opioid infusion are dangerous, and especially so in morbidly obese patients, and the elderly. Most grossly obese patients have problems moving their upper body mass to breath normally. Many also suffer from *obstructive sleep apnoea*, and some have *central sleep apnoea* too. If a patient obstructs their airway when they are asleep at night at home, then they are more likely to do so in hospital where they have received drugs such as opioids (even in epidurals). Using opioids is particularly hazardous in morbidly obese patients. There is a danger when sedated obese patients, with reduced respiratory drive, are propped up in bed. When they fall asleep and their head flops forward to obstruct their airway they quickly and silently die (*Ondine's curse*).

Sleep apnoea is a cause of unexpected postoperative death.

Notes

1. Baker N, King D, Smith EG (2002) *Journal of Hospital Infection* 51:153–4.
2. Sessler DI (1997) *New England Journal of Medicine* 336:1730–7.
3. Harper CM, NcNicholas T, Gowrie-Mohan S (2003) *British Medical Journal* 326:721–2.
4. Van der Berghe G, Wouters P, Weekers F *et al.* (2001) *New England Journal of Medicine* 345:1359–67.
5. Adams JP, Murphy PG (2000) *British Journal of Anaesthesia* 85:91–108.
6. A report by the American Society of Anaesthesiologists (2000) *Anesthesiology* 92:1168–92.

24

Chronic disorders

Diseases covered in this chapter are not found elsewhere in this book. They were chosen because they are either common, like alcoholism, important, because errors in management can cause harm, for example hepatorenal syndrome, or the disease represents useful principles applicable to many other diseases.

The ASA classification

Unfit patients frequently come to surgery. Their illness may be a result of their lifestyle of smoking, drinking or over-eating, or an acquired or inherited disease. In the 1940s the American Society of Anesthesiologists published a scale known as the ASA class to grade the fitness of patients presenting for anaesthesia. The classification has proved remarkably robust and remains one of the better predictors of surgical and anaesthetic outcome.

ASA I   Fit for their age.

ASA II   Mild systemic disease not interfering with daily activities.

ASA III   Severe disease interfering with daily activities.

ASA IV   Severe disease that is a constant threat to life

ASA V   Moribund. Submitted for surgery in desperation.

E.   The letter E is added if the operation is an emergency; eg. ASA IV E

AIDS/HIV

Those at high risk of HIV/AIDS include homosexual and bisexual men and their partners, older haemophiliacs, intravenous drug users and children of affected mothers. Heterosexually transmitted HIV is common in many countries. In some poorer countries it occurs tragically, because of inadequately sterilized medical or dental equipment and where syringes and needles are reused.

HIV (*human immunodeficiency virus*) is the quiescent phase of the disease. Most of these patients are taking immunosuppressive drugs and are at risk of acquiring nosocomial infections. Use standard precautions to protect the patient and yourself. The biggest risk to staff is through needle stick injuries.

AIDS (*acquired immune deficiency syndrome*) is the active phase of the disease where the patient is infected with one or more of a bizarre variety of organisms. These patients are usually frail, often with severe lung infections and recent weight loss. Patients with end-stage AIDS seldom come to surgery and are rarely encountered in the recovery room.

Alcoholics

Alcoholism occurs when a person's drinking is either damaging their health, or causing disruption to their lives, or the lives of their families and associates. It is a hidden disease and far more prevalent than suspected. In Australia and the UK it affects about 15 per cent of the adult population, and the elderly are not exempt. In the league table, just behind cardiac disease it is the next most major cause of perioperative morbidity. It hides behind diseases such as hypertension, dilated cardiac myopathy, atrial fibrillation, dementia, postoperative delirium and liver disease.

People who drink more than four standard drinks a day tend to be tolerant to many sedative drugs. As they emerge from anaesthesia they may be restless, and move about in a semi-purposeful manner before they awake properly. They may try to sit up, and open their eyes before spitting out their airway. During this time they appear dazed, will not respond when you speak to them, and occasionally become violent. Do not remove their airway; let them take it out themselves.

Alcoholics are susceptible to spontaneous hypoglycaemia, especially when physiologically stressed after surgery. If they remain mentally obtunded, or become sweaty or restless then check that their blood glucose level is greater than 4 mmol/L. If not, give 20 ml of 50% glucose slowly through a freely running drip into a large vein.

Thin alcoholics can become hypothermic during surgery. Do not discharge them until their temperature is greater than 36°C.

Drug addicts

Marijuana

Marijuana smokers tend to cough excessively after general anaesthesia. This settles quickly with one or two puffs of salbutamol.

Heroin

Following general anaesthetics heroin addicts are susceptible to respiratory depression in the recovery room. Their respiratory centres remain partially insensitive to rising carbon dioxide levels for 3 or more months after their last 'hit'.

If you give naloxone to a using heroin addict it may trigger acute *opioid withdrawal syndrome*. This presents with abdominal cramps, sweating, itch, and lacrimation and simulates all sorts of postsurgical disasters. Addicts too, are entitled to good postoperative analgesia. Titrate opioid analgesics intravenously to achieve an effect. Some recovering addicts are apprehensive that perioperative opioids will reignite their addiction. In this case substitute opioids with NSAIDs or local blocks.

Cocaine and amphetamine

Cocaine and amphetamine (speed, ecstasy) users can become alarmingly hypotensive after surgery. Continual use of these drugs depletes neuronal stores of noradrenaline. Consequently with the stress of surgery there may not be enough noradrenaline stored in the nerve endings to maintain the blood pressure. The blood pressure of cocaine and amphetamine users responds readily to normal doses of direct-acting vasopressors such as noradrenaline, but they may need additional hydrocortisone supplements to sustain the response. If they are regular users of cocaine they may not respond to indirect-acting vaspopressors, drugs such as ephedrine or metaraminol.

Intravenous drug users often have hepatitis C (or occasionally hepatitis B). Chronic liver dysfunction prolongs the sedative effects of anaesthetic drugs, which may require patients to stay longer than usual in the recovery room. They also have an increased risk of bleeding, and a higher susceptibility to infection.

Epilepsy

Epilepsy is caused by uncoordinated, spontaneous and uncontrolled neuronal discharge somewhere within the brain. The type of seizure depends on where the abnormality occurs. To prevent perioperative seizures epileptics should take their usual medication on the day of surgery.

There are two types of seizures: a one-off *isolated seizure* associated with fevers, head trauma, hypoxia, hypoglycaemia; and *recurrent epileptic seizures*. An isolated seizure may occur in men after transurethral resection of the prostate if water from the irrigation fluid enters their circulation.

Epileptics may fit in the recovery room, and the seizure can take many forms. Frank seizures are obvious, but a subtle seizure in a semicomatose or paralysed patient may only be revealed by twitching around the mouth. Seizures cause brain damage and must be controlled quickly. All seizures respond well to thiopental. The anaesthetist may use thiopentane to stabilize seizures while assessing the situation and starting other measures such as a phenytoin infusion.

Facial twitching in a comatose patient
may indicate an epileptic seizure.

Drugs that may trigger seizures are propofol, sevoflurane, methohexitone, pethidine, and anti-cholinergics. Pethidine, with its neurotoxic metabolite nor-pethidine, is a major offender, particularly if the patient has renal impairment.

Intellectually impaired

Caring for the intellectually impaired patient after surgery can be quite a challenge. Careful preoperative planning involving the patient's carers, their family, recovery room staff and the ward avoids a lot of problems. The patients have the same needs in the recovery room as children or a demented elderly person. In the recovery room they need the sole attention of a dedicated nurse who can communicate at the patient's level of understanding. It helps if someone they know and trust accompanies the patient. Often these patients cannot verbalize their needs. They cannot use pain scales, but they require the same pain relief as a normal patient. Assess their pain as you would in a child.

Liver disease

The liver is the largest organ in the body. It is a factory for many biochemicals including coagulation factors and it is the headquarters for carbohydrate, fat and protein production and breakdown. Its enzyme systems metabolize many drugs, and toxins. The liver only needs about 20 per cent of its metabolic capacity to fulfil its day-to-day functions. The remaining, or spare metabolic capacity, is reserved to break down lactic acid produced during exercise. Postoperatively the liver mobilizes essential glucose from protein and glycogen stores.

In patients with liver disease spontaneous hypoglycaemia can occur without warning. Check their blood glucose levels when they are admitted to the recovery room.

The liver's oxygen supply comes from the hepatic artery. During general anaesthetics the hepatic artery blood flow may halve reducing the liver's oxygenation, which a diseased liver tolerates poorly. After general anaesthetics it is not surprising that those with liver disease are slower to metabolize drugs and this prolongs their recovery.

The liver metabolizes many anaesthetic drugs. When tourniquets or vascular clamps are released large amounts of lactic acid from hypoxic tissues flood into the circulation. The liver is impressively able to metabolize lactic acid, but not if it is acidotic, hypoxic, hypoglycaemic or cold, or the patient has been taking metformin for diabetes.

Metformin-induced lactic acidosis

Metformin, used to treat type 2 diabetes, blocks the liver's ability to metabolize lactic acid. Usually metformin is withdrawn 36 hours before surgery where it is anticipated that tourniquets or vascular clamps will be used, or large amounts of tissue damaged.

An acute lactic acidosis can present in the recovery room. If it occurs it is potentially fatal and more than half the patients die. Lactic acidosis is more likely if the liver is already affected by cirrhosis, jaundice, gallbladder disease, Gram-negative sepsis, or where volatile anaesthetic agents have reduced liver arterial blood flow during long operations.

Patients with a developing lactic acidosis have a rising respiratory rate, they feel breathless, and want to sit up to get their breath. They develop a tachycardia, skin flushing and may start to sweat.

Send blood for blood gas analysis, lactate levels, electrolytes and urea, blood glucose concentration, and full blood examination. Lactic acidosis becomes severe once lactic acid levels rise higher than 3 mmol/L.

The patient will need to go to ICU. Management of metformin-induced lactic acidosis includes correcting hypovolaemia, and oxygen therapy. Using bicarbonate to correct the acidosis is hazardous.

Managing patients with liver disease

Principles include:

- Keep patients well oxygenated, and if necessary maintain tissue perfusion with an inotrope such as dobutamine.
- If opioids are given, watch for respiratory depression. This may cause acidaemia and hypoxia, which are not well tolerated by a sick liver.
- Keep patients with liver disease warm.
- Suspect clotting factor deficiency when a patient with liver disease has prolonged bleeding from venous or arterial puncture sites, or the surgical site.

Hepato-renal syndrome

To avoid renal failure in jaundiced patients (hepato-renal syndrome) the aims of management are to:

- keep their urine output above 1 ml/Kg/hr;
- insert a urinary catheter to monitor the urine output;
- ensure hydration is adequate. Give at least 2 litres of crystalloid at 6-hourly intervals;
- treat systemic infection with appropriate antibiotics.

Neither mannitol nor furosemide improve the prognosis and may be harmful.

Multiple myeloma

Multiple myeloma is a relentlessly progressive bone marrow plasma cell tumour. Patients often have fragile vertebra and ribs, so move and position them gently. The excessive protein they excrete can damage their kidneys, so keep their blood volume normal, and do not allow them to become hypotensive or dehydrated. Their plasma is often syrupy and protein-laden, placing them at risk of deep vein thrombosis. Prophylaxis against deep vein thrombosis depends principally on adequate fluid replacement, doing stir-up exercises to prevent venous stasis, and giving a low molecular-weight heparin, such as enoxaparin. Graded compression stockings are helpful.

Musculoskeletal disease

Patients with a wide variety of musculoskeletal disease and myopathies are susceptible to malignant hyperthermia. This may present in the recovery room so monitor their temperature, and watch for the signs of sweating, rising respiratory rate (reflecting hypercarbia) and tachycardia.

Patients with muscular dystrophy are weak. They require smaller amounts of all anaesthetic agents than normal patients and are especially vulnerable to the residual effects of muscle relaxants. Make sure they can sustain a 5-second head lift from the pillow, and that they can deep breathe and cough before the anaesthetist leaves the recovery room. Where possible, use regional blockade for pain relief. If you need to use opioids then give increments of about one-fifth of the estimated dose and watch for slowing respiratory rate and depth before repeating.

Normal doses of muscle relaxants may overwhelm patients with low muscle mass. Watch for signs of inadequate reversal; this is especially likely to occur as the neostigmine wears off about 45 minutes after it was given. You may need to give a second dose of neostigmine. Start with a half dose of neostigmine and atropine and monitor the effects with a 5-second head lift.

Patients with connective tissue disorders often have thin atrophic skin and pressure sores are common especially if they have been lying on the operating table for some time. It is so easy to tear their fragile skin if you drag them across a bed sheet, or tear off adhesive dressings carelessly.

Myaesthenia gravis

Myaesthenia gravis (MG) is a chronic autoimmune disease characterised by episodes of muscle weakness. It is caused by an autoimmune attack on acetylcholine receptors, so that nerve impulses cannot reach the muscles. It mainly affects muscles innervated by the cranial nerves. It is treated with anticholinergic drugs such as pyridostigmine.

Occasionally patients with rapidly progressing MG undergo a thymectomy in order to relieve the symptoms of the disease. Usually these patients need ventilatory support for a few days after surgery and are transferred directly from the operating theatre to ICU.

Many patients with MG are intermittently treated, over the years, with huge doses of prednisolone. They may need hydrocortisone supplement if their blood pressure falls while they are in the recovery room.

Avoid benzodiazepines, such as midazolam or diazepam, in patients with MG. These drugs make patients extremely weak, and at risk of aspiration. Opioids are safe, but reduce the dose in line with their reduced muscle mass. Other drugs likely to exacerbate MG symptoms are gentamicin, β-blockers, and calcium channel blockers. If a patient with MG drops their blood pressure, then consider giving a 100 mg of hydrocortisone.

The weakness in patients with MG is treated with one of the anticholinesterase drugs. These drugs include pyridostigmine, neostigmine or physostigmine. If a patient becomes weak while in the recovery room, it is difficult to know whether they are having a *cholinergic crisis* caused by too much anti-cholinesterase, or a *myaesthenic crisis* where the patient has not received enough anti-cholinesterase. The two conditions can be separated if the anaesthetist gives the ultra-short-acting anti-cholinesterase, edrophonium 10 mg IV slowly over 5 minutes. If the patient gets stronger then it is a myaesthenic crisis, if they get weaker then it is a cholinergic crisis. In the latter case the anaesthetist may need to support the patient's breathing with a *bag and mask* for a few minutes until the drug has worn off.

Eaton—Lambert syndrome

Eaton—Lambert syndrome is an immune mediated disease, with similar features to myasthenia gravis that occurs in some patients with small-cell carcinoma of the lung. It occurs if *acetylcholine* is not released from nerve terminals and the muscle weakness does not respond to anti-cholinesterases.

Multiple sclerosis

Multiple sclerosis (MS) is a slow progressive episodic disease caused by patchy demyelination of nerve fibres in the brain and spinal cord.

The main problems in the recovery room with patients with MS are laryngeal incompetence predisposing to aspiration, and autonomic instability causing erratic fluctuations in blood pressure and pulse rates.

Fever trigger severe relapses; even a rise in temperature as small as 0.5°C causes their condition to worsen dramatically. Warn ward staff to monitor postoperative temperatures carefully, and treat fever aggressively.

Although general and neuraxial anaesthesia are safe in patients with MS, spinal and epidural anaesthesia are usually avoided. MS often worsens temporarily after surgery, and these neuraxial blocks will be inevitably blamed even though there is no evidence to support this assumption.

Myotonic dystrophy

Myotonic dystrophies are a group of inherited genetic disorders that cause selective muscle weakness. They tend to progress as the years pass. The most common is myotonic dystrophy (*Steinhart's disease*) can occur at any age and predominately affects distal muscles. Patients with muscular dystrophy are susceptible to malignant hyperthermia. Monitor their temperature and report it to the anaesthetists immediately if their temperature rises beyond 37.4°C. Patients suffering from myotonic dystrophy are highly sensitive to muscle relaxants and may develop signs of residual paralysis in the recovery room. They also have great difficulty in coughing effectively.

Paget's disease

Paget's disease is a chronic disease that causes the bones in elderly adults to become honeycombed. Localized areas of bone become hyperactive, and are replaced with highly vascular porous bony tissue. Since most patients have no symptoms, the diagnosis is easily missed on preoperative assessment. These people usually have a prominent forehead, and a prominent tibial ridge. They shunt large volumes of blood from their arteries straight to their veins, bypassing tissues. They need a high cardiac output simply to maintain their blood pressure. Patients with Paget's disease become hypoxaemic easily, so continue supplemental oxygen in the ward. Be prepared for overwhelming blood loss following orthopaedic surgery.

Parkinson's disease

Parkinson's disease is a slowly progressive degenerative CNS disorder usually affecting older men. It has three main features: slow movement, muscular rigidity, and resting tremor. Because they cannot move quickly to readjust their posture, people with Parkinson's disease are particularly prone to falls, and often come to surgery to repair the damage. In the recovery room these patients are at risk of aspiration and are unable to mount an effective cough. Those with advanced disease are usually frail.

Severe Parkinson's disease is often treated with the dopaminergic drugs, L-dopa and carbidopa. They may develop arrhythmias or hypertension in recovery room, because their adrenergic nerve endings are chocked full of noradrenaline, waiting to be released when triggered even by a trivial stimulus. Their blood pressures can surge without warning. Monitor them with an ECG and be prepared to give a β-blocker, such as metoprolol, to control tachyarrhythmias.

A common error is to give drugs with antidopaminergic activity, such as metoclopramide, droperidol or prochlorperazine, to control nausea. These drugs will render the patient rigid and unable to move (*acute Parkinsonian crisis*). This is treated with intravenous benztropine.

Peptic ulceration

Peptic ulcer disease (PUD) is often exacerbated by surgery. Over the perioperative period patients with peptic ulcers or reflux oesophagitis should be covered with a proton pump inhibitor such as pantoprazole. Ranitidine, a 5-HT3 antagonist, is often used because it can be given intravenously, but it is not as effective as protein pump inhibitors.

In the recovery room keep patients with PUD in the recovery position until they are fully conscious and able to care for their own airway.

Phaeochromocytoma

Phaeochromocytomas are tumours that secrete catecholamines. The main problem following their resection is that patients may be hypovolaemic and become hypotensive in the recovery room. They sometimes need a surprising amounts of colloid or blood to maintain their blood pressure. If the tumour has been active for more than a few months the patient may also have a cardiomyopathy. In this case the blood pressure and cardiac output may need to be supported with dobutamine or even noradrenaline.

Uncommonly a patient my come to surgery with an unsuspected phaeochromocytoma. Induction of anaesthesia is an unintended and sometimes alarming provocative test. Patients abruptly develop the traditional signs of hypertension, pallor, and palpitations. Their systolic blood pressure may exceed 300 mmHg. The operation is usually postponed and they will be sent to the recovery room for further management, where they may need nitroprusside and β-blockade to control the heart rate and blood pressure.

Porphyria

Porphyrias are a family of inherited diseases of errors in the synthesis of haeme, the porphyrin unit of haemoglobin. It is more common in Nordic people who have carried it with them as they migrated to other parts of the world. The biochemical precursors of haeme are toxic, and cause a plethora of confusing symptoms: acute abdominal pain, vomiting, neuropathies, epilepsy, psychiatric disturbance, and even coma. Surgical stress, and anaesthetic drugs, especially barbiturates, such as thiopental, may trigger all three types of hepatic porphyria.

Psychiatric disease

Brains get sick too. At some time in their lives more than 20 per cent of the population suffer from some form of mental illness (including dementia) and 4 per cent are severely disabled by it. Many patients are taking psychotropic medication that interacts with anaesthetic drugs and analgesics.

Anxiety is part of a spectrum of emotions that blends into fear, agitation, panic and terror. Do not dismiss these emotions lightly. They are associated with neurohormonal responses that trigger hypertension, myocardial ischaemia, and arrhythmias. Acutely anxious patients profit from an anxiolytic premedication such as temazepam 10 mg orally 50 minutes before coming to theatre.

For very anxious patients, oral lorazepam 4 mg 75 minutes before coming to theatre is extremely effective, but for a benzodiazepine-naive patient it tends to persist well into the postoperative period. ("Goodbye Tuesday, hello Thursday … where did Wednesday go?"). For day case procedures do not discharge home (Stage 3 recovery) patients who have taken lorazepam unless they are accompanied by an adult who can protect them.

Patients with chronic anxiety disorders are often taking psychotropic medication and there is a high comorbidity with other psychiatric conditions especially alcohol, cigarette and drug abuse, which they use to self medicate to numb their anxiety.

Phobias are disproportionately severe responses to a potentially threatening stimulus. Needle phobias and mask phobias are common, and can cause panic ending in a *vasovagal reaction* where the patient develops bradycardia and faints. There is no point in trying to overcome phobias with logical reasoning; it never succeeds. In the recovery room do not challenge a patient's mask phobia; they will often accept nasal prongs for oxygen therapy. Better still cut the top third, including the metal shaper, off a plastic face mask and use this. Most mask-phobic patients will accept a mask as long as they cannot see it.

Similarly, needle phobias are overcome if the patient cannot see the needle. Obscure the patients view so that they cannot see what you are about to do and ask the patient if they will now accept a sharp slap to the puncture site to disguise the prick of the needle to follow.

Management

In the recovery room most anxious patients respond to gentle words of reassurance and a compassionate touch.

Agitation is not a defined medical term, but describes a state of acute high anxiety. Patients do not hallucinate, and are oriented in time and place, however they may behave in an irrational manner. A small dose of 2–5 mg of intravenous midazolam usually settles agitation. Always remember that agitation is a cardinal sign of developing hypoxia. Other causes include awareness under anaesthesia, youth, preoperative anxiety, mutilating operations; or occasionally acute withdrawal from heroin, benzodiazepine or alcohol.

Depression

Depression is an overwhelming and pervasive feeling of despair, sadness and pessimism with an inability to get enjoyment out of life. We are not talking about a mood here, certainly not sadness or grief: we a talking about an illness.

> The only reason I got out of bed this morning was that I hadn't died during the night. There is no pleasure to be found in anything. I have lost music and birdsong, sunsets and my daughter's blue eyes … and I grieve terribly for the loss.

It is hard to imagine a more profound cry of despair.

The brain in a depressed person functions slowly, and repercussions are reflected throughout the body. Depression adversely affects many physiological processes causing autonomic dysfunction, insulin resistance, increased platelet aggregation, and decreased cellular immunity. Depressed patients metabolize drugs slowly, especially opioids and benzodiazepines; they heal poorly, their immunological systems malfunction and they are six times more susceptible to infection and wound breakdown, and have a threefold higher incidence of ischaemic heart disease and venothromboembolism. Depressed patients are four times more likely to die in the postoperative period than a patient without mental disease.

Most surgeons do not do elective operations on depressed people until they are treated; and this is a most treatable disease.

Electroconvulsive therapy

Electroconvulsive therapy (ECT) is used on profoundly depressed people who are not responding to drug treatment. ECT is astoundingly effective and a few sessions can turn a patient who is in a semi-vegetative state into a functioning individual. ECT is a very safe procedure, but requires a trained anaesthetist to administer the anaesthetic and a psychiatrist to apply the electrodes and give the shock. You may be asked to care for them afterwards.

Following preoxygenation, the patient is given an induction dose of propofol, a small dose of atropine, and a short-acting muscle relaxant. Then an electro-convulsive shock is applied to one hemisphere (usually the left) to induce a seizure. The seizure causes a tonic spasm, followed by a series of convulsive fits. The patient has a profound parasympathetic response, with bradycardia and salivation, and recovers consciousness within several minutes.

Once the fitting has stopped turn them on to their left side, and give them oxygen. Check their vital signs. If patients continue to salivate and their heart rate is less than 50 beats/min then you may need to give further atropine.

Patients with pacemakers can safely have ECT. They need ECG monitoring. Have an appropriate magnet nearby to convert the pacemaker to a fixed mode if the patient gets a bradycardia.

Schizophrenia

Schizophrenics have *psychotic thought disorders* affecting the way they feel and behave. Untreated, the patient's mind and personality slowly disintegrates. Withdrawn schizophrenics are so wrapped up with their delusions and halluci-nations that they cannot communicate with anybody else. Anti-psychotic drugs allow patients to lead fairly normal lives. Acutely disturbed schizophrenics are highly delusional, and may become physically combative to protect themselves from perceived dangers. They must take their medication on the day of surgery. Almost all their anti-psychotic medication interacts adversely with pethidine and tramadol, however morphine and fentanyl are safe. Ketamine, propofol and fentanyl seem to decrease emergence confusion in schizophrenic patients.

Do not discharge schizophrenic patients from the recovery room if they appear unsettled, or agitated. In this case the anaesthetist may use a small dose of haloperidol to relieve their distress. They may not verbalize their fears, but their faces betray their feelings.

Bipolar disorder

Bipolar disorder was once called manic depression. Patients swing between episodes major of depression, curled up in a miserable ball on a bed, and flights of frenetic activity where the patient's exuberance precludes sleep, and normal prudent judgement is lost. Awaking one morning the patient might buy a several sports cars, or not sleep for several days on end. Bipolar patients must take their lithium as usual on the day of surgery. Ensure that their lithium levels were checked before surgery.

As in patients with schizophrenia, avoid pethidine, and tramadol. Do not give patients on lithium either haloperidol or droperidol, because the combination can cause a fatal encephalopathy.

Table 24.1 Possible problems with anti-psychotic drugs

Drug	Possible problems
Tricyclic antidepressants, e.g. amitriptyline, doxepin	Exaggerated response to catecholamines. Avoid ketamine, tramadol and pethidine.
Serotonin reuptake inhibitors, e.g. paroxetine, sertraline	Serotonin syndrome with tramadol and pethidine. Mild antiplatelet activity.
Monoamine oxidase inhibitors, e.g. tranylcypromine, isocarboxazid	Possible fatal response with pethidine and tramadol
Lithium	Avoid droperidol, metoclopramide and tramadol.
Phenothiazines, e.g. promethazine, prochlorperazine, chlorpromazine	Excessive sedation with pethidine. Possible hypotension with metoclopramide, tramadol.
Quetiapine	Avoid pethidine and tramadol.
Risperidone	Avoid tramadol and pethidine.
Valproate sodium	
Zaprazadone	Avoid pethidine and tramadol.

Antipsychotics and the ECG

Many of the anti-psychotic drugs cause prolonged QT interval on the ECG. These patients have abnormal functioning calcium channels in their cardiac cell membranes, and may flip into a serious form of ventricular tachycardia called torsades de points if given trigger drugs such as pethidine, tramadol or the butyrephenones (droperidol or haloperidol). If a patient who is routinely taking antipsychotics is given one of the trigger drugs, then monitor them with an ECG while they are in the recovery room, and organise for them to have a full 12-lead ECG when they return to the ward.

Quadriplegics and hemiplegics

Patients who are partially or completely paralysed have unused peripheral nerves innervating muscles, and underused autonomic fibres serving blood vessels. These nerve endings are packed with noradrenaline and other neurotransmitters.

In the recovery room pain or hypoxia can cause the nerves to abruptly dump all these transmitters into the circulation (*autonomic hyperreflexia*) to cause fulminating hypertension and cardiac arrhythmias. Once the hypertension is treated the arrhythmias usually resolve spontaneously.

Rheumatoid arthritis

Rheumatoid arthritis is characterized inflammation of peripheral joints with progressive destruction of articular and periarticular connective tissue. It affects about one per cent in the general population. Women are affected three times more often than men.

Patients with rheumatoid arthritis are more susceptible to opioid-induced respiratory depression than normal people. They are more prone to respiratory obstruction, and particularly sleep apnoea.

They have stiff necks and brittle bones, so be careful when turning them or transferring them from the trolley to the bed. Their cervical spines are frequently unstable, so extend their necks gently, or you may damage their spinal cords and render them quadriplegic.

They often have thin, atrophic skin that tears easily when you remove adhesive dressings. Similarly their veins are fragile; so make sure drip cannulas cannot move up and down in the veins. Do not put needles in the backs of their hands. They often have temporomandibular joint destruction, so be careful, when inserting or removing airways, and do not over-extend their lower jaw.

Because patients with severe rheumatoid arthritis are often thin, hypothermia may become a problem: keep them warm.

Many sufferers are moderately anaemic and some have pulmonary fibrosis. Consequently they tend to have a higher resting respiratory rate than normal, and find it difficult to cough or deep breathe effectively. They may be taking steroids and need hydrocortisone to support their blood pressure.

Sickle cell syndromes

Sickle cell syndromes are a serious problem, and patients occasionally die in the perioperative period unless they are carefully managed.

Sickle cell syndromes included a cluster of inherited autosomal recessive diseases causing chronic haemolytic anaemia. It occurs almost exclusively in African Negroid people and those people from the malaria belt of Africa, Central America and around the Mediterranean Sea. Those who inherit one gene (*heterozygotes*) get sickle cell trait (HbAS), and those who inherit a gene from both parents (*homozygotes*) get sickle cell disease (HbSS). The full-blown sickle cell disease (HbSS) occurs in about 0.4 per cent of Negroid people who are usually anaemic, have multiple bone painful infarcts and are severely affected. In contrast about 6 per cent have heterozygous sickle cell trait are not anaemic, have no painful episodes, or thrombotic complications and may be unaware they have a problem. All patients from affected parts of the world must have a Sickledex® screening test before surgery, and if necessary a confirmatory haemoglobin electrophoresis.

> *Most patients with sickle cell disease have
> slightly yellow sclera.*

Problems occur, either with the trait or the disease, if patients' become *hypoxaemic* (that is where their arterial oxygen tensions fall below 60–70 mmHg (8–9.3 kPa)). If patients' oxygen saturations fall below 93% their haemoglobin molecules deform into spiky tactoids. The tactoids deform the red cell into their distinctive sickle shape, and eventually destroy them.

Less obviously, hypoxaemia can occur in just one limb if a tourniquet is applied, or the blood pressure is repeatedly measured with a non-invasive blood pressure monitor. It also occurs if the patient becomes febrile or hypothermic, or acidotic.

The sickle-shaped red cells clog the microcirculation causing multiple organ and tissue infarcts. Then as red cells rupture they release haemoglobin into the circulation. This *haemolytic crisis* can precipitate renal failure, particularly if the patient is also septic.

Patients may present for surgery because of complications of their disease, for instance to graft leg ulcers or debride dead bone from their limbs.

Those patients with the full sickle cell disease (HbSS) presenting for elective surgery usually undergo a series of preoperative exchange transfusions to raise their haemoglobin levels above 100 gm/L and are treated with hydroxyurea to reduce the number abnormal circulating red cells.

In the recovery room never let patients with sickle cell syndromes become hypoxaemic, acidotic or cold. Keep their inspired oxygen high, keep them warm.

Continuously monitor their perfusion status. Do not allow them to develop signs of poor peripheral perfusion. Replace blood loss early. Monitor them with a pulse oximeter, and test their urine for haemoglobin before discharge.

To guarantee red cell oxygenation patients with sickle cell syndromes should return to the ward; and remain on oxygen for at least 4 hours. Manouevres such as the routine use of anti-coagulants, or anti-platelet agents, giving high concentrations of oxygen or alkalyzing their blood with sodium bicarbonate, or magnesium glutamate do not improve the outcome.

Smokers

Elderly smokers usually have ischaemic heart, cerebrovascular and peripheral vascular disease. Smokers often cough uncontrollably especially after bronchoscopy. Persistent cough can often be controlled by lidocaine 1.5 mg/Kg made up to 5 ml in saline and given by a nebulizer.

On the other hand some older smokers make no effort to cough. They seem oblivious to the sputum rattling in their airways, or are unable to muster the lung reserves necessary to cough it up. Unless the sputum is cleared it will dry into thick plugs, block the airways and go on to cause segmental lung collapse or pneumonia. Give them humidified oxygen. Encourage them to deep breathe and cough. If necessary, gently use a laryngoscope to help you suck sputum from the upper airway. It is better to use regional blockade for pain relief, because morphine depresses the desire to cough, and pethidine dries out the sputum making it difficult to cough up.

Strokes

Cerebrovascular disease is common; it has the same risk factors as ischaemic heart disease: smokers, aged over 60 years, hypertension, diabetes, dyslipi-daemia, obesity, and sedentary lifestyle. There are two forms of stroke: embolic and haemorrhagic. Embolic stroke is more common, and occasion-ally occurs during surgery especially after carotid endarterectomy. In the worst cases, the patient develops localizing signs, such as weakness down one side, or may not even regain consciousness.

Major surgery with 3 months of a stroke or transient ischaemic attack increases the risk of a further stroke or cardiac ischaemia in the early postop-erative period. Usually elective surgery is deferred until the danger period has passed, but if not then monitor these patients carefully for signs of cardiac ischaemia.

Patients who are disabled by previous strokes may have difficulty coughing, problems in adjusting their position, telling staff they are in pain or that their bladders are full. Make a small signboard, so that patients can point to simple pictures representing pain, nausea, full bladder and so forth. You can also use this board for patients who do not speak English.

Thyroid disease

Hyperthyroidism

Hyperthyroidism occurs when the thyroid gland produces excessive hormones called (T3 and T4). Although not as common as hypothyroidism overt hyperthyroidism is usually easy to recognize, but subtle undiagnosed hyperthyroidism may cause problems in the recovery room. Suspect hyperthyroidism in a patient who comes to theatre with atrial fibrillation with a pulse rate exceeding 100 beats/min. Many symptoms of hyperthyroidism are similar to adrenergic excess. The patients are thin, heat intolerant, and almost invariably have a resting tachycardia.

In the recovery room, with the postoperative stress of emerging from their anaesthetic, they may develop rapid ventricular tachycardias or atrial fibrillation.

Think of thyroid disease if the patient is taking amiodarone.

In the frail and elderly the diagnosis of hyperthyroidism is sometimes missed. It may present as a wasted, elderly woman with an agitated dementia (*thyrotoxic madness*) and atrial fibrillation or a resting tachycardia.

Hypothyroidism

Hypothyroidism occurs when the thyroid gland produces insufficient thyroid hormones. Subtle hypothyroidism occurs in 10 per cent of elderly women, and frequently the diagnosis is overlooked for years. Typically the patient feels 'tired and run down', but the diagnostic hint is their dislike of the cold. Occasionally unsuspected hypothyroid patients undergo anaesthesia.

If the diagnosis of hypothyroidism is missed at preoperative assessment patients come from theatre cooler than expected, be slower to wake up, and become unduly sleepy with sedative drugs or opioids. Think of hypothyroidism if an older woman is 'difficult to wake up'.

Myxoedema

Myxoedema is a severe form of hypothyroidism. It is easily overlooked during the pre-anaesthetic work up since the patient is a slow thinker and consequently classed as 'a poor historian'. They are usually obese elderly women, but may not have the classic dry, coarse hair, podgy features and a large tongue described in textbooks. Typically they come to recovery room cold, comatose, with a bradycardia, hypotensive and are 'slow to emerge'.

In patients with myxoedema all drugs are metabolized slowly. Muscle relaxants are difficult to reverse and the patients may have to go to ICU for further management. These patients are particularly sensitive to opioids and normal doses may cause profound respiratory depression.

Trauma

Trauma patients present a host of diagnostic, treatment and nursing challenges. Usually, a specialist trauma team has stabilized their condition as much as possible before they come to the operating theatre. By the time the patient reaches the recovery room their cardiovascular and respiratory status is usually acceptable. The anaesthetists, surgeons and trauma team will supervise their care. Usually trauma patients are immediately transferred back to ICU, but less severe cases remain in the recovery room before returning to the ward.

Principal problems

Frequently little is known about the trauma patients' medical history; they are often affected by alcohol, and every physiological system is in disarray. The four immediate problems are head and neck injuries, haemorrhage, renal failure and still undiagnosed injury.

In the early stages the aim of surgery is to save the patient's life; to do as little as possible as quickly as possible, and to return later to do the reparative surgery. Initial surgery involves stopping the bleeding, and putting in appropriate surgical drains. The patient returns to ICU to stabilize their condition. Trauma patients may come to theatre many times in the subsequent days or weeks.

Full stomach

Trauma patients are at risk from a full stomach. Following trauma the stomach may take 36 hours, or more, to empty once they are admitted to hospital.

Assume that all trauma patients have a full stomach.

Trauma patients usually come to the operating theatre with a full stomach. The anaesthetist inserts a nasogastric tube and tries to aspirate the stomach during the procedure, and leaves it in place. Aspirating the stomach and the presence of a nasogastric tube does not guarantee the stomach is empty. Trauma patients often vomit or regurgitate while in Stage 1 recovery before their protective reflexes have returned fully, so nurse them in the recovery position and keep someone to help nearby, and a hissing sucker ready.

Alcohol

Many trauma cases are affected by alcohol and some gravely so. If you have any doubts whether your patient is affected send blood to the lab for a blood alcohol level. Alcohol reduces patients' tolerance to many drugs, especially *phenothiazines*, sedatives and opioids. Blood alcohol levels greater than 0.1% are a potent cause of postoperative hypotension. Not only does alcohol cause peripheral vasodilation, and aggravate heat loss, but also in higher doses suppresses cardiac contractility. In the recovery room these effects can confounded the diagnosis of bleeding, cardiac tamponade and delayed recovery.

Thoracic injuries

Patients with large segments of flail chest should not be extubated. They need ventilation in ICU for some days postoperatively until their flailing segment has stabilized. It is a common error to extubate them early. A thoracic epidural is an ideal way to control pain.

Tension pneumothorax or cardiac tamponade may cause the trauma patient to collapse abruptly in the recovery room.

Concealed haemorrhage

Keep in mind patients may have unsuspected concealed haemorrhage compromising their circulation. Litres of blood can be lost into the abdomen or pelvis without any signs of swelling. Typical blood loss from a fractured pelvis is 4–6 litres, and 2 litres from a fractured femur.

Blood loss presents in the recovery room with a persistent tachycardia and a tendency for the blood pressure and urine output to fall. If the patient's blood pressure falls by more than 20 mmHg when you sit them up at 45° you can be almost certain they are hypovolaemic.

Head injury

Occult head injury may cause diagnostic confusion if the patient does not fully recover consciousness after the anaesthetic. If the skull fractures during a head injury, some of the shockwave is dissipated away from the brain. This has a protective effect. Beware of the patient who has lost consciousness at the time of injury, and recovers consciousness, but whose conscious state is clouded while in the recovery room. Preoperatively, those with significant head injuries invariably have a headache.

Coma

Patients who do not open their eyes when their name is called, and are not roused by a gentle shake of the shoulder are defined to be comatose. Their airways are in grave danger should they regurgitate or vomit. In a comatose patient who is spontaneously breathing, even a subtle change in the pattern or rate of breathing indicates a change in their conscious state. Notify the anaesthetist.

Glasgow Coma Scale

The Glasgow Coma Scale (GCS) is the most widely used system for quantifying conscious level after traumatic brain injury. Its advantages are that it is simple and widely known. To get a score use the best eye-opening response, the best verbal response and the best motor response.

Do not use the GCS to describe coma in recovery room patients unless they are post-trauma.

Table 24.2 Glasgow Coma Scale

	Response	Score
Eyes opening (E)	Spontaneous	4
	To voice command	3
	To pain	2
	No response	1
Verbal response (V)	Normal conversation	5
	Disorientated	4
	Words (incoherent)	3
	No words – only moans	2
	No response	1
Motor response (M)	Normal	6
	Localizes to pain	5
	Withdraws to pain	4
	Decorticate posture	3
	Decerebrate response	2
	No response	1
Score out of is		

Its disadvantages are that the GCS is only intended for head-injured patients. It is not intended to describe patients' emergence from their anaesthetic. Many of the clinical features of traumatic brain injury are modified or absent in other forms of coma. For instance it is unusual for patients with drug-induced coma to develop decerebrate or decorticate response unless there has been hypoxic brain damage. Furthermore, the result can be skewed by alcohol intoxication, drugs and metabolic disturbances.

If a patient is intubated they cannot talk; so for this reason it is best to document the best response by its individual components; so that a normal patient with the maximum score of 15 would be recorded E4, V5, M6. An intubated patient would have a score E4, V intubated, M6. The GCS is of limited use in the recovery room. Use the modified Guedel levels instead.

Cervical spine injury

Trauma patients are assumed to have cervical spine damage, until this has been eliminated. A useful sign is of cervical spine damage is that bleeding behind the posterior pharyngeal wall causes it to bulge forward slightly. The anaesthetist may see this during intubation.

If there is any doubt whatsoever about the stability of patients' cervical spines then must be fitted with a hard collar neck protection device before they are moved to the recovery room.

Multisystem organ failure

Multisystem organ failure (MSOF) is a hazard after major trauma. The syndrome occurs when major tissue damage releases a zoo of cytokines into the circulation, along with cell debris, marrow fat, and high levels of circulating catecholamines (particularly noradrenaline), cortisol and other stress factors. All this affects heart, lung, liver and kidney function. The lungs develop *acute respiratory distress syndrome*, the liver struggles on, cardiac contractility may decrease, and *disseminated intravascular coagulopathy* is a risk. The kidneys are particularly susceptible to injury, and their function usually deteriorates during the first few postoperative hours. If the kidneys fail then the prognosis is bad; renal failure in the presence of MSOF carries at least 60 per cent mortality.

In the recovery room record the patient's urine output half hourly. Ideally, try to maintain urine output above 1 ml/Kg per hour. If urine output falls below 0.5 ml/Kg/hr, then the anaesthetist needs to act quickly to prevent acute renal failure. A threatened kidney does not tolerate hypoxia, hypotension, or hypovolaemia.

Acute respiratory distress syndrome

Acute respiratory distress syndrome (ARDS) is a form of respiratory failure arising from a variety of insults on the lung and is part of the spectrum of multisystem organ failure. The clinical signs are those of pulmonary oedema including dyspnoea, refractory hypoxaemia, diffuse pulmonary infiltrates increasing the stiffness of the lungs. About 30 per cent of patients who get ARDS die.

The recovery room's role in preventing ARDS is to filter and warm blood when transfusing trauma or septic patients, avoid excessive intravenous crystalloids, humidify inspired oxygen, and where possible to turn the patient every half hour to prevent raised vascular pressures in the dependent lung. Further steps include minimizing the patient's stress response by avoiding hypotension, treating pain, and preserving renal perfusion.

How to transport trauma patients

Most patients with severe trauma are transferred on their beds straight from the operating theatre to the intensive care unit. Move them quietly and gently lest you destabilize their blood pressure, or rip their lines out. Many hands make light work. If you do keep them in the recovery room, make a list of all their problems on a board where they can be seen by all the staff.

25

The bleeding patient

Blood is composed of red cells (erythrocytes), white cells (granulocytes and lymphocytes), and platelets suspended in honey-coloured plasma. Plasma contains clotting factors, proteins for transporting various substances, and electrolytes. As a clot forms into a jelly-like blob, the clotting factors are removed from the plasma, leaving behind serum.

A patient who is bleeding on the operating table or in the recovery room is at risk of harm from a myocardial infarction or stroke. Blood transfusion is life-saving therapy. If a patient is bleeding and you expect that you will need more than two units of blood then give ample warning to your hospital's blood bank and haematologist. Delegate one member of the staff to organize the blood transfusion and liaise with the blood bank technicians and the haematologist.

Anaemia

Blood transfusions are used to prevent tissue hypoxia in patients who are either anaemic or bleeding.

Red blood cells contain haemoglobin molecules, which carries oxygen. *Haemoglobin* (Hb) is a tangled ball of protein chains with a ferrous *ion* in a cleft. The ferrous ion slides out of its cleft to bind oxygen as the blood passes through the lungs (turning crimson in the process), and slides back releasing it in the tissues' capillaries (turning a bluish hue). When fully saturated with oxygen, haemoglobin inside red cells carries 650 times more oxygen than is dissolved in plasma.

Anaemia occurs when the total *mass* of haemoglobin is less than normal for the patient's age and sex. The normal concentration of Hb in blood is about 140 gm/L. For practical purposes patients become anaemic once the level falls to less than 110 gm/L, although this does not automatically require treatment.

Of the many causes of anaemia, the most common in the recovery room is blood loss. Some patients are anaemic because their bone marrow is suppressed by diseases such as chronic infections, chronic inflammatory disease (particularly rheumatoid arthritis), cancer or long-standing kidney disease.

With acute blood loss, both plasma and red cells are lost together so the haemoglobin concentration (haematocrit) changes little. Gauge blood loss using observations such as pulse rate, urine output, central venous pressure and perfusion status. If you give a crystalloid or a colloid to restore the blood volume to patients who are bleeding they will develop a dilutional anaemia.

Physiology of oxygen supply

Our core responsibility in the recovery room is to ensure sufficient oxygen is delivered to patients' brains and hearts to prevent hypoxic damage.

While resting, an adult uses 3.5 ml/Kg/min of oxygen for basal metabolic needs. During exercise, or with shivering, fever or emotional stress, the amount of oxygen the body uses increases many fold. Damage quickly occurs if the heart or brain are even temporarily deprived of their oxygen supply.

To identify potential problems we need to understand the chain of events involved in getting a molecule of oxygen from the inspired air all the way to a cell's mitochondria where it is used. As a person breathes in, oxygen is carried into their lungs in the inspired air. Oxygen diffuses from the alveolus into the bloodstream where it is taken up by the haemoglobin inside red cells and then transported to the tissues where it used. This seems simple but each step is a link in a chain, and if one or more steps are not functioning properly the tissues will become hypoxic.

There are four causes of tissue hypoxia

1. *Anaemic hypoxia* occurs where there is insufficient haemoglobin.
2. *Hypoxic hypoxia* occurs where the lungs are diseased, causing *low blood oxygen saturations.*
3. *Stagnant hypoxia* occurs when the cardiac output is insufficient to pump the red cells through the tissues fast enough.
4. *Metabolic hypoxia* occurs when there are metabolic disturbances such as hypothermia, alkalosis or electrolyte imbalance that alters the way haemoglobin takes up and releases oxygen.

How oxygen gets to the tissues

The volume of oxygen delivered to the cells depends on the amount of haemoglobin present in blood, and how fast the circulation carries the red cells to the tissues.

How oxygen gets to the tissues *(continued)*

Oxygen content of blood

The oxygen content of haemoglobin (Hb) depends on the:

- number of grams of haemoglobin in each litre of blood;
- percentage oxygen saturation of haemoglobin;
- number of millilitres of oxygen carried by each gram of haemoglobin.

In other words haemoglobin acts as a 'container' for oxygen. The total volume of oxygen carried in the blood depends on the number of containers, how full of oxygen each container is, and the size of the containers.

The laboratory measures haemoglobin concentration, and we can measure oxygen saturation with a pulse oximeter. The carrying capacity of haemoglobin remains fairly constant at about 1.34 ml of oxygen for every gram of haemoglobin.

$$\begin{array}{l}\text{Oxygen content} \\ \text{of blood}\end{array} = \begin{array}{l}\text{Hb} \\ \text{concentration}\end{array} \times \begin{array}{l}\text{Hb} \\ \text{saturation}\end{array} \times \begin{array}{l}\text{Hb capacity} \\ \text{for oxygen}\end{array}$$

$$= 150 \text{ gm/1000ml} \times 98/100 \times 1.34 \text{ ml O}_2\text{/gm of Hb}$$

$$= 200 \text{ ml of oxygen carried by each litre of blood.}$$

How fast the heart can deliver blood to the tissues depends on the cardiac output. In a resting adult the cardiac output is about 5000 ml/min. In healthy young adults can increase fivefold with exercise or to cope with other physiological stresses, however many elderly people, or those heart disease, can only increase their cardiac output a little.

Putting it all together we can calculate the oxygen supply to the tissues.

Oxygen supply to the tissues = volume of oxygen carried by blood × how fast it is delivered

$$\begin{array}{l}\text{Oxygen supply} \\ \text{to the tissues}\end{array} = \begin{array}{l}\text{oxygen content} \\ \text{of blood}\end{array} \times \begin{array}{l}\text{cardiac} \\ \text{output}\end{array}$$

$$= 200 \text{ ml/L} \times 5 \text{ L/min} = 1000 \text{ ml/min}$$

Of the 1000 ml of oxygen delivered to the tissues each minute, an adult at rest uses only 250 ml. The remaining 750 ml of oxygen remains bound to haemoglobin. In the extreme circumstances of shock, extreme exercise or hypoxia, an extra 250 ml of oxygen can be extracted from the haemoglobin. This means that the usable amount of oxygen in fully oxygenated blood is only about 500 ml/min. So if your patients' oxygen delivery falls to a *critical point* of about 500 ml/min they will be near death.

All else being equal, if a patient's haemoglobin concentration decreases by half, say from 140 gm/L to 70 gm/L, then the amount of oxygen delivered to the tissues falls by half from 1000 ml/min to 500 ml/min.

The critical point

In a normal person at rest the heart delivers about 1000 ml/min to the tissues, but in a bleeding patient there is less haemoglobin to carry the oxygen. Once the volume of oxygen delivered to the tissues falls to 500 ml/min the patient in grave danger of dying. Healthy young people readily withstand a haemoglobin of 70 gm/L because they can easily compensate by doubling their cardiac output from 5000 ml/min to 10 000 ml/min. You will recognize the higher cardiac output by their rapid heart rate. Their high stroke-volume causes the typical bounding pulse of anaemia. However, older or less fit people may not be able to achieve the increase in cardiac output and will go into shock.

A useful rule is that patients can only cope with one disturbance of either anaemia, or low oxygen saturation or a low cardiac output. If two of these factors combine then the tissues will become hypoxic; and the combination of all three factors is often lethal. For example bleeding patients can cope quite well with the developing anaemia provided they are not hypoxic, but if they also have low oxygen saturations and cardiac failure they are likely to die.

Physiology of coagulation

Bleeding occurs when blood leaks away from damaged blood vessels. *Haemostasis* is the process that stops bleeding. The hole in the blood vessel is plugged with a fibrin clot. Once blood starts to clot there has to be a mechanism to stop it, otherwise the whole circulation would clot. There are two processes that stop clots forming in places they are not needed: fibrinolysis and inhibition of coagulation. Despite decades of investigation the process is still a bit of a mystery, but most haematologists agree with the following facts: haemostasis needs four things:

1. coagulation factors and calcium ions;
2. sufficient numbers of functioning platelets;
3. endothelial factors;
4. fibrinolysis.

With the help of vitamin K the liver makes coagulation factors VII, IX, and X and prothrombin that circulate in the plasma in an inactive form waiting to help a clot form. The liver also makes a stringy protein called fibrinogen.

Platelets circulate in the bloodstream. These microscopic plate-shaped packages are packed with granules containing adenosine diphosphate, prostaglandins, serotonin, factor V and other compounds needed to form clots.

When a blood vessel is damaged little strands of collagen fibrils from the wound poke out into the blood stream and flap about like water-weeds.

When passing platelets collide with the collagen they instantly discharge their granules, and shrivel into burr-shaped grappling hooks that catch on to and *adhere* to the collagen fibrils. The platelets also *aggregate* together in clumps. Passing fibrinogen strings get entangled in the hooks and are converted to fibrin.

Circulating coagulation factors use calcium ions to convert prothrombin in the plasma into an enzyme called *thrombin*. Thrombin turns inactive fibrinogen into strings of *fibrin* that quickly mesh and ensnare more passing platelets, red and white cells. In this way the process snowballs to form a gelatinous tangled clot.

Once a gelatinous clot has formed, factor XIII shrinks the mesh into a tight dry fibrin plug that blocks the hole in the vessels. It takes about 6 minutes for the vessel to stop bleeding, but some hours for the clot to mature into a tight plug.

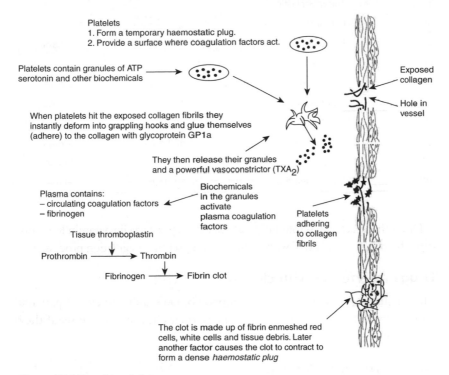

Figure 25.1 How blood clots

Normally, blood neither clots unless it needs to, nor in places where it should not. *Prostacyclin*, one of the prostaglandins, stops the process snowballing out of control. It is secreted by vascular endothelium, preventing platelets from sticking to undamaged vessel walls so that unwanted clots do not form there.

If clots form in places where they are not wanted, a circulating *proteolytic* enzyme called fibrinolysin, breaks down stray fibrin into little bits called fibrin split products (FSPs), and fibrinogen into fibrin degradation products (FDPs). Fibrinolysin is switched on by factor XII and thrombin.

Table 25.1 Blood clotting factors

Factor		Half-life	Stability
I	Fibrinogen	4 days	Stable
II	Prothrombin	2–5 days	Stable
III	Thromboplastin		
IV	Calcium		
V	Proaccelerin	12 hours	7 days
VI	Activated V		
VII	Proconvertin	300 min	Stable
VIII	Anti-haemophilic	17 hours	7 days
IX	Christmas	40 hours	Stable
X	Stuart–Prower	40 hours	7 days
XII	Hageman		Stable
XIII	Fibrin stabilizing	12 days	Stable

Drugs that react with serotonin, prostaglandins, prostacyclin, vitamin K, or any other biochemicals involved with clotting will upset the coagulation process.

Drugs interfering with clotting

Many patients are taking drugs that impede blood's ability to clot. If patients continue to bleed after surgery then check their clinical notes to see if they have been taking any of these drugs.

Drugs affecting platelets

Aspirin

Low-dose aspirin (60–150 mg) is used principally in patients who are at risk of stroke or myocardial infarction. Aspirin inhibits prostaglandin synthesis, which is needed for platelet to aggregate to form clots. It permanently disables the affected platelets for their entire 10-day life span.

Aspirin is usually stopped four days before major surgery. This allows blood to clot effectively enough for most surgery. Bleeding with neuro- or urological surgery is so serious that most surgeons stop aspirin 7–10 days before the operation. Platelet transfusion given 12 hours after the last dose of low-dose aspirin readily reverses its anticoagulant effects.

Clopidogrel

Clopidogrel is an anticoagulant used in patients who have coronary stents implanted. It is not as effective as warfarin. Clopidogrel permanently prevents platelets aggregating, and thus lasts for the whole of the platelet's 10-day life span. Clopidogrel is usually withdrawn 7–10 days before surgery. However, if it is withdrawn in patients who have recently had a cardiac stent that has not yet had epithelium cover the lumen, the risk of the stent clotting and causing myocardial infarction is unacceptably high.

Clopidogrel and aspirin

When used together, the synergistic combination of clopidogrel and aspirin is a highly effective anticoagulant. Both agents block platelet aggregation for the whole of their 10 day lifespan. Even if the last dose of the combination was given more than 5 days ago consider them as a potent cause of bleeding. Platelet transfusion will generally correct bleeding if it is given 8–12 hours after the last dose of the combination.

Dipyridamole

Dipyridamole inhibits platelet function. It is occasionally used in patients with mechanical heart valves, or a secondary prevention of embolic strokes. It is readily reversed by platelet transfusion. Its vasodilating properties can cause hypotension.

Others

Other drugs that affect blood clotting include all the NSAIDS, and all the SSRIs. Even glyceryl trinitrate (GTN) has a transient anti-platelet effect. Their individual effects are equivalent to low-dose aspirin, but when used together their effects are amplified.

Streptokinase given for acute myocardial infarction activates *plasminogen* to plasmin, causing fibrinogen to break up, not only in thrombi, but also haemostatic fibrin plugs. Postoperatively it causes uncontrollable bleeding from the surgical site.

Sometimes haemorrhage is treated with antifibrinolytics agents such as aprotinin, or acid.

Drugs affecting clotting factors

Coumadin (Warfarin)

Warfarin is the most widely used anticoagulant. Usually warfarin is stopped 5 days before surgery. Warfarin's effect is monitored with an INR. The INR needs to be more than 1.5 for most surgery. The effects of warfarin can be reversed over 18 hour with vitamin K, or immediately with fresh frozen plasma.

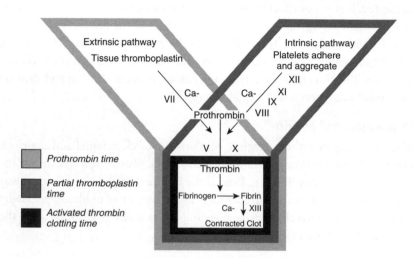

Figure 25.2 The clotting cascade and its tests

Heparin

Unfractionated heparin (UH) is often used during vascular surgery to prevent clots forming. Its clinical half-life is 50 minutes, but this is prolonged if the patient is hypothermic. The anaesthetist usually reverses the effects of heparin with protamine before the patient leaves the operating theatre.

If patients continue to bleed the anaesthetist may give an additional dose of protamine. Protamine 1 mg IV will reverse the effects of approximately 100 units of heparin. Give protamine slowly (over 10 minutes), otherwise it may cause hypotension and pulmonary artery vasoconstriction. Paradoxically, excessive protamine depresses platelet function and so aggravates bleeding.

Low molecular weight heparins (LMWH) are used perioperatively in patients who are at risk of developing deep vein thromboses. The two most commonly used are enoxparin (Clexane®) and dalteparin (Fragmin®). Remember these LMWHs are given subcutaneously and not intramuscularly.

Bleeding disorders

Disorders causing bleeding fall into the groups:

- Platelet disorders cause immediate prolonged bleeding during surgery.
- Coagulation disorders caused bleeding after surgery. Haemophilia causes bleeding later in the ward, where as von Willebrand's disease may cause bleeding in the recovery room.
- Disorders of small blood vessels cause bleeding during surgery.

Coagulation disorders

Most chronic coagulation disorders are inherited genetic diseases. Usually they are well known to the patients and their families.

von Willebrand's disease

von Willebrand's disease (vWD) is more common than haemophilia. Patients with vWD have a normal platelet count, but defective platelet adhesiveness and a deficit of factor VIII. Routine coagulation profiles are usually entirely within the normal range.

There are many variants of this genetic disease. Mild forms of vWD are difficult to diagnose, consequently patients may be unaware they have inherited it. However, they may have bled after tooth extraction, or had menorrhagia and know of 'bleeders' in their family.

Fortunately, patients with vWD who are surgically stressed have other changes in their blood that make them clot more than usual, so often bleeding is not a problem. However, if they do bleed postoperatively, then bleeding typically occurs in the recovery room.

Pressing on the bleeding site with a sterile pad generally controls superficial bleeding. If this fails then a haematologist or anaesthetist will prescribe specially derived factor VIII, which contains von Willebrand's factor. In the past cryoprecipitate was used, but should now only be given if a suitable virus-inactivated concentrate is unavailable.

Desmopressin (DDVAP®) is often given before surgery. This drug may make the patient feel nauseated, and turn impressively pale.

Haemophilia

The *haemophilias* are a group of inherited bleeding disorders caused by clotting factor deficiencies, usually involving factors VIII, IX or XI. Usually haemophiliacs have been treated with factor VIII and XI concentrates before coming to surgery. Virus inactivated cryoprecipitate or fresh frozen plasma can be used as a substitute. Haemophiliacs usually do not bleed immediately after surgery, but may do so in the ward some hours later. Bleeding from superficial wounds, although staunched by pressure, resumes when the pressure is released. Do not give intramuscular injections. Some older haemophiliacs have HIV or hepatitis C, because they received blood transfusions before effective screening for these diseases were in place.

Disseminated intravascular coagulation

Disseminated intravascular coagulation (DIC), sometimes called consumption coagulopathy, causes uncontrollable bleeding. It may occur in patients who have suffered acutely life-threatening disasters where a lot of tissue is damaged; such as multiple trauma, severe systemic sepsis, and obstetric emergencies. Patients with DIC may come from intensive care for emergency surgery, and still be bleeding when they arrive in the recovery room.

The underlying problem is that these patients spontaneously form clots everywhere. The clots plaque out like cobwebs along the inside of blood vessels, snaring red blood cells and damaging them. The mangled red cells seen under a microscope appear as *microangiopathic haemolytic anaemia*.

Meanwhile the fibrinolytic system is trying to dissolve all the cobweb clots. As they dissolve the clots release fibrin degradation products (FDP) and fibrin split product (FSP) into the plasma. Elevated levels of FSP and FDP with a falling platelet count are signposts to the diagnosis. Eventually, the patient runs out of clotting factors and platelets, and starts to bleed uncontrollably. A warning sign of developing DIC occurs when old venipuncture sites start to bleed. DIC is a life-threatening problem that needs expert advice from a haematologist. The only way to manage DIC is to identify and treat the underlying cause; for example using antibiotics to treat sepsis, or evacuation evacuating the uterus of retained necrotic tissue.

Platelet disorders

The normal platelet count is 150 000–300 000/ml. Platelets are put out of action by drugs, such as aspirin, clopidogrel, NSAIDs, SSRIs and dipyridamole. The platelet count is normal, but the platelets do not functioning normally.

This condition is sometimes called *thrombasthenia*.

A lack of platelets, *thrombocytopenia*, rarely causes spontaneous bleeding, although it may do so after surgery. Patients tend to have lots of superficial bruises on their arms and legs.

There are many causes of thrombocytopenia including:

- idiopathic thrombocytopenic purpura (ITP);

- alcoholic with liver disease;
- patients with bone marrow suppression.

Patients with ITP may come to theatre for splenectomy with the aim of preventing the spleen from removing platelets from the circulation. As soon as the spleen is removed, the patient is transfused with platelets. This transfusion may be continued in the recovery room.

A platelet count of 60 000 or more is sufficient for most surgery, but surgeons prefer it to exceed 100 000. Anaesthetists prefer a platelet count of at least 100 000 before using spinal or epidural anaesthesia.

Table 25.2 Special transfusions

Disease	Haemostatic defect	What to use
Haemophilia A	Absent/low factor VIII	Desmopressin
Haemophilia B	Absent/low factor IX	Factor IX concentrate
Von Willebrand's	Defect in vWF	Desmopressin

Diseases of blood vessels

Many diseases weaken blood vessels so that they bleed more easily or fail to retract properly to prevent bleeding. Common diseases include scurvy, amyloidosis, vasculitis, and connective tissue disease such as rheumatoid arthritis. Patients on long-term prednisilone therapy often have bruises on their arms and legs, and thin skin that tears easily. Take care not to tear their skin while moving them or removing dressings.

Blood transfusion

The spread of HIV, Hepatitis C and other diseases transmitted by blood transfusion has altered the way we use blood, during and after surgery. Anaesthetists are more reluctant to give blood, and patients are more reluctant to receive it. Advances in understanding the physiology of tissue oxygenation makes it possible to reduce the amount of blood transfused, and in many cases avoid it completely. Intraoperative salvage and reinfusion of blood enables many major operations to be done without blood transfusion.

Transfusion is life-saving therapy, and when properly screened is safe. If you need blood to save a life, do not withhold it because of fear of transfusion-transmitted disease. Blood transfusion is ultimately needed to prevent your patient having a myocardial infarction, a stroke, or developing cardiac failure.

Haemorrhage causes three problems:

1. Hypovolaemia, an imprecise colloquial term that clinicians use to describe a situation where the circulation contains less blood than normal.

2. Anaemia.

3. Coagulation disorders.

Where to find more information

- The Australian Red Cross has an excellent manual, *Transfusion Medicine*, freely available over the Internet, that covers all aspects of blood transfusion.

- In New Zealand the NZ Blood Service publishes the *Transfusion Medicine Handbook*.

- In the UK the Blood Transfusion & Tissue Transplantation Services publish the *Handbook of Transfusion Medicine*, 4th edn, 2007. There is also a Department of Health toolkit, *Better Blood Transfusion*. Regional Authorities publish their own guidelines.

- In Canada the multidisciplinary Canadian Society for Transfusion Medicine sets standards for hospital transfusion services.

Transfused blood is a tissue transplant

Transfused blood is an expensive and limited resource. It is a living tissue transplant, and like all transplants the donor' blood must be immunologically compatible with the recipient blood otherwise transfusion reactions occur. Serious transfusion reactions are always dangerous and sometimes lethal.

*A patient with Group O blood
must always receive Group O blood.*

Blood groups

There are four principal blood groups: O, A, B and AB. Each of these blood groups can be further divided into two main rhesus subgroups: Rh positive and Rh negative. The recipient's serum may have antibodies against many other antigens in donated blood. These antigens reside on the donor's red cell membranes. There are many antigens with names like Lewis, Duffy, and Kell.

Typing and cross-matching

To prevent transfusion reactions donor blood is first typed and then cross-matched against the recipient's blood before infusion.

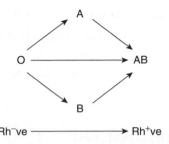

Figure 25.3 Blood or platelet groups theoretically safe to give

Blood typing

Patients must receive compatible blood. Before issuing blood your hospital's blood bank will type the patient's blood into its respective blood group and rhesus group. The technician will hold a sample aside, in case more blood is needed later. The typing process takes about 10 minutes.

Blood cross-match

After grouping the patient's blood the hospital laboratory then tests it against the donor's blood to make sure that they are compatible. Blood cross-match ensures that the many other antigens that may be either in the donor's or recipient's blood is not going to trigger an antigen–antibody reaction in the patient. This cross-match takes about 50 minutes.

In an emergency you can use typed blood without going through the whole cross-match. Typed blood is less than one per cent likely to cause a transfusion reaction.

Table 25.3 Blood groups

Blood group	Red cell antigen	Serum antibodies	Prevalence in population (%)
O	None	Anti-A	45
		Anti-B	
A	A	Anti-B	43
B	B	Anti-A	10
AB	A and B	None	7

Useful facts

- For grouping and cross-matching collect 10 ml of blood in EDTA tube.
- Grouping blood takes about 5 minutes using an automated machine.

- Automated cross-matching blood takes about 20 minutes.
- If it is done by hand then cross-matching takes at least 50 minutes.
- If the patient has unusual antibodies in their serum, which react against the donor's red cells, then cross-matching blood may take 4 or more hours.

How blood is cross-matched

Typing blood

First the patient's blood is typed to see which of the four major blood groups it belongs. This is done by adding the patient's serum to four little white dishes containing a solution of special reference red cells of blood groups A, B and AB and O. If the patient's serum causes the red cells to clump together then it contains antibodies to the antigens stuck on the surfaces of the reference red cells. For instance, if the patient's group is O then the patient's serum will clump the red cells of groups A, B, and AB, but not O. In contrast, if the patient's group is AB, then it will not clump any of the cells.

Then the patient's red cells are mixed with both rhesus positive serum (containing Rh antigen) and rhesus negative serum (containing no Rh antigen) to see which reference serum causes the red cells to clump.

Cross-matching blood

Cross-matching blood is a miniature trial transfusion in a test tube to see if the patient's (recipient's) blood is compatible with the donor's blood.

Next the donor's red blood cells are mixed with the recipient's serum to detect whether the recipient has antibodies that would cause a transfusion reaction.

Up to this point the process takes about 20 minutes.

Then a full cross-match is done, where the recipient's serum is incubated against a bank of donor red cells to check for other antibodies.

If the full cross-matching is done by hand it takes about 50 minutes in total.

Allogeneic blood

Allogeneic blood comes from a blood donor. Although this carries more risks than autologous blood, improvements in processing and storage have reduced the problems to a minimum. Allogeneic blood is cheaper to process, and in the long run more cost-effective.

Autologous transfusion

Autologous blood is blood collected from the patient, which is then stored in case they need a transfusion at a later date. It can be stored for up to a month before surgery. This pre-deposited blood eliminates the risk of transmitting viral disease, or causing immunologically mediated reactions. Sadly more than half the autologous blood collected is wasted. It is inconvenient to collect and more expensive to process than donor blood. Intraoperative red cell salvage has largely replaced the need for pre-deposited autologous blood.

Normovolaemic haemodilutiion

Occasionally several packs of blood are withdrawn at the beginning of the anaesthetic, and replaced with colloid. The collected blood is later reinfused during the operation, or more often in the recovery room.

Bleeding

Patients may bleed either quickly or slowly. Rapid blood loss is easier to recognize, however microvascular ooze is, like a dripping tap, slow but the blood loss eventually mounts up.

Revealed haemorrhage is easy to recognize; it is either coming out of the wound or is in the drain bottles. On the other hand, *concealed bleeding* into the peritoneum, thorax, or big muscle beds is less obvious. Concealed bleeding following a total hip replacement can exceed 1500 ml before local swelling becomes obvious; but with a fractured pelvis or bleeding into the abdomen many litres of blood collects before the abdomen distends. Once patients become hypovolaemic their life is in danger.

Slow bleeding – microvascular ooze

Microvascular ooze occurs slowly enough for the body to compensate. The cardinal sign is a decreasing haemoglobin and packed cell volume. Microvascular ooze is caused by either metabolic disturbance or more usually hypothermia. Some drugs lingering in the body aggravate ooze.

- Check if the patient is taking any anticoagulant drugs.
- Treat hypothermia.
- Then give 4 units of platelets.
- Now check the coagulation profile.
- If that ooze continues then use fresh frozen plasma.
- The ultimate, but rarely used, therapy is a direct blood transfusion from a compatible donor directly into the patient.

Rapid blood loss

Rapid blood loss causes hypovolaemia. Treat ongoing rapid blood loss with blood transfusion. Such *pre-emptive transfusion* in an actively bleeding patient reduces the incidence of problems later.

There are large differences in the techniques of managing *controlled bleeding* during surgery, and the more complex problem of managing *uncontrolled bleeding* associated with trauma, haemorrhagic shock, or failure of blood clotting.

Rapid blood loss after an operation is usually arises from problems with surgical haemostasis: either a vessel has started to bleed, or a surgical tie has slipped off a blood vessel.

Hypothermia is the cause of most microvascular ooze.

What to do immediately

Bleeding from the surgical site may occur as the patient's blood pressure rises in the recovery room. Monitor wounds and especially drain bottles for excessive loss. If they drain more than 100 ml in 30 minutes then inform the surgeon. If the bleeding is coming from the wound, then apply direct pressure on the bleeding site. Put on a pair of sterile gloves, pad the site and press firmly. Pressure dressings are not effective, and often cause venous congestion which aggravates the problem. You can temporarily *isolate* a limb by applying a blood pressure cuff and then inflating it above the systolic pressure.

- Stop bleeding and restore the blood volume.

- Do not delay transfusion. The sooner haemorrhagic shock is treated, the better the outcome.

- Preferably use blood, but any colloid plasma expander or even crystalloid solutions will suffice while you wait for blood to be cross-matched.

- If you are desperate then use typed but uncross-matched blood.

- If the patient continues to bleed suspect hypothermia. First rewarm your patient, and then give six units of platelets.

Acute bleeding

How to manage bleeding

- Lay the patient flat.
- Give oxygen by mask at 6 L/min.
- Call for help.

- Lift their legs on to a pillow. This runs about 400 ml of blood into their central circulation. Never tip them head down; not only is it distressing for the patient but it alters the distribution of blood flow within the lungs, and pushes abdominal contents up against the diaphragm reducing the patients *functional residual capacity*. This severely impairs oxygen uptake.

Figure 25.4 Place legs on pillow

- Start basic monitoring: ECG, pulse, blood pressure, attach a pulse oximeter and measure their core temperature.
- Check the intraoperative blood loss, and replacement. Are they balanced? From this you will get an idea of how much blood you will need to give.
- Give blood. If available use the patient's own blood type, or else use low titre O-negative blood.
- Continue using blood until fully cross-matched blood arrives.
- If blood is not available then use any plasma expander at hand. Preferably use a colloid rather than a crystalloid.
- Warm all fluids with an in-line blood warmer such as the Level 1®.

Aim to maintain:

- Systolic blood pressure >100 mmHg;
- Pulse rate < 100 bpm;
- Hb > 80 gm/L or the haematocrit > 25%.

If you are giving more than 2 units of blood then use a microfilter to prevent post-transfusion lung injury. Give each unit in less than 60 minutes. Do not allow it warm in its bag because it will deteriorate rapidly at room temperature

How much blood to give

Give colloid or blood until the patient's jugular venous pressure (JVP) rises, or they no longer feel faint when they sit up. At this point the patient will probably still have poor perfusion status with cold hands and a low urine output, but their pulse rate should be slowing, and their mean blood pressure rising. It may take up to an hour before perfusion to their hands and feet improves. You will need to top-up their blood volume as their vasculature dilates.

Giving blood? Give oxygen too!

How to manage ongoing bleeding

- Use the central line to assess continued bleeding and to guide your fluid therapy.
- Aim to keep the CVP in the range of +5 to +8 cm H_2O.
- If you are not certain whether the patient's blood volume is roughly normal then rapidly infuse 5 ml/Kg boluses of blood, or colloid. If the CVP rises for a minute or two and then falls again keep repeating the boluses until the CVP remains above 5 cm H_2O.
- Listen to the lung bases. Crackles, followed by a wheeze, indicate the patient's blood volume is becoming overloaded.
- You will know when you are gaining on the blood loss if the pulse progressively slows over the following 5 to 10 minutes, and the urine output increases beyond 1 ml/Kg/hr.

*Blood is a living substance. It deteriorates quickly at
room temperatures.*

How to use coagulation profiles

- Coagulation studies help you work out why the blood does not clot, and what to do next.
- Send blood for INR, aPTT, haemoglobin, platelet and fibrinogen levels.
- If the INR is >1.8 then clotting factors are less than 30% of their normal levels. This is the minimum acceptable level; below this level microvascular bleeding (ooze) is almost certain to occur.
- Other useful predictors of microvascular bleeding are platelets < 50 000 × 10^3/L, fibrinogen < 0.75 gm/L, and an aPTT > 1.5 its normal time.

Do not give platelets, fresh frozen plasma, or clotting factors in anticipation of bleeding. The coagulation system is remarkably robust and will form clots with as little as 10 000 × 10^3/L platelets. The vascular endothelium quickly promotes clotting providing the patient is warm, and has a well oxygenated liver.

Warming blood

If you anticipate giving more than 100 ml/min, or more than two units of blood in an hour, then use an in-line blood warmer to warm the blood to 37°C. Warm blood for those at risk of hypothermia: the young, the elderly, and the infirm; and those patients who have *cold agglutinins*. If you give cold blood at 4°C, each unit will decrease the patient's core temperature by about 0.25°C. Cold blood is painful to infuse through peripheral veins. It may cause red cells to clump, impeding flow through the microcirculation, and it is a major cause of bleeding. Do not transfuse cold blood rapidly through a central venous line; it is likely to cause arrhythmias and the cardiac output to fall.

It is extremely dangerous to warm the pack of blood in warm or hot water, because this will cook the blood, haemolyse the red cells and destroy the clotting factors.

Never put blood in a microwave oven, because microwaves do not heat uniformly. They concentrate intense heat in separated small areas, boiling the red cells.

In-line blood warmers are essential for massive transfusions. Warming blood from 4°C to 37°C decreases its viscosity 2.5-fold, and dilates the patient's veins allowing transfusions to run faster.

Blood transfusions run slowly through standard blood warmers. To overcome this difficulty there are a number of newer systems such as the Level-1™ which delivers 500 ml/min, while the Rapid infusion System™ delivers 1500 ml/min.

Water bath blood warmers are less commonly used now. Dry heat blood warmers such as the Atom™ do not require dedicated disposables and accept any standard giving set.

Every blood warmer should indicate the temperature, have a thermostat control and warning alarms. The temperature must never exceed 41°C. Blood warmers can be dangerous if they malfunction so they need maintenance checks every 12 months.

Drugs used to promote haemostasis

A number of drugs are used to reduce bleeding during surgery and in the recovery room. These include tranexemic acid, aprotinin, protamine, and desmopressin (DDVAP®). Other agents promote local coagulation including applied fibrin (Tisseal®), and spray on albumin/gluteraldehyde (Bioglue®) and procoagulant swabs.

How to minimize the need for transfusion

Patients who are at risk of bleeding such as those taking anticoagulants, those with congenital abnormalities of haemostasis and those undergoing major blood-loss surgery should be identified preoperatively and given alternative regimes.

During surgery the anaesthetists may use techniques including: salvaging autologous blood, intentional haemodilution and pharmacological manipulation of haemostasis with drugs such as desmopressin or aprotinin.

Transfusion threshold

Before the operation the anaesthetist considers the oxygen delivery equation to help decide the value of the lowest safe haemoglobin (Hb) concentration or *packed cell volume* (PCV) for that patient. This lowest safe value is called the *transfusion threshold*. Once the PCV or haemoglobin concentration falls below the transfusion threshold, then it is time to start a blood transfusion.

You can easily measure either the haemoglobin concentration or the PCV in your operating suite's mini-laboratory.

Table 25.4 Transfusion threshold

Criteria	Start blood transfusion when PCV falls below	Start blood transfusion when Hb falls below
Young healthy people	0.22	70 gm/L
Age > 50 years	0.25	80 gm/L
Age > 60 years	0.28	90 gm/L
Age > 70 years	0.31	100 gm/L
IHD or CVD*	0.31	100 gm/L
IHD + respiratory disease	0.33	110 gm/L

*IHD, ischaemic heart disease; CVD, cerebrovascular disease.

Principles of blood transfusion

Transfusion thresholds are useful and save unwarranted blood transfusion, but they are merely a guide. Do not delay transfusion until the transfusion threshold is crossed if the patient is showing signs of hypoxia including confusion, ST changes on their ECG, a tachycardia greater than 100 beats/min, their blood gases reveal an acidosis, or they have a poor perfusion status.

Blood and blood products should not be used for trivial reasons. Every unit carries an inherent risk, and the aim is to use as little as possible. Make sure that the reason for giving blood is documented on the patient's chart.

When to transfuse blood

Blood transfusion may be necessary in patients who are hypovolaemic, anaemic or have coagulation disorders.

Signs of hypovolaemia are:

- continuing bleeding;
- persistent tachycardia;
- cold extremities with a poor perfusion status;
- postural hypotension where the patients blood pressure falls > 200 mmHg when you sit them up;
- angina;
- breathlessness;
- decreasing urine output;
- confusion, anxiety or a deteriorating conscious state.

Patients who cannot tolerate a low haemoglobin include those with:

- coronary artery disease;
- myocardial ischaemia;
- congestive cardiac failure;
- a history of transient ischaemic attacks or suspected cerebral ischaemia;
- symptomatic valvular heart disease such as severe aortic stenosis;
- a history of previous ischaemic stroke.

Patients who have acute or chronic problems with bleeding or anaemia including those with:

- disseminated intravascular coagulation;
- inherited bleeding disorders such as haemophilia or von Willebrand's disease;
- thrombocytopenia;
- bone marrow failure.

Therapeutic goals

The therapeutic goals are to maintain patients' blood pressure within 20 per cent of their preoperative levels, keep the pulse rate between 60 to 80 beats/min, and maintain a urine output of more than 1 ml/Kg/hr.

It is sometimes a difficult decision to know when to transfuse blood, or when to use other fluids. Even in the operating theatre it is difficult to measure fluid or blood loss accurately. Blood is lost on to drapes, runs under the table, and moisture evaporates quickly from open abdomens. Weighing swabs and measuring the amount in suction bottles only gives an estimate.

Which fluid to use first

It is not yet certain whether albumin solutions (or other colloids) are superior to crystalloids in resuscitation, but there is an increasing preference for albumin solutions because much larger quantities of crystalloids are needed. Whether to use crystalloids or colloids first in bleeding patients has caused much emotional debate over the past 10 years.

> *Fluid of choice, crystalloid or colloid?*
> *This debate is unresolved and ongoing.*

There are important differences between the safety of the colloids available. Albumin 5% seems to cause less anaphylactoid response than other colloids. Compared with albumin the polygelines cause 12 times as many reactions, hydroxyethyl-starches 4 times and dextrans 2 times.[1]

Most anaesthetists start with 1–2 litres of Hartmann's solution, then use albumin 5%, and if necessary follow this with blood.

Infusion of large amounts of crystalloids can cause problems. They seep into the tissues causing peripheral oedema, and may migrate into the lungs later to cause pulmonary oedema. Over the coming days the kidneys need to excrete this excessive fluid.

Limit the infusion of synthetic colloids, such as poygelines (Gelofusin™ and Haemaccel™), dextran, or hydroxyethyl-starches (Hetastarch™) to no more than 25 ml/Kg in any 24-hour period.

Table 25.5 Normal blood volume

Age	Blood volume
Neonates	100 ml/Kg
Children < 12 years	80 ml/Kg
Adults	70 ml/Kg

Hypovolaemia

Hypovolaemia occurs when the circulation does not contain enough blood to fill it adequately. The body progressively compensates by mounting a predictable sequence of responses – the first of which is to activate the sympathetic nervous system.

The single most useful sign of early hypovolaemia is postural hypotension. If a patient feels faint (or their BP falls by > 20 mmHg) when you sit them up, they are almost certainly hypovolaemic. Severe postural hypotension makes the patient nauseated.

Look for a deteriorating perfusion status. An early sign of hypovolaemia is subtle vasoconstriction of the arterioles. To detect this squeeze a fingernail bed. Blood should flush back within 2 seconds. The next sign is when the hands begin to cool.

Tachycardia usually occurs. Look for a rising pulse rate, and be especially concerned if it exceeds 90 beats/min. If the patient has recently taken a β-blocker the pulse rate may not rise, but the blood pressure falls in line with the blood volume.

Especially in younger people, the blood pressure does not fall with haemorrhagic shock until shock enters the decompensated stage.

> *Do not rely on hypotension as a warning sign of developing shock.*

Once the urine output falls below 60 ml/hr then consider hypovolaemia as a cause. In the recovery room if urine output falls to less than 30 ml/hr then you must look for and exclude haemorrhage.

Elderly people do not vasoconstrict as effectively as younger people. Consequently the elderly tolerate blood loss poorly, and their blood pressure will fall earlier.

Sweating, air hunger, alarm and confusion are signs the patient is entering the phase of *irreversible shock*.

Table 25.6 Clinical signs of haemorrhage in a 70 Kg adult male

Severity	Mild	Moderate	Severe	Critical
Class	Class 1	Class 2	Class 3	Class 4
Blood loss (ml)	< 750	750–150	1500–2000	> 2000
Blood loss %	0–15	15–30	30–40	> 40
Pulse rate	80–110	> 110	> 120	> 140
Blood pressure	Normal	Normal	Decreased	Decreased
Pulse pressure	Normal	Decrease	Decreased	Decreased
Respiratory rate	12–20	20–30	30–40	>40 (gasping)
CVP (cm H_2O)	2 to 5	–2 to 2	–2 to –5	< –5
Urine output ml/hr	>30	20–30	5–15	Minimal or none
Perfusion	Cool hands	Pale hands	Cold hands	Sweating
Capillary return	Normal	< 2 seconds	> 2 seconds	Undetectable
Conscious state	Normal	Anxious/agitated	Cofused	Lethargic or coma

Based on the American College of Surgeons Classification of Haemorrhagic Shock.

How to estimate the amount of blood loss
How to replace blood if you know the volume lost

Most of the time it is difficult to know how much blood or fluid has been lost. In this case use other criteria such as clinical signs, haemoglobin concentration, and give blood once the transfusion threshold has been crossed.

Table 25.7 What to transfuse

Blood Volume lost	What to do
15% (750 ml) in an adult	No need to transfuse
15–30%	Transfuse crystalloids or colloids
20–40% in an adult < 50 years	Rapid volume replacement with crystalloids or colloids
20–40% in an adult > 50 years	Rapid volume replacement with crystalloids or colloids and red cell replacement according to haemoglobin
> 40%	Rapid volume replacement with crystalloids or colloids and blood

How to replace blood if you do not know the volume lost

Some hints for managing patients who are bleeding slowly:

- Check the haemoglobin or haematocrit frequently.
- Start giving blood once the haemoglobin falls to the *transfusion threshold*.
- Treat hypovolaemia separately from anaemia.
- Replace blood volume first.
- Prepare to give blood if the patient pulse rate rises above 100 bpm.
- If a patient is developing an acidosis then use blood straight away.
- Notify the blood bank early about the situation.

  Aim to maintain:

- the systolic blood pressure > 100 mmHg;
- pulse rate < 100 bpm;
- Hb > 80 gm/L or the haematocrit > 25%.
- if giving more than 2 units of blood then use a microfilter to prevent post-transfusion lung injury;
- give each unit in less than 60 minutes. Do not allow it warm in its bag because it will deteriorate rapidly at room temperature.

Massive blood transfusion

The generally accepted definition of a massive blood transfusion is where the patient's blood volume is replaced within a 24-hour period. This is impractical, because most bleeding occurs quickly, and problems arise once you give more than 5 units of blood per hour. A better definition of massive transfusion is where half the patient's estimated blood volume has been replaced within the previous 4 hours.

In an emergency you can use typed but uncross-matched blood of the same blood group as the patient's. There is less than one per cent chance of a severe reaction. Most operating rooms keep four units of low antibody titre Rh-negative blood to use in emergencies. Where possible do not give Rh-positive blood to an Rh-negative patient, however you may give Rh-negative blood to an Rh-positive patient.

After eight units of blood:

- use the freshest blood (< 10 days) available;
- measure the FBC, whole blood clotting time, INR, aPTT;
- give Fresh frozen plasma (FFP) to maintain the INR and aPTT < 1.5 times normal;

- if the aPTT or INR >1.5 normal then measure fibrinogen, fibrin split products, and fibrin degradation products;
- give platelets once the count < 50 000 × 10³/L or you see microvascular ooze;
- if there is catastrophic bleeding (> 8 units per hour) serial coagulation studies will not help. In this case give 8 units of platelets after the 8th unit of blood and 8 units of FFP. Then use 2 units of platelets and one unit of FFP for each successive unit.

Figure 25.5 Set up for a massive blood transfusion

How much O-negative blood to use

Once the patient has received more than 4 units of group O-negative blood you will need to continue with O-negative blood. If, at this stage, you revert to the patient's own group the O-negative blood you have used may contain antibodies to the cross-matched blood you get from the blood bank.

When the laboratory has the time to carefully cross-match a fresh blood sample from the patient you can revert to the patient's own blood group.

Figure 25.6 Improvised pressure bag

The laboratory needs to prove there are no detectable passive haemolysins in the blood they issue.

You can make an improvized pressure infusor. Carefully cut open one end of the tough outer plastic container in which many bags of intravenous fluid are delivered. Reinforce the container with non-stretchable cloth surgical adhesive (such as zinc oxide tape or Sleek®) so that it can withstand pressure. Then attach a blood pressure cuff inflation bulb to an empty litre bag. Slip the litre bag inside the reinforced outer bag to act as inflatable bladder. Insert a bag of blood or other fluid with its giving set attached. As you inflate the bladder the bag of fluid is compressed against the reinforced outer container.

How to know if the coagulopathy is severe

After about 10 units of blood 40 per cent of patients develop a severe coagulopathy (INR or aPTT double normal) with thrombocytopenia (platelets less than 50×10^9/L). However, you cannot predict the severity of the coagulopathy from the number of units of blood you have transfused. Haemostasis is affected by many factors, particularly: hypothermia, liver blood flow, acid-base status, the mass damaged tissue, and tissue oxygenation.

Tips about massive blood transfusion

- To avoid confusion allocate one person to liaise with the technicians in the blood bank, the haematologists, and other back-up services.

- Give the blood bank ample warning because large blood transfusions tax the resources of most blood banks. Even in a teaching hospital it takes about 30 minutes to deliver type-specific uncrossed matched blood.

- Use the freshest blood possible. To avoid storage lesion, and multi organ failure avoid transfusing blood collected more than 10 days ago.[2]

- Warm blood with an in-line blood warmer such as the Level 1™

- To prevent the lungs becoming clogged with microemboli, filter blood through special 20–40 μm microfilters to remove cellular debris from the blood bag. Packed cells flow through micro-filters much faster if they are diluted with 0.9% saline.

*The blood pressure does not necessarily fall in
early haemorrhagic shock.*

- Use a Y-giving set with 0.9% saline on one arm and the blood pack on the other. Run saline into the blood pack, and then use a pressure infuser to run it into the patient. Take all connectors out of the line as they impede flow.

- Site at least two drips and 'piggy-back' them. This allows you to continue pouring blood into the patient through one line, while you are replacing the bags of blood on the other.

- Use the largest gauge, shortest intravenous cannula in the biggest vein you can find.

- Use blood to prevent tissue hypoxia and not simply to expand plasma volume.

- Give blood on a unit-by-unit basis. Even one unit of blood may be enough to improve tissue oxygenation.

- Where possible use leucocyte-depleted blood for patients undergoing bowel surgery, in those with cancer, as well as in those who are already immunosuppressed, and those with intercurrent infections.

Problems with massive transfusion

Potential major complications of massive transfusions include:

- hypothermia – blood will not clot effectively if the core temperature < 35°C;
- acid-base abnormalities – immediately a metabolic acidosis, 36 hours later
- a metabolic alkalosis;
- citrate toxicity – usually only a problem if the patient is hypothermic;
- hyperkalaemia.

Practicalities

Blood should either be running into your patient or stored in the special blood fridge at 2–6°C. Blood deteriorates rapidly as it warms. Do not leave it lying around on bench tops. Most blood packs have a temperature-sensitive label to indicate if this has happened. Never store blood in an ordinary household refrigerator. Frozen red cells are dead red cells. If they are transfused into a patient they will rupture, releasing their haemoglobin to clog the kidney.

Cold hands = poorly perfused kidneys.

How to identify patients

Giving the wrong blood is given to the wrong patient is the commonest cause of serious or fatal adverse reactions to blood transfusion. Such clerical errors are totally avoidable.

Every hospital should have a Blood Transfusion Committee. It is their responsibility to formulate a policy to document and trace a unit of blood on every step of its journey beginning with its collection from the vein of the donor, to its infusion into the vein of the recipient. To reduce the risk of clerical error many hospitals use portable barcodes to ensure the right blood gets to the right patient. Because of the problems with vCJD legislation in many countries requires that all blood and blood components must be traceable to the recipient for 15 years.

Two trained staff must independently check each unit before it can be transfused. Meticulously check each unit of blood before giving it. Check the labels on the blood pack, the transfusion slip accompanying it, the patient's identification bracelet, and the patient's record. EVERY detail must match exactly. The blood's identification number, the blood group, and its expiry date must exactly match the details on the transfusion slip.

Tips about technique

- Do not directly mark intravenous bags with solvent marking pens because the ink penetrates the plastic and contaminates the solution.
- Do not vent plastic containers with needles.
- Wear gloves and eye protection when putting up blood.
- Be careful not to put your fingers on the needle in such a way that it may carry contaminants into the bag.
- Before putting up blood, invert the bag a few times to mix the components.
- Use a standard (170–260 µm) filter to remove clots and macroaggregate debris. To avoid the chance of bacterial colonization, change the giving set every 12 hours.
- Microaggregate (20–40 µm) filters are not necessary for routine blood transfusions. Use if you plan to give two or more units of blood in one transfusion

A common mistake when setting up a drip. Note the forefinger contaminating the sterile needle as it is being inserted into the bag of intravenous fluid.

Figure 25.7 An error

episode, or for massive blood transfusion. Microfilters prevent trash from the bags of blood embolizing to the lungs. They reduce the risk of adult respiratory distress syndrome, non-haemolytic febrile reactions and thrombocytopenia.

- *Leucocyte reduction filters* are round flat filters used for red cells. They remove 99.9% of the white cells from the blood, which otherwise might cause febrile non-haemolytic transfusion reactions. They also greatly the reduce the transmission of cytomegalovirus.

- Non-filtered giving sets can be used for 5% Albuminex® 30% Albuminex®, or polygelines.

- Apart from 0.9% saline do not add anything whatsoever to blood or components. This includes drugs.

- Crystalloids (Hartmann's solution or Ringer's lactate) and polygeline colloid solution (Haemaccel™ or Gelofusion™) contain calcium ions, which reverse the citrate anticoagulant, and the blood will clot in the lines. Dextrose 5% solutions cause red cells to aggregate and will eventually cause haemolysis.

- Cold blood infused faster than 100 ml/min may cause cardiac arrest. Use a blood warmer if you are giving more than two units in one hour, or in patients who have cold agglutinins. Blood must not be warmed above 41°C.

Blood and its components

Whole blood

Packs of whole blood usually contain about 400 to 500 ml. Except for autologous transfusion, whole blood, either stored or fresh, is rarely used.

Packed cells

Red cell concentrates (packed cells) come in bags of about 300 ml. They contain no effective clotting factors or platelets. The sticky viscous packed cell concentrate does not pass easily through microfilters. To make them run through a filter more quickly you can dilute them in 0.9% saline. Do not use Ringer's lactate or Hartmann's solution, since calcium ions in the solutions cause blood to clot in the intravenous line.

One pack of blood in a 70 Kg adult raises the haemoglobin by about 1gm/L (or 100mg/100ml). Red cells should be infused rapidly. Most patients easily tolerate a unit in 60 minutes, and no infusion should take longer than three hours.

Storage lesion

Blood can be stored in a special refrigerator at 2–7°C for up to 35 days. During storage potassium continuously leaks out of the red cells into the plasma, and may cause arrhythmias if infused too quickly down a central line. After rewarming the red blood cells quickly take up the potassium.

After a few days in the refrigerator blood starts to suffer *storage lesion*; platelets disintegrate, and clotting factors degrade. Stored red cells pick up oxygen readily enough, but they will not release it to the tissues. It may take up to 18 hours for the surviving red cells to start functioning properly.

If bleeding will not stop, then ask for fresh four-day old blood.

Boutique blood

Special types of blood are available for specific patients. Cytomegalovirus (CMV) seronegative blood is used for cytomegalovirus seronegative patients who are on immunosuppressive chemotherapy, have lymphoma or leukaemia, or are pregnant. Gamma radiation kills white cells (T-lymphocytes). Use irradiated blood for immunosuppressed patients. Prestorage leucocyte-depleted blood is used for those who have had previous febrile non-haemolytic transfusion reactions. If these latter patients are taking ACE inhibitor medication they may be unexpectedly hypotensive.

Platelets

Surgical bleeding is most unlikely to be a problem if the platelet count is greater than $50\,000 \times 10^6$/L, but they must be working. In some cases of chronic thrombocytopenia surgery can be performed with counts as low as $10\,000 \times 10^6$/L.

Platelets come in packs of 70 to 100 ml and are stored at room temperature. They are issued in O, A, and B groups only. If Rh-positive platelets are used in

Rh-negative women then give them anti-D immunoglobulin. Give each unit of platelets through a fresh standard blood-giving set. Each unit should be infused in no longer than 30 minutes, but may be given rapidly over 5 minutes if necessary. One unit of platelets usually raises the platelet count by about $10\,000 \times 10^3/mm^3$.

Store platelets at 22°C (room temperature), and not in the refrigerator. Treat them gently. Their role in life is to burst, which they readily do at the slightest provocation. Do not suck them into a syringe through a needle, or slap the packs around on the bench.

When to use platelets

Indications for platelet transfusion in recovery room are:
- Continued bleeding after surgery when the platelet count is $< 50\,000 \times 10^3/mm^3$.
- Continued diffuse microvascular bleeding (ooze) when the platelet count is $< 50\,000 \times 10^3/ml^3$.
- Dysfunctional platelets where the patient has been taking drugs such as aspirin, NSAIDs, calcium channel blockers, SSRIs, β-blockers, or local anaesthetics.

Five per cent albumin

Five per cent human albumin (50 gm/L) is a purified, sterile, colloid derived from human plasma. It does not need to be cross-matched. It is most useful as a plasma expander in resuscitation while you wait for blood to arrive. Rarely, it may cause hypotension. Although never reported there is a theoretical risk of transmitting Creutzfield–Jakob disease (CJD), but not HIV or hepatitis viruses.

Fresh frozen plasma

Fresh frozen plasma FFP contains all the clotting factors (especially factor VIII). Normally the body contains the equivalent of about 12 units of FFP. Even in extreme cases, 12 units should restore coagulation factors to normal levels.

Reserve Group O plasma for Group O recipients.

FFP is stored at -25°C. It is delivered in 150–300 ml bags of beige ice. Usually the blood bank defrosts them for you. Use the ABO group compatible with the recipient's red cells.

Fresh frozen plasma can be infused rapidly, although some say this increases the risk of adverse reactions.

When to use fresh frozen plasma

- To restore labile coagulation factors in massive transfusions once the INR or aPTT is > 1.5 time, or when factors V and VIII are < 25% of normal.
- To immediately reverse the effects of warfarin.
- To treat DIC where there is active bleeding.
- With surgical bleeding in patients with severe liver disease.

Do not use fresh frozen plasma simply to expand plasma volume, or before coagulation studies have demonstrated it is needed, or when the patient is hypothermic, or before you have seen the effect of a few units of platelets. If specific therapy is available, such as cryoprecipitate, factor VIII, or other specific factor concentrates, then use these in place of fresh frozen plasma.

Do not defrost fresh frozen plasma in a microwave oven, or in hot water, because you will denature the enzymes. Use FFP within 6 hours of thawing.

The biggest risk of blood transfusion is iatrogenic pulmonary oedema.

Cryoprecipitate

Cryoprecipitate is prepared from a single donation, frozen at minus 30°C and takes 30 minutes to thaw. Cryoprecipitate contains fibrinogen, factor VIII, factor XIII and von Willebrand's factor.

When to use cryoprecipitate

Microvascular ooze is likely if fibrinogen is greater than 50 gm/L. Consider using cryoprecipitate when the fibrinogen values are trending towards 0.75 gm/L.

Start with 1–1.5 donor units per 10 Kg body weight. Cryoprecipitate is not treated to remove viruses. Do not use it to treat haemophilia or von Willebrand's disease, if alternative therapies are available. Use the correct ABO group.

Recombinant factor VIIa

Factor VII is one of the enzymes in the clotting pathway. In severe haemorrhage the body may not be able to make Factor VII fast enough. Although only approved by the makers for treating haemophiliacs, recombinant human factor VIIa (rhFVIIa or NovoSeven®) is increasingly being used *off-label* to treat uncontrollable haemorrhage.[3]

Drugs decreasing transfusion requirements

Desmopressin (DDVAP™), a synthetic analogue of vasopressin, causes intense vasoconstriction – the patient goes 'white as a ghost'. It releases factor VIII from endothelium and *procoagulant* components of factor VIII. It is useful when patients with von Willebrand's disease bleed following surgery, and where bleeding is caused by platelet abnormalities associated with *uraemia*. It is sometimes used where large blood losses are expected, such as the insertion of Harrington's rods.

Antifibrinolytics

Tranexamic acid and epsilon-aminocaproic acid stabilize existing clots, and prevent primary fibrinolysis.

Aprotinin (Trasylol™) inhibits fibrinolysis and also kallikrein-induced activation of the clotting cascade. It diminishes postoperative blood loss. Antifibrinolytics occasionally promote pathological thrombosis.

Problems with blood transfusions

Risk of transmitting disease

The risk of transmitting disease from allogeneic (donor) blood is now very low indeed. The risk of transmitting HIV is far less than 1 in 5 million, and the risk of hepatitis B or C is approaching this level too.

Table 25.8 Estimated risks of blood transfusion[1,2]

Risk	Frequency per unit transfused (estimated)	Deaths per million units
Acute haemolytic reactions	1:12 000 to 1:40 000	0.67
Delayed haemolytic reactions	1:1000 to 1:10 000	0.8
Bacterial sepsis	1:500 000	< 0.25
Hepatitis B	1:1 339 000	< 0.5
Hepatitis C	1:3 636 000	< 0.5
HIV	1:7 299 000	< 0.5
Syphilis	< 1:1 000 000	
TRALI	1:5000 to 1:100 000	0.67
Variant CJD	Possible	

To put these risks into perspective, the risk in any single year of an urban dweller being killed in a car accident is 1: 10 000. For people who live in rural areas, the chance of being killed by a bolt of lightning is about 120 000 in a given year. It is worth noting that, in a teaching hospital, the risk of giving too much blood to a patient and causing pulmonary oedema is about one per cent.

Blood transfusion reactions

Microbial contamination

Sepsis is the leading cause of transfusion mortality. Bacteria can get into the blood as contamination from skin organisms when the blood is collected from the donor. If the bag of blood is frothy, or chocolate brown or is distended, it is probably infected. Do not open it! Return it to the blood bank.

Because platelets are stored at room temperature they are more likely than blood stored in a refrigerator to be a culture medium for bacteria.

Variant Creutzfeldt–Jakob disease

Variant Creutzfeldt–Jakob disease (vCJD) is a human *prion* disease, which is an abnormal host-encoded glycoprotein that accumulates in the brain. Another form of the disease is bovine-spongioform encephalopathy (BSE, or 'mad cow disease' which can be passed on by blood transfusion. Because of this concern most blood banks will not accept blood donors who have lived in the UK for a period prior to 1992. There is no known reliable test for this disease but processes are being developed to remove prions from blood component.

Acute haemolytic transfusion reaction

The most tragic transfusion reactions occur when ABO-incompatible blood is accidentally given to a patient. These accidents are usually caused by clerical lapses – giving the wrong blood to the wrong patient. Almost everyone has naturally occurring antibodies (including anti-A and anti-B) in their blood. If challenged these *autoantibodies* activate a special plasma protein called complement that rapidly ruptures circulating red cells to cause shock and renal failure. This can be fatal, even if only a small volume of incompatible blood was transfused.

ABO-Rh typing alone results in a 99.8 per cent chance of a compatible trans-fusion. This means that in an extreme emergency you are fairly safe giving typed but uncross-matched blood.

Signs

Signs of blood transfusion reaction are those of haemolysis and an acute immune reaction. Mild reactions present with: fever, tachycardia, sweating, and urticaria. Severe reactions occur with additional: back and chest pain, hypotension, oliguria, haemoglobinuria and progress to disseminated intravascular coagulation, renal failure, and sometimes death.

Management

Turn off the transfusion. Monitor vital signs, and perfusion status. Give high-flow oxygen by face mask. Change the drip sets and continue the infusion with 0.9% saline. Re-identify the patient and blood pack. Inform the blood bank and return the unused blood and pack. If the patient starts to wheeze then treat them for anaphylaxis. If the patients' urine turns dusky brown they may be developing haematuria; treat this with mannitol 1.5 gm/Kg IV to promote a diuresis. Mannitol works within minutes and lasts for 2–3 hours.

Febrile non-haemolytic transfusion reaction

A *febrile non-haemolytic transfusion reaction* (FNHTR) is defined as a rise in body temperature of 1°C or more during a transfusion. It usually occurs towards the end of the transfusion. It is the most common adverse effect of transfusion occurring in about one per cent of transfusions. Bioreactive substances, such as interleukins or complement fractions that accumulate when blood is stored, usually cause FNTHR. These reactions are seldom dangerous and are treated by simply stopping the transfusion. If the patient has had a previous febrile reaction use leucocyte-depleted blood for subsequent transfusions.

Allergic reactions

Transient hives (*urticaria*) and itching occur in about 1–3 per cent of transfusions and indicate a minor allergic reaction to the donor's plasma proteins. Treat it by stopping the transfusion. However if the patient also starts to wheeze, or becomes hypotensive, then you are dealing with much more serious anaphylaxis.

Anaphylaxis

Anaphylactic reactions occur rarely; in about 1:50 000 transfusions. Coughing is usually the first sign, followed shortly by wheeze, urticaria, hypotension, and abdominal cramps. They begin immediately or as late as 45 minutes of the start of the transfusion. The less serious anaphylactoid reactions can be delayed by 2–3 hours after the start of the transfusion. The shorter the time it takes for symptoms to develop after the start of the transfusion, the more serious the reaction. Anaphylaxis is treated with adrenaline and cardiorespiratory support as usually required.

Transfusion-related lung injury

Transfusion-related lung injury (TRALI) is an immune mediated life-threatening syndrome with symptoms and signs similar to acute respiratory distress syndrome (ARDS). Transfusions of fresh frozen plasma (FFP) are the main culprit. In most cases, there is an antibody in the donor's plasma that reacts with the recipient's white cells. TRALI presents with respiratory distress, hypoxia and fever, which progresses over several hours to a chest X-ray revealing a bilateral white-out with diffuse alveolar and interstitial infiltrates. More than 80 per cent of patients with transfusion-related lung injury recover with appropriate management.

How to manage transfusion reactions

If, shortly after starting a blood transfusion, your patient starts to cough or develops an itchy rash all over their body that looks like hives, then they are having a blood transfusion reaction.

Immediately turn off the transfusion. Reassure your patient and record their pulse, blood pressure, respiratory rate and oxygen saturation. Give oxygen by mask. Summon help. Notify the anaesthetist. Set up a saline infusion using a new intravenous giving set. Take the giving set that has the blood in it and seal both ends so that the laboratory can sample blood in the IV line. Return the patient to Stage 1 recovery care – they will possibly needing double nursing care.

Recheck the data label on the unit of blood with the blood cross-match form and the patient's wrist name band. Notify the hospital's blood bank. Take three samples of blood from the arm opposite the infusion. Put a sample of blood in each of three tubes: a white capped (*serum*) tube: in a blue capped (*citrated*) tube and a pink capped (*EDTA*) tube. Fill out a pathology request slip labelling it: 'Transfusion reaction investigations'. Send the three specimens of blood, the sealed IV line and any previously empty bags to the haematology laboratory in a large sealed plastic bag.

If the patient develops only a slight fever (< 1°C rise) then the reaction is probably a febrile non-haemolytic reaction. If they develop rigors, chills, shivering, or they become restless or short of breath, or their temperature rises higher than 38.5°C then the reaction is more severe. Patients with very severe life-threatening reactions go on to develop one or more of loin or back pain, hypotension, tachycardia, blood oozing from drip sights or wounds, or hypotension and collapse. These reactions indicate one of the following: a haemolytic reaction, bacterial contamination, anaphylaxis, or developing hours later, a transfusion-related lung injury. To survive the patient will need skilled specialist care from the anaesthetist, haematologists and other medical and nursing staff.

Notes

1. Barron ME (2004) *Archives of Surgery* 139:552–63.
2. Flores JM, Jimenez PI *et al.* (2001) *Injury* 32:5–12.
3. Roberts H, Moore D, White G (2004) *Blood* 104:3858–64.
4. Report presented at the Strategic Blood Forum in Syndey, 30 August 2006.

26

Surgical issues

Drains and catheters

Surgical drains are inserted to stop fluid accumulating in potential spaces. They drain away collections of unwanted fluids such as blood, pus, gastric fluids, and lymph.

The question of whether to routinely drain sites where fluids may accumulate remains controversial.[1] There is no doubt that some drains are useful, such as T-tubes used in biliary surgery and nasogastric tubes after oesophageal surgery.

Drains are usually made from biological inert silicon rubber (Silastic®) and they cause little tissue damage. Red rubber drains can cause intense inflammatory response, setting up a track along which fluid can escape after the drain is removed.

Figure 26.1 Mini-concertina drain

Drains can be open to the air or closed to prevent contamination. They can drain passively or be actively sucked. Open drains include corrugated sheets of rubber or plastic. The fluid collects in gauze, or a stoma bag. There is a risk of infection with these drains. Closed drains allow fluids to escape into bottles or packs – these include chest and abdominal drains. There is less risk of infection with closed drains.

Nasogastric tubes

Handling bowel reduces gastrointestinal mobility for a few days and during this time fluid transudates into the stomach and bowel. Nasogastric tubes drain the fluid accumulating in the stomach and proximal small bowel after abdominal surgery, reducing the risk of postoperative distension, regurgitation and aspiration pneumonia. There is little evidence to support the routine use of nasogastric tubes after uncomplicated abdominal surgery and there is evidence they increase the risk of pulmonary aspiration. They are of proven benefit after oesophageal resection, gastric surgery, and for decompressing the bowel in intestinal obstruction.

Figure 26.2 Fastening the nasogastric tube

Usually nasogastric tubes are left to drain freely. For their siphoning action to work properly, keep the bag below the level of the bed. Sometimes the surgeon will request 4-hourly aspiration. Aspirate these tubes very gently. The fluid should almost flow freely into your syringe with little or no suction. Never apply vigorous suction to the tube because you will damage the stomach's delicate mucosa. Do not kink off the nasogastric tube 'to prevent air flowing back into the stomach' – it won't. (Consider the consequences of applying the same amount of suction to the mucosa in your mouth.)

Urinary catheters

Urinary catheters are another form of drain. They are used to relieve or prevent urinary retention and bladder distension, or to monitor urine output. Most are inserted through the urethra, but where this is impractical the patient may need a suprapubic catheter. Urinary catheters are usually made of a form of silicon plastic, or occasionally latex rubber. Men need 38 cm long catheters, and women need 22 cm long catheters. Their diameters range from 10 Fr to 24 Fr, but 14 Fr is the most useful size. There are many different types used for specialized purposes, including whistle-tipped, Gibbon, Tiemann, Malecot, and Nelaton catheters.

To lower the risk of introducing infection, use an aseptic technique to insert catheters. Use ample lubricant. If you select the appropriate size they should simply glide in. Do not inflate the balloon until you see urine flowing from the catheter. Never use force when inserting a catheter. If you have difficulty then the patient may need a suprapubic catheter. Do not use a catheter introducer unless you have been trained in its use. When you first place the catheter, make a note of the residual urine volume in the patient record.

Laparoscopy

Laparoscopic surgery is the treatment of choice for cholecystectomy, and many gynæcological procedures. It is also used for herniorrhaphy, vagotomy, lumbar sympathectomy, and as a partial procedure for large bowel resections, nephrectomy, and even oesophagectomy.

The advantages of laparoscopy are a smaller wound with less tissue damage. The result is less postoperative pain, less physiological disturbance, and shorter hospital stays.

Problems with laparoscopic surgery include accidental damage to intra-abdominal structures, and the risks of introducing carbon dioxide under pressure. Under pressure gas can escape into the tissues causing subcutaneous emphysema, or even enter blood vessels, causing gas embolism.

Absorption of carbon dioxide can cause hypercarbia and acidosis resulting in cardiac tachyarrhythmias. Patients may come to recovery room flushed, with a tachycardia and a wide pulse pressure.

In the recovery room the patient may still be breathing-off the excess carbon dioxide and consequently feel short of breath. This resolves within a few minutes. The insufflated carbon dioxide has to be excreted eventually through the lungs.

Following abdominal laparoscopy the gas may irritate the diaphragm causing referred pain to the shoulder tip. Typically patients feels as though some-one has wrenched their shoulders. The pain resolves with conventional analgesia.

Abdominal surgery

General principles

Postoperative hypoxaemia is common after abdominal surgery. This is partly a result of pain stopping the patient from taking deep breaths and coughing effectively. The best pain relief is provided by epidural analgesia, although this is not without hazard. Some anaesthetists use intercostal blocks to give temporary relief for a subcostal incision. Once your patient has adequate pain relief you can safely encourage deep breathing and coughing. You may need to support their wound while they do so.

The closer the incision is to the diaphragm,
the more painful it becomes.

For 3 to 5 days after major bowel surgery, such as a Whipple's procedure, large amounts of fluid *transudate* into atonic bowel. Unless the fluid is replaced the patient will become hypovolaemic. The hidden fluid in the bowel is called *third space loss*. To help monitor fluid balance the anaesthetist usually inserts a central venous catheter to guide fluid therapy.

To avoid urinary retention most patients need a catheter after major surgery on the lower abdomen such as hysterectomy or abdominal perineal resection.

The sick laparotomy

A *laparotomy* is a procedure to open the abdomen so that the surgeon can explore the cavity to find out what is wrong.

Emergency laparotomies for intra-abdominal catastrophe are a greater risk than elective laparotomies. Patients are often hypovolaemic and additionally may have systemic sepsis, hypothermia, hypotension, myocardial depression, renal impairment and malfunctioning lungs. Following the procedure patients are usually transferred directly from the operating theatre to the intensive care unit. Recovery room nurses often accompany the anaesthetist on the journey to the intensive care unit.

Moving such a patient from the operating table is fraught with hazard. There are lines, and wires and tubes and drains everywhere begging to be pulled out. Many hands make light work. Do it gently. As soon as the patient is on their bed stop everything and check their vital signs. The simple act of moving sick patients often destabilizes their blood pressure.

Use a plastic slide sheet such as a PatSlide® to gently move the patient from the table. Never use the "one, two three ... heave!" technique where patients are bounced across on a sheet or canvas from the operating table to a trolley or bed. Drips, drains and tubes easily get ripped out, and rough handling will destabilize the patient's blood pressure.

During transfer to the ICU make sure you have an emergency box containing everything you might need on the way. Carry a spare oxygen cylinder.

One difficulty is keeping the multitude of lines, cables, tubes and drains from tangling. Do not disconnect or try to sort the lines. Just move them in bulk. Do make sure they are clearly labelled, both where they leave the pumps, and where the other end of the line enters the patient. A useful technique is to use white sticky paper labels and fold them in half around each line then sort them out and unravel them later. One common error is to spend 10 minutes sorting out the lines, during which time the patient is virtually ignored.

It is well worthwhile, at some convenient time, to spend an hour or so planning and practising how to transfer these sick patients; where to put the pumps, how to carry the infusions, what to do with the monitors and where to hang the drains and so on.

Splenectomy

Splenectomy is an operation to remove the spleen. Splenectomy is used to treat some types of thrombocytopenia; but occasionally, being delicately friable, the spleen is damaged during incidental surgery, starts to bleed and has to be removed. A simple elective splenectomy causes few problems in the recovery room. Apart from pain control, concealed bleeding is the principal immediate risk. Watch for deteriorating skin perfusion, and tachycardia. Do not depend on hypotension to warn you of haemorrhage. Following splenectomy the platelet count increases dramatically, and 2 to 3 days later may reach $750\,000 \times 10^3/mm^3$. This predisposes the patient to forming clots in their great veins.

Colon and rectal surgery

Colon and rectal surgery is usually for cancer and involves opening the abdomen and operating deep inside the pelvis. It is painful so many patients return to the recovery room with epidural analgesia. Test the upper level with ice.

If they have a colostomy or ileostomy, note the volume and nature of the drainage. If there is profuse loss of small bowel content from the stoma, it may intensify the patient's metabolic derangement in the recovery room.

Abdominoperineal resection

During abdominoperineal resection the lower sigmoid, rectum and anus are removed. The ends of the proximal colon are exteriorized to form a permanent colostomy. Check the colour of the colostomy to make sure it is pink. If it looks blue, or congested tell the surgeon. Abdominoperineal resection is a formidable procedure, with considerable tissue damage and blood loss. Patients frequently become hypothermic.

The final phase of the operation, the excision of the rectum, is done with the legs in the lithotomy position. When the legs are lowered blood re-enters the capacitance veins from the central circulation revealing hypovolaemia. Usually the anaesthetist will give the patient a colloid load just before the legs are taken down. Carefully watch the patient for signs of developing hypovolaemia for the first 20 minutes after they return to the recovery room.

Whipple's operation

Whipple operation is major surgery to resect a carcinoma of the head of the pancreas. It is sometimes called a *pancreaticoduodenectomy*, which involves the removal of the gallbladder, common bile duct, part of the duodenum, and the head of the pancreas.

For 3 to 5 days after major bowel surgery large amounts of fluid transudate into atomic bowel as a hidden third space loss. Unless this fluid is replaced as it is lost the patient will become hypovolaemic. The anaesthetist will insert a central venous line to guide fluid replacement.

Cholecystectomy

Cholecystectomy is the surgical removal of the gall bladder when it is inflamed or obstructed, if gallstones have caused pancreatitis, or where cancer is suspected.

Laparoscopic resection is the commonest way of removing the gallbladder. However, about 10 per cent of patients, usually the very obese or those who have had previous abdominal surgery, require a laparotomy. Following this laparotomy the most common complication is right lower lobe atelectasis. In the recovery room encourage deep breathing and coughing to prevent this complication. Coughing is painful and your patient needs excellent analgesia. Morphine can precipitate biliary pain in patients who have had a cholecystectomy. Use pethidine instead.

Internal bleeding can occur, especially if a tie slips off the cystic artery or there is an unnoticed minor laceration of the liver. Back in the ward concealed haemorrhage remains undetected until the patient becomes severely shocked. In the recovery room be suspicious if the patient develops a tachycardia, or their peripheral perfusion deteriorates. Confirm your suspicion by testing for a postural drop in systolic blood pressure.

Abdominal lipectomy

Abdominal lipectomy sometimes called an *apronectomy* or 'tummy tuck', is a traumatic operation. The long incision traverses the lower abdomen, large masses of fat are removed, and the incision is closed under tension. Sometimes blood loss exceeds a litre. The patients are obese, and have similar problems to all obese patients. Pain is often the first sign of a developing haematoma. Check that there is no swelling or wound ooze before giving analgesia. If she wishes to sit up raise both the foot and the head of the bed into the 'banana position' to take the tension off the stitches.

Figure 26.3 Banana position for recovering after abdominal lipectomy (cot sides would normally be in place)

Perineal surgery

Operations on the perineum, such as haemorrhoidectomy, are painful. Often this is usefully controlled with a caudal block, but they tend to wear off abruptly. Warn the patient to ask for analgesia when they first start to feel pain.

Thoracic surgery

General principles

Many patients having thoracic surgery are elderly, and debilitated with malnutrition; some have cancer, others severe lung disease. They need skilled staff to monitor them closely during their stay in the recovery room.

The patient's posture and position affects the ventilation and perfusion of their lungs. If the patient is on a ventilator, the uppermost areas of the lung are better aerated. If the patient is breathing spontaneously then the dependent areas of the lung are better aerated. In both situations the dependent areas of the lungs get more perfusion. To achieve the best outcome you need to position your patient so that aeration matches with perfusion of their lungs. A spontaneously breathing patient in the recovery room has better gas exchange if they are nursed semi-sitting at 45° in Fowler's position.

After thoracic surgery there are four principal acute threats: concealed bleeding, pneumothorax, pneumomediastinum, cardiac tamponade and arrhythmias. A chest X-ray will help with the diagnosis. Pneumothorax presents with dyspnoea, sometimes with pleuritic pain, and a deviated trachea. Tension pneumothorax progresses rapidly to abrupt cardiovascular collapse. With cardiac tamponade the patient first develops a tachycardia, followed by a falling blood pressure, and their JVP rises.

Pneumomediastinum occurs when air leaks into the mediastinum. The air can track into the neck. So feel for crackles (*crepitus*) under the skin in the sternal notch. If you feel crepitus notify the surgeon because the patient may need to return to the operating theatre to patch the leak.

If the pericardium is damaged during surgery the patient may develop cardiac arrhythmias, particularly atrial fibrillation, while in the recovery room. Unrecognized hypomagnesaemia may contribute to this.

Figure 26.4 Set-up for continuous three-bottle low-pressure drainage of the thoracic cavity. Note how the principle of the three-bottle drainage is incorporated into a plastic drainage system moulded to form three chambers

Check that the drain tubes are patent and swinging correctly. Never tie drain tubes to beds, the linen or anything else: if patients roll over they may pull them out. To avoid damaging delicate lung never apply high-pressure suction to the drains or 'milk' the tubing with an old-fashioned roller pump clamp. Never clamp thoracic drains, particularly if they are bubbling or the patient is being ventilated. Air that is unable to escape will quickly build up to cause a tension pneumothorax. Do not lift drain bottles on to the bed. Keep the drain bottles below the patient otherwise fluid in the bottle may drain back into the patient.

Occasionally air leaks occur, and the patient becomes acutely breathless. Notify the surgeon and prepare to return the patient to theatre to control the leak.

If the surgeon opens both the peritoneal and the thoracic cavity or divides the diaphragm, then the patient usually remains intubated, and will be extubated later in ICU. Otherwise patients come to recovery room extubated. As soon as possible sit them up. This improves their oxygenation and ability to breathe and cough effectively. They should return to the ward on continuous humidified supplemental oxygen overnight.

Bronchoscopy

Bronchoscopy is used to inspect the airways and to help diagnose lung disease, also, to take a biopsy, or remove a foreign body, and occasionally to insert airway stents. Occasionally it is used to treat certain lung conditions. Fibreoptic bronchoscopy is usually done under local anaesthetic as an outpatient procedure, whereas rigid bronchoscopy requires a general anaesthetic because an instrument resembling a 40 cm pipe is passed into the trachea.

If the patient returns to the recovery room still unconscious after a bronchial biopsy then nurse them on their side with the biopsy side down so that if they bleed, the blood will not enter the unaffected lung on the opposite side. As soon as they are awake sit them up, and support them on two or three pillows.

Following rigid bronchoscopy patients often cough uncontrollably. The anaesthetist will probably have sprayed the throat and larynx with lidocaine before the patient comes to the recovery room; but despite this they may cough violently, become hypoxic and distressed. The anaesthetist may suggest controlling this with lidocaine 1 mg/Kg made up to 5 ml in saline and given by a nebulizer. Take care that nothing the patient coughs up touches any part of you. Wear a gown, gloves and goggles.

Mediastinoscopy

The *mediastinum* is the space that separates the lungs and lies between the sternum and the spinal column. It contains the heart, oesophagus, trachea, large blood vessels, the thymus, and lymph nodes. During mediastinoscopy a lighted instrument called the *mediastinoscope* is inserted through a small incision in the neck. This enables the surgeon to directly view the structures in the upper thorax. Mediastinoscopy enables examination of the lymph nodes in a patient with lung cancer, and if necessary a biopsy of suspect areas is used to stage their disease.

Patients come to recovery room with a small wound and no drains. However, their thoracic cavity may conceal much mischief, such as massive occult bleeding from a damaged great vein or pneumothorax from a breached lung. Watch for signs of airway obstruction, deviation of the trachea and developing dyspnoea. A chest X-ray will reveal widening of the mediastinum or air outside the lungs. Air can track into the neck, so feel for crackles (*crepitus*) under the skin in the sternal notch or neck. If you feel crepitus notify the surgeon and prepare to insert a chest drain. The patient may need to return to the operating theatre.

Oesophagectomy

Oesophagectomy involves the surgical removal of part of the oesophagus for cancer, or high-grade dysplasia of the lower oesophageal mucosa (*Barrett's oesophagitis*). This procedure is usually performed with laparoscopic and thorascopic instruments, reducing the extent and severity of the surgery. If the chest and abdomen are opened this becomes a major, long and often bloody exercise. A length of bowel with its blood supply replaces the excised oesophagus. The principal risk is disruption of the anastomoses followed by frequently fatal mediastinal infection. Worldwide the peri-operative mortality rate is about 10 per cent but is less than 2 per cent in specialized units.[2]

Most patients remain intubated after surgery, and are then transferred to ICU for a short period of ventilation. Their stay in recovery room is usually brief. Those who do stay in the recovery room need intensive and experienced nursing. Plan to allocate two nurses to care for them. Watch the ECG carefully. About 60 per cent of patients develop postoperative cardiac arrhythmias (particularly atrial fibrillation) and 20 per cent get major respiratory complications.

If patients are extubated in the recovery room, wait until their temperature is greater than 35.8°C. Check that you can hear normal breath sounds over the right side of the chest, and the underwater seals on the chest drain tubes are swinging or bubbling correctly. Check that the nasogastric (NG) tube is stitched through the frenulum of the nose so it cannot be accidentally pulled out. The NG prevents accumulating fluid distending the relocated bowel and tearing the stitches out. Make sure the NG tube is draining freely. Aspirate it gently.

Thymectomy

Thymectomy is excision of the thymus gland that lies in the upper mediastinum. This is usually done in an attempt to relieve the symptoms and modify the progress of myasthenia gravis. Thymectomy is typically done through a sternal split. Postoperatively there is a slight risk of pneumomediastinum.

Myaesthenics commonly take the anticholinergic drug (pyridostigmine) to counteract the muscle weakness. Pyridostigmine is often omitted for a few hours before surgery and recommenced in the recovery room. Some patients need postoperative ventilation until they are able to breathe and cough adequately. Those who have had respiratory failure in the past, or who are taking more than 750 mg of pyridostigmine a day are likely to require postoperative ventilation. Do not extubate them until they can sustain a 5-second head lift. They must return to their maintenance anti-cholinesterase drugs as soon as possible. If necessary give these drugs down a nasogastric tube.

Sometimes neostigmine is used as an alternative to pyridostigmine. For every 30 mg of pyridostigmine they are taking preoperatively, use intravenous neostigmine 1 mg postoperatively. You will need to give atropine with the neostigmine to prevent bradycardia, salivation, abdominal cramps and bronchorroea. Start with intravenous neostigmine 2.5 mg and atropine 1.2 mg given over two minutes. Continue giving neostigmine in 1 mg boluses every 3 minutes until you reach the equivalent dose of pyridostigmine. For instance, if the patient is taking a 120 mg pyridostigmine, the maximum dose of neostigmine is 4 mg. You may need to repeat the neostigmine in 2 to 4 hours time depending on their ability to lift their head off the pillow.

Vascular surgery
General principles

Vascular surgery is used to repair major blood vessels, damaged or obstructed by trauma or disease. Vascular surgery is physiologically stressful. Major vessels are clamped diverting blood flow through unaccustomed routes. Blood loss may be large, renal and gut blood flow is often abruptly compromised, the operations are long, and the patient usually has associated illnesses, such as ischaemic heart disease, cerebrovascular disease, and frequently diabetes.

Intensive monitoring

Many patients are intensively monitored with an arterial line, triple lumen central venous catheter, 5-lead ECG, and possibly a pulmonary artery catheter in their right subclavian or left internal jugular vein, and a urinary catheter.

These patients need close observation in the recovery room. They are at high risk of coronary ischaemia, and more than half do not get the warning chest pain.

Major aortic surgery

Abdominal aortic aneurysm repair is the commonest major abdominal vascular procedure. An aneurysm occurs when a blood vessel swells, stretching its walls and ballooning abnormally outward. The normal diameter of the aorta is about 2.5 cm. If the lumen swells to more than 6.5 cm the aorta is likely to acute rupture and the patient will probably bleed to death.

At the end of major vascular surgery patients appear haemodynamically stable. As soon as they are moved on to their bed for transport, they drop their blood pressure and central venous pressure, revealing that they are hypovolaemic.

If they are not transferred directly to ICU or HDU postoperatively, they may remain in the recovery room for a lengthy time.

Potential problems

- Hypothermia. Patients will fare better if they are electively ventilated until their temperature rises beyond 36°C.

- Myocardial ischaemia is common. Monitor closely for ST changes using a 5-lead ECG (leads II and V5).

- Cardiac support. The patient may well be receiving ionotropes or vasodilators delivered through syringe pumps.

- Renal hypoperfusion. Up to 25 per cent of patients develop renal impairment after aortic surgery. Closely monitor urine output. If urine output is < 30 ml/hr, then try a fluid challenge of 5 ml/Kg of saline.

- Pain. Analgesia is best achieved with a T6–T11 epidural infusion preferably with diamorphine, which is more effective than fentanyl. Those who do not have an epidural will need patient-controlled analgesia.

- Ongoing bleeding. Hypothermia is the usual cause. Check the preoperative transfusion threshold and give blood if it has been exceeded. Check the activated clotting time; it should not exceed 140 seconds. Use platelets first and fresh frozen plasma only if needed.

- Spinal cord ischaemia causing paraplegia is a rare and devastating complication.

Carotid surgery

Carotid endarterectomy is a surgical procedure to open the lumen of the internal carotid artery and remove plaque so that blood flow can be restored to the brain. It is usually performed when carotid stenosis is greater than 70 per cent or the patient is experiencing neurological symptoms.

The danger is not over once the surgery is completed. The two most likely complications are stroke and myocardial infarction. Complications can appear within minutes, so keep patients under close observation in the recovery room for at least 3–4 hours postoperatively rather than transferring them to ICU.

Postoperatively about 5 per cent of patients develop a blood clot on the raw lining of the artery, usually within two hours of surgery. This causes signs of a stroke. If the artery is unblocked within 30 minutes the stroke will, most likely, resolve.

Patients should be able to lift each leg off the bed, and strongly grip two of your offered fingers with each hand. Ask patients to show you their teeth, and watch for asymmetry in their grin.

Watch for bleeding causing swelling in the neck; it may progress to cause respiratory obstruction. Check the drain tubes are allowing blood to escape. Notify the anaesthetist and surgeon if the patient develops noisy breathing, or stridor.

Because of trauma to the baroreceptors up to 65 per cent of patients become hypertensive and up to 35 per cent become hypotensive. Hypertension forewarns of deterioration in cerebral function or stroke, and also cardiac ischaemia. Notify the anaesthetist if the systolic blood pressure exceeds 160 mmHg. Use short-acting nitroglycerine to control blood pressure, and avoid longer acting agents such as hydralazine.

Cerebral hyperperfusion syndrome may cause a migraine like headache. As the blood supply is restored the weakened cerebral vessel walls stretch; they may even burst, causing stroke.

Watch for signs of cerebral hypoperfusion, such as nausea, and deteriorating conscious state. Stroke tends to cause unilateral signs. In contrast whereas cerebral hypoperfusion causes more global dysfunction with agitation, clouding of consciousness, seizures, and unless relieved, stroke. The patient must return to the ward with meticulously defined postoperative orders.

Breast surgery

Mastectomy

Mastectomy involves the surgical removal of an entire breast, usually to treat serious breast cancer.

There are four types of mastectomy: subcutaneous mastectomy; total or simple mastectomy; modified radical mastectomy; and radical mastectomy.

It most cases, breast cancer is treated by limited mastectomy with identification of a sentinel node, and selective lymphatic resection. However, radical mastectomy is a much larger procedure involving removal of the chest wall pectoral muscles in addition to the breast and axillary lymph nodes. In the past this operation was the standard for women with breast cancer, but fortunately it is rarely necessary today.

After mastectomy nurse patients on their back with their heads turned to one side in case they vomit. If they are obese sit them up as soon as they are fully conscious. Tight breast-binding dressings achieve little. The pressure they exert is insufficient to stop bleeding or prevent haematoma, and they severely impede the patient's ability to deep breathe and cough effectively.

On the side of the operation elevate the patient's arm on two pillows. Extension of surgery into the axilla may impede venous return causing the arm to become congested and blue. If this happens notify the surgeon. To avoid putting tension on her stitches, help her to change position if she is uncomfortable.

Figure 26.5 The mastectomy position

Breast reduction surgery

Breast reduction surgery is done for women to reduce the bulk of their massive breasts. Sometimes kilograms of breast tissue are removed, and 1500 ml or more blood can be lost. Pain can be a problem.

Gynaecology
General principles

Gynaecological surgery is pelvic surgery conducted on women's reproductive organs. It may involve opening the abdominal cavity, but many operations can be done through the vagina.

Higher risk of deep vein thrombosis

Gynaecological surgery often subtly disturbs venous blood flow back from the legs. These women are at a higher risk of deep vein thrombosis. Most deep vein thromboses start in the recovery room, so encourage leg movements. Make sure they are written up for suitable thromboprophylaxis.

Patients who have had their legs in lithotomy position for more that 30 minutes frequently become hypotensive when their legs are laid flat again. When their legs are elevated about 400–600 ml of blood runs down into their central veins. As their legs are let down, the blood re-enters their legs, their central venous returns falls, and they become abruptly hypotensive. Nurse these patients with their legs elevated on pillows for the first hour, and give them 5 ml/Kg of intravenous fluid during that time.

Nausea and vomiting

Because surgery on the uterus and ovaries stimulates the vagus nerve, nausea and vomiting are common. This form of nausea usually responds to metoclopramide.

Vaginal surgery

Vaginal surgery is performed with the legs in lithotomy. Over-abduction of the legs causes postoperative hip or knee pain. If the patient has hip or knee pain, then record this fact in the notes and notify the surgeon. Check their pads for continued vaginal bleeding.

Hysteroscopy

Hysteroscopy involves a visual inspection of the lining of the uterus with a fibreoptic hysteroscope. To allow a view, irrigation fluid is instilled into the uterus opening up the cavity. Some of this fluid may be absorbed. Irrigation fluid causes the same problems as the *TURP syndrome*. Unlike men, premenopausal women and children risk fatal cerebral oedema if their serum sodium falls abruptly below 130 mmol/L, whereas men and postmenopausal women do not run this risk until their serum sodium falls below 125 mmol/L. In the recovery room cerebral oedema first shows up as a headache which is made worse when patients move their head around.

Tubal surgery

Cauterization of the Fallopian tubes is painful. Some surgeons drip 0.5% bupivacaine into the cut end of the tubes, which provides excellent pain relief for the first hour. Nausea and vomiting can be troublesome. If the pain is spasmodic it may respond to pethidine more than morphine.

Surgery on the limbs

Hand surgery is often done under regional blockade. The usual local anaesthetic used for brachial plexus blocks is lidocaine because it has 2–3 hour action. If the anaesthetist has used bupivacaine then reassure the patient feeling will return eventually though it may take a day or more. Since the arm is both numb and paralysed, warn the patient not to try to move their hand because it can fly about uncontrollably. Patients have hit themselves in the face while attempting to investigate their new plaster; some have even broken their noses. Following hand surgery the arm is usually splinted, with at least a plaster back-slab. Elevate the arm in a box-sling to reduce swelling. Monitor the perfusion of the fingers.

Figure 26.6 Box sling

Amputations

Amputation of a lower limb is occasionally performed for trauma, but more often for arterial insufficiency. In the latter case the patients are usually old, sick and frail with a combination of ischaemic heart disease, malnutrition, diabetes, and the accumulated ravages of decades of smoking. Apart from the diabetics, who are protected by numbness from peripheral neuropathy, most patients have considerable pain, and have received high doses of opioids over the preceding days or weeks. This means they need proportionally higher doses of opioids that you would otherwise expect.

Amputation is best done under spinal anaesthetic or epidural anaesthesia, as this reduces the risk of postoperative *phantom limb pain*. Having protracted, excrutiating pain in a limb that no longer exists affects about 65% of amputees, and the pain is refractory to most therapy. This pain is a form of chronic pain. To help alleviate this problem patients require outstanding analgesia postoperatively.

Send patients back to the ward with an Esmark's bandage taped to the top of their bed, so that should a ligature come off a major artery a tourniquet can be applied immediately before they bleed to death.

Orthopaedic surgery

General principles

Operations on bones are painful. Do not be alarmed if young patients especially need more than the usual amount of opioids to control their pain. It is best to start analgesia before they reach the recovery room, and use a multimodal technique. Fortunately much lower limb orthopaedic surgery is now performed under either spinal or epidural technique that effectively controls pain.

Tourniquets

Operations done under tourniquet, such as knee replacements, may bleed vigorously, up to a litre or more, while the patient is in the recovery room. Monitor the drain bottles for blood loss. Check the patient's records for a cause such as aspirin, NSAIDs, SSRIs or even herbal remedies. Also check that blood is available should a transfusion become necessary.

Type 2 diabetics who take metformin are at risk of severe lactic acidosis unless this drug has been ceased at least 36 hours before surgery. Metformin prevents the liver metabolizing the huge flood of lactic acid which suddenly enters the central circulation when the tourniquet is released. If the patient starts to hyperventilate or their pulse rate rises, then notify the anaesthetist immediately.

Arthroscopy

Arthroscopy is painful. It is usually done as a day case procedure. Most surgeons put a small dose of morphine into the joint, which controls pain for 24 hours or more. If the patient complains of pain in the recovery room it may indicate bleeding into the operation site. Notify the surgeon.

Hip surgery

Patients having hip replacement surgery tend to lose blood, and they continue to bleed into the surgical site for some time after they have left theatre.

Several litres of blood can be lost during hip replacements and after fractures of the femoral neck. Blood spilled on the floor and drapes make it difficult to estimate the loss, and the patient may come to recovery room either hypovolaemic or fluid overloaded. Often patients continue to bleed in the recovery room. The loss may be concealed inside the wound, and unless detected the patient may be discharged to the ward still bleeding. This has been the cause of a number of deaths. Up to 1500 ml of blood can be lost into a thigh before it starts to swell noticeably.

Hypoxia is a constant threat to elderly orthopaedic patients.

It is usually the elderly, with all their concurrent medical problems, who have hip surgery. Elderly patients with fractured necks of femurs are almost always hypoxic before they get to theatre; and the hypoxaemia becomes worse postoperatively. Following hip surgery patients often become hypoxaemic in the recovery room, especially if they have had a general anaesthetic. Periodic hypoxaemia can recur for up to five days after surgery. "Grandma was never the same after she broke her hip." Hypoxaemia usually occurs at night during sleep, and remains mostly unrecognized. It contributes to postoperative confusion and the residual cognitive damage may be permanent. This tragedy is avoidable. Mandatory supplemental oxygen, especially for the first few nights, reduces the risk substantially.

Contributing factors to the risk of hypoxia are opioid infusions, fat emboli; and although not often considered malnutrition contributes to muscle wasting so that these elderly patients cannot cough or deep breathe effectively.

Abduction pillow

After hip replacement surgery, a Charnley (*abduction*) pillow is used to keep the legs apart, strapped in the abduction position. Before you put on the pillow check the circulation to the feet. Put the wide end between the ankles. Apply the straps in such a way that you can easily slip your fingers between the strap and the skin. Be careful not to compress the peroneal nerve with the straps.

Routine orthopaedic observations

- Check the drain tubes every 15 minutes. Make sure they are patent. Record the volume of drainage, and its colour and nature: serous, clotted blood, or bloodstained fluid.
- Check the neurovascular status every 15 minutes. This includes: volume of peripheral pulses, limb colour and temperature, rate of capillary refilling; as well as occurrence of numbness, tingling, swelling and if possible movement.
- Keep the limb in the correct position set by the surgeon.
- Check for evidence of fat emboli.

Plaster checks

If a patient has a plaster applied check the exposed limb distal to the plaster to see that circulation is not impaired.

Observe and record:

- Warmth, colour and capillary refilling.
- Movement of fingers or toes.
- Sensation and presence of pain, numbness or tingling.
- Pulses.
- State of plaster; whether it is showing signs of bloodstains or seepage.

Hints about plasters

- Elevate the arm or leg on a pillow to help prevent swelling.
- You cannot rely on numbness or tingling to warn of nerve compression if the patient has had a regional anaesthetic.
- Capillary refill is the most useful sign. Gently squeeze a finger or toenail bed. Blood should flush back pink within 2 seconds.
- Pain in a plastered limb is an ominous sign of ischaemia. Tell the surgeon immediately.
- Occasionally, muscles cramp or spasm inside the plaster. This usually responds to a small dose of diazepam 2 mg given intravenously.
- Outline any oozy stains on the plaster with an indelible pen. Put the date and time on the boundaries.
- Always ask the surgeon to review the plaster before the patient returns to the ward.

Surgery of the head and neck

General principles

Following head and neck surgery, the principal worry is the patency of the patient's airway. Bleeding behind the deep fascia in the neck can obstruct lymph and venous drainage from the surgical site without much obvious swelling on the outside, however the swelling inside may rapidly obstruct the airway. Check the drain tubes are draining. The first sign of airway obstruction will be noisy breathing. Notify the anaesthetist immediately.

The vagus nerve is often disturbed during surgery, and this predisposes to nausea and vomiting. Surgery around the bifurcation of the carotid artery can disturb baroreceptors, so that blood pressure may be unstable for some hours after the operation.

Blepharoplasty or meloplasty

After facelifts or eyelid surgery sit the patient up. The eyes are sometimes bandaged. If the patient complains of pain it may mean a haematoma is developing beneath the dressings. Sterile iced water-soaked pads help reduce the swelling. Do not disturb these patients, or encourage coughing. Let them recover quietly. Before discharging patients back to the ward check for double vision, a sign of a developing haematoma.

Faciomaxillary procedures

Major jaw surgery may take 4–6 hours. These patients are often young, the surgery is painful and they require deep anaesthesia. It may take some time to for them to wake up. They sometimes come to the recovery room still intubated. The anaesthetist can not extubate the patient until they are sufficiently awake to look after their own airway. After mandibular surgery the teeth may be fixed together with elastic bands.

Nasal surgery

Following nasal surgery the nose is usually packed with stuffed glove fingers, gauze, silk, or yellow BIP paste. Partially conscious patients find it difficult to breathe through their mouths, and are distressed at having their airway blocked, they may become restless and thrash about. The anaesthetist should remain with patients until they are fully conscious. Sit them up as soon as possible. This helps reduce venous bleeding into the soft tissues around the eyes, and postoperative facial swelling.

Opioids are best given intra-operatively and NSAIDs postoperatively. Pain is not usually a problem as the surgeon injects local anaesthetic. Opioids, if they are used, may suppress ventilation. They can also cause the patient to get a very itchy nose, which he may attempt to rub vigorously. A small dose of promethazine 6.25 mg IM usually resolves the problem. Naloxone will remove the itch, but plunge the patient into pain.

Sometimes a piece of tissue or blood clot will fall on to the vocal cords causing laryngospasm, coughing or a hoarse voice. If you suspect this has happened the anaesthetist may check the larynx, and pharynx with a laryngoscope.

A large blood clot can easily be hidden in the nasal pharynx where it cannot be seen. This *coroner's clot* can be aspirated without warning into the trachea, to totally block the airway. After surgery on the upper airway gently use a dental sucker to explore the nasopharynx.

Figure 26.7 The coroner's clot

An excessively dry throat may make patients restless. Once they are fully conscious, give them a piece of wet gauze to suck or little sips of water.

Sometimes small bits of plaster get into the eyes and irritate them. If this happens, notify the surgeon, and record the fact in the history. Irrigate the eyes with sterile 0.9% saline. Check the eyes are not red before discharging the patient to the ward. Cold wet swabs to their eyes are comforting, and help prevent peri-orbital bruising.

Tonsillectomy

Following tonsillectomy bleeding into the pharynx is a grave danger. Nurse these patients in the *recovery position* without a pillow until they are conscious. With patients weighing less than 50 Kg put a pillow under their hips and tilt them slightly head down so that the blood can drain from their mouth.

Tonsillectomies are painful, but there are problems if the patient is deeply sedated after this operation. Check with the surgeon or anaesthetist before giving additional opioids. Patients with sleep apnoea are at particular risk of obstructed airways, and silently become apnoeic. Always have a working sucker tucked under their pillow. Use soft plastic catheters, which will not dislodge stitches, or damage friable surgical site, rather than the standard metal sucker.

A bleeding tonsil is a major recovery room emergency. Ensure every patient has freely flowing intravenous infusion sited, just in case it is needed. If it is accidentally pulled out replace it immediately. Most tonsillectomies need intravenous fluids for 24 hours. If you are continually aspirating blood from the pharynx notify the surgeon. Remember that babies and infants are seriously compromised with as little as 10 per cent blood loss. This may only be two well-soaked small swabs in infants.

Figure 26.8 Tonsillectomy position

Cleft palate

After repairing a cleft palate the surgeon may put a loose looping suture through the tongue. To clear the airway, gently pull the loop forward. Leave the suture in place for 36 hours until the facial swelling subsides. Pain can be a problem, so give analgesia early. Keep the face clean and watch for oozing from the nose or mouth. Notify the surgeon if it continues. It may be necessary to splint the arms of children so they cannot suck their fingers. Monitor their oxygenation with an oximeter. Never turn your back on children, because respiratory obstruction may occur quickly, silently and without warning. You will find it easier to monitor the child's heart rate by feeling the apex beat, rather than the carotid or radial pulse.

Dental surgery

Many of the problems with the care of postoperative dental patients are those of tonsillectomy. Hypoxaemia and airway problems remain a risk. Nurse the patient in the recovery position. Check that those with valvular heart disease have received antibiotic prophylaxis against endocarditis. In dental patients diclofenac or ibuprofen gives better pain relief than paracetamol and codeine.

Intellectually disabled patients

It is almost impossible to do dental procedures in intellectually handicapped patients under local anaesthetic. These patients need general anaesthesia for even minor procedures. Many will have Down's syndrome; of these 40 per cent have valvular heart disease and need antibiotic prophylaxis against endocarditis. People with Down's syndrome have a lower intelligence than normal, and are easily confused by unfamiliar routines. They may become frightened when away from people they know and trust. Adult patients can be very strong indeed, and some become combative when frightened or in pain.

Sometimes they have 'security blankets' – a favourite object – these can come to theatre and recovery room with the patient.

Intellectually disabled patients require one nurse dedicated to the patient. You may need strong attendants. Midazolam quickly controls agitation, but the effective dose is highly variable. Some are easily sedated with a small dose, while others are quite resistant. Patients with Down's syndrome are particularly sensitive to opioids, and require about half the dose of a normal person. Their biggest risk is airway obstruction. They have short stiff necks and large tongues, and are particularly susceptible to laryngeal stridor. Some patients have unstable atlanto-occipital joints. Be especially gentle when extending their bull-necks, because you may dislocate their cervical spine and render them quadriplegic.

Thyroid and parathyroid surgery

After thyroid or parathyroid surgery, sit the patients up as soon as they regain consciousness. Check and resecure their dressings. These patients are frequently nauseated because the surgeon has retracted on, or near, the vagus nerve in the neck. Check which anti-emetic they have received during their anaesthetic, and choose another from a different group. Suitable alternatives are prochlorperazine 12.5 mg IM, or metoclopramide 15 mg IV, or ondansetron 4–8 mg IV. If they have received preoperative instruction, properly applied acupressure is surprisingly effective in these patients.

Concealed bleeding, usually from the superior thyroid artery, beneath the deep fascia in the neck, blocks lymphatic and deep venous drainage, and can quickly cause airway obstruction. The problem is not tracheal compression, but rather obstruction of veins, and especially lymph drainage, which rapidly causes submucosal oedema. If you look in the mouth you will find the mucosa of the pharynx ballooning into the lumen. If the patient develops noisy breathing or stridor then notify the anaesthetist immediately.

The internal swelling generally makes re-intubation either hazardous or impossible. In this case sit the patient up. Give high concentrations of oxygen. Wherever possible the patient should return to the operating theatre for the surgeon to control the bleeding. If not, you must act alone. Take out the skin clips or sutures and the wound will fall open. Using sterile instruments take out the deep sutures running transversely across the deep fascia at the bottom of the wound. Blood will gush out, and the tissues will fall away exposing the trachea. If necessary you can push a percutaneous tracheostomy tube beneath the first tracheal ring to gain an airway. Usually this will not be necessary. Opening the wound can do no harm, and you may save the patient's life.

Management of stridor after thyroid operation

Step 1. Put the patient on high inspired oxygen, and sit him up.

Step 2. Take out the skin clips or sutures. The wound will fall open

Step 3. Using sterile instruments take out the sutures running transversely in a straight line in the bottom of the wound. The tissues will fall open, and allow the blood to drain out. No harm can be done by this procedure, and it may save the patient's life.

Remove
these stitches

Figure 26.9 The stitches to remove should stridor occur

Send the patient back to the ward with a sterile pack containing all the instruments needed to take out the stitches. The pack should be fastened to the head of the bed so that the instruments are available immediately should the stitches need to be removed in a hurry.

Radical neck dissection

Radical neck dissection is a traumatic operation for cancer of the oropharynx or salivary glands. It involves en-bloc resection of all the lymph nodes and vessels from the mandible to clavicle along the course of the jugular vein. Airway obstruction is a major risk, and most patients will return to recovery room with an elective tracheostomy, and a number of drains inserted to allow blood to escape. Watch for swelling in the operative field indicating bleeding below the deep fascia. The risk of swelling in the neck is similar to that of a thyroidectomy.

Operations on the left side of the neck may damage the thoracic duct, in which case milky *lymph* may appear in the drain bottles.

Pneumothorax can follow major neck surgery. Suspect it if the patient develops stabbing chest pain or difficulty in breathing. The larynx may be pushed away from its midline position toward the affected side. Percuss the chest. A pneumothorax has the same deep hollow quality you will hear if you percuss a pillow.

Urological surgery

General principles

Patients undergoing urological surgery are usually elderly people with multiple intercurrent diseases. They are prone to developing complications in the first 2 hours after surgery. Keep them a little longer, and do not discharge them until you are sure they are stable. Just because they are awake does not mean trouble is not looming.

Because common urological operations have long names they are usually abbreviated:

- Transurethral resection of the prostate = TURP.
- Transurethral bladder tumour resection = TURBT.
- Percutaneous nephrolithotomy = PCNL.

Sepsis

A urinary tract can host a variety of bacteria. During TURPs, or when the surgeon relieves a chronic obstruction, a shower of bacteria may enter the blood stream. The cell membranes of Gram-negative bacteria contain incredibly potent *endotoxins*. This endotoxic shower manifests as a short episode of hypotension, sometimes with severe chills, and flushing. If the temperature starts to rise then it indicates septicaemia. Gentamicin 2 mg/Kg is the usual prophylaxis against this event. A single dose of gentamicin will do no harm, but another dose should not be given until the patient's creatinine clearance is calculated; otherwise there is a risk of kidney damage and irreversible deafness. Furosemide greatly accentuates gentamicin's toxicity.

Transurethral resection of the prostate

Those who have had a spinal anaesthetic for TURPs are especially vulnerable to complications. They have been flooded with irrigation fluid, sometimes 20 litres or more, some of which they may have absorbed and they have had their legs raised in lithotomy position for a long time.

Hypothermia is a big problem. Patients can get very cold. The elderly do not tolerate this well. Prevention is better than cure. Warm all irrigating and intravenous fluids. Use convection warming blankets on the patient in the recovery room. Do not discharge the patient back to the ward until his temperature is greater than 36.5°C.

When the patient's legs are taken down from the lithotomy position, up to 800 ml of blood can rush back into the leg veins and the blood pressure may suddenly fall. To prevent this elevate the legs on pillows while the patient is in the recovery room. Give intravenous colloid continuously until the patient is stable.

TURPs are not particularly painful. If the patient complains of pain then suspect clot retention or even a ruptured bladder.

TURP syndrome

TURP syndrome is a serious problem. It occurs when irrigation fluid enters the circulation causing a combination of acute hyponatraemia and acute fluid overload. The most usual irrigating solution contains 1.5% glycine in water. If the patient has had more than 15 litres of irrigation fluid, or has been on the table for longer than 45 minutes then expect problems. On the patient's arrival in the recovery room send blood to check the haemoglobin levels and serum sodium concentration.

Acute hyponatraemia causes the conscious state to deteriorate. The patient initially describes tingling or numbness around the mouth, and then may find it difficult to form thoughts and talk coherently. Headache, vomiting, confusion soon follow. Finally the patient may have convulsions and lose consciousness. Symptoms appear when the serum sodium (Na^+) drops below 130 mmol/L, becomes severe when Na^+ concentration is less than 125 mmol/L and is often fatal when less than 120 mmol/L.

Acute volume overload presents first with a rising respiratory rate, decreasing oxygen saturations, then cough, then wheeze; and finally overt pulmonary oedema. At this stage the patient is unable to lie flat and is coughing up frothy pink fluid.

Once the central nervous system is affected, consider using hypertonic 3% saline. Using this requires judgement and experience, and is better done in an intensive care unit.

Glycine toxicity

Glycine toxicity occurs if sufficient glycine enters the circulation. This may cause transient blindness with or without cardiac failure. Other signs are a sequential progression of nausea, vomiting, slowing respiratory rate, confusions, and convulsions.

Burns

Managing patients with burns is a challenge. After surgery they are physiologically unstable and may respond unpredictably so assign your most experienced staff to look after them.

Burns oedema and limb ischaemia

The patient becomes oedematous about 18 hours after major burns. As oedema develops, circumferential burns on a limb act like a non-flexible tourniquet. Regularly check peripheral capillary return, if a limb becomes congested, or white, an *escharotomy* is urgently needed. This involves cutting the tight band of dead tissue strangling the limb. It is a relatively painless procedure, and does not require an anaesthetic, but it may bleed vigorously so be prepared to give a rapid transfusion.

Airway burns

Patients with facial burns always have airway burns too, and probably smoke damage to bronchi and lung tissue. As the airway becomes progressively oedematous and swollen, wheezing, or noisy breathing warns of impending airway obstruction. Watch for agitation, or restlessness heralding hypoxia.

If the lips and tongue swell to close the airway you may need to gently insert a soft nasopharyngeal airway as a temporary measure. Lubricate it well with 2% lidocaine gel. Even in a conscious patient these airways are well tolerated. Avoid rigid plastic tubes, which can damage tissues, rupture nasal cartilages, and introduce infection into the paranasal sinuses.

Burnt face = burnt airway.

Monitoring

It can be difficult to find somewhere to put the ECG dots, or blood pressure cuffs. The ECG dots can go anywhere on the limbs, and they can even be put on the head if necessary. Just place them so they form the corners of an equilateral triangle around the heart. If the arms are burnt then use a large blood pressure cuff on the thigh to measure blood pressure.

Pain

With full thickness burnt skin the nerve endings are destroyed so the burn is painless. Debridement of burns, especially the hands or feet, is very painful. Donor sites are more painful than the grafted area. If the debrided areas are extensive local blocks are impractical.

Patients with acute burns are often in a lot of pain. Their pain is made worse because they are frightened. Take time to comfort and reassure them. As you remove their anxiety much of their pain will dissipate. One remembers the compassionate nurse who stroked a burnt man's forehead –his pain disappeared and he fell asleep.

If high doses of opioids are ineffective, or only give short periods of pain relief, supplement it with ketamine. Use a loading dose of ketamine 0.1 mg/Kg followed by an infusion of 1–4 mg/Kg/hr. Use the larger dose in a young person, and lower in the elderly. To reduce the chance of hallucinations, keep the environment quiet, and do not disturb the patient. Use a small dose of diazepam or diazamul to reduce the chance of hallucinations; midazolam is too short-acting to be useful.

Hypothermia

Hypothermia is a grave problem. In the operating theatre the ambient temperature is low and the evaporative losses are high. Burnt patients are invariably hypothermic on their return to the recovery room. To minimize further heat loss, increase the ambient air temperature to above 30°C. Cover the patient with a warm air blanket, space blanket and warm towels. Warm all intravenous or dialysate fluids. Heat and humidify the inspired air if possible. Monitor the patient's core temperature with a temporal artery infra-red scanner, oesophageal probe, or tympanic membrane sensor.

Fluid balance

Monitor central venous pressure and urinary output. It is well known that patients with burns lose a lot of fluid, but over-enthusiastic resuscitation risks pulmonary oedema. Conversely, renal failure and shock occur if fluid replacement is not adequate. Maintain the central venous pressure 9–12 cm of water above the level of the right atrium. Avoid diuretics, because the hourly urine output is a useful guide to volume replacement in the early stages of burns resuscitation.

Bleeding

Grafted and donor sites can bleed extensively. Watch the bandages carefully for signs of further blood or fluid loss. Monitor the patient for signs of impending hypovolaemia: tachycardia, a urine output less than 30 ml/hr and poor peripheral circulation.

If a burnt patient becomes sweaty and hypotensive consider either septicaemia or hypovolaemia.

Notes

1. Menon MA, Menom B, Menon MI (2002) *Hospital Medicine* 63:282–8.
2. Sherry KM (2001) *British Journal of Anaesthesia* 86: 611–13.

27

Infection control

In Britain, hospital acquired infection kills 5000 patients a year, and consumes the resources of twenty-seven, 400-bed hospitals. The cost is phenomenal.[1]

Transmission of infectious diseases between patients and staff, and between one patient and another is preventable. There are two main issues: keeping yourself safe from infections the patients may be carrying, and keeping the patients safe from infections carried by other patients or health care workers. If staff do not adhere to strict protocols they place everyone at risk.

How infections occur

There is a clearly recognizable chain of events that lead to infection. Each link in the chain is necessary, and the more links we remove the less likely cross-infection can occur.

The chain comprises:

- a source;
- a mode of transmission;
- a breach in body defences;
- leading to infection.

The chain of infection

1. There must be an infectious agent: virus, bacteria, fungi, protozoa or prion.

2. An infectious agent needs a source or reservoir where it can thrive and replicate; or at least settle. Patients are a good reservoir, especially as they are a source of pus, blood, faeces, or flakes of skin (called *squames*). Some organisms remain for long periods on equipment, linen, benches and stethoscopes simply waiting to hitch-hike to a suitable host. Hepatitis B can survive for 7 days, and hepatitis C for 13 days or more at room temperature on dried blood. HIV is fragile and survives outside the host for only a few minutes.

3. If a patient is infected, then there has to be some way the micro-organism can leave their body. The vehicle may be droplets from a sneeze or cough, or secretions, blood, skin squames, urine, or faeces.

4. The micro-organism then has to travel to the next person. This can occur through direct contact, or indirect contact (e.g. hitch-hiking on a stethoscope, blood pressure cuffs or your hands). It can be airborne spread; transmitted through a vector (such as a malarial mosquito, or house fly), ingested in contaminated food, or it can be inoculated through a breach in the skin (needle stick injury) or absorbed through a mucous membrane (influenza).

5. People vary in their susceptibility to infection. While some are already immune, others are immunologically compromised in the presence of disease. Many elderly patients are suffering from severe degrees of unrecognized malnutrition, which leaves them open to infection.

Important organisms

Some infections are more hazardous to staff, such as HIV or Hepatitis B or C, whereas others are more dangerous to sick patients such as methicillin resistant staphylococcal aureus (MRSA) or vancomycin-resistant enterococcus (VRE). Staff and patients may unwittingly and without ill effect be colonized with MRSA or VRE.

HIV/AIDS

The human immunodeficiency virus (HIV) is a blood borne retrovirus first described in 1981. It had probably been around for many years before this. In industrialized nations, about 1:350 people carry it, but the prevalence rises to more than 40 per cent in some parts of Africa. After a short illness with symptoms similar to infectious mononucleosis (glandular fever), people with HIV have no further symptoms for many years, and often do not know they have the disease. Eventually, as the immune system breaks down the patient is infected with uncommon infections such as herpes zoster, or cryptosporidiosis; or they develop a lymphoma. In this later symptomatic stage the disease is called acquired immunodeficiency syndrome (AIDS).

HIV is diagnosed with serological testing. *Seroconversion*, where anti-HIV antibodies appear in the victim's blood, occurs about 3 months after the initial infection.

HIV is transmitted by blood, and other body fluids from infected people. The virus can be transmitted horizontally through sexual intercourse, blood donations, and donated organs, or sharing infected needles. It can also be transmitted vertically from mother to child.

Needlestick injuries

HIV has been transmitted to health professionals, but worldwide this is fortunately rare. The main risk to staff is through needle-stick injury. Fortunately seroconversion is uncommon, and is estimated to occur on about 1:300 needle-sticks.

About 75 per cent of needle-stick injuries are potentially preventable.[2] Recapping needles is the commonest cause of needle-stick injury. A feeling of being hurried, tired or ill also puts you at risk. A needle should either be in the patient, or in the sharps' container. Never put a used syringe and needle down. Never remove a used needle from its syringe; drop the whole unit into a sharps container. Do not allow your sharps containers to become so full that people need to stuff objects into it.

For injuries with needles, sharp instruments, bites or deep scratches encourage bleeding, but do not suck and do NOT squeeze the wound. Wash well with soap and water. Immediately report the injury to your hospital health service unit for management. Most hospitals have forms for you to fill in and a protocol for both you and your patient to follow for blood testing.

Early treatment with antivirals can prevent infection becoming established in people exposed to HIV and HBV and can eradicate evidence of viruses in more than 90 per cent of people with acute hepatitis C virus infection.

To be effective a combination of the anti-HIV drugs indinavar, lamuvudine and zidovudine is best administered within 72 hours of exposure, and continued for 4 weeks.

What is the long-term risk?

The estimated mean risk for a full time nurse working for 30 years in the operating theatre suite of contracting HIV is 0.049 per cent, and for hepatitis C is 0.45 per cent. This means that for every 1000 recovery nurses working for 30 years about 5 may contract HIV from a contaminated percutaneous injury (PCI). Statistically you are six times as likely to be killed in a car accident in any given year.

Hepatitis B

Hepatitis B (HBV) is a DNA virus spread via blood products, sexual intercourse, intravenous drug users, health care workers and substandard sterilization of surgical instruments in developing countries. Seroconversion after a needle-stick is about 3 per cent. The incubation period is 60–120 days. It progresses to chronic liver disease in 2–10 per cent of people. The surface antigen Hbs-AG is present from 1–6 months after exposure. A genetically engineered vaccine is 95 per cent effective and should be offered to all staff working in the recovery room. Passive immunization (anti HBV antibody) can be given to non-immune contacts after high-risk exposure.

Hepatitis C

Hepatitis C (HCV) is an RNA virus spread by blood transfusion, drug addicts sharing needles, tattoo needles, skin piercings, and barber shop razors. It is not spread by sneezing, coughing, oro-faecal routes or through intact skin.

One serious and major source of infection is substandard sterilization of surgical and dental instruments in developing countries (where more than one per cent of the population are affected), but in 40 per cent of cases the cause remains unknown.

Seroconversion after a needle-stick is about 30 per cent. About 15 per cent of those infected progress to chronic infection. About 20 years after the initial infection for every 100 people infected: 15 get cirrhosis, 10 die of liver failure, and 10 develop hepatocellular carcinoma. Treating the acute infection with double combination therapy with interferon and ribravirine now gives a 50 per cent cure rate.

There are no tests available to differentiate acute, chronic or resolved infection; however a persistently elevated ALT level suggests chronic disease. There is no vaccine for hepatitis C.

Other hepatitis viruses

Hepatitis D (HDV) co-habits with HBV. Hepatitis E (HEV) is similar to HBA, and may be encountered in patients from the Indian subcontinent. Hepatitis GB causes usually asymptomatic post-transfusion hepatitis, but HGB-C may cause acute liver failure.

Tuberculosis

Pulmonary tuberculosis (PTB) is making a comeback in the community. Some strains are now resistant to all antibiotics – multiple drug *resistant tuberculosis* (MDRTB). *Tuberculosis* (TB) is an airborne bacterium (*Mycobacterium tuberculosis*) transmitted as an aerosol by coughing or sneezing, and common in most developing countries. It most commonly occurs in the lungs but it may occur in other sites of the body (e.g. kidney, lymph nodes, liver, abdomen, brain, and bone). Adults with non-pulmonary tuberculosis are regarded as non-infectious, and outside the operating theatre are safe to treat as normal patients, but treat as infectious aerosol-generating procedures such as wound irrigation, and abscess incision.

Patients with MDRTB require special precautions outside the capabilities of most hospitals.

Recovering tuberculous patients

Use disposable anaesthetic circuits and bacterial filters. Immediately after use, put all contaminated articles in designated infectious waste containers. Wear gown, disposable gloves, and N95 mask and cover your head. This is particularly important for the staff who may encounter sputum, bronchial secretions or aerosol droplets from coughs or sneezes.

Ideally, only those with a BCG inoculation will look after the patient with TB. The patient must be recovered in the operating theatre, and not in the recovery room. Do not accompany the patient back to their isolation unit. Leave all your potentially contaminated clothing in the operating room, and shower yourself and wash your hair.

Notify your Occupational Health Authorities of the names of all staff who were exposed to the patient, or handled infectious material in any way.

MRSA

Methicillin resistant staphylococcus aureus (MRSA) bacteria are resistant methicillin, flucloxacillin and other beta-lactam antibiotics. MRSA are commonly found in hospitals, but found far less commonly in the wider community. MRSA seem no more virulent than antibiotic-sensitive organisms, but because of their resistance they are more difficult to treat. They are spread around the hospital on people's hands, and for this reason these infections are largely preventable. Some health care workers become *reservoirs*, because they carry MRSA as part of the resident skin flora.

Risk factors for developing the disease are prolonged hospital stay, severe underlying disease, and malnutrition. These bacteria enter the body through open wounds, drain tubes, skin lesions and pressure sores.

When perfectly healthy people come into a hospital ward their skin becomes transiently colonized within hours. This is the reason that orthopaedic surgeons prefer patients for major joint surgery to be admitted on the day of their operation, go straight to the operating theatre, and not pass through the ward first.

N95 mask

The National Institute of Occupational Safety and Health (NIOSH), which is part of the United States Center for Disease Control, sets standards for respirators and masks. Air must pass through respirators, but can leak around the sides of masks. However the terms are used casually to mean the same thing. The number (95, 99, 100) refers to the efficiency the devices filter particles. An N95 respirator filters out 95 per cent of the particles that attempt to flow through the device. Similarly an N99 respirator filters out 99 per cent of the particles and an N100 respirator filters out 100 per cent of the particles that attempt to flow through it. N means not resistant to oil. Many viruses are small, from 0.04–0.8 μm in diameter. Particles of this size readily pass through an N95 filter, however airborne micro-organisms are carried on water droplets generated when someone sneezes or coughs. These 5 μm droplets are far too large to pass through an N95 respirator.

VRE

Vancomycin-resistant enterococci (VRE) are causing troublesome wound infections in some surgical units. VRE is resistant to all antibiotics apart from rifampicin. This disease is transmitted from a colonized individual's faeces to a surgical patient by hitch-hiking on the hands of a member of staff. This cross-contamination is easily prevented if staff wash their hands after coming into contact with potentially contaminated material, including bed sheets.

Barriers to transmission

Innate defences

Humans have evolved elaborate and efficient defences against invading micro-organisms. Every day each of us shrugs off an assault by micro-organisms with no ill-effect. However, if our defences are compromised by malnutrition, or disease, or our natural defence barriers are breached by surgical incisions, intravenous infusions, drains or catheters then we run the risk of being overwhelmed.

Cross-infection in hospitals occurs where pathogenic micro-organisms migrate from one infected patient to another. Hospitals tend to breed particularly virulent *nosocomial* bacteria, which invade readily and are resistant to antibiotics.

Protect your own skin

If you are using good-quality handwashing lotions then skin cracks should not be a problem, but if they do occur skin cracks may get infected. Cover small wounds with occlusive membrane dressings such as Tegaderm® or Op-Site® to provide a good barrier. Gloves will easily slip on and off over the plastic dressing. Use them on knuckle-scrapes too instead of Bandaid®-type dressings which tend to come off under gloves. Change the membrane at the end of the shift or your skin will become macerated. Also change it if it starts to lift off.

You can contaminate your hands by merely taking the patient's pulse.

Skin

Your most important piece of protective equipment is your skin. Intact skin is a superb barrier to infection. Look after it even when you are not on duty. Most bacteria and other micro-organisms do not survive long in its acid environment, and the resident flora such as micrococci, Staph. epidermitis and diphtheroids crowd out newcomers.

Bacterial colonization is measured by counting *colony-forming units*. Different areas have different bacteria counts. The scalp has an average of 1 000 000 colony-forming units cm^2 (CFU cm^2) whereas hands range between 40 000 and 4 000 000 CFU cm^2.

Bacteria on the hands can be divided into two groups: resident and transient. Resident flora live in deeper layers of the skin, and they are usually benign. Transient bacteria colonize the superficial layers. They are usually picked up by staff during direct contact with patients or contaminated objects. Resident bacteria are not removed by normal hand washing, but transients are. Unfortunately some staff pick up pathogenic bacteria, such as MRSA, which then become part of their resident flora population. MRSA like warm wet places: the nose, groin and axilla. Some patients are taking broad-spectrum antibiotics. These can selectively kill parts of the resident population, which makes way for antibiotic-resistant bacteria to set up home. Once the skin is disrupted by surgery, these antibiotic-resistant bacteria can invade to cause serious wound infections.

Respiratory tract

Most inhaled micro-organisms are entrapped in mucus secreted by the mucous membranes lining the respiratory tract. The mucous membranes are guarded by a variety of white cells, macrophages, complement, and by special immunoglobulins called IgA. Bacteria rarely penetrate these defences, but some airborne viruses may; the recurring epidemics of influenza are an example.

Gut

Our gut houses more bacterium and micro-organisms than there are cells in our body. Most are harmless commensals, some help by producing vitamin K, and excluding unwelcome bacteria, but others are pathogenic. If ordinary commensal bowel flora contaminates the peritoneum, say after colon surgery, the resulting peritonitis and septicaemia is frequently fatal.

Urinary tract

The one-way flow of urine usually flushes unwelcome bacteria out of the urinary tract, but indwelling catheters can provide nooks and crannies where pathogenic bacteria can survive and grow.

How to prevent transmission

Bacteria are everywhere. In non-medical offices high bacterial counts can be found on light switches, telephones, computer mice, and other work surfaces, while the communal coffee cups revealed a 40 per cent contamination with faecal bacteria.[3] If an ordinary office is such a cesspool, then consider the organisms lurking in the nooks and crannies of your recovery room.

Hand hygeine

Hand hygiene is the essential core for *Standard Precautions*. It is the most ignored, but most effective way of reducing cross-infection. It is tempting to take short cuts in personal hygiene when working in a busy recovery room, but lapses not only cause increased infection rates among patients, but increase your risk of infection too.

In 2002 the Centers for Disease Control and prevention in the United States produced a detailed 48-page document, *Guidelines for Hand Hygiene in Health Care Settings*. Every one should read this clearly written, and excellent report.

Essentially, its recommendations were:

- When your hands are visibly dirty wash them with soap and water, and then decontaminate them with an alcohol-based hand rub.
- If your hands are not visibly dirty decontaminate them with an alcohol-based rub.
- Alcohol-based hand rubs must be available at every patient site.
- If your hands come into contact with any bodily fluids or potentially contaminated sites such as dressings or mucous membranes, then wash your hands with antimicrobial soap to decontaminate them.

Decontaminate your hands:

- before you touch patients or their surroundings;
- before putting on gloves to do any sterile procedure;
- when moving from a contaminated body-site to a clean body-site;
- after touching medical equipment in the area of the patient;
- after removing your gloves.

Alcohol-based rub kills almost every germ.
Soap and water merely cleans them.

Additional tips

- Post the maker's directions above the alcohol-based rubs dispenser.
- Do not top-up dispensers. Replace the bottles with new ones when they are empty.
- The best-alcohol rubs contain n-propanol because they *denature* proteins (n-propanol is not widely available in the US).
- Although dermatitis caused by alcohol rubs is rare,[4] this is no place for false economy. Use good-quality rubs that are acceptable to the staff. Avoid those rubs containing perfumes because they are more likely to cause allergies and skin reactions.
- Avoid bar soaps, because they are warm wet places where bacteria can grow.
- Take off hand jewellery, and bracelets.
- Wash your hands with soap for at least 30 seconds (put a clock above the sink to time it).
- For sterile procedures you may need a surgical forearm scrub. This takes 2–5 minutes. Long scrubs are unnecessary.
- Scrub your nails.
- Pat your hands dry with paper towels. Do not rub them dry because you will damage the skin.
- Use a dry towel to turn off the tap.
- Do not install hot air-blowers because they contaminate the whole room.
- Alcohol-based rubs are flammable. Bulk-store them safely, because they have *flash points* when they spontaneously ignite between 21–24°C.

Fingernails

Keep fingernails short and clean. Do not wear artificial nails because they shelter a zoo of potentially pathogenic micro-organisms, even after hands have been washed[5]. Freshly applied nail polish does not seem to be a problem, but there is a potential for chipped nail polish to harbour organisms.

Jewellery

Wedding rings and hand jewellery are better off than on, because they interfere with hand hygiene, collect *microbes*, damage gloves, and tear patient's skin.

Overshoes

There is little evidence overshoes reduce theatre contamination from micro-organisms carried on the footwear. Overshoes help prevent staff footwear being contaminated with blood or body fluids; and this is especially so where there is a risk of blood-borne viruses. Get your own footwear. Make sure it is impervious to blood, body fluids, and falling needles, and can be decontaminated if necessary. For high-risk situations, thick-soled Wellington boots are best.

Aprons

Wear an appropriate plastic apron whenever you are dealing with fluids, or there is a chance of being contaminated with blood, secretions or other body fluids, or dealing with infectious patients.

Table 27.1 Plastic aprons' colour code

Colour	Function
Red	In contact with blood, or bowel secretions
Blue	Directly dealing with patients, changing beds etc.
Yellow	Dealing with patients in isolation
White	For doing clean procedures, e.g. wound dressings

Gloves

Where possible use latex gloves because they give better protection than non-latex gloves.

Choose the type of glove worn appropriate to the task, as follows:

Sterile gloves are worn to protect the patient. They must be worn for invasive and aseptic procedures requiring a sterile field, involving normally sterile areas of the body.

Non-sterile gloves are worn to protect staff members. They are worn for non-sterile procedures where there is a perceived risk of contaminating your hands hand through contact with blood or body fluids, secretions (excluding sweat), contaminated patient care items, non-intact skin or mucous membranes.

General purpose non-sterile utility gloves are worn for housekeeping chores including *cleaning*. These rubber gloves are worn to protect the wearer's hands from cleaning agents and prolonged immersion in water.

> *Each time you change your gloves, decontaminate your hands.*

Masks, goggles, spectacles and visors

Wear protective eye guards whenever there is a risk of body fluids splashing into eyes or mouth.

Hats

Theatre caps prevent hair and skin squames from escaping, and to stop your hair being contaminated by splashes of body fluids. Although there is no need for non-scrubbed staff to wear caps, it is a good thing to keep your hair covered while in the theatre block.

Standard precautions

Universal Precautions against transmission of infection were introduced more 25 years ago when HIV/AIDS was first recognized as a hazard to hospital staff. Universal Precautions are now called Standard Precautions. *Standard Precautions* requires all health care workers to assume that all body substances from all patients be treated as potential sources of infection regardless of diagnoses or perceived risk.

> *All staff are to assume all patients are always infectious.*

Safe working practice demands standardized procedures to protect staff, other patients, and visitors from cross-infection.

Standard precautions include policies on hand hygiene, gowns, gloves, face protection, safe use and disposal of sharps, safe handling of specimens, safe handling of linen, safe disposal of clinical waste, and decontamination of spills and accidents. If you have cuts or abrasions then cover them with waterproof dressings.

Staff with breaches in their skin such as dermatitis, psoriasis, eczema, skin wounds or other skin disorders must not come into contact with potentially contaminated material.

> *All body fluids are potentially infectious.*

Wear clean latex gloves whenever you are touching potentially infective substances, and change them between tasks.

Table 27.2 A Standard Precautions checklist

Question	
Do staff wear gloves appropriately?	Yes/No
Do staff wash their hands appropriately?	Yes/No
Are the following available?	Yes/No
– Aprons	Yes/No
– Face-protection goggles, and visors	Yes/No
– Gloves (including non-rubber latex ones)	Yes/No
– Masks	Yes/No
Are single use items ever reused?	Yes/No
Is linen dealt with appropriately?	Yes/No
Are stethoscopes, and blood pressure cuffs cleaned regularly?	Yes/No
Are sharps handled safely?	Yes/No
Is there a formal policy for handling biological spills?	Yes/No
Is there a formal policy for needle-stick injuries?	Yes/No

Hazardous health care workers

In 2001 the Department of Health (UK) set up a committee to assess the potential for health care workers to be a hazard to patients. Accordingly they proposed that new health care workers be tested for blood-borne viruses (BBV): HIV, hepatitis B, hepatitis C; and tuberculosis, and those who are positive be excluded from doing exposure-prone procedures (EPP). This did not exclude such workers from working in the NHS, but restricted them to working in clinical areas where they posed no hazard to patients. These tests are not compulsory, but health care workers new to the NHS who decline to be tested are not cleared to perform EPP.

Spills

Quarantine all spillages of blood and body fluids, and deal with them immediately. Make the area safe. Wear a red disposable apron. Soak up the spill with paper towels and wash the area with neutral detergent. For blood spills on hard surfaces throw sodium hypochlorite solution on the area, leave it soak for 10 minutes, and then rinse the area with neutral detergent and water and allow it to dry. Discard contaminated articles: paper towels, gloves and apron into the yellow clinical waste container. Do not use hot water because it coagulates proteins, which then sticks to surfaces offering shelter for micro-organisms.

Waste

All clinical waste contaminated with body fluids or tissue must be discarded in yellow waste bags and sealed securely. Never transfer clinical waste from one container to another.

Use transparent plastic bags for household waste only. Some hospitals use black plastic bags for this purpose, however these can conceal inappropriately jettisoned waste.

Linen

All linen is infectious, but the risk of transmission is low. Use standard precautions. Contaminated linen goes into red bags. If the linen is wet, put it in double bags, so that contaminated fluids cannot seep through to the outside.

Additional precautions

Fortunately in the operating theatre and recovery room the risk of transmission from one patient to another is small, and if it does occur then, it is almost always because of a lapse by a member of staff.

Standard Precautions are a basic risk minimisation strategy. Use Additional *Precautions* when Standard Precautions are not enough to prevent transmission of infection. *Additional* Precautions are used for highly transmissible pathogens including airborne transmission or droplet of highly contagious agents such as influenza, chickenpox, tuberculosis, and pertussis; and direct or indirect contact with dry skin or contaminated objects colonized by multi-antibiotic resistant Staphylococcus aureus (MRSA) or vancomycin-resistant enterococci (VRE).

Microbes don't fly. They hitchhike.

Additional Precautions include using personal protective equipment such as a particulate filter respirator for tuberculosis, or assigning already immune staff to attend a patient, for example those who had chickenpox (varicella) in the past.

All blood and body fluids, tissue, secretions, and products, are potentially infective regardless of the perceived risk of the source.

Screening and isolating patients only work if people tending the patient are not carrying the bug.

Table 27.3 Sources of contamination

Potentially infectious body fluids	
Major	**Minor**
Blood	Urine
Faeces	Nasal secretions
Wound ooze	Gastric secretions
Pus	Peritoneal dialysis fluid
Sputum	Ascitic fluid
Saliva	Pleural and pericardial fluid

Potentially infectious body sites	
Major	**Minor**
Wounds	Nasal passages
Skin lesions	Mouth
Drainage sites	Intravascular access sites Peri-anal area Armpits

Ten sensible precautions

1. Most hospitals have an Infection Control Unit as part of the administration structure. Its duty is to set standards, write protocols and enforce them with regular quality assessment procedures.

2. Staff in the recovery area should wear theatre gear. Do not wear your street clothes. Visitors should wear a gown, not necessarily for infection control, but to reinforce the idea that they are in a restricted area.

3. Ensure your recovery room has the minimal possible flat surfaces such as shelves. Do not allow the room to become a storage area.

4. Have a regular cleaning schedule.

5. If a member of staff has an infectious illness such as a 'cold' then they must stay at home. It is easy to transfer airborne viruses to already compromised patients with disastrous consequences. Postoperatively a patient

who has picked up a cold from a sniffling member of staff is highly likely to get pneumonia.

6. Ensure every site has facilities for washing hands.

7. Nebulizers can be a source of infection because they spray a fine aerosol into the air which may disperse infective particles.

8. Neutral detergent is adequate to make surfaces biologically safe.

9. Insist on immediate repairs to cut linoleum or broken woodwork, chipped surfaces. These places harbour pathogens.

10. Never clean, wash or place instruments in handbasins.

If an item cannot be cleaned, then it cannot be disinfected or sterilized.

Cleaning

Cleaning involves washing with water, *detergents* and scrubbing or using ultrasound to dislodge foreign material such as dust, blood, secretions, excretions and micro-organisms from objects and people. Cleaning simply removes, but does not inactivate, micro-organisms. Cleaning keeps things looking good, and is one of the most cost-effective procedures a hospital can do. Organic residue shelters micro-organisms and prevents sterilizing agents or disinfectants from coming into contact with the surfaces of the item being sterilized. Protein in particular inactivates some chemical disinfectants.

Disinfection

Disinfection is a process for removing all organisms except bacterial spores from an object.

Points to note:

- Automated thermal washer-disinfectors are effective, but make sure you select the appropriate cycle.
- Make sure you use a properly certified instrument-grade disinfectant. Usually these are used alone or in an automated chemical washer-disinfector.
- Disinfection is not a sterilizing process.
- Disinfection is not simply a convenient substitute for sterilization. Do not use thermal disinfection for instruments that need to be sterile. However, thermal disinfection is more effective than chemical disinfection.

Table 27.4 Which disinfectant to use[6]

Disinfectant	Indication
Alcohol	
70% alcohol impregnated wipes	Wiping down dressing trolleys, stethoscopes.
Hypochlorite solutions	
Sodium hypochlorite solution 1 in 20 dilution (500 ppm available chlorine)	Decontamination of environmental surfaces (e.g. after a blood spill).
OPA (orthophthaladehyde)	High-level disinfection for heat-sensitive equipment that is unsuitable for autoclaving, e.g. transoesophageal echo transducer probes, thermistors.
Peracetic acid	High-level disinfection of heat-sensitive equipment that is unsuitable for autoclaving, e.g. endoscopes in a washer/disinfector machine

How to use disinfectants

- Use sachets of antiseptics and disinfectants once only, and then throw them away.
- Before using any disinfectant or antiseptic check that the solution is clear and there is no particulate matter visible.
- If you open a flask of a water-based solution, such as aqueous chlorhexidine, then it must be discarded within 24 hours.

Antiseptics and their use

Antiseptic agents are substances that are rubbed on the hands or applied to surfaces to reduce the population of micro-organisms.

Table 27.5 Antiseptic agents

Antiseptic name	Indication
Aqueous chlorhexidine solutions	
Chlorhexidine 2% (green)	Handwashing before an aseptic procedure.
Chlorhexidine 4%	Surgical handwashing in OR.
Aqueous chlorhexidine 0.1% (blue)	Urinary catheter insertion, perineal wash-downs.
Chlorhexidine and cetrimide (yellow)	Perineal wash-downs. Lacerations.

Table 27.5 (continued) Antiseptic agents

Antiseptic name	Indication
Alcoholic chlorhexidine solutions	
Chlorhexidine 0.5% in 70% alcohol (pink)	Skin preparation where an alcohol swab is inappropriate (e.g. blood cultures, IV insertion).
Chlorhexidine 1% in 70% alcohol (pink)	Decontaminating hands that are not visibly soiled.
Alcohol	
Microshield (61% ethanol & emollients white)	Decontaminating hands that are not visibly soiled.
Alcohol swab – saturated with 70% isopropyl	Preparing small areas of skin
Povidone iodine solutions	
Povidone iodine scrub (0.75% povidone iodine)	Handwashing (in specialist areas)
Povidone iodine solution (10% povidone iodine)	Skin preparation for surgery

Sterilization

Sterilization is a process that eliminates or destroys all forms of microbes including, virus, bacterial spores and fungi.

Principle techniques for sterilizing equipment include:

- moist heat using steam under pressure;
- dry heat;
- ethylene oxide;
- automated sealed low-temperature peracetic acid, hydrogen peroxide plasma and other chemical sterilant systems;
- ionizing radiation.

All of these give a minimum sterility assurance level (SAL), but the process must be validated to make sure it has worked properly.

Do not use, or trust ultraviolet light units, incubators, microwave ovens, domestic ovens and pressure cookers, because they do not guarantee sterilization.

Keep permanent records so that, if necessary, you can trace the source of an infection to at least a batch level, and preferably to an individual patient.

Notes

1. Plowman R, Graves N Griffin M (1999) London: Public Health Laboratory Service.
2. Raghavendran S, Bagry H S, Leith S (2006) *Anaesthesia* 61:867–72.
3. Meer RR Gerba R *et al.* (1997) *Dairy Food and Environmental Sanitation* 17:352–5.
4. Widmer AF (2000) *Clinics of Infectious Diseases* 31:136–43.
5. McNeil SA, Foster CL, Kaufmann CA (2000) *Clinical Infectious Diseases* 32: 367–72.
6. *The NHS Healthcare Cleaning Manual* (2004).

28

Design of the recovery room

Location of the recovery room

Shortly after the first anaesthetic was given in 1846, Florence Nightingale recognized the need for a special area, and special nursing care of patients recovering from ether anaesthesia. She wrote in her book *Notes on Hospitals* that the patient should be placed in a small room near to the ward, with clean fresh sand on the floor, clean bedclothes, and windows to admit the sunlight and fresh air.[1]

Figure 28.1 Plan of a typical recovery room

The recovery room is part of the operating theatre suite, located close to the operating theatre, but it should be readily accessible to medical staff who are in their street clothes. The staff tea room should be nearby so that the doctors having a break at the end of a case can quickly come to the patient if needed. It is also useful if there is a communicating window or door between the recovery room and the holding bay where patients arrive for theatre with their escorting nurses. Patients who are ready to leave can then be sent back with these nurses. It is best to have the intensive care unit on the same level and close to the recovery room.

Ideally there should be restricted as well as public access, and a separate entrance for goods delivery so that supplies do not take the same route as patients.

There should be adequate space for administrative offices and a mini-laboratory to do simple procedures such as measuring blood gases or urinary sodium levels. A computer-assisted drug narcotic dispensing unit saves a lot of time.

Consider incorporating an isolation room for managing patients with infections, contaminated wounds, and those who are immunosuppressed. This room needs to have both negative- and positive-pressure air conditioning.

In hospitals with fewer than 200 beds it is useful to have the ICU adjacent to the operating theatre. The recovery room can then be a functional part of the ICU but remain a separate area away from the unit. Such an arrangement means that staff, facilities and equipment can be shared between the two areas. A further advantage is that after hours when there are less staff on the wards patients can be recovered in the ICU. The disadvantage is the risk of transferring infection from ICU patients to the surgical patient. This transmission of nosocomial infection is preventable but requires scrupulous care and iron-tight discipline. Wearing gowns and handwashing are crucial to this.

Plan for the recovery room

Many recovery rooms are poorly designed because they are built, almost as an afterthought, to fit into an operating theatre suite design, rather than to fit the needs of the staff and patients.

The minimum size of a recovery room should not be less than 164 m^2 for a department of eight theatres.[2] Square recovery rooms are more efficient than long rectangular ones, because they keep traffic paths as short as possible and allow nurses to talk easily with each other. Plan an open and uncluttered room with no support structures obstructing your view. Avoid swing doors if possible.

The total overall area of the recovery room should be 18 square metres for every trolley bay. Depending on the workload and expected turnover most hospitals will find that 1.5–2 trolley bays for each operating theatre is sufficient. However, those with high turnover and short cases (such as tonsillectomies) will require up to three beds per operating theatre.

There must be provision for rapid evacuation of the recovery room in an emergency. The provisions need to include strategies for evacuating comatose or unstable patients. Many hospitals have recovery rooms in places that would be almost impossible to evacuate in times of peril.

Standards

There are many things to consider when planning and building a recovery room. Fortunately architects and engineers have access to help in the form of standards.

Standards are sets of specifications that cover almost everything to do with construction, design, safety, purchase and applications of buildings and equipment used in hospitals. Many countries, including Australia, the United Kingdom, the European community, and the USA have their own standards that specify such things as the design of buildings, the supply of piped gases, the quality of lighting, uniformity of fittings for anaesthetic apparatus, the formulation of drug names, electrical safety, hospital signage, medical records and so on. The International Organization of Standardization (ISO) based in Switzerland is slowly gaining consensus between the various national standardization bodies and bringing them into line. In the European Community the Comité Européen de Normalisation has made rapid progress towards standardization. One notable recent advance has been the standardization of the generic names of drugs. Eventually apparatus designed and used in one country can be used equally safely in another; and the various fittings, pipes, and colour codes are uniform.

Make sure that anything you design or build or buy complies with the accepted standards in your area. We have drawn freely on various standards to list ideas that may help you.

Trolley bays

The minimum number of trolley or bed spaces is 1.5 for each operating room. Operating suites with rapid turnover will require more spaces. There are statistical methods, such as the theory of queues, for helping decide the appropriate number of recovery room bays for each operating room.

Each recovery room trolley bay should be identical, with the same items of equipment in the same places. Do not design bays that are mirror images of each other, they are confusing to work in. Consistency ensures easy access to equipment and safe practice.

Each trolley bay should be visible from anywhere within the room. If you design a central island for your nurses' station make sure the bench top is low enough for staff who are sitting down to see over the bench top. Keep flat surfaces to a minimum.

Make sure that patient trolleys can move easily around the room with the minimum number of corners to negotiate. Have two wide doors for access; one from the operating theatre and one to the wards, ideally these should be on opposite sides of the room. However, the recovery room should not become a shortcut for people going to and from the operating theatres.

As a rule trolley bays need to be at least 3.5 metres long with at least 2 metres on each side to allow equipment such as portable X-ray equipment, ventilators, and warming blanket, to be brought to the patient. Nine square metres is the absolute minimum. Each trolley bay needs at least 1 cubic metre of storage space within the room, and at least 3 square metres of shelving and storage space outside the room, but nearby.

Common mistakes when planning recovery rooms are to have too little storage space, insufficient power points (general power outlets), insufficient suction outlets and not enough room on either side of the patient for all the services that may need to be brought to the trolley side. It is wise to consider provision for future technological advances.

Each recovery room trolley bay needs its own service utilities mounted on the wall at the head end of the patient trolley.

Trolley bay fixtures

Equipment needed for each trolley bay should include:

- two high-pressure oxygen outlets equipped with flow meters and nipples;
- two high-vacuum, high-flow suction outlets including receiver, tubing, rigid handpiece, and a range of suction catheters. These must conform with relevant national standards;
- two high-pressure medical air outlets;
- eight mains electric (*general*) *power outlets*;
- an emergency red panic button alarm on the wall above the patient's head;
- overhead runners similar to curtain rails with hooks are preferable to drip stands;
- one mobile examination light that can be swung to provide light at any point on the patient.

Appropriate electronic monitoring facilities mounted on the wall at eye level such as:

- ECG;
- carbon dioxide monitors;
- pulse oximeters;

- large under floor conduits to carry communication cables to the central nurses' station;
- a blood pressure monitor attached to the wall at eye height to prevent errors caused by parallax;
- privacy screens;
- two shelves with slightly raised edges to prevent things falling on the floor;
- handwashing facilities for scrubbing up, one between two is ideal;
- somewhere to keep the patient's chart;
- storage space or bins for a day patient's belongings.

Within the trolley bay keep:
- a good-quality stethoscope;
- oropharyngeal and nasopharyngeal airways;
- sterile disposable gloves (powder free);
- unsterile disposable protective gloves in all sizes;
- a pressure infusion bag for giving IV fluids rapidly;
- oxygen tubing with connectors;
- T-piece or T-bags® for delivering oxygen to spontaneously breathing patients who have a laryngeal mask or endotracheal tube in place;
- self-inflating bags (Laerdal® or Ambu®); and a Mapleson C circuit;
- bowels and kidney dishes;
- paper tissues;
- a good-quality reliable torch with spare batteries;
- scissors;
- tape; gauze and mouth swabs;
- sealable plastic bags for transporting potentially infectious material;
- containers for haematology and pathology specimens;
- blood gas syringes;
- a range of needles, syringes, and skin cleaning preparations.

Within the recovery room keep:
- a 12-lead ECG machine;
- a neuromuscular function monitor;
- a warming cupboard for blankets;
- a procedure light;

- basic surgical tray;
- bronchoscopy equipment;
- a ventilator;
- provision for inserting chest drains;
- blood gas and electrolyte measuring equipment;
- a refrigerator for storing heat-labile drugs.

Design your recovery room
so that you can see all the patients, all the time.

Emergency station

Establish an *emergency station*, where the defibrillator and trolleys (*crash carts*) for managing cardiac arrests and other emergencies are kept. Keep this in an easily accessible place. The emergency station needs a mains power supply to keep the portable equipment's batteries charged.

Emergency trolleys (crash carts)

Keep trays and trolleys set up for anaphylaxis, malignant hyperthermia, emergency airway care, emergency bronchoscopy, insertion of thoracic drains, minor surgical procedures, and vascular access. Attach the relevant protocols to the trolley. It helps to have a large, clear colour photograph of each set-up so that the trays can be checked quickly and are always put together in the same way. Photographs will tell you immediately what is missing. Consider sharing infrequently used trolleys such as those for malignant hyperthermia and bronchoscopy with the anaesthetic department.

Isolation rooms

Plan to incorporate isolation rooms into your recovery room; sterile ones to manage immunosuppressed patients, and non-sterile ones to manage patients with highly contagious airborne diseases such as TB. Sterile isolation rooms, with airlocks, are kept at *positive pressure* with highly filtered air, so that organisms are not able to enter, whereas those where patients with infectious diseases are treated are kept at negative pressure so that organisms cannot escape.

Other facilities

Air conditioning

Air conditioning should maintain the temperature of the recovery room between 21° and 24°C with the capability of increasing it to 26°C. The relative humidity should be between 40–60% under all conditions with at least 12 air changes per hour, which is the same as the operating theatres. Anaesthetic gas pollution can be high in the recovery room, because patients continue to exhale gases, especially the volatile vapours, for some time after leaving the operating theatre.

Clocks

A clock with a sweep second hand should be visible from all over the recovery room. Include battery replacement as part of your routine maintenance programme.

Use the 24 hour clock when noting time on charts and in the records.

For example:

$$Midnight = 0.00 \ hr$$
$$10.20 \ a.m. = 10.20 \ hr$$
$$Noon = 12.00 \ hr$$
$$8 \ p.m. = 20.00 \ hr$$

Cylinders

The gas in a cylinder is at extremely high pressure of 120 000 kPa or 2000 pound per square inch. Handle cylinders with care. Do not drop them. They have been known to explode like a bomb. Use chains to make sure large cylinders stay upright and cannot fall over. Store them in a cool place well away from direct sunlight. Do not accept delivery if they show signs of rust.

Make sure you have the right key to turn them on and off. Cylinders have to be cracked before use. To *crack a cylinder*, gently turn it on for an instant to blow out any dust or grit that may be lodged in the cylinder's neck; otherwise the particles may damage apparatus.

Oxygen cylinders

Oxygen is neither explosive nor flammable, but it vigorously supports combustion. There are four sizes of oxygen cylinders normally available.

Table 28.1 Gas cylinders

Cylinder size	Litres	Cubic feet
G cylinder	7000	250
E cylinder	3500	125
D cylinder	1400	49
C cylinder	400	14

Defibrillator

Defibrillators are an essential piece of equipment. They are used to treat cardiac arrest and some forms of arrhythmias. In a small hospital it may be necessary to share one defibrillator with the whole theatre block. Keep it with the resuscitation trolley in the recovery room. There are many types, but the most useful are portable, lightweight, run on mains power or rechargeable batteries, and have an internal ECG monitor. Include its routine check in your maintenance plan.

Defibrillators put out large amounts of current; as much as 7000 volts at 4 joules. They are dangerous if they are not handled properly. Staff have been electrocuted while demonstrating its use. Practise using the defibrillator, but not while it is charged up. Defibrillators need special conductive jelly or conductive pads. Store these on the same trolley as the defibrillator. In hot climates slightly moisten the pads with saline if they are dry. Do not allow the saline to leave the area of the pad, or a short-circuit may occur. Do not use a non-conductive jelly (such as KY Jelly®) or water because it will cause a deep burn during cardioversion.

Emergency power

A reliable power supply is crucial. An emergency power generator is essential in case the mains supply fails. This should automatically switch on if there is mains power failure. As an additional back-up in case both systems fail and the recovery room is plunged into total darkness fit one or more emergency battery-powered torches that automatically switch on when mains power fails.

If there is a fire in any part of the hospital the fire brigade may cut off the electricity supply so they can use water to put the fire out.

Most cases of macroshock occur when someone touches a live electrical wire, and the full mains current flows through their body to earth. Their heart goes into ventricular fibrillation (VF), which causes them to die from electrocution.

In contrast microshock occurs when tiny currents of a few millivolt passes through an electrolyte infusion or pacemaker wire to cause VF. Isolation devices protect against macroshock. Proper flooring, adequate humidity and properly earthed electronic devices guard, but do not completely protect, against microshock.

Emergency button

Site a large red panic button on the wall above each trolley bay to call for help. The best buzzer is one with an urgent repeating sequence that can be heard throughout the theatre complex, including the changing rooms. To prevent them being accidentally activated design them to pull on rather than push. Identify them with clear signs, and test them daily.

Electrical protection devices

Ordinary wiring used in domestic houses has its electrical protection (Class A) limited to fuses, an earth wire in the cord or two levels of insulation (double insulation).

Recovery rooms are a *Body Protected Area* (Class B) giving protection against macroshock in the event of an accident. Macroshock protection is provided, preferably with an isolation transformer, or less preferably with core balance earth leakage devices.

Isolation transformers are fitted to the mains power supply and prevent a person being electrocuted if they touch an electric live (*active*) wire in the power supply while they are in contact with the earth. Such an event can easily happen for instance if someone accidentally spills fluid into an electrical device. Isolation transformers are expensive and require regular checking and maintenance.

Core balance earth leakage devices are a cheaper alternative, It detects a current flowing to earth and shuts down all the power on that circuit before enough current has passed to electrocute the person. For most recovery rooms this is sufficient, but it has the disadvantage of interrupting the power supply, which needs to be switched on again manually. To ensure that core balance works properly all earth points in the circuit need to have a common heavy copper grounding cable.

Modern recovery rooms are now designed to conform to cardiac-protected areas (Class Z). Class Z areas are similar to Class B areas but include special wiring to ensure that no exposed surfaces of plumbing, electrical equipment, or anything that can conduct electricity in the vicinity of the patient can create an electrical gradient sufficient to cause microelectrocution.

Flooring

Lay non-slip flooring with a non-absorbent surface of uniform colour that can easily be cleaned. Patterned or speckled flooring hides dirt, and makes it difficult to find small objects that fall on the floor.

Fire equipment

Fit fire-control equipment and smoke detection alarms in the recovery room.

Ensure fire extinguishers, fire hoses, and fire blankets, are installed in prominent places. Get advice from your local fire department. Remember to budget for regular maintenance of the equipment.

The best type of fire extinguisher for the recovery room is one that uses compressed carbon dioxide. This copes with fires involving wood, paper, burning plastic, live electrical equipment, flammable liquids, and oil.

Fire safety

Put up notices in conspicuous places giving clear instructions about what to do in case of fire.

R	Rescue	Remove patient to a designated safe place.
A	Alarm	Sound alarm.
C	Contain	Close windows and doors to isolate the fire.
E	Extinguish	Only attempt to put the fire out if you know what you are doing.

Appoint specific staff as fire monitors, and take their photographs. Display their names, photographs, and duties at the entrance to the recovery room. These people will be in charge if a fire breaks out. All staff need regular training in case a fire does break out. Every member of staff should have written instructions on the back of their identification labels about what to do in the case of fire, or other emergencies requiring evacuation. Hold evacuation practices twice a year.

Hospitals do burn. And people do die.

Put Anglia® or similar evacuation sheets under each trolley mattress. These tough sheets have handles, straps, and buckles to wrap the patients in a protective shell. It is easy to drag this shell along the floor, even down stairs if necessary.

Glucose meters

Glucose meters are small electronic devices that measure blood glucose concentrations from a drop of blood from a finger or heel prick. Keep their instructions with the meter. They use special reagent strips. Store them in a cool dry place. Do not take blood from the toes or feet of diabetics, or patients with vascular disease, because the puncture site is likely to get infected. Serious infections can cause the patient to lose a limb.

Handwashing basins

Ideally there should be one handbasin with hot and cold water running through an adjustable mixer system, liquid soap, paper towels, and a waste bin between adjacent trolley bays. Avoid hot air dryers because they are noisy, and spray germs and squames all over the room.

Haemoglobinometers

These compact cheap and accurate electronic devices read the concentration of haemoglobin on a reagent strip. Most are easy to use, but the microcuvettes used in some makes are damaged by humidity giving inaccurate results.

Humidifiers

Humidity is a measure of the mass of water vapour in a gas. Humidifiers increase the amount of water vapour in inhaled gases, helping prevent the tracheobronchial mucosa from drying out, and preserving the action of surfactant in the lungs. Humidification of inspired gas is especially important in those with acute or chronic respiratory disorders.

There are three principal types of humidifiers:

1. Condenser humidifiers. These are also known as heat and moisture exchangers (HME). They are effective, cheap and disposable. As the patient breathes out, the expired water vapour collects on baffles of the humidifier. When the patient breathes in, the dry air rushes over the baffles and becomes partially saturated with water vapour. Use HME only on patients who are on a ventilator. They are not designed for patients spontaneously breathing through an endotracheal tube or laryngeal mask because they are easily blocked by sputum and may then suffocate the patient. Special HMEs are available for tracheostomies. If their baffles become blocked with sputum the ends blow off so that the airway cannot obstruct.

2. Heated humidifiers are useful to help warm ventilated hypothermic patients. They deliver gas at 37–40°C at a relative humidity of 100%. They are expensive, need close attention and require regular maintenance. Only fill them with sterile water rather than tap water, because of the risk of transmitting pathogens such as *Legionella*. These humidifiers have a probe near the patient's airway to warn of overheating, because temperatures above 42°C cause tracheal burns.

3. Bubble-through humidifiers, where the gas passed through cold water are ineffective. Use only sterile water especially in warmer climates because tap water carries the risk of aerosol-acquired infections.

Infusion sets

Blood transfusions require special infusion sets with 120 micron filters. A useful type has an in-line squeeze pump for rapid transfusion. A Y-giving set is particularly useful for high-volume transfusions. These sets have an internal diameter of 3.2 mm. Special trauma sets for rapid transfusion have a 5.72 mm bore.

Infusion pumps and syringe drivers

Syringe drivers (such as the Atom®, Graseby®, Ohmeda® and Terumo®) use a turning screw to accurately deliver small volumes of fluids from a syringe. They are used to give small, but precise amounts, of concentrated fluids. Because of the compliance in the tubing, at flow rates of less than 10 ml/hr most have a slow start up time, and it may take 10 minutes or more before they are a delivering a steady flow. Inadvertently giving excess drug can occur if the fluid siphons into the patient, or if an obstructed line is suddenly released. To avoid errors only use the syringe recommended by the makers. Fatalities have occurred when syringe drivers are incorrectly set at the wrong flow rate. The most frequent error is wrongly setting the decimal point. Good syringe drivers have clearly marked figures with different-coloured marking on each side of the decimal point. Always get two trained staff to independently check drugs, dilutions and pump settings.

Infusion pumps

Infusion pumps (such as the IMed®) are drip-set regulators and deliver a set number of millilitres per hour through an infusion set. Always use them with a dedicated line. If you attach anything else to the line you must insert a one-way valve to prevent back flow. Multi-lumen central venous catheters are useful for running up to three separate infusions through a single catheter. However these catheters are more likely to be colonized by pathogenic micro-organisms. If infusion pumps are not set up correctly they can deliver unintended amounts of fluid.

Imprest system

An imprest system for drugs and disposable items makes restocking easy. Under this system commonly used items are held in the recovery room. It is the duty of the pharmacist and supply officer to check and restock them to the agreed quantity every day.

Drugs

Recovery rooms need a wide range of drugs. Sometimes they will be needed in a hurry. A set of recessed shelves with a door that can be rolled down is ideal. Organize your drug cupboard in alphabetical order according to generic name. Post an alphabetical list of both the trade names and generic names on the door. Consider having a third list of drugs arranged under their pharmacological actions, for instance a list of antibiotics, cardiac drugs etc.

Laryngoscopes

Laryngoscopes are essential equipment. Buy the same make and model, so that the blades, handles, batteries and globes can be interchanged. The parts of different brands are not interchangeable and if you get the bits mixed up, it becomes a jigsaw puzzle to reassemble them. Choose a brand with a detachable blade so that it can be easily washed, and cleaned. Do not autoclave blades with fiberoptic components because they will be destroyed. The handle may rust, so do not autoclave it; merely remove the batteries, wash the outside and dry it carefully. Sometimes the electrical contact between the blade and the contact on the handle corrodes. Clean it with a piece of steel wool or sandpaper until the brass contacts shine.

Part of your morning check should be to see that all the laryngoscopes lights shine white and bright. If the light is dim or yellow check the batteries are fresh, and the brass electrical contacts are clean. A dim light is not due to a faulty light bulb: they either work, or they don't. Keep a supply of spare bulbs nearby because they blow easily especially if knocked or dropped.

The most useful blades are:

- MacIntosh curved blade. This comes in three sizes: child, standard and large. The standard is the most useful, but have at least one each of the others available.
- Kessel blades. These are essential for fat patients with short necks.
- Paediatric blades are straight. Choose a brand with the light as close as possible to the tip of the blade.
- A right-handed blade is useful if patients who need to be intubated are lying on their side.

Library and Internet access

Have an unlocked bookcase built to house a small library of reference books, and your guidelines and protocols. Consider purchasing a practical reference book on drugs, a textbook of medicine such as *The Merck Manual*, and an ECG reference guide.

Internet access and a computer at the nurses' station will enable you to go online to check authoritative sources for certain problems.

Lighting

Consider the advantages of windows and natural light for both the patients and the staff. If natural daylight is not available, light the room with special colour corrected fluorescent tubes. Do not use blue-light fluorescent tubes or incandescent light bulbs because these make it difficult to judge the patient's colour, and delay the diagnosis of cyanosis. The lights should provide 100 *candela* for every 10 square metres of floor space. Effectively this is enough light to read the printing on a drug ampoule at arm's length with one eye covered. For most purposes two 25-watt fluorescent tubes are enough to cover 10 square metres.

Linen and laundry

Make provision to collect soiled linen, and other contaminated waste. Plan for the orderly disposable of paper and clean plastic. Clear plastic bags for clean are preferable so that staff can easily see the contents.

Music

The recovery room should be kept as quiet as possible. Do not play music in the recovery room. Not only is music distracting, but it substantially delays the time it takes for staff to respond to alarms or other abnormal sounds such as a patient developing a wheeze. The human ear is excellent at detecting small changes in sound in the environment (like things that go bump in the night). Music, because it is constantly fluctuating, abolishes that ability. Patients say that waking from anaesthesia in a noisy environment is distressing.

Nerve stimulators

Nerve stimulators are used to assess the degree and type of neuromuscular block in patients who remain paralysed at the end of an anaesthetic. Do not use them in awake patients as they are painful. Test for muscle strength by asking the patient to squeeze your fingers.

Notice boards

It is useful to have a large white board and erasable pens for teaching, immediate notices and planning patient management at the nurses' station.

Oxygen concentrators

In regions where bottled oxygen is expensive or difficult to obtain oxygen concentrators can provide an economical supply of nearly pure oxygen from air. If you are working in an isolated hospital, oxygen concentrators are a most worthwhile proposition. The purchase price of a concentrator is about half the cost of a year's supply of the same amount of oxygen from cylinders. The compressors in these units run on mains electric current but in emergencies they will run on the output from a small generator. The power consumption of a concentrator is only 350 watt, even a petrol generator or a truck battery fitted with an oscillator will give 600 watt.

Room air is basically a mixture of two gases: 21% oxygen and 79% nitrogen. This air is drawn into the machine through a series of filters and compressed to a pressure of 4 atmospheres. It is then passed into a canister of manufactured zeolite (a form of aluminium silicate) which acts as a molecular sieve. Nitrogen binds to the zeolite and oxygen passes on to a storage tank. After about 20 seconds the zeolite sieve becomes saturated with nitrogen, and the supply of compressed air is automatically diverted to a second canister where the process is repeated. This gives a constant output of oxygen. While the pressure in the second canister is at 138 kPa the pressure in the first is reduced to zero. Most of the nitrogen then comes off the zeolite, and is released to the atmosphere. A small back flow of oxygen from the alternative cylinder assists the process.

The life of the zeolite crystals is about 20 000 hours, or about 10 years. The gas emerging from the two cannisters and into the reservoir chamber is about 95% oxygen. This oxygen can be drawn off at about 4 litres/minute without any loss in concentration. Higher flows result in lower percentages of oxygen. The concentrators are not suitable to drive ventilators or compressed gas anaesthesia machines such as a Boyles machine. Remember, if the power fails there is only 2–3 minutes oxygen stored in the machine.

Servicing is required about every 5000 hours, it is not difficult and can be carried out by the user. Make sure you are given all the instructions for this when you purchase the machine. You should also be given at least 2 years' supply of spare parts.

If you are investing in oxygen concentrators you should buy two. Keep them clean and assign responsibility for them to one, named, person.

Decor

Paint walls and ceiling light neutral colours. Avoid colours such as blues, greens, pinks and yellows because they reflect misleadingly on patients' skins.

Patient trolleys

An absolute minimum of four patient transport trolleys are needed for each working theatre: one for attending to the patient in theatre, one for the patient in recovery room; and one for transporting the patient back to the ward and one in reserve. Only use trolleys built to the specification required by international standards.

Trolleys should:

- be quickly able to be tilted head or foot down by at least 25° from the horizontal;
- enable the patient to sit up with support;

and have:

- a frame to house portable monitoring equipment for transport;
- an adjustable footrest or bed-end to stop the patient sliding down;
- a firm base and mattress that will not sag should cardiac massage be needed;
- easily manoeuvred trolley sides or rails to stop the patient falling off;
- removable poles to carry drips;
- have large castor wheels with easily applied brakes;
- provision for portable suction and oxygen;
- a tray for carrying small articles such as the patient's history, dentures, and other belongings;
- provision for transporting ventilators, monitoring equipment, and drain bottles, and urine bags.

It is unnecessary to transfer patients from 'a sterile trolley' on to a 'non-sterile trolley' in the theatre block.

If your hospital has suitably designed beds, then patients having major surgery can be brought to the recovery room on their beds, although it is preferable for them to be on a narrower trolley.

Refrigerators

You will need two refrigerators: one for storing heat labile drugs, and other items, such as ice for testing the efficacy of local blocks, and another thermostatically controlled *blood fridge* for storing blood and vaccines. The blood fridge should have a clock-chart and an alarm to warn if the temperature has risen or fallen below set limits. If the alarm goes off check with the blood bank because you may need to discard all the biological items.

Security

The recovery room needs to be in a secure location so that passers-by cannot gain access. This is particularly important at night when there are not so many staff about. Usually the whole theatre block, including the recovery room, is secured by electronic sliding doors that are opened with a swipe card or numeric keypad.

Space blankets

Space blankets® are thin shiny metallic sheets made of Mylar®. This material is an exceptionally strong (but easily torn) plastic sheet, which has a layer of silver a few molecules thick adsorbed on to it. Put the silver side next to the patient. They minimize radiant heat loss, however they conduct heat easily and need to be separated from the patient's skin by a sheet or blanket, which seals a layer of insulating air around the patient's body. They conduct electricity so keep them away from electrical apparatus. They are highly flammable and burn with intense heat to melt into a small red-hot plastic ball.

Spirit levels

Spirit levels are used for levelling transducers with the isophlebotic point on the body. You can easily make one from a 1.8 metre length of plastic tube whose ends are joined to make a loop. Half fill the tubing with coloured water (use ink), join the ends, seal it with tape, and label so it is not discarded.

Suction

A totally reliable high capacity, high volume suction system is lifesaving. In order to cope with blood and sticky mucus each sucker must be capable of sustaining a free flow of at least 80 L/min and achieve an occluded suction pressure of at least 60 kPa (460 mmHg) even if nearby suckers are working too.

To prevent the suction inlet from becoming blocked include a fluid trap (usually a 3 litre plastic container) between the sucker and the wall outlet. The tap collects the secretions, blood and other fluids and prevents the system becoming clogged with muck. The wall outlets are usually protected with a sintered brass filter. Unless these filters are cleaned daily they soon become clogged and the suction pressure falls.

Change the tubing between patients and replace the suction bottles as soon as they are contaminated.

Suction is your lifeline. Establish a maintenance routine where the hospital engineers clean, test and maintain the system daily.

Telephones

Noisy telephones disturb patients and demand to be answered. Use a quiet ring tone. The theatre receptionist or a secretary should filter trivial incoming calls.

Mobile phones are safe to use in the recovery room. It remains an urban myth that they generate sufficient electromagnetic fields to disrupt equipment.

If you are still concerned, then don't use them within one metre of electronic monitors.

X-ray screens

Many hospitals are switching over to electronic data transmission, but you will still need X-ray viewing screens for old sheet X-rays.

Isolated hospitals

Additional considerations

Nominate one member of your department to be in charge of the purchase, care and maintenance of equipment. This is an important and time-consuming job.

Work out why you need the equipment in the first place.

- Will it improve patient safety? For example a pulse oximeter.
- Will it help staff work more efficiently by doing routine chore better? For example a non-invasive blood pressure machine.
- Can it do something that was impossible before? For example an oxygen concentrator.
- Does it need a special power source? A gas-powered ventilator is useless unless there is a reliable and cheap source of compressed gas to run it. Many isolated hospitals have to work with an erratic and unreliable power supply.

Equipment must be robust and reliable. Robustness is important, and reliability essential. Equipment is useless if it constantly needs maintenance, or has to be sent a long distance for repairs. Before purchasing any piece of equipment, find out how often it breaks down. In engineering terms this is known as the *mean time between failures* (MTBF). The best of the oxygen concentrators have an MTBF of 6000 hours of operating time.

What happens when your piece of equipment does breakdown? Does it break down in a safe way?

If in doubt about the reliability of the equipment, or its suitability for the task, telephone your nearest university teaching hospital and consult either the Biomedical Engineering Department or the Department of Anaethesia. They should be able to give you helpful and unbiased advice.

When buying expensive equipment, such as electronic monitors or ventilators; involve the engineering staff in the planning phase. Consider their advice on technical matters about the choice of equipment, and what sort of training they need; and particularly, the manufacturer's ability to provide support such as manuals, maintenance contracts, spare parts, and training films or familiarity courses.

Servicing equipment in a remote hospital

Of all the areas in which the isolated hospital has problems servicing equipment causes the most difficulty. Lying around departments of most isolated hospitals is broken down or unusable equipment. Thoughtful planning avoids such waste.

Sending equipment away for repairs or servicing can take many months and is expensive. Often a local technician can do the work if he has access to the workshop manuals. Do not buy equipment unless the company is willing to release circuit diagrams, and detailed workshop manuals of the equipment. Get at least two copies of the operator's manual and the maintenance manual; one for the hospital's biomedical engineers, and one to keep in the department. Check the manuals are complete, relevant, clearly written and illustrated (surprisingly often, this is not the case). Poor instruction manuals indicate that the company selling it is not reliable.

Where do spare parts come from? Importing spare parts from another country can take months. Make sure there is an after sales' service, with a reliable supply of spare parts. It is a good idea to order appropriate spare parts when the equipment is purchased. Even with normal wear and tear some pieces will begin to break down almost immediately; for example the rubber bulbs on blood pressure machines, or rubber straps on an electrocardiograph, and blood pressure cuff bladders. This is especially true in tropical climates where rubber perishes quickly.

Most equipment requires simple servicing by the people who use it. Establish a regular program of checking the equipment with clear order on what is to be done, and enforce them or else it may not happen! Every time a service is carried out, enter it in a book kept with the equipment.

This includes:

- daily, or pre-use checks;
- routine calibration;
- daily or pre-use cleaning and the reporting of faults;
- ensuring accessories are serviceable and complete;
- consumables are available.

Regular checks should be done by the biomedical engineers. To make things proceed smoothly the following questions need to be considered:

- what is to be maintained?
- how is it to be maintained?
- when is it to be maintained?
- is the maintenance effective?

To answer the first question draw up an inventory or register of equipment that needs maintenance. Commission equipment before putting it into use. Commissioning involves setting up a maintenance programme and training staff to use and care for the equipment. The regular maintenance schedule must balance the manufacturer's recommendations with how often the equipment is used. The more often the equipment is used, the more frequently it should be checked.

Documentation is crucial, and card index systems are best in a smaller hospital. We hesitate to recommend computer-based systems in an isolated hospital because they require expert staff to run them. If the computer breaks down (and proper back-ups have not been made) all your data can be lost.

Some items of biomedical equipment such as blood gas machines require periodic calibration by an outside agency. Try as far as possible to calibrate the apparatus on the spot to avoid long periods without the equipment, and the risk of damage during transport. Bring the technician to the machine, try not to send the machine to the technician.

If servicing and maintenance is beyond the resources of your biomedical engineers it is possible for regions or even countries, to co-operate to share a technician at regular intervals. This reduces cost, and increases efficiency.

If it cannot be repaired, then condemn broken biomedical equipment. Do not leave it lying around in your department. Ask the Supply department to organize its disposal, and attend to the proper inventory and accounting procedures. Consider modifying the equipment to extend its useful life, or using parts of it for other things.

Disposables

It is tempting to buy disposable items, because they release staff from the chores of cleaning and sterilization. Disposables save wages, and time, and reduce the chance of cross-infection. However, they are expensive, and need lots of storage space. If you are working in a isolated hospital think carefully before you discard, or stop using reusable items such as stainless steel dishes, metal suckers and linen drapes. Circumstances can make disposable unobtainable. Once the routines for cleaning and sterilizing reusable items are abandoned, it is hard to start again.

An inventory system is needed to automatically re-order disposables. Delegate this clerical function to either the pharmacy, or the supply office.

Reusing disposable items is a controversial issue. Many disposable items which have not been exposed to blood, or body fluids, can be washed, and then sterilized and safely reused. In many countries, medicolegal problems make the reuse impracticable.

Budgets

Most hospitals require every service area, such as the recovery room to have their own budget with the freedom, within set limits, to purchase and maintain their equipment. Until you are familiar with the budgets it is worthwhile sitting down with a hospital administrator to check through the figures to see how the department is managing financially.

Notes

1. Nightingale F (1863) *Notes on Hospitals.*
2. English Department of Health (NHS Estates) (2002) *Revised schedules of accommodation.*

29

Working with people

Perioperative care

In 2000 it was reported that of the 50 000 perioperative adverse events reported to the Australian Incident Monitoring System (AIMS) each year, one in eight can be ameliorated or prevented by a coordinated preadmission process.[1]

Over the past decade integrated perioperative practice has developed into a specialty in its own right. One way to avoid problems is to have a careful production line approach to routine surgical procedures. This involves an orderly sequential process of preoperative assessment and optimisation, operative care, recovery room, the surgical ward, rehabilitation, and all the paramedical support programmes (such as social work, occupational therapy, pharmacy, and counsellors) are assembled in a production line to make sure the patient gets the best care and nothing is omitted or overlooked.

Preoperative assessment clinics

Preoperative assessment clinics now routinely prepare patients for surgery, to make sure they arrive at the operating theatre door in the best possible physical and psychological shape. The process requires identifying potential problems, optimizing intercurrent disease, and especially discussing with the patients each step and procedure they will undergo during their hospital stay. For instance if patients are to receive spinal or epidural anaesthesia they need to know in detail what to expect. Informed consent includes discussion of both the perceived benefits and the possible harms of the procedure.

Study the preadmission assessment.

Clinical pathways started in the preadmission clinic guide the patient's care through a standardized sequence of best practice protocols. The patient's post-operative care is planned from the time they first consult the surgeon to the time their rehabilitation is complete and their welfare is handed back to their local doctor and local health facility. The aim is to ensure that the patient's hospital stay is free from unexpected adverse events, and they recover from their surgery and are able to resume their normal lives as quickly as possible.

Preoperative assessment clinics are multidisciplinary involving medical staff, anaesthetists, perioperative nurses, physiotherapists, and occupational therapists. Other specialists are co-opted as needed; these include pharmacists, dieticians, and diabetic educators. Over 70 per cent of patients aged 65 years or more who attend the Preadmission Clinic at Box Hill Hospital have sub-optimally controlled or undiagnosed disease, or are taking inappropriate medication, or taking their medication inappropriately. If such things are missed then problems may arise in the recovery room.

Cultural and religious issues

Recovery staff need to be sensitive to customs of patients from diverse cultural, ethnic and religious backgrounds. Under some circumstances recovery room staff find it frustrating to have to change their usual practice to incorporate patients' traditional methods or religious beliefs.

Sometimes patients' beliefs seem to be not in their best interests. For instance Jehovah's Witnesses have sincere and deeply held beliefs that do not allow them to accept any blood or blood product under any circumstance. To staff faced with a patient bleeding to death in front of them this is a challenging and painful dilemma. Jehovah's Witnesses believe that personal commitment to their faith is more important than their family or their own life. They may refuse surgical or medical intervention for themselves or their children. In some countries the law will not allow treatment to be withheld from minors under a certain age. If you foresee conflict or have doubts about the situation involve your hospital's legal and ethical consultants immediately.

Jews from a European background regard family involvement of ultimate importance. They feel more comfortable if they have had three or four opinions before they decide on treatment.

Some cultures require all messages to be transmitted through the oldest male member of the family; others preclude men caring for women in the recovery room or women caring for men.

It is easy to accidentally offend some patients by the way you say things, or with non-verbal communication. Direct or prolonged eye contact in some cultures (such as North American Indian, and some Australian aborigines) is considered aggressively disrespectful, whereas in some other cultures (South American and European) to avoid eye contact is a sign of a lack of interest. Some Vietnamese or Thais are deeply offended if you touch their head without their permission. A warm smile, gentleness, genuine concern and a respectful soft voice, will ease the path through this cultural minefield.

Some cultures and religions have certain articles of clothing or jewellery they wish to wear, or have nearby. As far as possible accommodate their wishes.

Interpreters

If a patient is not fluent in English you may need an interpreter in the recovery room. Use medically trained interpreters, and as far as possible avoid using family members. A good interpreter copies (or if necessary interprets) your body language, and translates your words. Talk directly to the patient, and use the interpreter only as an instrument to translate what you are saying. Keep your sentences short and pass on one fact at a time. Although the face-to-face method is best, in some complex or sensitive situations it is better to explain to the trained clinical interpreter exactly what you want to tell patients or their families, and then leave them to do it for you.

Staffing recovery room

Standards for the levels staffing of recovery room vary from country to country, and according to the workloads, the type of surgery and the fitness and age of the patients. Many countries have set standards and guidelines on these matters. Each recovery room must establish its own staffing protocols, and insist that they are given the resources to adhere to them.

Staff must be proficient in cardiac life support.

Every member of staff working in recovery room must be proficient in *basic life support*, but additionally specialist recovery room nurses need to be proficient with *advanced cardiac life support*.

It is difficult to lay down firm rules about the ratio of specialist to non-specialist staff working in the recovery room. Clearly, if patients are physiologically unstable or potentially may become so, then a one to one ratio of specialist staff to patients is needed. However, if the patients are stable, the surgery is minor and the anaesthetic uncomplicated then such intense supervision is not warranted.

Recovery stages

We have divided recovery from anaesthesia and surgery into three stages: Stage 1, Stage 2, Stage 3 recovery. There are also the special cases of Extended Stage 1 and 2 recovery. We believe that if these stages are precisely defined it will increase the safety of patients treat them in a holistic manner.

To define the stages the boundaries between each stage must be absolutely clear. The stages also recognize that the patient's stay in recovery room is just the first step in a process that may take months or years to complete.

Stages 1 and 2 recovery are determined by the immediate availability of one or other of the two levels of *cardiac life support* should anything go wrong.

Basic life support includes the basic ABC of resuscitation: maintenance of a clear airway, support of breathing and external cardiac massage.

Advanced cardiac life support includes all the other procedures needed to deal with a cardiac arrest (including defibrillation) or emergency airway problems at least up to (and in some cases including) intubation.

The defining question is: "Is it likely that the patient may encounter an incident that would cause harm?" If the answer is "yes", then they are in Stage 1 recovery, if the answer is "no", then they can step down to Stage 2 recovery.

Stage 1 recovery

Stage 1 recovery includes physiologically unstable patients, and those patients who potentially could become unstable and are consequently at a risk of harm.

Staffing

Patients in Stage 1 recovery must be attended by *specialist nursing staff* who are proficient at advanced cardiac life support. Specialist nursing staff means nurses who are fully qualified and certified as recovery room nurses.

An anaesthetist should remain within the operating suite while there are any patients in Stage 1 recovery in the recovery room.

Known unstable patients

Stage 1 recovery includes patients whose *vital signs* deviate significantly from their preoperative baseline values. These patients may still be:

- comatose;
- receiving ventilatory support;
- intubated, or require a laryngeal mask to preserve their airway;
- receiving vasoactive drugs;
- hypothermic;
- bleeding;
- or have a major metabolic disturbance.

Supervision

Stage 1 recovery requires at least one specialist recovery room nurse be present in the recovery room for each non-specialist nurse.

Double care = two nurses to one patient

Patients require *double care* if one or more of the following:

- physiologically unstable;
- critically ill;
- being ventilated;
- agitated or combative.

Dedicated care = one patient to one nurse

If the patient is one or more of the following:

- unstable with vital signs outside their preoperative baseline;
- intubated with either an endotracheal tube or laryngeal mask (including ventilated patients);
- receiving vasoactive drugs;
- is receiving a transfusion or blood or blood products;
- under the age of 8 years whether conscious or not.

Shared care = two patients to one nurse

If:

- one patient is conscious and stable, and the other is unconscious and stable;
- both patients are conscious and stable.

All patients who have unstable vital signs remain in Stage 1 recovery.

Potentially unstable patients

Whether a patient will become physiologically unstable in the future is not easily quantified, but specialist recovery room nurses will readily recognize factors that put the patient at risk.

As a guide potentially unstable patients have one or more of a combination of the following:

- cardiovascular instability;
- respiratory insufficiency;
- metabolic problems (such as diabetes, acid-base disturbance, or hypothermia);
- or where the patient bled during the surgery (raising the possibility of functional anaemia).

Any one of these components alone is unlikely to cause worrying physiological instability. However, should one or more other components intervene there is the potential for a cascading chain reaction that may result in the patient suffering cerebral, cardiac or tissue hypoxia.

Extended Stage 1 recovery includes patients discharged to ICU or coronary care unit, or other high-care units where the specialist nursing staff caring for the patients have equivalent training and abilities of specialist recovery room nurses.

Stage 2 recovery

Stage 2 recovery includes stable patients who are conscious and competent (although they may still have residual effects of a local anaesthetic or neuraxial block). The patients should have stable vital signs comparable to their preoperative baseline for at least 30 minutes before they are discharged to the ward.

Patients may be attended by non-specialist nursing staff who are proficient at basic life support.

In the ward (Extended Stage 2 recovery)

Here the patient will be cared for by staff who have equivalent skills and training of a non-specialist recovery room nurse.

During Stage 2 recovery at least one specialist nurse should be immediately available, but the care of patients can be left with non-specialist qualified nurses.

Supervisory care = one nurse to three patients

If the patients are:

- over the age of 8 years;
- under the age of 8 years but with a parent present.

Special supervisory care = one nurse to two patients

If the patients are one or more of the following:

- under the age of eight years;
- receiving intravenous fluids;
- at potential risk for some untoward event to occur such as bleeding;
- require plaster checks.

Standard care = one nurse to five patients

Standard care is the level of care normally available on a surgical ward. This should never be less than one nurse for every five patients.

Stage 3 recovery

Stage 3 recovery applies to patients who have yet to recover fully from the effects of their surgery or anaesthetic no matter how long this takes.

After day case procedures *Stage 3 recovery* applies patients who are discharged into the care of a competent and informed adult who can intervene in the case of untoward events. This carer may have no skills in cardiac life support techniques, or any medical knowledge, but must be capable of recognizing problems and know what to do about them. The carer must have clear written instructions of what to do about pain, nausea and vomiting, continued ooze from the wound site, or attacks of faintness. In case problems arise the carer needs a phone number to call, and a plan in place to bring the patient back to the hospital (or day care centre) if necessary. In other words do not send a patient to a remote location without a telephone and transport to bring them back should it become necessary.

Stage 3 recovery also applies to those who have been discharged from hospital, but remain at risk from complications of their surgery or anaesthetic, no matter how remote. Hospital staff tend to assume that once a patient leaves the hospital, even after days or weeks in the ward, they have recovered and all will be well. As any family doctor will tell you this is not necessarily so because of the occasional wound breakdown, deep vein thrombosis, or pulmonary embolism occurring after the patient has gone home. Recent surveys have shown a surprising number of elderly people die in the first 6 weeks after discharge from major surgery, some without ever coming to the attention of the hospital. Furthermore the psychological repercussions of serious illness, such as depression, can haunt patients for months to years. For this reason *Stage 3 recovery* involves a holistic view of the patient, and their family, as part of a continuum of health care and welfare, and not merely simply their stay in the recovery room.

Who must be present in the recovery room

Every member of staff working in recovery room must be proficient in basic life support, but additionally specialist recovery room staff must be proficient with advanced cardiac life support including defibrillation. As a basic requirement someone proficient in advanced cardiac life support must always be present in the recovery room while any patient is in Stage 1 recovery.

Specialist perioperative nurses

One advance in perioperative practice has been the evolution of *specialist perioperative nurses* (SPN)[9]. These nurses work as a member of a specialist surgical team such as orthopaedics, urology, or thoracic surgery. A specific nurse meets their patient when they first attend for preoperative assessment. The SPN then accompanies them through every step of their hospital stay until they 'wave goodbye at the hospital gate'. Even then the SPN telephones their patients for up to 6 weeks after their discharge. SPNs are also involved in educating patients, troubleshooting, discharge planning, administrative responsibilities and social welfare.

Often the specialist perioperative nurse is the only health care worker who is with the patient every step of the way. It is hard to overstate the value of this bond for the patients' emotional well-being, in having someone they know and trust for the continuum of care, and to identify and prevent clinical and organisational errors.

It is prudent for the surgical unit's SPN to brief the recovery room nurses on the patients about to arrive under their care.

Should the recovery nurse do preoperative visits?

It would seem ideal for recovery room nurses to see their prospective patients before surgery. The patients would then know what to expect during their stay in the recovery room, and be reassured by a familiar face when they emerge from anaesthesia. The nurse, knowing the patient's condition, would be able to make a nursing plan before the patient arrives. Preoperative visiting schemes have been tried many times, but few have lasted for more than a month or two. The reasons for their failure includes changing nursing shifts, irregular operating schedules, patients being admitted through a surgical services unit only a few hours before surgery and not going to the ward first. It has fallen on the nurses in the preadmission clinic to explain the recovery room procedures. A well-planned preadmission clinic has ex-theatre nurses on their staff.

The main reason that the visiting schemes do not work is that there is not enough time or resources. In a hospital doing 10 000 surgical procedures a year, if a recovery room nurse spends 20 minutes with each patient and 10 minutes making notes, this amounts to 5000 hours, or an additional 2.5 full-time nursing equivalents. The administrators in most hospitals are reluctant to allocate resources in this way.

Administration

Administration of a recovery room is a large topic; so we will only touch on it here.

The recovery room is usually supervised by either the Nursing Director of the Operating Theatre Suite or the Director of the Department of Anaesthesia. A trained and certified nurse should manage the area. Clerical staff are needed to answer phones, take messages, keep track of supplies, handle medical records and so on.

Planning is usually delegated to an Operating Theatre committee composed of nurses, medical staff, and administrators. Some tips to make this committee run smoothly are that it should:

- be small with no more than six members;
- hold regular meetings;
- have defined written responsibilities;
- have an agenda circulated some days before each meeting.

One of the principal roles of the committee is to establish guidelines and protocols.

Protocols and guidelines

Protocols are designed to be followed precisely, whereas *guidelines* allow latitude for commonsense. *Policies* lay out a course of action for the future. Protocols ensure everyone does the same thing in the same way. Most clinical and administrative problems occur again and again, and every hospital has its own way of dealing with these issues. It is not easy or appropriate to transplant routines from one hospital to another, so develop your own policies and protocols. Protocols, policies and guidelines make auditing performance easier.

You will need protocols for:

- checking equipment and drugs;
- transferring patients from one area to another;
- handover of patients from one area to another: from theatre to recovery room staff, and from recovery room staff to ward staff;
- documentation;
- emergency procedures;
- discharge criteria;
- and responsibilities of the various categories of staff.

Routines and protocols help prevent mishaps and errors. Written guidelines help staff manage the more complex postoperative problems such as epidural catheters, or airway problems after thyroidectomy.

Protocols need to be concise, well-written and helpful. Keep them in the recovery room where everyone has access to them. You will know if they are being consulted because a good set of guidelines will soon look well thumbed and dog eared.

Do not make them too long, because no one will read them. The *Peri-operative fasting in adults and children* guidelines issued in 2005 by the Royal College of Nursing is an erudite 266 page document, whereas their summary is only 30 pages. It would be more helpful and probably read more often if it was summarized on one sheet of paper.

Reference books

A small library with a set of reference books is useful. Do not lock them away after hours. You never know when you may need to consult them. Reference books on practical pharmacology and nursing procedures help cope with situations that might not be covered by your protocols or guidelines.

Message book

A message book is useful to pass messages on to staff on following shifts. Use it to keep track of equipment you have loaned to other parts of the hospital, to follow up good ideas, and even staff requests for roster changes.

Maintenance books

Maintenance books ensure the weekly check of equipment, such as the defibrillator, has been done properly.

Weekly meetings

Weekly meetings should be part of your quality assurance programme.

Audits

Audits are part of the quality control process. They help you find potential problems, and may reveal information to improve patient care. They also provide a benchmark so that you can compare your performance with that of other equivalent recovery rooms in your area. Once you have corrected a problem, repeat your audit to make sure it really was solved. This check is called *closing the audit*. Audits can be a tedious chore, but they really do make a difference.

Risk management

Clinical governance

One in ten patients suffers an adverse event while in hospital.[2] Simply being in an acute care hospital in Australia carries a 40-fold greater risk than travelling in a car.[3] Preventing or controlling these adverse events is the role of risk management. Risk management is merely one large cog in the much larger wheel of clinical governance.

Clinical governance is a *system* designed to integrate education, clinical audit, best practice, risk management, research, and effective communication.

It is necessary to identify and document each one of these factors to detect when things go wrong, analyse what went wrong, fix the problem, and try to make sure that it does not happen again. All this sounds simple, reasonable and logical, but it is difficult to implement on a large scale. Difficulties arise when a single component of a complex system is modified. This throws the rest of the system into disarray. So it is tempting to simply patch each problem as it arises, and leave an outdated or hazardous *system* intact. Think about the implications of closing the recovery room for a week to install a better suction system: lists cancelled, staff not working, urgent cases transferred elsewhere, political ramifications, dust, dirt and much more. It is easier to put a patch on the problem by installing inferior portable suckers.

Risk

The recovery room is a high-risk area because there is ample opportunity to accidentally harm otherwise well people.

Risks arise whenever you do something that might have an uncertain outcome. Where risks are present adverse events are eventually inevitable.

Adverse events are those that cause unintended harm to patients through any action, either directly or indirectly, by a member of hospital staff. These unintended complications or injuries either prolong hospital stay, or require additional measures to manage them. Complications of surgery, such as wound infection or deep vein thrombosis, are adverse events. There are two things to look at when analysing adverse events: was it predictable, and could it have been better managed? Each component can be rated on a scale from low to high. For instance the risk of a patient vomiting could be predicted as high, but even though it was predicted the subsequent management of the vomiting may have been suboptimal.

Not all adverse events are preventable, but those that are preventable are called *errors*. Just because an adverse event occurs does not mean anyone has been negligent or that it was avoidable. All medical care entails risk and bad things happen despite the most scrupulous, rigorous and conscientious care.

Near misses occur when something goes wrong, but the event is detected and averted before anyone is harmed. For instance someone notices that the wrong drug is about to be given to the patient before it occurs.

Incidents occur when an event has occurred that harms or could harm someone within the hospital precincts. (This includes staff, patients and visitors.)

Sentinel events are serious clear-cut events that occur because of errors made by health care workers, for instance amputating the wrong leg, or giving blood of the wrong group to a patient causing a haemolytic transfusion reaction, or intravenous gas embolism by detaching a central venous line.

Sentinel events occur when protocols are not followed. These events need thorough investigation using the techniques of *root cause analysis.*

Routines and protocols

Routines and protocols are designed to minimize the effect of adverse events when they do occur. Unsafe *systems* and poorly planned protocols cause needless harm. Sadly some hospital administrators ignore this truth, because as we have seen, changing systems is very difficult indeed.

Types of risk

Risk management falls into two categories: proactive and reactive risk management.

Preventative (*proactive*) risk management involves identifying risks before they occur, and then putting in place strategies to prevent them happening. Preventative strategies include such things as preoperatively identifying patients who are likely to vomit in the recovery room, so that they can be given prophylactic anti-emetics during their anaesthetic, or washing your hands to prevent cross-infection.

Responsive (*reactive*) risk management involves dealing with adverse events once they have occurred. Examples include policies and protocols to deal with death in the recovery room, aspiration of stomach contents, or needle-stick injuries to staff.

Reasons why things go wrong

1. *Slips* result in an unintended action and are usually caused by human error.

2. *Lapses* are caused by rule-based mistakes. That is by applying a bad rule or failing to apply a good rule.

3. *Knowledge-based mistakes* occur because you don't know what you are doing.

4. *Violations* occur when rules are deliberately broken.

5. *Mishaps* are unpredictable events, statistically certain to occur.

6. *System errors* occur when the managerial frameworks are flimsy.

7. *Communication errors* occur when people don't pass the message on.

(These terms are adapted from an excellent reference: *Human Error* by James Reason. Publisher: Cambridge University Press (October 26, 1990).)

Why errors happen

We all make mistakes: humans do. But in some jobs mistakes can harm, injure or kill. Working in recovery room is one of these jobs. No one ever makes mistakes intentionally. Good people do not come to work in the morning saying: "I'm going to purposely harm someone today."

Errors are preventable adverse events.

Mishaps are not preventable

Mishaps are not preventable, but they are inevitable. Sooner or later you will encounter a patient who has an anaphylactic reaction despite having no known drug allergies, or a patient who becomes violent on emerging from an anaesthetic. Where patients or staff are harmed the outcome is called a *serious adverse event*.

Errors are preventable

Slips, lapses, poor training, violations or protocols, system errors and communication errors are all preventable. Errors occur at all levels of care, not only with high-risk procedures. Good governance prevents errors.

Human error causes slips

Slips are caused by human error. Many slips occur because of absent-mindedness or lack of concentration. Slips are preventable, but they rarely occur simply because of one single factor. Slips tend to occur in familiar and routine settings where staff are preoccupied or distracted.

Brains on autopilot

Our brains can only cope with so much information without going into meltdown. Slips occur if our attention is constrained by something else going on around us, or some worry on our mind. Have you ever done something like putting salt in your tea, or a grapefruit skin in the dishwasher? These slips are not as stupid as they might first appear. One rarely thinks about automatic tasks. Your brain was simply on autopilot.

These virtues of economy, of delegating attention to autopilot while doing routine tasks, free up our mind to think of other things. It's part of our make-up. You rarely play close attention to what you are doing while having a shower before going out for the evening; your mind is off elsewhere.

If the same error occurs more than once, then look for a system error. Do not blame the individual.

If you are on autopilot while tending patients in the recovery room then slips are likely. Two most common slips in the recovery room are giving the wrong dose of a drug, or allowing an intravenous infusion to run in too quickly. One way to avoid the autopilot phenomenon is to vary your tasks during each shift as much as possible: recover a patient, go to the ward with the next, and teach, and so on.

Efficient brains fill in the gaps

Our barins are vrey eficifeint. Tehy do as lttile wrok as pssoilbe to prferom ritoune tasks in the rceoevry room.

As we read those sentences, our brains look at the first letter, the last letter and the length of the word, and then fill in the gaps. If our brains did not fill in gaps we would be flooded by sensory inputs. To avoid be overwhelmed we direct our attention to what is important. Are you wearing a watch? What colour are the walls? However, such economy of neural processing makes it easy not to notice when things that are normally routine, are now going wrong.

Causes of errors

Human errors

Knowledge-based errors occur where training is inadequate, experience is lacking, or facts are unknown or unavailable. A common preventable error is to prescribe two or more drugs without realizing that they may interact with each other, such as giving metoclopramide to someone on a dopamine infusion. The facts are well known, but unless the knowledge is remembered, and then applied – an error occurs. Computer systems for dispensing drugs reduce the risk of such lapses.

Fatigue is a common cause of error. A member of staff who is sleep deprived or has been working too long without a break cannot think quickly and will inevitably sooner or later make a mistake.

Working in unfamiliar environments or settings, or having to cope with time pressures, or with complex clinical problems also creates situations where errors are more likely to occur.

Lapses occur when protocols are not followed.

Adverse events increase logarithmically as patient to nurse staff ratios increase. Things are missed, short cuts taken: harried staff make mistakes.

Lapses occur where protocols and rules, for one reason or another, are not followed. This is rarely due to laziness, or incompetence. The protocols and guidelines used in recovery rooms are part of an integrated and extremely complex *system*. Protocols and guidelines cannot possibly cover every situation, and when they do not, then staff are tempted to improvise or take short cuts. No one error, no one technical failure causes disaster. It usually takes a diabolical combination of factors aligning each other through tiny windows of opportunity for a lapse to cause a problem. This phenomenon is sometimes called the '*Swiss Cheese Effect*'. Think about a stack of slices Swiss cheese; the holes in the cheese may not align, but as circumstances change and holes overlap then gaps in the system are revealed.

Disasters are always predictable – in hindsight!

Most errors are systematic

Honest analysis of an adverse event will probably reveal up to 20 or more factors contributing to the disaster. Many of the factors are systematic such as inappropriate rostering, insufficient staff or supervision, lack of knowledge, high workloads, time pressures, inadequate equipment, tired or distracted, or out-of-sorts staff, and almost inevitably poor communication.

Proper training and ongoing education help prevent errors.

Good recovery rooms are not necessarily the ones where errors never seem to occur, because errors happen every day. If there seem to be no errors, then the slips and lapses are probably being concealed. Good recovery room managers recognize error-prone situations, detect adverse events when they occur, and have contingencies in place to correct them.

Lack of communication causes disasters

A common system error occurs where there are unclear lines of authority for doctors, nurses, and other health care workers. Unless there are clearly defined lines of responsibility and authority about patients' care, the recovery room can become a high-risk zone where the surgeon and the anaesthetist give conflicting instructions, or worse still think the other is taking the responsibility. This is a scenario for a disaster. Under these circumstances it is easy for the recovery room nurse to end up in a void, and enticed to act independently without knowing the full surgical or anaesthetic implications of the case. This puts the nurse in an untenable position. As a general rule the anaesthetist is the head physician responsible for the patients' medical care in the recovery room. If an adverse event occurs notify the anaesthetist immediately.

Poor communication is a root cause of many problems. This is one reason to employ specialist perioperative nurses. They know their patients. They know the system. The patient's specialist perioperative nurse has information, much of which is not in the patient's notes.

Why handwashing may be a system problem[4]

Hospital-acquired infection can be halved if staff wash their hands appropriately. The bacterium *Legionella pneumophilia* grows in warm water. In the early 1980s scares about *Legionella* forced hospitals to increase hot water temperatures so that the bacteria could not survive. This made hand washing difficult. Many hospitals do not have mixer-taps, and when staff were confronted with scalding water from one tap and freezing water from the other they stopped washing their hands, and the incidence of hospital-acquired infections soared.

Audits and quality of care

Audits collect and record data about outcomes. Good practice demands this is done regularly, and systematically. Good governance gives us the resources to do so. Audits are designed to improve practice and the care of patients. For this reason the data must be recorded honestly. Apart from helping identify adverse events the data may well be used in confidential enquiries. It is not about how good we are, but about how bad we are. If we can stop bad things happening then what remains is better than it was. Each little improvement is a step towards better care for our patients.

Quality assessment

Quality assessment answers the question, "Is what we are doing in the recovery room working properly?" This involves identifying risky situations, evaluating them, assessing the available resources, determining a course of action, and planning for contingencies.

Quality assurance

Quality assurance answers the questions, "Are we achieving what we set out to achieve? And if not; then why not? And what are we going to do about it?"

Risk management

Risk management relies on identifying risky situations, and then putting in place measures to counteract them. These measures include creating policies, protocols and guidelines; while other measure includes appropriate education, proper training, repeated practice and regular review of outcomes.

The secret of risk management is to create successive layers of defence involving checking, and rechecking and checking yet again. Other examples of multiple layers of defence include coloured labels for syringes, two staff independently checking drug doses, patients having labels on both wrists and ankles, different coloured containers for different levels of waste, or fail-safe alarms on monitors.

Quality assurance involves continuous monitoring, and regular review.

Policies, protocols and guidelines

Policies set down the general principles of what you are to do under defined circumstances. For instance hospital policy does not allow you to disclose medical information about your patient to other persons, without the patient giving written and signed permission.

Protocols set down the details of procedures to follow under specific circumstances. These procedures are not optional; they are rules to be obeyed. The rules are usually laid out in a step-wise manner.

Guidelines are suggestions of what to do under certain circumstances. They do not carry the weight of compulsion, but are there to guide you. Guidelines require that you use common sense. However, common sense is not always a common commodity. Ultimately common sense relies on *education*, which enables you to understand why you are doing something; *experience* in that you have seen and done it before and can quickly recognize it again; and *training* so that you can respond rapidly and uniformly to the circumstances.

To be effective protocols and policies must be clear, brief, objective and unambiguous. Recently, we came cross a 12-page protocol on "how to empty a urine bag" filled with jargon, and with 21 references. Busy staff are unlikely to read it, students will ignore it, and sadly the message is lost.

To formulate a protocol you need:

- up-to-date and accurate information on the topic;
- practical ideas on how to modify or control risk;
- clear ideas on how to implement the protocol;
- to regularly review and revise the protocol.

Good protocols set out in the simplest and clearest language:

- the purpose of the protocol;
- the medical/nursing/administrative reasons for the protocol;
- how to do it – equipment and resources required;
- special rules – who can do what, and where;

- precautions and contraindications;
- where to get help if things go wrong;
- definitions – explaining the meaning of the technical words;
- where to get more information;
- a future date when the protocol will be reviewed.

  Problems with protocols:
- the information may not be current or accurate;
- protocols might not be applicable to a particular individual;
- they may not allow for flexibility in clinical practice.

Risk management and the law

Some hospital policies are mandated by statute law. For instance a patient who dies in recovery room becomes a coroner's case. Some are subject to common law and precedent, such as what constitutes patients' consent to decisions about their care, and how their consent must be obtained.

Nurses are not immune from their legal responsibilities.

How to protect yourself from legal problems

You must keep your knowledge and skills up-to-date. This includes your knowing the laws and statutory regulations affecting the way you practice.

- Ignorance of the law is not a legal defence.
- Preferably join both a professional nursing association, and a union.
- Maintain adequate indemnity insurance. This is especially important if your employer does not cover aspects of your practice.
- Keep your patients' records conscientiously. Write everything down. If an event is not in writing, then it effectively it did not occur. You will have difficulty, perhaps in five years time, proving events in a courtroom.
- Do not use abbreviations in the patient's medical record unless they conform to your hospital's guidelines.
- Write only what you see, do and hear in the patient's record. Clearly separate opinion from fact. Do not pass judgment. "The patient was rude and stupid" is not acceptable. "I feel the patient was impolite and ignorant of the facts", is barely acceptable. "The patient appeared upset, and I believe does not understand what I told him", is an acceptable observation.
- Never criticize colleagues or the hospital in front of patients, and never in the medical record.

- If you disagree with hospital management, or disgree with your colleagues then, as soon as possible, write everything down, and date it. Keep your notes as a personal record.
- Follow your hospital's policies and procedures. If you feel they are inadequate then work through appropriate channels to address your concerns.
- Foster relationships. Be considerate, polite, respectful and truthful.
- Treat your colleagues fairly. Do not allow your views on their lifestyle, religion or culture to prejudice your professional relationship with them.
- Talk to your colleagues because communication breakdown is the most frequent and serious cause of errors.
- Take legal threats against you seriously. Seek help immediately.

Risk management is everybody's responsibility.

Table 29.1 How to classify adverse events

Category	Definition	Example
A	No error	
B	Error, but no harm	
C	Error with no harm, but needs watching	
D	Error, with harm, but the harm was only temporary	
F	Error and harm. Requires intervention	

Managing people

We all have strengths and weaknesses, and not everyone is suited to manage people. Managing people is partly an innate gift, and partly training. Simply being good and competent at one's job is not a qualification for a managerial position.

It is difficult to be popular and a good manager. For this reason, in the long run it is far better to be fair than nice. It is the manager's job to ensure that all their staff understand their personal and collective duty for patient safety.

Managing risk

How to get feedback

Risk management involves managers listening to patients, and staff, and carefully considering what they have to say: their criticisms, suggestions, solutions and ideas.

Good managers listen with their ears of their heart,
but analyse with the logic of a computer.

Good managers are realistic, and non-critical, and able to temper enthusiasm with experience. They need to cultivate an easy non-threatening relationship with their staff and patients. They avoid micromanaging staff under their control by allowing competent people to get on with their job, and give them the resources to do so.

Good communication is the key. Managers need tact and empathy to tell their staff what is expected of them, and correct them when they are wrong. Managers need to establish formal structures, for reporting adverse events and, just as importantly, near-misses (slips and lapses).

Compliment in public.
Criticize in private.

Ensuring compliance and accountability

Once policies and protocols are in place it is essential to check compliance to find out if staff are following them, and if not, then why not. If there is a system problem it may be that the protocols are impracticable.

Sometimes staff feel that a change in direction is unwarranted. To counteract this requires a change in the culture of the unit. For fear of criticism, ostracism, or ridicule staff may be reluctant to report adverse events, or near misses. Possibly there is a culture of covering up mistakes, or taking shortcuts.

Direction and strategy

It is management's role to set direction, and establish strategies. *Direction* is a statement of intent; it defines exactly and precisely where we want to go in the long term. *Strategies* are the plans we make to get there.

To put strategies in place you will need to clearly determine your objective, have sufficient data to make sensible decisions, identify possible obstacles, have the necessary resources (knowledge, human resources, and finance), and develop a timetable to implement your plan. At each step you will need to re-evaluate your progress.

An organization may change direction when existing strategies are hazardous, or no longer work; or because new superior techniques come along. A change in direction occurred with the move away from general anaesthesia for Caesarean section to spinal anaesthesia. The strategies put in place to achieve this included setting up a climate for change by educating patients and staff.

Our goal might be to reduce to reduce the level of pain patients have when they are discharged from the recovery room. The strategies include a wide variety of analgesic techniques. For most problems there is no one simple answer; instead you will need many different strategies to achieve a satisfactory outcome. For example, consider all the different ways to control pain in the recovery room. No one strategy suits every patient.

Elegant solutions evolve from collaborative problem-solving.

Changing the culture

As anyone who has tried to get doctors to wash their hands before and after touching a patient will know, changing culture requires many qualities including patience, empathy, tact, discretion, reason, coercion, and humour.

To change hospital or unit culture, means to change the way people think. If we can change the way people think then they will change the way they act.

Ethics and morality

Even in recovery room we sometimes we have to make extremely difficult decisions: what to do about a Jehovah's Witness who has just had a Caesarean section and is now bleeding to death. We know that a couple of units of fresh frozen plasma will save this young mother's life; how to cope with death in the recovery room; how to deal with dangerously incompetent colleagues. These are difficult and serious questions. The study of ethics and morality helps guide us in dealing with such quandaries.

Morality

It is the privilege of our profession to care for people. Our patients trust us with this care; they have faith in us to honour their welfare. The privilege of this trust, this honour, sometimes gets lost in the busy-ness of our day. Often the office politics, problems and personalities of the moment are more prominent in our thoughts. But they are not more important. Without continually reinforcing feelings for morality and ethics, it becomes tempting to take short-cuts in our work, or to become disrespectful to others, or be inconsiderate or even unkind to our patients.

Ethics

Ethics is about the proper and moral conduct of our profession. To be ethical we need to be competent, have integrity, and conform to professional etiquette.

It is our patients' welfare that, and above all else, is our first consideration. Over the years, academics, philosophers, lawyers, theologians, politicians and others have argued and debated and tried to lay down principles of what this means. But it is simple. It means: "treat others as you would have them treat you or those you love". It is as basic as that.

The most important person in the room is the patient;
any room, at any time and any patient!

Although this is a simple notion it is not always possible to achieve if our morals and beliefs get in the way. Take abortion for instance. Some regard this practice as heinously repugnant, while others see it as a woman's basic right. We must treat patients with all the care and concern we can summon; to nurture their physical, mental, psychological, spiritual and emotional welfare, and put this care above our feelings.

There are four principals to help us find the way to do this:

1. *Autonomy* is the right of individuals to make decisions on their own behalf.

2. *Beneficence* is the duty, where possible, to do good.

3. *Non-maleficence* is the duty to do no harm.

4. *Justice* is a broad concept that includes ideas of equity and fairness.

Treat every patient as you would your sister,
parent or child, and demand that others do too.

Don't blame the individual

When adverse events do occur, it is almost instinctive to find the person who caused the problem and load the responsibility on them – to blame them. Blaming one person for an adverse event is a delicious emotion.[5] Naming, shaming and blaming is easy, satisfying, and extremely unjust. When we do load blame on someone else, then bad things follow. Blame nails responsibility on one individual. Everything becomes their fault. This lets the rest of us off the hook. Blame ignores the circumstances leading up to the event, and unless we dispassionately analyse these circumstances, nothing will be done about it.

Competent administrators understand this. It then becomes their job to do a rigorous *root cause analysis* to find out why the adverse event occurred in the first place, and the resolve to put good systems in place to ensure that it does not happen again. Unfortunately the term root cause suggests there is simply one single cause behind an adverse event. This is almost never the case.

Don't shoot the messenger

There have been many tragedies over the years because the administrative framework, procedures, equipment, or facilities have been inadequate. Competent hospital administrators are aware of this too, but if they do not have the facts they cannot deal with the problem.

Sometimes things are not as they should be. If you have sound reason to think your ability to manage your patients safely is compromised by inadequate staffing levels, equipment or other resources then draw the matter to the attention of the management. Keep written records with dates, times and names about your concerns, and what steps have been taken to try and resolve them.

Respect the skills and work of your colleagues, but if you have well-founded fears about the performance or conduct of either yourself or other staff members then you are obliged to bring them to the attention of the management in a respectful, and private way. Most hospitals have contingency plans to deal with such matters. They have done so in the past, and they will do so in the future.

Whistleblowers

It would be comforting to believe that administrators, senior staff and government authorities always respond appropriately to reports of inadequacy or incompetence, but there have been terrible disasters either because staff at the coal face have been afraid to speak up, or because they have been ignored, and regrettably at times even persecuted and forced to leave their work.

Every country has its problems. For six years doctor and nurses at the Bristol Royal Infirmary in the UK knew that babies were dying or being injured during cardiac surgery – yet did nothing about it until a young anaesthetist blew the whistle. He was demonized and told that it was easier to sack a junior anaesthetist, than two eminent cardiac surgeons; so he emigrated to Australia.[6]

Recently some Australian operating theatre nurses complained about the incompetence of a senior surgeon in a Queensland hospital.[7] They were ridiculed and humiliated, and eventually left their employment. With commendable courage they pursued their claims outside the system. The nurses were eventually vindicated; the surgeon fled the country. But tragically a number of patients had already died because of the surgeon's alleged incompetence. Was it all the surgeon's fault? Why did the anaesthetists not intervene? Were there other failures in the system that allowed such a tragedy to happen? How was such an incompetent person appointed in the first place? Has the system been changed to prevent such events in the future?

Notes

1. Runciman W (2000) Preoperative Assessment and Planning. A paper presented to the Australian New Zealand Society of Anaesthestists, 22 July 2000.
2. Ross Baker G, Norton P (2004) *Canadian Medical Associaton Journal* 170(11):1678–85.
3. Runciman WB, Moller J (2001) *Iatrogenic Injury in Australia*. A report prepared by the Australian Patient Safety Foundation.

4. Moore A (2000) Editorial in the online journal Bandolier, www.ebandolier.com
5. Emeritus Professor James Reason in a paper presented to the Royal Australasian College of Surgeons in 2005.
6. Retrieved September 2006 www.abc.net.au/rn/healthreport/stories/1997/10683.htm
7. Retrieved September 2006 www.abc.net.au/rn/healthreport/stories/2005/1417427.htm

30

Working with facts

In this chapter we will examine some very basic ideas in the science of statistics, and then see how to use them to help our patients (at least not harm them) by applying these techniques in evidence-based practice.

Statistics

We cannot cover the full scope of statistics in a few paragraphs, but instead let us browse through some of common concepts you might encounter in journals and books.

Statistics is the study of the methods of collecting and analysing data. We collect data by taking *samples* from *populations* of individuals. Statistical analysis measures what is happening in a few people and then *extrapolates* the results to make predictions about what is happening in the population as a whole. To increase our *power* to get to the truth, and to reduce *bias*, which may confound us, our samples are usually collected randomly from a defined group (called a *set*) of the population.

Let us do a study on the effects of morphine on blood pressure. Seems simple? But selecting good samples and collecting valid data is difficult. To prevent *errors* we need to research and define exactly what we want to do. For example it is not generally known that men and women respond to morphine analgesia differently.[1] Additionally, if you measure blood pressures simultaneously in your right and left arm the readings may differ by up to 20 mmHg. So our study needs to take these factors into account.

For the most part statistics is a study of *probability*. If you think about it, probability is the only way to deal with uncertainty. We are uncertain whether it will rain today. Looking at the low grey clouds we might predict that it probably will.

Statistical analysis can never prove something to be true, it can only estimate how likely (or unlikely) it is to be false.

There are two main branches of statistics: *descriptive* and *inferential statistics*.

Descriptive statistics describe how to summarise, organize and simplify data so that we can manage it more easily. For example: how to find the *mean* (average) of a number of measurements, or the *mode* (the most common value), or the *median value* (the middle of the range of series of values).

Inferential statistics allow us to determine the chance that a real difference exists between observations in one group, and another. Examples of inferential statistical techniques include *correlation* and *confidence levels*. We use correlation every day; for instance, cyanosis correlates with hypoxia and stridor correlates with respiratory obstruction. We use confidence levels to measure how confident we are that something hasn't happened simply by chance. When we look at the laboratory reports of electrolyte results we find that the normal range of serum sodium is 135–145 mmol/L. Studies using inferential statistical methods show that we can be confident that 95 per cent of normal people have serum sodium levels within that range (called a *confidence interval*), but 5 per cent of the sodium levels of perfectly normal people lie outside that range. The *normal* serum sodium concentrations are between 135–145 mmol/L. We can predict this with 95% *confidence* or with *confidence levels* of + 2.5% and – 2.5%.

Sensitivity and specificity

The terms *sensitivity* and *specificity* are widely used to make logical decisions about the diagnosis and management of patients. For example, some, but not all, bacteria make chemicals called nitrites. If we test urine with a dipstick and find that it contains nitrites and lots of white cells then it is almost certain that the patient has a urinary tract infection. The presence of nitrites and white cells gives this test 100% *sensitivity* for a urinary tract infection. The bad news is that about 50% of patients with urinary tract infections do not have both nitrites and white cells in their urine. Thus, the *specificity* of this dipstick test is only 50%. If we rely only on nitrites and white cells to find urinary tract infections then there is a 50% *false negative result*. Similarly *false positive* results can occur with many tests; in which case the test says something is wrong, when in reality nothing is wrong and everything is normal.

Number needed to treat (or harm)

In the past decade statisticians have introduced a number of new techniques. The *number needed to treat* (NNT) is one of the more useful. In adults the NNT with paracetamol 1000 mg for moderate post operative pain is 3.8. This means you would have to give almost four adults 1000 mg of paracetamol for one of them to get effective pain relief. Similarly, some drugs and treatments can be harmful (such as anti-cancer drugs) in which case we measure the *number needed to harm* (NNH).

Evidence-based practice

In our day-to-day practice it is easy to be led astray and either give unnecessary treatment or withhold effective treatment when it is needed. How do we know what is best for our patients? In the past doctors and nurses have relied on the opinions of experts to guide them on what to do. Too often that is all they were: merely opinions. Treatments were based on belief and experience, usually without solid evidence to support them. Sometimes these opinions were simply wrong, and occasionally tragically lethal. One of the saddest events occurred when doctors and nurses recommended that mothers place their sleeping babies on their stomachs instead of their backs. It seemed a good idea at the time, but tens of thousands of babies died from cot death before researchers showed how dangerous this practice was.

Every day recovery room nurses use harmful or ineffective treatments, such as tipping hypotensive patients head down (harmful), or using metoclopramide to treat opioid-induced vomiting (ineffective).

It is easy to be misled into believing some intervention works when it does not, especially when we base our ideas on incompletely understood physiological or pharmacological principles. Just because we have always done something in a particular way does not mean it is either beneficial or that it does no harm: nor does it mean that there may not be better options.

The only way out of this conundrum of doing good and preventing harm is, as far as possible, to do things that are proven to work. This is the basis of evidence-based practice (EBP). EBP is the process of making decisions about patient care based on the best available research evidence, and then integrating decisions with clinical expertise and the patient's wishes.

How the facts are discovered

Evidence comes from carefully conducted clinical trials. The most valid trials are properly conducted randomized controlled trials (RCTs).

Over the past decade tens of thousands of RCTs have been done, especially involving drugs. More recently other interventions have been evaluating nursing, surgery, physiotherapy, and even recovery room procedures and practices. Hard data about many aspects of our practice is slowly accumulating and the evidence is being weighed, but there is a long way to go yet.

How evidence is collected

There are more than two million papers and articles published in English-speaking medical and nursing journals each year. How can we possibly find ones that directly benefit our patients?

It takes skill and time to find and analyse available data critically. Has the study been properly conducted? Are the statistics appropriate? Is the sample large enough? How can we use the evidence? Answering these questions is not easy; so most of us have to rely on reputable journals and reviews, and special searches by organizations devoted to gathering and analysing evidence, and formulating guidelines. These organizations include the Cochrane Collaboration based in the UK, the McMaster University (Canada), the National Institute for Nursing Research in the US, and the National Health and Medical Research Council (Australia).

How evidence is analysed

It is easy to be influenced by our hopes, beliefs and prejudices, and even easier to be led astray by bias. *Bias* occurs when the information we have about something does not give an accurate picture of what is really going on. Bias is a systematic deviation from the truth. Occasionally rogue researchers intentionally introduce bias for profit, glory, honour or status, but most bias simply occurs because of haste, ignorance and ineptitude.

A *meta-analysis* is the mathematical synthesis of the results of two or more separate trials addressing the same hypothesis in exactly the same (*homogeneic*) way. This data is then statistically analysed, and the results compared. This process is called a systematic review.

A *systematic review* is a summary of the scientific evidence gathered from two or more randomized trials. The evidence it provides is stronger than the results from a single randomized trial. Preferably systematic reviews answer just one question, and present it in a manner we can easily understand. Systematic reviews need to fulfil specific requirements: they must be comprehensive, minimize bias, and use statistically valid information.

It is easier to understand a good meta-analysis than it is to plough through piles of original primary research papers. The downside of meta-analysis is that it is easier to be misled by faulty (or even fraudulent) methods. A weak point with meta-analysis *is* heterogenicity. *Homogenicity* means that each trial is done under exactly the same conditions, collects data in the same way and uses the same statistical techniques. *Heterogenicity* occurs when they are not. Homogenicity compares apples with apples. Heterogenicity compares apples with pink-footed gerbils; or the renal function of dehydrated greyhounds with human patients.

Table 30.1 Analysing evidence

Level of evidence	Where does the evidence come from?
1. Evidence with a high degree of reliability.	Studies that use well-tested methods to make comparisons in a fair way and where the results leave very little room for uncertainty. Trial design: usually Level 1 studies are systematic reviews or large, high-quality randomized controlled studies.
2. Evidence with reliability but open to debate.	Studies that use well-tested methods to make comparisons in a fair way but where the results leave room for uncertainty (for example, due to the size of the study, losses to follow-up or the method used for selecting groups for comparison). Trial design: usually Level 2 studies are systematic reviews without consistent findings, small randomized controlled trials, randomized controlled trials in which large numbers of participants are lost to follow-up, or cohort studies.
3. Some evidence without a high degree of reliability.	Studies where the results are doubtful because the study design does not guarantee that fair comparisons can be made. Trial design: usually Level 3 studies are systematic reviews of case–control studies or individual case–control studies.
4. Some evidence but based on studies without comparable groups.	Studies where there is a high probability that results are due to chance (for example because there is no comparison group or because the groups compared were different at the outset of the study). Trial design: usually cohort or case–control studies where the groups were not really comparable, or case–series studies.

Not all evidence is equally valid. Some evidence is obtained from randomized controlled trials, while other evidence is based on solid observation. For these reasons evidence is classed on its strength, as set out in the table.

There are several dozen classifications of levels of evidence. Some are more complex than others. The sensible one tabled above is used by the New Zealand Guidelines Group. The Oxford Centre for Evidence-based Medicine uses a similar system for evaluating the levels of evidence (LOE) with categories labelled A, B, C and D, while the USA uses a more complex one with six levels of evidence.[2]

How to ask the right questions

If you ask the following questions, then they demand an evidence-based answer:

- What are the options for treatment?
- What are the possible outcomes of those options?
- How likely is each of these outcomes to occur?

Are there any drawbacks to evidence-based practice?

For most of our nursing and medical practice there is little, and often, no hard evidence to support the way we do things. Unfortunately many clinical trials are performed so poorly that their data is worthless or misleading.

Hormone replacement therapy (HRT) was for years advocated to prevent heart disease and stroke in postmenopausal women. The evidence for its benefit came from a single trial that was not *powered* to look for these outcomes anyway. Millions of women were prescribed HRT. It took a huge US government survey - the Women's Health Initiative – to prove that HRT contributed to heart disease and stroke.

On the other hand some professionals argue that:

- the principles of evidence-based care discount clinical experience;
- qualitative trials also provide valid information;
- usually there are no trials or guidelines for the problems of a particular patient. It suppresses clinical freedoms;
- it opens the door for insurance companies to refuse to reimburse for procedures that have not been proven (yet) to be effective;
- it is unethical to have a placebo trial in diseases where effective therapy is available.

Much of our practice is obvious common sense. It is obvious folly not to have cot sides on trolleys, or to leave comatose patients unattended. However, other practices we take for granted are not so clear. Strangely, there is little direct data in the literature to prove that giving a general anaesthetic to a patient with an active respiratory tract infection predisposes to pneumonia, but every anaesthetist knows from experience that this is true.

Randomized controlled trials

Randomized controlled trials compare patients receiving one treatment for a particular disease with another group of patients who are receiving either a placebo (*sugar pill*), or a different treatment. Both groups contain patients selected at *random*, and the trials are done under tightly controlled conditions. Some trials are *double-blinded* in that neither the patients nor the people running the trial know which group is getting which treatment. Blinding increases the *power* of a trial.

Randomized controlled trials are designed to eliminate bias. When selecting samples to study, the data will be biased if, on the average, your samples do not accurately reflect what is going on in the population you are studying.

Suppose you wish to study the frequency of age groups in the general population. You could stand on a busy city railway station at 8.30 a.m., select people at random and ask their ages. But your sample would be biased. Young children are at school, and the retirees are probably still in bed. Your survey would be biased towards office workers who probably do not own cars.

Randomized trials need to be properly powered to extract the data you are seeking. If you were doing a study on weight loss, but chose to measure people's weight in 100 Kg increments, then a weight loss of few kilos would be missed. Your study is insufficiently powered to give meaningful results. However, if your survey is designed to find the proportion of the population who weigh 100 Kg or more, then the power of your study is sufficient.

Notes

1. Aubrun F, Salvi N, Coriat P, Riou B (2005) *Anaesthesiology* 103:156–60.
2. NHMRC (1999) *A guide to the development and evaluation of clinical practice guidelines.* Canberra, NHRMC.

Appendix 1

Trolley set-ups

Emergency trolleys are best prepared in advance and stored for easy access. Those that are rarely required, like malignant hyperthermia and bronchoscopy, can be shared with the operating theatre. Photograph the layout and tie the photograph, encased in plastic, to the trolley. This makes it easy to check the set-up each day. Discourage people from borrowing from these trolleys. Keep the trolleys as near as possible to the fridge and the defibrillator. If you are a small hospital without piped oxygen you will need to keep a full cylinder and regulator close too.

Trolleys include:

- IV access;
- reintubation – these two, which are most frequently required, can be combined into a general emergency trolley;
- cardiac arrest;
- paediatric – this can be a tray on the bottom shelf of the main trolley which can be lifted up when required;
- anaphylaxis;
- thoracic aspiration and chest drain insertion;
- malignant hyperthermia;
- bronchoscopy;
- local anaesthetic trolley.

General emergency trolley

If you have a small recovery room you may wish to combine your main trolley.

A typical set-up for a general emergency trolley would include:

- an intravenous tray with all sizes of cannulas, spirit wipes and gauze;
- tubes for taking blood studies and a key to their coding;
- tubes for blood gas studies;
- boxes of non-sterile gloves, all sizes;
- two laryngoscope handles with batteries;

- extra batteries;
- laryngoscope blades (all sizes);
- stylettes and guide wires (malleable metal or plastic);
- water soluable lubricant;
- oropharyngeal airways, all sizes;
- nasophyngeal airways, all sizes;
- laryngeal masks (including an intubating laryngeal mask);
- cricothyroidotomy kit;
- retrograde intubation kit;
- self-inflating manual resuscitation bag, such as Ambu® or Laerdal®;
- face masks to fit this bag;
- oxygen tubing to connect the bag to the oxygen source;
- bronchoscopes with their light source: small, medium and large;
- cuffed endotracheal tubes, all sizes;
- catheter mounts and tight connections;
- 20 ml syringe for inflating tracheal cuffs;
- Magill forceps;
- wooden mouth-gags.

Drugs should be kept on the trolley or in the fridge, as appropriate. Leave a list of the drugs kept in the fridge on the trolley.

The following drugs are suitable for the trolley, you will probably add others:

- two ampoules of thiopentone, with water to dilute them;
- ketamine;
- propofol;
- suxamethonium, put out two ampoules each day and keep the main supppply in the fridge;
- diazepam or diazemuls;
- midazolam;
- atropine 0.6 mg;
- lidocaine 1% and 2%;
- dextrose 50%;
- adrenaline 1:1000 and 1:10 000;
- hydrocortisone 100 mg;
- intravenous fluids and drip tubing.

Local anaesthetic trolley

A local anaesthetic trolley should be ready at all times for the urgent insertion of a spinal or epidural. This should include:

- gown and sterile gloves, all sizes;
- four sterile drapes;
- sterile gauze;
- sponge holders;
- preparation solution such as cetrimide;
- local anaesthetic drugs;
- commercial packs for spinal and epidural procedures;
- spare needles and other individually packed sterile items if available;
- needles and syringes of various sizes;
- lignocaine 1% for skin analgesia.

Thoracic drain trolley

This trolley should hold the following:

- one medium stainless steel tray, or similar commercial packed tray;
- one small kidney dish;
- two small gallipots;
- one scalpel handle size 3;
- one toothed dissecting forcep;
- two pairs of artery forceps;
- one suture scissors;
- one needle holder;
- one 1/0 atraumatic silk suture;
- one scapel blade size 10;
- sterile packs of cotton wool swabs;
- sterile packs of gauze;
- three sterile drapes.

Add to this:

- lidocaine 1%;
- disposable syringes and needles;
- povidone (Betadine®) skin preparation;

- drain tubes of various sizes including children's sizes;
- trochars, Argyle® or similar.

Malignant hyperthermia trolley

This trolley should be kept right beside the fridge and a supply of Ringer's lactate and normal saline should be set aside in the fridge for use in this crisis, if it should occur. Also in the fridge, dedicated to this emergency, keep:

- nasogastric tubes;
- dantrolene sodium, at least 20 ampoules (shelf life is 3 years);
- regular insulin.

On the trolley keep the following:

- urinary catheter and insertion tray;
- a urinometer;
- fresh breathing circuit;
- temperature probe and recorder;
- cooling blanket (or note where this is stored);
- rectal tube;
- intravenous, central venous and pulmonary artery catheters;
- tubes for blood gas and haematological studies;
- equipment for administering high-flow oxygen;
- sterile distilled water, at least 2 litres;
- a sterile bowl for mixing dantrolene and this water;
- mannitol;
- frusemide;
- sodium bicarbonate 8.4% 100 ml;
- dextrose 50%;
- procainamide hydrochloride.

Requirements for rescuscitation of the newborn

These include:

- a high-sloping trolley;
- a radient heater;
- oxygen, a flow meter, limited to a flow of 4 L/min, and tubing;

- a suction which is set at 40 cm water pressure;
- suction catheters, sizes 5–10 F;
- a bulb syringe;
- a meconium aspirator;
- sterile gloves, all sizes;
- a stethescope;
- a laryngoscope with straight blades;
- extra bulbs and batteries;
- airways, sizes 000, 00 and 0;
- small masks;
- endotracheal tubes, sizes 2.5 to 3.5. Check that the tube has an end on it which will fit into the mask mount if you need to intubate;
- laryngeal mask, size one;
- a neonatal Ambu® or Laedal® rescucitation bag;
- pulse oximeter with appropriate sensor for a baby;
- ECG;
- umbilical catheter, 3–5 F;
- sterile umbilical vessel catheterization tray;
- needles and syringes, all sizes;
- three-way taps;
- IV giving set with a burette;
- 0.9% saline, 4% dextrose, 1/5 N saline;
- albumen 5%;
- dextrose 10%;
- adrenaline 1:10 000;
- naloxone 0.4 mg/ml;
- sodium bicarbonate mmol/L 10 ml ampoules;
- sterile water and saline 10 ml ampoules;
- adhesive tape;
- scissors.

Appendix 2

Infusions

Some drugs need to be administered at a constant rate for a number of hours or longer. This is best achieved by an infusion. A solution is prepared with a known concentration of drug. This is delivered at a rate calculated to keep the blood concentration of the drug at a fairly constant level. A loading dose is needed for most drugs. The advantages of an infusion are that the effect of the drug is smoother, a lower overall dose is required and the need for repeated injections is eliminated.

There are two ways to administer an infusion

1. *Syringe drivers* give small volumes of concentrated drug through a catheter placed in one of the large central veins such as the superior vena cava. The drugs are usually so concentrated that they will injure smaller peripheral veins and may cause severe tissue damage if extravasation occurs.

   Never infuse concentrated drugs through peripheral veins.

2. *Infusion pumps* give larger volumes of fluid. Generally the drugs are less concentrated and often it is possible to safely infuse them into smaller peripheral veins.

Prepare written protocols

Prepare written protocols for each drug used. In them, set down the dose of the drug and the required pump or syringe drive settings. Include details of the expected effects, complications and management of these complications. Staff should be familiar with all the effects and expected problems before the infusion starts. Establish clear written instructions about limits of the parameters of blood pressure, pulse rate, respiratory rate and other variables.

Each drug needs its own dedicated separate intravenous line. It is unwise to use one catheter for infusing a number of drugs. Do not 'piggy-back' lines by using multi-entry ports or plug infusions into intravenous lines carrying other intravenous infusions. For safety potent drugs should be infused through a multi-lumen central venous catheter, with each lumen carrying only one drug.

```
Patient's name _____ Unit record number _____
Ward _____ Date _____ Time prepared _____
Prepared by _____ Checked by _____
DRUG AND DOSE ADDED _____
_____
_____
_____
Concentration _____ Duration of infusion _____ Time to finish _____
```

To prevent errors, always have two trained staff independently check the drug concentration and the rate of infusion. The staff must understand how to use the equipment.

In the doses recommended below, the concentration of drug has been chosen so that the pump settings in millilitres per hour represent some simple numerical function of the drug dose in units per hour. For example if morphine is to be given then a setting of 4 ml/hr will give a dose of 4 mg/hr.

Attach an intravenous additive label to bags, flasks, or syringes containing drugs.

Use a central venous catheter

Many of these drugs are highly concentrated and cause severe thrombophlebitis and tissue necrosis if infused into peripheral veins. They should only be infused through a central venous line.

Multi-lumen catheters

Multi-lumen catheters are more expensive and are associated with more catheter complications. Each potent drug needs its own dedicated separate intravenous port.

Be careful of dead space

Be careful of dead space in lines and catheters. *Dead space* is the volume fluid you need to inject into the line before it reaches the patient's bloodstream. If you do not fill the catheter with the drug (prime the line) it will take some time to fill the dead space and reach the patient. Furthermore if you flush the line you may wash unwanted drug into the patient.

Check your doses with someone else

Always independently check your dose regime with another member of trained staff who understand the infusion pumps and how to use them.

What to monitor

If you are infusing vasoactive drugs, then monitor the patient with an ECG, and continuously record intra-arterial blood pressure.

Important notice

Most of the following drugs are highly concentrated and will cause severe thrombophlebitis and tissue necrosis if infused into peripheral veins. So infuse them into central veins only through a central venous catheter.

When infusing vasoactive or cardiac drugs always monitor cardiac rate and rhythm with an ECG and continuous record blood pressure, preferrably an intra-arterial blood cannula.

Patients receiving infusions need constant monitoring and careful nursing care. Patients must never be left unattended. Everyone needs to be familiar with the pharmacology of the drugs, their actions, and side effects. Written protocols are needed and patient cardiovascular and other parameters need to be carefully specified.

Drug	Dilution	Dose
Adrenaline Epinephrine in USA 1 ml of 1/1000 = 1 mg = 10 ml of 1/10,000 = 1 mg	Adrenaline 3 mg Make up to 5 ml in 5% dextrose	1 ml/hr = 1 µg/min 1–30 µg/min Increase dose by 1 µg/min until desired effect
Amiodarone	Amiodarone 300 mg in 50 ml of 5% dextrose. (Not stable in saline.)	Loading dose: 25 µg/Kg/min for 4 hrs May be given at 5 mg/Kg over 20 min if urgent Maintenance: 5–15 g/Kg/min
Dobutamine	Dobutamine 250 mg Make up to 41.5 ml in 5% dextrose	1 ml/hr = 100 µg/min 2.5–15 µg/Kg/min
Dopexamine	Dopexamine 10 mg Make up to 41.5 ml in 5% dextrose	1 ml/hr = 4 µg/min
Furosemide (Frusemide)	Furosemide 100 mg make up to 50 ml in normal (0.9%) saline	1 ml/hr = 2 mg/hr Loading dose: 0.5 mg/Kg Maintenance dose: 0.1–1 mg/Kg/hr Protect from light.

Important notice *(continued)*

Drug	Dilution	Dose
Glyceryl trinitrate GTN, nitroglycerine	Glyceryl trinitrate 100 mg Make up to 41.5 ml in 5% dextrose	1 ml/hr = 40 µg/min Maintenance dose: 1–5 µg/Kg/min Increase dose by 2–40 µg/min
Heparin 1 mg = 100 units	Heparin 25,000 units make up to 25 ml in 5% dextrose	1 ml/hr = 1000 units/hr Low dose: 75 units /Kg stat then 10–15 units /Kg/hr Full heparinization: 200 units/Kg stat then 15–30 units /Kg/hr
Insulin	Insulin 50 units Make up to 50 ml in 5% dextrose	1 ml/hr = 1 unit/hr
Isoproterenol (isoprenaline)	Isoproterenol 3 mg Make up to 50 ml in 5% dextrose	1 ml/hr = 1 µg/min 1–20 micro/min Increase dose by 1 µg/min until desired effect
Lidocaine (lignocaine)	Lidocaine 1000 mg Make up to 41.5 ml in 5% dextrose	1 ml/hr = 0.5 mg/min Run at: 8 ml/hr for 1 hr 6 ml/hr for 2nd hr 4 ml/hr for next 24 hrs
Morphine	Morphine 50 mg Make up to 50 ml in 5% dextrose	1 ml/hr = 1 mg/hr Loading dose: 0.1–0.5 mg/Kg Normal requirements 0.02–0.1 mg/Kg/hr
Noradrenaline Norepinephrine in USA	Noradrenaline 3 mg Make up to 50 ml in 5% dextrose	1 ml/hr = 1 µg/min 1–30 µg/min Increase dose by 1 µg/min until desired effect
Nitroglycerine	see Glyceryl trinitrate	
Verapamil	Verapamil 50 mg Make up to 50 ml in 5% dextrose	1 ml/hr = 1 mg/hr Loading dose: 1 mg/min up to 10 mg (10 ml of 10% calcium gluconate may be needed to control hypotension) or 0.1–0.1 mg/Kg IV over 10 minutes

Glossary

2,3-DPG 2,3-diphosphoglycerate. This biochemical molecule is normally found nested in a little hollow at the core of the haemoglobin molecule. 2,3-DPG lowers the force of attraction between haemoglobin and oxygen so that an oxygen molecule can escape more easily once the pressure of oxygen in the surrounding fluid falls.

Acetylcholine A neurotransmitter in the peripheral nervous system where it stimulates voluntary muscle fibres to contract, and in the parasympathetic nervous system, where it attends to house-keeping functions of the body, and in the central nervous system where it helps regulate memory. In the parasympathetic nervous system and central nervous system it has **muscarinic activity**, whereas in the peripheral nerve serving voluntary muscle it has **nicotinic activity**.

Acids Substances that donate hydrogen ions to chemical reactions.

Action potentials Action potentials occur when neurons are activated. A wave of electrical charge tumbles along the membrane of the neuron as ions enter through special ion channels. This temporarily reverses the electrical charge of the inside of the membrane from negative to positive. When the wave hits the end of the nerve it releases a **neurotransmitter**, and then the wave disappears. In muscles the action potential stimulates the muscles to contract.

Activated partial thromboplastin time (aPTT) tests the integrity of the intrinsic coagulation system, and common coagulation pathways. For most laboratories the normal range is 36–34 seconds (or < 6 sec above normal control values). Interpret this test cautiously. There is a poor correlation between the aPPT and a clinically significant coagulopathy. aPPT also rises with any inflammatory disease.

Acute coronary syndrome (ACS) A collection of signs and symptoms that suggest the patient has just had, or is about to have, a heart attack. ACS includes problems such as accelerating angina, ST changes on the ECG, rise in troponin or creatinine kinase (CK-MB) and ischaemic arrhythmias.

Acute pain Pain of recent onset and expected to have limited duration.

Acute tubular necrosis The end result of renal hypoxia or poisoning with toxins. The dying cells lining the kidney tubules swell to occlude the lumen of the tubule. Distressed endothelial cells lining the intra-renal blood vessels pile up on one another obstructing blood flow.

Adrenal cortex is an endocrine gland that secretes **corticosteroids**. These steroids are used for a wide range of long term metabolic responses that help restore homeostasis. Cortisol is secreted in large amounts just before dawn to help the body prepare for the day. Aldosterone aids in the reabsorption of sodium from the kidney, androgens for male sexual development, and oestrogens for female sexual development.

Adrenal medulla is an endocrine gland that secretes adrenaline and some noradrenaline. The adrenaline circulates in the blood stream to activate a **sympathetic response**.

Adrenaline is the hormone of exercise. In the USA it is called **epinephrine**. Adrenaline prepares the body for exercise and helps sustain exercise once it starts. In physiological amounts it increases cardiac output, increases the blood flow to skeletal muscle, and mobilizes stored glycogen to glucose in the liver to provide energy for exercise. Adrenaline in pharmacological amounts is used as a vasoconstrictor in local anaesthetics, in the treatment of anaphylactic reactions to increase the blood pressure, and as an **ionotrope**.

Adrenergic drugs stimulate the sympathetic nervous system. **Sympatheticomimetic** drugs mimic the effects of noradrenaline or adrenaline; and include ephedrine, metaraminol, phenylephrine, dopamine, and dobutamine

Adrenergic receptors Receptors for the two catecholamines adrenaline and noradrenaline. Some of their important functions are to regulate the blood flow through arterioles, and modulate blood pressure and cardiac output.

Aeration means to fill with ambient gas. Ambient means whatever the patient is breathing. It may be air, or air supplemented with oxygen.

Afferent and **efferent** arterioles. Afferent means to 'flow into', and efferent means to 'flow out of'.

Afterload is the pressure the heart needs to overcome to eject its stroke-volume.

Agonist An agonist is a neurotransmitter, a drug or other molecule that stimulates receptors on the outside of cell membranes to change the chemical reactions inside a cell.

Alcohol-based hand rub designed to rub on the hands to reduce the number of viable micro-organisms. The 60% solutions in a water-based emollient work better than the 90% solutions, because the proteins in **microbes** are not denatured in the absence of water.

Aldosterone A steroid hormone produce by the adrenal cortex. It acts on the distal tubules in the kidney, triggering them to reabsorb sodium and water. The effect on a person is similar to a saline infusion.

All-or-none response With this response either nothing happens, or the maximal outcome occurs. Nerve fibres either conduct an impulse or they do not. Another useful term for this response is a ballistic response.

Allodynia is pain caused by a stimulus that would not normally provoke pain.

Allogeneic means a tissue that is genetically dissimilar and therefore potentially immunologically incompatible with other members of the same species. In other words, an allogeneic transfusion is a blood transfusion from a person who is not an identical twin. It comes from a donor. Note the spelling allogeneic, not allogenic.

Alogenic describes some event causing pain.

Amino-acid transmitters These are the most prevalent neurotransmitters in the brain and spinal cord. They include glutamate and aspartate which excite (or stimulate) neurons into action, or glycine and gammahydroxybutyrate (GABA) which inhibit neurons from passing on an **action potential**.

Aminoglycosides are bacteriocidal antibiotics used predominately against Gram-negative bacteria. They have to be given by injection because they are not absorbed from the gut. They have two major disadvantages: in higher doses they damage kidney tubules, and cause deafness.

Anaemia is either a low haemoglobin concentration or a low total red cell mass. Iron deficiency, or chronic bleeding usually causes microcytic anaemias, while the macrocytic anaemias are caused by liver or bone marrow disease.

Anaerobic means in the absence of oxygen.

Anaerobic metabolism are metabolic processes that can proceed in the absence of oxygen.

Analgesia is the absence of pain in response to a stimulus that would normally produce it.

Android obesity Represented by the typical male beer-gut. The man has skinny legs and looks like an apple on two matchsticks. Android obesity carries a high risk of cardiovascular disease, stroke, and diabetes, as well as deep vein thrombosis.

Angiotensin-converting enzyme (ACE) is found in the lungs. It converts angiotensin I into angiotensin II. Angiotensin II is the most powerful vasoconstrictor of all.

Angiotensin-converting enzyme inhibitors These are a first choice treatment for certain types of hypertension. They stop angiotensin I being converted to angiotensin II by the angiotensin converting enzymes (ACE) in the lungs.

Angiotensin-receptor blocking drugs (ARBs). These are a group of drugs – the sartans, e.g. irbesartan and candesartan – that block the effect of angiotensin-II, and so prevent arterioles constricting. The ARBs are used when ACE inhibitors are causing unacceptable side-effects.

Angiotensinogen is a prohormone produced in the liver.

Anions are negatively charged ions. Usually they are formed from non-metals such as chloride (Cl^-), but may be more complex ions such as bicarbonate (HCO_3^-)

Anion gap The anion gap reveals the presence of ions in plasma that are not normally picked up on routine biochemistry. For example lactate ion, carrying a negative charge, is not included in the routine electrolyte tests; but a low anion gap may reveal its presence. Anion gap = (Na + K) – (Cl – Bicarb) normally lies within the range of 7–27 mmol/L.

Antagonist An antagonist is a drug or molecule that occupies a **receptor** so that an **agonist** cannot latch on to it to trigger a response.

Antidiuretic hormone (ADH) is also called **vasopressin**. It is a nine-peptide hormone released from the posterior pituitary gland. ADH makes the collecting tubules in the kidney permeable to water so that water is retained.

Apnoea The complete absence of breathing.

aPTT see **Activated partial thromboplastin time**.

Arachidonic acid is an unsaturated fatty acid, an essential component of cell membranes, which is a precursor for the production of prostaglandins.

Arginine vasopression see **Vasopressin.**

Arrhythmias are abnormalities in the heart rate or rhythm.

Aspartate An amino acid derivative used in the central nervous system as a neurotransmitter.

Asystole means the heart has stopped (a cardiac arrest). The ECG shows a straight or gently undulating base line with no electrical activity.

Atrial ectopic beats occur when the impulse arises in odd places within the atria and not in the SA node.

Atrial fibrillation (AF) occurs where the atrial excitation wave is uncoordinated and atria ceases to contract. No P-waves can be seen on the ECG and the ventricles contract irregularly. If the chest is opened the atria look as though they are shivering or writhing like a bag of worms.

Atrial flutter occurs where the atria are contracting ineffectively fast. It is seen as a saw-toothed picture between each QRS complex.

Autoantibodies are antibodies that occur naturally in people. They do not need an antigenic stimulus to produce them. Examples are naturally occurring antibodies against blood groups, and **cold agglutinins**.

Autonomic nervous system (ANS) is part of the peripheral nervous system. It regulates the activity of internal organs. Traditionally the ANS was divided into **sympathetic** and **parasympathetic nervous systems**. More recently the term **sympathetic response** has been replaced by addressing its components: a **noradrenergic response** (mediated by **noradrenaline**) and an **adrenergic** response (mediated by **adrenaline**). In contrast, the term *parasympathetic response* is now more often called a *cholinergic response*, because it is mediated by the neurotransmitter *acetylcholine*.

Autoregulation is the ability of an organ to regulate its blood flow to keep it constant despite changes in the blood pressure. The kidneys autoregulate their blood flow to keep it constant between mean arterial blood pressures of 80–160 mmHg.

Axial and **non-axial airways**. Between the lips and the terminal respiratory units the airways branch approximately 22 times. Most airways branch gently from the line of airflow and are called axial airways. While other branches leave the main pathway at sharp angles and are called non-axial airways, because air does not readily divert from its natural course to flow through them. Air flowing down airways tends to take the line of least resistance preferring to flow through the axial airways. This preferential flow is the reason why the lower parts of the lungs are better aerated than the upper lobes.

Axons are the long fibre-like extensions leading to or from a neurone's cell body. Myelinated axons are covered in an insulating sheath made of Schawnn cells and carry nerve impulse rapidly. Unmyelinated axons are naked, and transmit information more slowly.

Bag and mask A commonly used expression that means to use a resuscitation bag (such as a Magill circuit) and an anaesthetic mask to ventilate a patient who is not breathing.

Baroreceptors Sensors that detect stretching of the walls of blood vessels. The ones in arteries are called *high-pressure baroreceptors*, while those in veins are the *low-pressure baroreceptors*.

Basement membranes Thin layers of collagen matrix on which a single layer of endothelial or epithelial cells lie. The basement membrane anchors these sheets of cells in place, and acts as a barrier to substances escaping through to the underlying tissue. Providing the basement membrane is not disrupted, epithelial and endothelial cells can regenerate and then migrate across the membrane to repair damage.

Bases Substances that accept hydrogen ions and in so doing release water.

Benzodiazepines A group of psychoactive drugs that depress the brain's arousal systems by potentiating the inhibitory effects of the neurotransmitter GABA. Midazolam is the most common one used for sedation and amnesia in anaesthesia. Their effect may take many hours to wear off, particularly in elderly patients. They may have paradoxically stimulant effects in some patients who can become abruptly violent in the recovery room. Taken over the long term they are drugs of dependence with severe withdrawal effects.

Body water is an imprecisely defined term often used informally to mean all the fluids in the body, both outside and inside the cells. Strictly speaking these fluids are not water, but are isotonic solutions of dissolved salts or **ions**.

Bradykinins are group of peptides found in the blood and tissue fluid that provoke inflammation. They are produced when special enzymes split globulins in the blood.

Breathing is the mechanical act of moving air in and out of lungs. Strictly used the term breathing is different from the term *respiration*.

Buffers are compounds in a solution that resist a change in hydrogen ion concentration when an acid or an alkali is added to the solution. It is a sort of chemical storage box that can either hold hydrogen ions or release them to keep their concentration in the surrounding fluid constant. When you add a hydrogen ion to the solution the box accepts one into storage. If you take a hydrogen ion away, then the box releases one into the solution to take its place.

Bacteraemia occurs where living bacteria can be isolated from blood's plasma. **Primary bacteraemia** occurs where there is no identifiable focus of infection. **Secondary bacteraemia** occurs where there is an identifiable focus of infection. Bacteria do not have to be present in the blood stream to activate the massive inflammatory response in severe sepsis. Fewer than 50 per cent of septic patients have a bacteremia, the rest have a focus of infection somewhere outside the bloodstream.

Bacteriocidal substances kill bacteria.

Barotrauma refers to lung injury caused by gas delivered under too much pressure causing structures to rupture, tear and burst.

Basal ganglia are a cluster of neurones deep in the forebrain. They play an important part in controlling movement, and include structures such as the caudate nucleus, putamen, globus pallidus, and substantia nigra. If certain cells in the substantia nigra die, the person gets Parkinson's disease.

Beta lactams A group of antibiotics that include penicillins and cephalosporins. A beta lactam ring contains three carbon atoms and one nitrogen atom.

Bier's block is a form of regional anaesthesia. The arm is emptied of blood with an elastic bandage, an arterial tourniquet applied to the upper arm, and the arm veins filled with 40 ml of 0.5% prilocaine. This block gives excellent analgesia for up to 40 minutes, although the tourniquet can become intolerably uncomfortable unless an intercostobrachial nerve block is also inserted.

Bougie A bougie is a long thin flexible rod that can be passed through an endotracheal tube to enable the tube to be moulded to a shaped that can be guided through the laryngeal opening. They are made of gum-elastic, or occasionally silicon-coated stiff wire.

Bradycardia A heart rate less than 50 beats per minute.

Brainstem The brainstem is like the stalk on a mushroom where the forebrain spreads out at the top of the stalk. Everything passing through the spinal cord to, and from, the forebrain passes through the brainstem. The brainstem also contains, among other things, the vital centres of respiratory and cardiovascular control.

Bundle branch blocks are defects in the left or right major branches of the conducting system of the heart that impede the spread of the cardiac impulse.

Calcium channels Gates in the cell membrane through which calcium can flow.

Candela (cd) The SI base unit of luminous intensity.

Capillary return time (CRT) The time taken for blood to flood back into a fingertip, or nailbed, once you stop squeezing on it. Ideally it should be about 1 second. It is a sign of poor peripheral perfusion if the CRT takes more than 3 seconds. CRT is particularly useful in neonates and small children.

Carboxyhaemoglobin Forms when the poisonous gas carbon monoxide (CO) binds to haemoglobin and displaces oxygen. Under certain circumstances carbon monoxide is generated in the anaesthetic machine if soda lime reacts with some of the volatile agents.

Cardiac failure Occurs when the heart does not function properly.

Cardiac impulse A small electrical current that washes like a wave over the surfaces of cardiac muscle cells causing them to depolarize. Depolarization triggers the cardiac myocytes to contract.

Cardiac index (CI) Allows cardiac output to be compared between people of different sizes and weights. It is the standardized cardiac output relative to body surface area. The normal CI at rest is 3000 ml/m^2/min.

Cardiopulmonary unit Refers to the heart and lungs functioning together to supply oxygen to, and remove carbon dioxide from, the tissues.

Cardiomyopathy Means there is something wrong with heart muscle. Many things damage heart muscle, such as congenital malformations, chronic ischaemia, alcohol, infiltrations with amyloid, fat, or iron, viral infections, or simply working too hard and wearing out (as occurs with hypertension).

Carina The anatomical landmark that marks the bifurcation of the trachea into right and left main bronchi. It is easily seen on a chest X-ray.

Catabolism Involves the breakdown of tissues to provide the body with the energy it requires. The essential feature is that more energy is expended faster than it is replaced and tissues simply waste away. Frequently after surgery this amounts to a muscle protein loss of up to one kilogram a day. Feeding the patient slows, but does not halt, the process.

Catalysts Molecules, including enzymes, which speed up chemical reactions, but do not become part of the final product. They can be used over and over again.

Cations Positively charged **ions**. Usually they are ions formed by metals such as potassium (K^+), sodium (Na^+), but they may be more complex ions such as ammonium (NH_4^+).

Catecholamines Amine derivatives of a basic chemical structure called catechol. They include adrenaline, noradrenaline, dopamine, and isoprenaline. They include a group of three neurotransmitters: dopamine, adrenaline (USA = epinephrine) and noradrenaline (USA = norepinephrine). They activate both the peripheral nervous system and the brain. These three molecules have similar structures and are part of a larger class of neurotransmitters called the monoamines. They are all involved with the sympathetic nervous system.

Ceiling effect Means that even if you give a higher dose of the drug, it has no further effect.

Central sleep apnoea see **Sleep apnoea**.

Cerebral cortex The outermost layer of the cerebral hemispheres of the brain. It is responsible for all the conscious experiences that go into making you who you are and what you feel. The cortex receives data from your senses, and assembles the electrical impulses into facts or observations you can deal with. It pulls together facts into knowledge, processes them, and stores them as memories. The cortex generates emotions and allows you to reason. Emotions are autopilot responses to complex situations. It takes longer for the cortex to integrate knowledge into understanding (much of this happens while you are asleep). Eventually your experiences and understanding coalesce into insight and finally wisdom. With insight you can plan, invent and create things to give you some control over your environment, and with wisdom you can anticipate, analyse and avoid bad things happening to you.

Cerebral hemispheres The two halves of the forebrain. The left hemisphere is specialized for speech, writing, language and sequential reasoning such as calculation or following a map; the right hemisphere is specialized for spatial abilities, face and shape recognition, and the perception of music and patterns.

Cerebral perfusion Refers to the adequacy of cerebral blood flow (CBF). The CBF is the volume of blood passing through the brain every minute. Usually this is about 15% of the cardiac output, or 750 ml/min. Cerebral blood flow is autoregulated, and thus remains constant with mean blood pressures between 70 and 170 mmHg. If cerebral perfusion is stopped for more than 15 seconds the patient loses consciousness.

Cerebrospinal fluid (CSF) About 150 ml of colourless fluid that bathes, supports and protects the brain and spinal cord. It is held in a container formed on the outer side by the dura mater, and on the inside by the arachnoid mater. The CSF regulates the brains extracellular fluid, containing ions and buffers, but almost no protein.

Chronic kidney disease (CKD) is A term given to degenerative or pathological disease, which causes either a reduction in the glomerular filtration rate, or the inability of the kidney to concentrate urine. CKD is graded into 5 stages.

Chylothorax Occurs when lymph leaks into the thorax. Lymph is usually a clear amber colour, but after a meal it may be milky from the absorbed fat.

Cleaning A process that removes micro-organisms and biohazardous materials from the surface of an object.

Clearance That volume of plasma from which a drug is completely removed in a given time. Note the drug is extracted from **plasma** and not blood. Its units are expressed as millilitres per minute (ml/min). Clearance is really the sum of all the processes that eliminate a drug from the body. Clearance depends on how efficiently the kidneys and liver metabolize and excrete a drug. Clearance of a drug, or other substance, is decreased if a patient has renal or liver disease.

Clinical pathways (chemoreceptors are specialized cells that respond to changes in the chemical composition of body fluids) A roadmap of every aspect of patients' care from the time they first attend the hospital to the time they finally return to the care of their local doctor. Good clinical pathways document a treatment goal, define the intended objectives at any instant, and review whether the targets have been achieved. The clinical pathway includes a nursing plan, necessary medical interventions, documentation and communication strategies, psychological support of patients and their families, and a discharge plan. In a surgical case the pathway includes the patient's preoperative medical and nursing assessment, psychological preparation, education, perioperative and postoperative care and review after discharge from hospital.

Cold agglutinins *are* **Autoantibodies** that occur in some people (especially if the patient is septic). The autoantibodies cause red cells to burst (haemolysis) if their body temperature falls below 35.5°C.

Colony-forming units Bacteria are cultured on special agar plates kept in an incubator. Each bacterium rapidly replicates to become visible dots on the plate. The number of these colony-forming units gives an estimate of the number of bacteria present at the site where the sample was gathered.

Coma A state of unresponsiveness where patients have their eyes closed, and do not respond when their name is called, or when shaken by the shoulder. This may seem a strange definition, but some people with severe brain damage who are deeply unconscious, will react with a dramatic reflex rigidity (*opisthotonos*) to painful stimuli, and some otherwise unresponsive patients may spontaneously open their eyes or smack their lips.

Complete heart block Occurs where none of impulses generated by the sino-atrial node reach the ventricles. The atria are beating independently of the ventricles.

Compliant Refers to the ease at which the lungs can be inflated. Compliant lungs are more readily inflated than incompliant lungs.

Complement is a proteolytic enzyme system in plasma that punches holes in certain bacteria causing them to rupture.

Cor pulmonale Occurs when pulmonary hypertension causes right heart failure.

Core temperature The temperature of the blood in the pulmonary artery and reflects the temperature of the major central organs: the brain, liver, kidneys, heart and lungs.

Creatinine Formed from phosphocreatine at a more or less constant rate as muscle protein is turned over. The kidney steadily removes the creatinine from the blood, and excretes it in the urine. As the GFR slows creatinine accumulates in the blood. A raised serum creatinine indicates renal dysfunction. Once filtered creatinine stays in the urine, where it can be collected to measure GFR.

Creatinine clearance is a crude measure of the **glomerular filtration rate (GFR)**. Creatinine clearance has been replaced with an *estimated glomerular filtration rate (eGFR)*.

Critical pathways see **Clinical pathways**.

Cyanosis A blue tinge to the skin or mucous membranes. It is usually a sign of severe hypoxaemia, but can also be caused by other agents. For hypoxaemia to cause cyanosis at least 30 gm/L of haemoglobin must be in its deoxygenated form.

Cytokines Biochemicals produced by nucleated cells that allow cells them to 'talk' to each other. Cells produce cytokines whenever their welfare is in danger. The stimulus can be sepsis, trauma, ischaemia, or anything causing inflammation. After surgery patients are a stew of circulating cytokines produced by injured cells to signal white cells to come to help clean up the damage.

Dalton's law of partial pressure States that in a mixture of gases the partial pressure of a particular gas is the pressure that gas would exert if it alone occupied the space available to it.

Day case procedure A procedure done in one day and does not require the patient to stay overnight or longer. Sometimes non-invasive investigations such as colonoscopy are referred to as day procedures.

Decontaminate hands means using an antiseptic hand-rub to reduce the bacterial counts on the hands.

Dehydration Imprecise jargon, which usually means loss of water, but not isotonic fluids, from the body. A term that is better avoided.

Delirium is an acute confusional state. The patients do not know where they are, cannot concentrate enough to remember what you have just told them, and will not consistently obey commands. You cannot reason with a delirious patient. For instance they take off their oxygen mask having, just a moment before, agreed to keep it on. They may hallucinate, talk in a garbled manner, or become belligerent.

Demand pump is one that changes its output to match the oxygen demands of the tissues. When we exercise our tissues demand more oxygen, so our cardiac output rises to meet it.

Denatured To structurally change or destroy proteins.

Depolarization Occurs as the electrical voltage across a myocyte's or nerve cell membrane abruptly reverses. In muscle the change in voltage causes an electric current to flow, and this current triggers the muscle fibre to contract. The voltage change occurs as charged ions flood back and forth through special ion channels in the cell membrane. Many of the channels require energy to pump the ions, while other in other channels the ions simply flow back and forth without help.

Desmopressin A synthetic analogue of the hormone **vasopressin**. Its trade name is DDVAP.®

Detergents Compounds which, when added to water, penetrate grease and oils and cause them to go into solution.

Dextrose The name used in the USA for glucose. It is a cyclical 6-carbon monosaccharide.

Diaphoresis A pompous word meaning sweating (or perspiring).

Diastole The phase of the cardiac cycle of contraction and relaxation when the heart relaxes.

Diastolic dysfunction Characterized by a stiff non-compliant ventricle which needs to be stretched before it will contract properly. Once stretched it contracts harder. So for a few beats at the beginning of each inspiration positive pressure ventilation helps distend the ventricle, making it contract harder.

Diastolic pressure The minimum blood pressure in the arteries during the cardiac cycle.

Disseminated intravascular coagulation (DIC) Occurs when the clotting system is so deranged that microscopic clots start forming spontaneously throughout the circulation. Unless treated it is usually fatal.

Dissociative anaesthesia Occurs when the cortex is chemically isolated from the brains lower centres. Ketamine is the only dissociative anaesthetic used clinically.

Diuresis To produce urine at a rate exceeding 1.3 ml/Kg/hr or for an adult 100 ml/hr.

Dynamic equilibrium Occurs when a process that is forming something is exactly balanced by a process that is undoing the same process. It generally refers to chemical reactions, however an analogy is adjusting the rate of water flowing into the top of a bucket to exactly balance the rate at which water drains out a hole in the bottom of the bucket.

Dyslipidaemia A term covering a wide range of abnormal lipid concentrations in the serum. The term includes high cholesterol levels, and also abnormalities in the balance between high-density lipoproteins (HDL) and low-density lipoproteins (LDL).

Dysphoria means the patient outwardly appears calm and tranquil, but inwardly feels jittery, agitated, and fearful. Colloquially it is known as the 'heebie-jeebies'

Dyspnoea Describes what patients feel when they cannot get their breath. Health care workers call it dyspnoea, while patients say they are breathless.

ECG is the accepted abbreviation for electrocardiogram. This device measures the tiny electrical currents generated by the muscles of a beating heart.

Echocardiogram Two-dimensional echocardiography which uses high-frequency **ultrasound** to measure the movement of the anterior and posterior walls of the ventricles. It calculates the stroke-volume by assuming the ventricle is ellipsoid in shape (which is not always the case). Three-dimensional echocardiography gives better results.

Ectopic means 'out of place'.

Ectopic cardiac beats Those arising from parts of the heart that normally would not initiate a beat.

Ectopic pregnancy occurs when the embryo implants somewhere outside the uterine cavity.

Efferent – see **Afferent**.

Electroencephalograph (EEG) A device measuring the electrical activity of the brain.

Ejection fraction The proportion of blood ejected from the ventricle with each contraction. In a healthy heart it should be more than 50% of the volume of blood in the ventricle at the end of diastole.

EKG is a variant (usually used in Europe) of the abbreviation ECG.

Elastin is the connective tissue of youth and suppleness; it is coiled like a spring. As we age, elastin gradually uncoils to become collagen. Collagen is stiff fibrous non-elastic connective tissue. Young skin has a lot of elastin in it – hence no skin wrinkles. The elastin in the lung is responsible for its natural springiness.

Electromechanical dissociation (EMD) Occurs where a formed wave can be seen on the ECG, but there is no detectable peripheral pulse. Always check that the patient has not bled. If the patient is not hypovolaemic then EMD is usually fatal. EMD is now called pulseless electrical activity.

End-organs Organs that are at the end of an arterial supply, such as kidney, spleen and brain, but not organs which blood flows through on its way to somewhere else, such as the heart, lungs or gut.

Efferent – see **Afferent**.

Endogenous Something that is manufactured inside a person's body which does not come from somewhere else.

Endorphins are a group of naturally occurring chemical compounds synthesized in the body that interact with opioid receptors in the central and peripheral nervous system.

Endotoxins are lipopolysaccharide peptide complexes produced by Gramnegative bacteria. All Gram-negative bacteria produce similar endotoxins which in absolutely minute amounts damage **basement membranes** all over the body, causing protein-rich fluid to ooze out of the bloodstream into the tissues. Clinically this is most apparent in the lungs where it causes low pressure pulmonary oedema.

Energy is the capacity of a system to do **work**.

Enzymes Proteins that clamp biochemical molecules together to produce a bigger compound, or tear compounds asunder into their components. They do this without the enzyme being damaged in the process. Enzymes are biochemical **catalysts**.

Epidural space Also called the extradural space or peridural space.

Epinephrine – see **Adrenaline**.

Exposure-prone procedures Procedures where there is a risk of injury to a health care worker (HCW). This injury can be caused by needles, sharp instruments or sharp tissues (teeth and spicules of bone) piercing the HCW's gloves, and allowing their blood to bleed back into the patient. The definition includes procedures where the operator's hands cannot be seen at all times. This would apply to surgeons, or those people working under drapes, but does not necessarily prevent workers affected by blood-borne viruses from taking blood samples.

Extracellular fluid (ECF) is the fluid bathing all the tissues in the body. There are two main compartments: the blood (whose volume is 80 ml/Kg), and the interstitial fluid (which accounts for 15 per cent of body weight).

Exudates Outpourings of fluid as a result of inflammatory processes. They contain more than 30 grams of protein per litre of fluid.

Facilitate To enhance or make easier.

Fat-soluble hormones see **Hormones.**

Feedback Using the output of a system to control its input. Positive feedback reinforces the output. A well-known example is in a public address system where the microphone picks up the output from the loudspeaker and amplifies it producing a howl. Negative feedback weakens the output.

If the temperature in your refrigerator falls to low, then the refrigerator stops cooling, until the temperature has risen to a preset range.

Filtrate Sometimes called **ultrafiltrate**, this is the fluid that enters the urine after the blood has passed across the glomerular sieve.

Force In 1685 Sir Issac Newton elegantly pointed out that something at rest, such as a brick, will remain at rest until some sort of force causes it to move; while on the other hand if it is moving it will continue to move (in a straight line) until some force stops it or changes the direction in which it is moving. If the stationary brick moves, then a force is accelerating it from rest to its final velocity, and the force needed to do this can be calculated by the equation:

$$\text{Force} = \text{mass} \times \text{acceleration}$$

The SI unit of force is appropriately the **newton**, which is the amount of force necessary to increase the velocity (accelerate) a mass of one kilogram at one metre per second every second.

Functional residual capacity (FRC) is the volume of air left in the lungs at the end of quiet expiration. At FRC the pressures distending the lungs equal the forces tending to collapse them. The FRC in a young adult is about 2.8 litres. It is a useful store of air that enables us to speak or hold our breath.

GABA is the acronym for the inhibitory neurotransmitter gamma-amino butyric acid.

General power outlet (GPO) is the formal name for that electric power outlet in the wall, which you plug devices into and then switch on.

Generic A generic drug is one where the name identifies its ingredients rather than its brand name. Generic names remain constant all over the world, whereas brand names tend to change from country to country. For instance aspirin is a generic name recognized world wide, whereas its brand names vary from place to place.

Glitazones are a group of drugs used to treat type 2 diabetes. They regulate the genes involved with fat and glucose metabolism.

Glomerular filtration rate (GFR) The volume of filtrate entering the collective proximal tubules every minute. Of this volume almost all is reabsorbed by the kidney tubules.

Glomerulus Forms the kidney's sieving mechanism. It is an invaginated bulb at the entrance to the nephron, which houses a tuft of about 20–40 capillaries.

Glucocortricoids are steroid hormones involved with metabolism and which have anti-inflammatory actions.

Glutamate An amino-acid derivative used by the central nervous system as a neurotransmitter.

Glyceryl trinitrate Also known as nitroglycerine, a potent vasodilator. Because it dilates arterioles by relaxing their smooth muscle, it reduces the force the heart needs to produce to eject its stroke-volume. It may also vasodilate coronary vessels improving the blood flow through them.

Gold standard A term used to describe the most practical and most accurate way to obtain a clinical measurement. A benchmark is the standard or reference point against which things can be measured, but it may not be practical.

Gynaecoid obesity The typical woman's pattern with most of the fat around her bottom and upper thighs. Think pear-shaped. It is not as hazardous as android obesity.

Haematocrit (HCT) Similar to packed cell volume. As blood is centrifuged the heavier red cells sink to the bottom forming a layer underneath the plasma. The proportion of red cells when compared to the total volume is called the haematocrit. It is usually expressed as a percentage. The normal haematocrit is about 45%. In patients who have been resuscitated with colloids or crystalloids the haematocrit tells whether there are enough red cells in the blood. Once the haematocrit falls below 35% the patient is said to be anaemic.

Haemolytic crisis Occurs when red blood cells burst, releasing their haemoglobin into the blood stream. Free haemoglobin clogs up the glomerulus in the kidney causing renal failure.

Half-life The half-life of a drug is the time taken for the blood concentration of a drug to fall by half. *Context-sensitive half-life* is how long it takes for half the drug's effects to wear off.

Heart blocks Defects in the conduction of the cardiac impulse from the atria to the ventricles. You can see this on an ECG where P-waves are further away from the QRS complex than normal. They might be a constant distance from the QRS complex (serious) or they may vary in distance (dangerous).

Heat A form of energy. The amount of heat produced, or lost, is measured in either kilocalories (Kcals) or kilojoules (KJ). If you extracted the heat from a litre of boiling water it would contain just over 1000 useable kilocalories before it turned to ice. A normal person uses about 1800–2000 kcal a day to live their humdrum sedentary lifestyle. A breastfeeding mother or manual labourer may use 3500 kcal or more each day.

HELLP Haemolysis, elevated liver enzymes and a low platelet count.

Hemiblocks Defects in the lesser branches of the conducting system of the heart that impede the spread of the cardiac impulse. The most common is a left anterior hemiblock. A left posterior hemiblock is more serious and suggests extensive cardiac disease.

HEPA masks High-efficiency particulate air-filtering masks.

Heparin-induced thrombocytopenia A life-threatening immune-mediated destruction of platelets. With exposure to heparin, antibodies are formed against platelet factor IV. It is associated with increased propensity to form clots, and may cause strokes, limb ischaemia, bleeding or death. Worry if the platelet count drops by 30–50% about 4 days after exposure to heparin.

Hepatic impairment Not well defined. Arbitrarily it occurs when one or more of the liver enzymes (ALT, AST or GGT) exceed three times its normal levels. Dying hepatocytes release these enzymes into the circulation. The liver is remarkably resilient, and at any age will repair itself if the noxious stimulus is brief, and the damage not excessive.

Hepatitis A generic term for inflammation of the liver. The inflamed liver cells release marker enzymes into the bloodstream, which can be detected on liver function tests. The most common cause of liver inflammation is alcohol, followed by prescribed medication.

Heterogenicity is a term used in statistics. When grouping things together for statistical **meta-analysis** (that is, analysing data from many diverse sources) you must group apples with apples, and oranges with oranges. This is called homogenicity. If you try to lump apples and hamsters together then you will have problems with heterogenicity.

High-pressure baroreceptors see **Baroreceptors**.

High-pressure pulmonary oedema see **Pulmonary oedema.**

Hormones Chemical messengers secreted by endocrine glands. They regulate the activities of their target organs. There are two functional groups of hormones: *water-soluble hormones*, which in tiny amounts act rapidly and then quickly disappear such as **anti-diuretic hormone** (ADH), and fat-soluble hormones ones which are produced in much greater amounts, and act over long periods such as oestrogen, testosterone and thyroxine to guide the development of the organs.

Humidity A measure of the **mass** of water vapour in gas. Humidification is the process of increasing the moisture content of air, and a humidifier is the device that does this.

Hypercarbia Occurs when the arterial $PaCO_2$ > 44 mmHg (> 5.79 kPa). It is the result of **hypoventilation**. Physicians generally use the term hypoventilation rather than hypercarbia.

Hyperchloraemia The concentration of chloride ion in the ECF is higher than the normal range of 95–105 mmol/L.

Hyperexcitable state Occurs when nerves fire with a trivial stimulus that would normally not cause any response.

Hyperventilation The arterial $PaCO_2$ is below the lower limits of normal (< 36 mmHg) (< 4.75 kPa)). Hyperventilation is not the same thing as breathing. To use the term hyperventilation correctly requires that either you know the end-tidal CO_2 or the $PaCO_2$.

Hypocarbia Occurs when the arterial $PaCO_2$ < 36 mmHg (< 4.75 kPa). It is the result of **hyperventilation**. Physicians generally use the term hyperventilation rather than hypocarbia.

Hypokalaemia Occurs when the serum potassium levels fall below 3.5 mmol/L. It becomes severe if it falls below 3 mmol/L and will eventually cause cardiac arrhythmias.

Hypothalamus A complex structure nestling deep in the underside of the brain at the upper end of the brainstem. It regulates the activities of the internal organs, monitors information from the autonomic nervous system, and controls the pituitary gland.

Hypoventilation Failure of the lungs to eliminate carbon dioxide. It is measured by a rise in the partial pressure of carbon dioxide in the arterial blood.

Hypovolaemia A term that is not well defined. Hypovolaemia usually means an insufficient blood volume, which if untreated leads to shock. In contrast dehydration usually means insufficient body water.

Hypoxaemia Occurs when the arterial PaO2 is < 60 mmHg (< 7.79 kPa). It reflects what is going on in the bloodstream. Severe hypoxaemia causes **hypoxia**.

Hypoxia Occurs when there is not enough oxygen to allow the cells to carry out their normal function. Oxygen-deprived tissues release lactic acid into the bloodstream. Blood gas analysis reveals a *metabolic acidosis*. It reflects what is going in the tissues. A patient can be hypoxaemic without being hypoxic, such as with opioid-induced respiratory depression. Or, more rarely is hypoxic without being hypoxaemic, such as with severe anaemia.

Idioventricular rhythms occur when all the heart's higher pacemakers are suppressed, and the ventricle contracts at its intrinsic rate of 25–35/min.

Infarction means the blood supply to a tissue has been cut off for so long that the tissue has died. Infarction is the end result of ischaemia.

Insensible fluid losses include those that we do not routinely measure; for instance: sweat, and water lost by the lungs. In a normal environment they amount to about 750 ml of fluid each day.

International Normalized Ratio (INR) This test is the same as the prothrombin time (PT) except that the test has been standardized so that all laboratories give consistent results. The normal INR is 1. INR is used to monitor warfarin therapy. For elective surgery the INR should be less than 1.5.

Interstitial nephritis is an acute allergic inflammatory reaction to drugs concentrating in the kidneys. The inflammation causes a damaging exudate into the area, usually around the glomerulus.

Ion channels are tailor-made pores or pumps in the cell membrane that only allow specific ions to pass.

Ionotropes Drugs such as adrenaline and dopamine, which increase the strength of cardiac contraction.

Ions Atoms or molecules that have lost or gained one or more electrons. This means the atoms now carry either a positive (such as Na^+) or negative charge (such as Cl^-).

Ischaemia Means there is not enough blood supply to maintain tissue metabolism. If a tissue remains ischaemic for long enough it will *infarct*.

Isophlebotic point A point on the skin that is level with the right atrium.

Isotonic means a fluid has the same osmotic pressure as extracellular fluid.

Kernicterus occurs when unconjugated bilirubin leaks into and damages neonates' brains.

Korotokoff sounds Generated by turbulence as blood flows through arteries partially compressed by a blood pressure cuff. You can hear them with a stethoscope.

Laparoscopy Using a laparoscope is to directly visualize the contents of the peritoneal cavity. In gynaecology it is used to inspect the ovaries, the outside of the Fallopian tubes and uterus. A laparoscope is an instrument, somewhat like a miniature telescope, with a built-in fibreoptic system to bring light into the abdominal cavity.

Lapses see **Slips**.

Laryngeal oedema Swelling of the mucosa in the larynx. There is a grave danger this will obstruct airfow.

Laryngospasm The reflex contraction of the muscles serving the vocal cords so that they shut tightly. Its function is to prevent foreign material entering the lower airway. It sometimes occurs when the larynx is irritated by something such as infection or an endotracheal tube.

Lean body mass The mass in kilograms of the richly perfused tissues of the vital organs, skin and muscle, but excluding poorly perfused fat. If we dosed obese patients on their total body mass, we would overdose them because the drugs do not enter the poorly perfused fat tissue readily.

For people over the height of 150 cm:

Lean body mass for men = height in centimetres − 100 Kg

Lean body mass for women = height in centimetres − 102 Kg

Limbic system A group of brain structures including the amygdala hippocampus, and basal ganglia that work together to generate and regulate emotion, process memory and coordinate fine movement.

Low-pressure baroreceptors see **Baroreceptors**.

Low-pressure pulmonary oedema see Pulmonary o**edema.**

Lymph Extracellular fluid with added white blood cells. The lymphatic system is similar to an agricultural drainage system used to drain swampy land. Lymph vessels drain all tissues except the brain, and finally end up in the body's main drain, called the *thoracic duct*. Lymph fluid in the thoracic duct usually is clear, but becomes milky after a fatty meal.

Lipoxygenases A group of enzymes that breakdown *arachidonic acid* into *leukotrienes*. These, and a number of other biochemicals initiate and sustain inflammatory responses.

Macrocytic anaemia see **Anaemia.**

Mannitol A non-toxic alcohol made from the sugars fructose or mannose. The body cannot metabolize mannitol: 20% mannitol solution is hypertonic, and exerts an **osmotic pressure** equivalent to four times that of 5% dextrose or 0.9% saline. It is excreted unchanged by the kidneys taking with it a large volume of water.

Mapelson circuits In 1954 William Mapelson classified semiclosed anaesthetic circuits into five types, of which the Mapelson A (the original **Magill circuit**) and C circuits are the two still in common use. In some places the Mapelson C circuit is also called the Magill circuit.

Mass A measure of the amount of matter in a body. Unlike weight it is not affected by gravity. The SI unit of mass is the kilogram.

Maximal sterile barrier precautions are a high level of aseptic technique. They require face mask, sterile gloves and sterile gown, and a large sterile drape to isolate the patient.

Mean A statistical term that describes the average of a range of values. There are a number of ways to describe how numbers are distributed over a range of numbers. Consider the numbers: 4, 4, 6, 8, 26. To get the mean value we add them up (sum them) and divide by 5. The mean value therefore is 50/5 = 10. The *median value* is the number in the middle of the range, in this case 6, and the *modal value* is the most common number; in this case 4.

Mercury-filled manometers An environmental and occupational health hazard. They have been removed from most clinical areas.

Metabolism The sum of all the physical changes and chemical processes that take place within an organism, including all the tiny steps where energy is transformed from one form to another inside cells. For instance chemical energy is transformed into electrical energy, or movement, or heat. Metabolism is the process of taking in a nutrient on a drug, breaking it down and reassembling it to repair and build body structures, and eliminating the wastes. Metabolism is the signature of life.

Methaemaglobinaemia occurs when the ferrous (Fe^{++}) ion in haemoglobin is oxidized to the ferric (Fe^{+++}) form. Oxygen, which binds loosely to ferrous ion, binds far more tightly to the ferric form so that it cannot escape from the haemoglobin. The blood becomes chocolate brown coloured, and the tissues may become hypoxic. The commonest cause of methaemoglobinaemia is an overdose of the local anaesthetic prilocaine. Ferric haemoglobin can be converted back to the ferrous form by methylene blue.

Micro-atelectasis Refers to the collapse of the smallest airways and alveoli in the lungs. It usually occurs when the terminal respiratory units fail to produce sufficient **surfactant**.

Microbes are living organisms that are too small to be seen with the naked eye. They include bacteria, yeasts, protozoa, and viruses. They do not include prions.

Microcytic anaemia see **Anaemia**.

Milli-osmol/Kg Milli-osmols per kilogram of water is a measure of the osmolality of the solution. Osmolality represents the number of osmotically active particles in a kilogram of water.

Minute volume (MV) is the volume of air moved into or out of the lungs in one minute. MV = RR × TV.

Mishaps see **Slips**.

mol Reflects the weight of a molecule. Molecules are very very small. Since we can't easily measure the weight of a single molecule physicists lump 6.023×10^{23} (62,300,000,000,000,000,000,000,000) of them together and measure the weight of the whole lot in grams. The weight of a mol of sodium is 23 gm and the weight of a mol of chlorine is 35.5 gm so that the molecular weight (or one mol) of sodium chloride (NaCl) is $35.5 + 23 = 58.5$ gm.

Multifocal premature beats Sign of a very irritable myocardium.

Muscarinic activity describes the effects of stimulating the parasympathetic nervous system: bradycardia, bronchosecretion, bowel movement, bronchospasm, and pupillary constriction. Muscarine is a biochemical found in some fungi, which if ingested in sufficient quantities causes the bowels to contract expelling their contents at both ends, the lungs to fill up with mucus so that the person drowns, and their heart to slow down and stop. A similar effect can be caused by excessive release of acetylcholine or an overdose of neostigmine (and some nerve gases). Atropine blocks the effect of muscarine (and neostigmine and nerve gases).

Myocardial contractility The force with which the heart contracts during systole.

Myogenic Smooth muscle in the walls of arterioles will contract when they are stretched. This elastic band-like reaction is called a myogenic response.

Naive A term sometimes used to describe patients who have not been previously exposed to a drug. For instance benzodiazepine-naive patients are usually sedated far more readily with lower doses of diazepam than those who take it regularly.

Nanomol This is one billionth of a **mol** (or one-millionth of a **millimol**). It is written as 10^{-9} mol. This small amount is roughly equivalent to finding one single pea in a cubic metres of peas, or roughly one pea in a pile of peas 30 metres high.

Narcotic An old imprecisely defined term indicating that a substance induces narcosis or sleep. It was a term applied to the opioids.

Neonates Babies in the first month of life.

Nephron The basic functional unit of the kidney. It is composed of a **glomerulus**, with its afferent and efferent arterioles, and the renal tubule.

Nephropathy Kidney disease where either the cause or its exact effect are unclear.

Neuroaxial block A block using local anaesthetics given into or around the spinal cord. This is a collective term for spinal and epidural anaesthetics.

Neuropathic pain Arises from damage to nerves along some part of their pathways from their origin in the periphery, to their integration in the CNS. It is caused by nerve damage due to compression, inflammation or direct trauma.

Neurotransmitter is a chemical released by neurones (such acetylcholine or noradrenaline) at synapses and neuromuscular junctions. It allows the effects of an **action potential** to be passed on to the next cell.

Newton not in (symbol: N) is a unit of force. It is the amount of force needed to accelerate a mass of one kilogram at one metre per second squared. One newton is roughly the amount of force exerted by gravity on an apple.

Nicotinic activity Acetylcholine is the neurotransmitter released at the neuromuscular junction in voluntary muscles, which makes them contract. In sufficient quantities nicotine (the same drug is in tobacco) causes similar effects. Excessive nicotine causes violent spasms of voluntary muscles. Muscle relaxants used during anaesthetics such as atracurium and vecuronium block the effects of acetylcholine (and nicotine) on voluntary muscle.

Nocioceptors detect pain arising from tissue damage, mediated by inflammatory biochemicals.

Nociceptors Pain receptors at the end of sensory nerves. They transduce the signal of pain. This means that they turn a painful mechanical stimulus into an electrical nerve action potential.

Nodal rhythms Occur where the AV node triggers the beat instead of the SA node. The pulse rate is usually 40–50 beats/min. The P-waves on the ECG are either absent (hidden in the QRS) or upside down.

Noise Occurs when an electronic signal is drowned out by unwanted stray signals from elsewhere. Examples of noise are muscle movement on an ECG, or 50-cycle AC hum from nearby mains current. To get a good trace you need as much signal and as little noise as possible.

Non-axial airways see **Axial airways**.

Noradrenaline One of the catecholamine-based neurotransmitters. It is secreted by sympathetic nerves to regulate blood pressure, and in the brain is involved in arousal, and reward stimuli, Noradrenaline regulates mood and sleep.

Noradrenergic response Part of the sympathetic response. As noradrenaline is released from sympathetic nerve endings it causes arterioles to constrict and the blood pressure to rise. The more life-threatening the event, the more noradrenaline is released. These events include hypoxia, hypovolaemia, sepsis, major tissue damage, and especially brain injury.

Normal The term normal has a number of different meanings. The most common meaning is average. A normal patient is a typical patient; one that does not deviate from the usual. A normal distribution curve is a graph which is distributed symmetrically about the average (or **mean**) value. Similarly normal biochemical results cover a range that applies to 95 per cent of healthy individuals.

Normal saline One that contains one gram of sodium chloride per litre; 0.9% normal saline therefore contains 900 mg of sodium chloride per litre.

Normovolaemia Implies the blood volume and the volume of the extracellular fluid are normal.

Nosocomial infections Infections acquired in the hospital.

Noxious stimulus One that damages tissue.

Obstructive sleep apnoea see **Sleep apnoea.**

Obtunded mental state A state of semi-consciousness where the patient only rouses when stimulated, or they are not fully conscious and cooperative.

Oedema Oedema fluid is a form of transudate. It collects in the interstitium of the ECF outside the cells.

Off-label drugs Registered drugs that are used in a way that has not yet been approved. Usually they are being used for a different indication than originally intended, or are given by a different route, or at a different dose to that recommended by the manufacturers. Using clonidine for pain relief, or **vasopressin** to support blood pressure are examples of off label drug use, but so is crushing drugs to form a suspension to pass down a nasogastric tube. When using drugs off-label the prescriber may have some liability should anything go wrong. The legal implications of this practice are unclear.

Ondine's curse A property peculiar to opioid drugs where although conscious the patient forgets to breath. Opioids depress the central response to a rising $PaCO_2$, which is one of the main physiological triggers to breathe. Ondine was an immortal water nymph in Teutonic mythology. She laid a curse on her wayward and mortal lover that he would have to remember to breathe. When he fell asleep, he died. Neither she, nor her lover, lived happily ever after.

Opiate An outdated term referring to the alkaloids derived from the opium poppy (*Papaveretum somniferum*). Morphine, codeine and heroin are still produced from poppies.

Opioids A diverse group of natural and semisynthetic alkaloid derivatives of opium. This definition includes endogenous peptides that interact with opioid receptors.

Orthopnea Occurs when patients get short of breath when they lie down.

Osmotic pressure The pressure (energy) that forces water to diffuse across a semi-permeable membrane (such as the cell membrane). Water tends to spread uniformly throughout a solution, so that its concentration is the same everywhere. It will pass through cell membranes to achieve this end.

Osmoreceptors are specialized cells that detect changes in osmotic pressure. They occur in the hypothalamus and in the kidneys and help regulate the body's fluid balance.

Packed cell volume Measured by spinning a sample of blood in a centrifuge so that the red cells pack down to the bottom while the plasma remains on the top. Normally the packed cells occupy about 45% of the volume (PCV = 0.45) and the plasma makes up the remaining 55%. Once the bleeding in young people has reduced the red cells to 22% (PCV = 0.22) they need a blood transfusion to prevent tissue hypoxia. The haematocrit is the same as the packed cell volume though it is quoted as a percentage not as a decimal fraction.

Paradigm Simply a different way of thinking about something. It involves a genuine change of attitude, or perspective. For example: orthopaedic surgeons wanting their patients to take aspirin preoperatively. This would have been unthinkable a few years ago.

Parasympathetic nervous system regulates housekeeping functions such as bladder and bowel control. Its neurotransmitter is **acetylcholine**.

Pascal (Pa) The SI-derived unit for pressure. It is equivalent to a force of one newton per square metre. A pascal is a tiny pressure; it as about the same pressure a grain of rice exerts on your hand. This unit is far too small to use in clinical work, so we measure pressure in units of 1000 pascals, which is a kilopascal (kPa). One kilopascal corresponds to about 1% of atmospheric pressure at sea level.

Peptides Strings of two or more amino-acids. Peptide chains join together to make proteins.

Peripheral shutdown A term used loosely by clinicians to describe a situation where the skin blood supply is poor. Patients with peripheral shutdown have cold hands, and poor capillary return. Their skin may be mottled or pale. It is a sign of excessive noradrenergic discharge.

pH A logarithmic scale used to measure the acidity or alkalinity of a solution. At 25°C a neutral solution, where the chemical and thermodynamic activity of the acid and alkali is equal, has a pH of 7.0. pH = 1 highly acidic and pH = 14 highly alkaline. The absolute extreme range for human life is pH 6.8–7.8.

Phantom limb pain A form of chronic intractable pain that occurs if acute pain has not been treated properly in the past. Severe unmodified pain causes neuronal wind-up in the dorsal horn of the spinal cord. The synapses transmitting pain become hyperexcitable so that the slightest stimulus triggers a huge response.

Phenothiazines A group of tricyclic drugs with anti-psychotic, major tranquillizing, and anti-emetic properties. They are competitive antagonists of dopamine (particularly D_2) receptors in the central and peripheral nervous systems. They also have anti-muscarinic activity (causing dry mouth, and urinary retention), antihistamine (sedation, anti-itch) and alpha1-adrenergic blockade (causing hypotension). Drugs include chlorpromazine (a neuroleptic) and prochlorperazine (an anti-emetic).

Phospholipids A group of compounds formed by chains of fatty acids and glycerol bound to phosphates. They have a fat (hydrophilic) head and a long stringy (hydrophobic) tail.

Plasma What is left behind when all the cells are removed from blood. Blood is normally composed of 45% cells and 55% plasma.

Plasma cholinesterase deficiency Used to be called pseudocholinesterase deficiency. This glycoprotein enzyme breaks down certain drugs, such as succinylcholine (succinyl choline), mivacurium and remifentanil. It is congenitally deficient or absent in about 1:1000 people.

Plasminogen A proenzyme in the blood. When activated to *fibrinolysin* it helps dissolve stray clots, and in doing so sometimes causes excessive bleeding. Fibrinolysin is the new name for *plasmin*.

Pons An identifiable swelling in the brainstem that, along with other structures, controls breathing, and regulates heart rate and blood pressure.

Polycythaemia Occurs when there are excessive red blood cells circulating. The blood may become so viscous that the blood fails to flow properly though the microcirculation, and becomes prone to clotting.

Polypharmacy Taking many drugs. It is a major cause of morbidity in the elderly. As a rule if a patient is taking more than seven different medications it is highly probable they will have a problem with adverse effects. Then it becomes a vicious cycle, as they take one medication to offset the side effects of another; for instance amitriptyline causes constipation, so they need a laxative, or an NSAID causes stomach pain and aggravates peripheral oedema so they take a diuretic and a protein pump inhibitor.

Positive fluid displacement (PFD) valve Attached to a central venous catheter to maintain a sterile closed system. They prevent tiny blood clots from plugging the tip of the catheter. When you disconnect a syringe after flushing the CVC a small quantity of fluid is forced through the catheter evicting any blood that might remain in the tip to form a clot. Unused lumens with these PFD valves need to be flushed only once a week; this greatly reduces the chance of bacteria coloni\ing an offending blood clot.

Positive pressure Pressure that is above the pressure of the surrounding atmosphere. Ventilators blow air into the patient's chest and in doing so exert a positive pressure in the lungs.

Positive end expiratory pressure (PEEP) A way of ventilating a patient so that at the end of their expiration the pressure in their airways remains above atmospheric pressure, usually by 2–5 cm H_2O.

Postoperative cognitive disorder (POCD) Cognitive function is about how well people solve problems, remember things, and anticipate events. Technically cognitive impairment is a blend of aphasia (language disturbance), apraxia (impaired ability to carry out motor activities despite intact motor function), agnosia (failure to recognize or identify objects despite intact sensory ability), and disturbance in the ability to plan, organize, sequence, and abstract. POCD is a real phenomenon affecting surgical patients over the age of 60 years (particularly men), 25 per cent of whom will have subtle impairment of their cognitive function 7 days after surgery, and 14 per cent will still be impaired at 3 months and 10 per cent at 2 years. Little is known about POCD – or its prevention. It is worse with longer anaesthetics. There is some evidence that periods of hyperventilation during the anaesthetic may contribute.

Postoperative nausea and vomiting (PONV) Customarily defined as nausea or vomiting occurring within 24 hours of anaesthetic. This is an unsatisfactory definition because anaesthetically induced nausea and vomiting usually occur almost immediately and certainly within 4 hours of anaesthetic. Vomiting occurring more than 12 hours after the last anaesthetic drug (including opioids) has been administered usually has a surgical cause such as gastric stasis or ischaemic gut.

Postural hypotension Occurs when a patients' blood pressure falls as they stand or sit up. The magnitude of the fall in blood pressure is measured as **postural drop**.

Postural drop A useful way of telling whether a patient's vascular volume is adequately filled. Measure the patient's systolic blood pressure. Now cautiously ease the patient into a semi-sitting (*Fowler's*) position. Measure the blood pressure again. If the systolic pressure falls by 20 mmHg or more then this is termed a postural drop. This is a reliable sign of hypovolaemia.

Pre-excitation Means that a part of the heart has been stimulated before it should have been.

Preload The length of a cardiac myocyte at the end of diastole. This depends on how far it has been stretched by blood flowing into the ventricle.

Premature atrial contraction Occurs when the atrial beat does not arise in the SA node, but somewhere else in the atria. Sometimes it is the result of a wave in the AV node taking a U-turn.

Premature excitations Ectopic beats arising from many different sites in the ventricles. It needs urgent treatment.

Pressure The force per unit area exerted by a substance perpendicular to its boundary with another substance. It is measured in newtons per square metre. The SI unit is the **pascal** which is a pressure of one newton per square metre. Atmospheric pressure is roughly 1000 Kpascals.

Primary bactaeremia see **Bacteraemia**.

Prions An abnormal form of abnormal host-encoded (PrP) protein found in the brain. Prions crumple adjacent normal protein (PrP) and turn it into another prion. Prions are not alive. They are responsible for variant Creutzfeldt–Jakob Disease (vCJD) the most common human form of bovine spongiform encephalopathy (BSE), also known as mad cow disease. No method of sterilization inactivates vCJD (except heating the object to red-heat). The abnormal proteins gum up the brain eventually causing dementia. There is no cure.

Pro-arrhythmias Drug-induced arrhythmias. They occur in about 10 per cent of patients on antiarrhythmic agents.

Procoagulant states Individuals with procoagulant states (**thrombophilia**) are prone to perioperative deep vein thrombosis (DVT) venous thromboembolism (VTE) and pulmonary embolism (PE). Thrombophilia is inherited, and 12 per cent or more of the Caucasian population are at risk.

Prostaglandins A large group of compounds derived from essential fatty acids in our diet. They are incorporated in the phospholipids that make cell membranes waterproof. When cell membranes are damaged they are released into the tissue fluid where they are turned into *inflammatory mediators* and other local messengers by COX enzymes.

Protamine A basic peptide derived from fish testes, which combines with acidic heparin forming a stable compound, thus inactivating the heparin. Protamine sulphate 1 mg neutralizes 100 units of heparin. Give it slowly – no faster than 50 mg in 10 minutes – because it causes systemic hypotension and severe pulmonary hypertension. Excess protamine acts as an anticoagulant in its own right.

Proteolytic enzymes Break down proteins into smaller bits.

Prothrombin time (PT) tests the internal coagulation pathway. In its standardized form it is called the INR (**International Normalized Ratio**) which is used to adjust the dose of warfarin, and guide the peri-operative use of drugs that modify clotting factors. The INR (and PTT) are prolonged in some bleeding disorders such as disseminated intravascular coagulation (DIC).

Pulmonary oedema Occurs when fluid accumulates in the interstitium or alveoli in the lung. It can be classified into two types: *high-pressure pulmonary oedema* occurs when the pressure in the pulmonary capillaries exceeds the oncotic pressure of blood forcing fluid into the interstitium and eventually the alveoli. This oedema occurs if the capillary vascular pressure exceeds 25 mmHg. *Low-pressure pulmonary oedema* occurs when the alveolar-capillary membrane is damaged in some way allowing fluid from the circulation to transudate into the alveoli. The pulmonary capillary pressure is normal.

Pulse oximeter An electronic device that measures oxygen saturation in the haemoglobin inside red blood cells (erythrocytes).

Pulse pressure The difference in pressure between the systolic and diastolic blood pressures. Pulse pressure = systolic pressure – diastolic pressure.

QTc The corrected QT interval on the ECG adjusted to the patient's heart rate.

Radiocontrast media Special dyes that are opaque to X-rays. They are injected to define blood vessels during radiological procedures. Some types contain iodine which may provoke an allergic response in susceptible individuals.

Receptor A cell or part of a cell, which is specialized to detect a stimulus or a change in its environment.

Recovery position The posture in which to place comatose patients to protect fluid or secretions entering their airway. Patient should be positioned on their side in such a way that their mouth is dependent and fluid can drain out freely. The position must be stable with no pressure on the chest to impair breathing. You need to be able to access the patient's mouth and nose should it become necessary.

Recovery – stages of see **Stages of recovery.**

Recruitment To summon help or aid.

Reflex An automatic response to stimulus. The same stimulus always produces the same response.

Remifentanil A new potent synthetic opioid rapidly broken down by non-specific enzymes in the blood and tissues. This gives it an ultrashort terminal half-life of less than 10 minutes which means its effects do not extend into the recovery room.

Rescue breathing used to be called mouth-to-mouth resuscitation (the kiss of life).

Resistance The resistance of the blood vessels to the forceful pumping of the heart is determined by their elastance and their diameter. The elastance is a measure of their ability to stretch with each pulse and then resume their previous shape.

Respiratory failure occurs when the patient becomes either hypoxaemic or is hypoventilating.

Respiratory rate (RR) The number of breaths taken each minute.

Re-uptake A conservation process whereby nerve cells reuse their neuro-transmitters by absorbing them back into the neuron.

Rhabdomyolysis Occurs when damaged muscle releases myoglobin into the blood. Myoglobin, being almost exactly the size of the holes in the kidney's sieve, soon blocks it. The myoglobin, which escapes into the urine, turns it brown. Myoglobinuria can be mistaken for haemoglobinuria.

Ringer's solution Formulated by a British physiologist, Sydney Ringer in the 1880s. Alex Hartmann added lactate to Ringer's solution to make it more suitable for children.

R-on-T phenomenon occurs when the R-wave on the ECG snuggles right up next to, or even inside the T-wave. This is a dangerous sign as the patient may flip into ventricular fibrillation, or a ventricular tachycardia. Treat this urgently.

Root cause analysis A method used in risk management of identifying a single cause for an adverse event. This is a bad concept, because there is very rarely, if ever, a single root cause of anything.

Saline overload and **saline depletion** are (for want of a better word) useful shorthand terms to describe the status of all the osmotically active ions in the extracellular fluid (ECF) volume. The ECF is composed of fluid containing the **cations** sodium, potassium, and calcium, and the **anions** chloride, bicarbonate, lactate and a little phosphate. This fluid is *isotonic* with the fluid inside cells. If patients have excessive ECF (saline overload) they become oedematous. If the patient has ECF depletion (saline deficit) they are 'dry', have a low urine output and develop **postural hypotension** if they sit or stand up.

Sensitization A process that produces an acute hyperawareness of an otherwise minor stimulus; for instance a slap on a sunburnt back.

Sepsis The term sepsis is tends to be used loosely to mean localized or generalized infection. More strictly, it is the presence of an infection and the subsequent physiologic responses to that infection including activation of the inflammatory cascade. Unchecked sepsis leads to the *systemic inflammatory response syndrome (SIRS)*. Severe sepsis causes end-organ dysfunction.

Series Blood flowing in series means that it flows sequentially down a single path from one point to the next. In contrast, if blood vessels are set in parallel, as they are in the lungs, then blood follows along a number of different paths to get from one point to another.

Serotonin A monamine neurotransmitter that plays a crucial part in events such as temperature regulation, sensory perception, alarm mechanisms, emotion and the onset of sleep.

SI unit An abbreviation for *Systeme internationale d'unites* or International System of Units which defines units used in measurement such as mass, length, time, ampere, mol, candela and so on.

Secondary bactaeremia see **Bacteraemia**.

Sick sinus syndrome (SSS) Refers to a collection of diseases arising inside the sino-atrial node. SSS does not affect the conduction of impulses through the atrial muscle. The characteristic ECG feature is an irregular pulse with normal PR interval. The SA node may stutter along firing intermittently, or alternatively it may speed up and slow down (**tachycardia-bradycardia syndrome**).

Sigh Every few minutes we take a deeper breath, a *sigh*, to re-expand collapsing terminal respiratory units. Ventilators too need this provision to prevent **micro-atelectasis**.

Sinus arrhythmia Occurs in young fit people where the heart rate slows on inspiration and speeds-up on expiration. In patients over the age of 55 years an alternating heart rate is more likely to be **sick sinus syndrome**, in which case it will have no correlation with breathing.

Sinus rhythm Occurs when the sino-atrial node dictates the heart rate at a regular rhythm between 50–100 bpm.

Sinus tachycardia A heart rate greater than 100 bpm. The P-waves and QRS waves are normal.

Slips, lapses and **mishaps** Slips and lapses are caused by human error, and mishaps are events that occur by chance. Slips occur because of system errors, inattention, fatigue, or inexperience. Lapses occur because procedures and protocols are, for whatever reason, not followed. Mishaps are inevitable, unpredictable (but not necessarily unforeseen) events such as an anaphylactic reaction.

Sleep apnoea *Obstructive sleep apnoea (OSA)* occurs especially in elderly obese men. Their airway collapses during deep sleep causing obstructive apnoea and frequently severe hypoxaemia. Some patients may have more than 30 episodes a night. There is a significant correlation between sleep apnoea and hypertension, dementia, cardiac failure ischaemic heart disease, stroke, and type 2 diabetes. *Central sleep apnoea* syndrome is the loss of respiratory drive when a susceptible individual is in deep sleep – they simply stop breathing until the noradrenergic nervous system is alerted. Usually their PaO_2 falls to damagingly low levels before this happens. These people are particularly susceptible to opioid-induced respiratory depression.

Somatic pain Comes from superficial structures such as muscles and skin, and is perceived through the spinal nerves. It is described as sharp, well localized, stabbing and is usually localized by one finger pointing at the source.

Specialist perioperative nurses (SPN) Sometimes known as clinical nurse consultant (CNC) or specialist perioperative practitioners (SPP). Others, rather than being confined to one surgical specialty cover many disciplines; for example integrated cancer coordinators (ICC) who care for cancer patients.

Spino-thalamic tracts Bundles of nerves passing from the spinal cord to the thalamus in the brain.

Squames Little flakes of shed skin. Like dust, they can float about in the air, and allow micro-organisms to hitch-hike from one place to another.

Stages of recovery Used to guide the care of patients in the recovery room, and determine their fitness to be discharged.

Stage 1 recovery Patients who need Stage 1 recovery are those who are physiologically unstable, or who potentially may become so.

Stage 2 recovery At this stage the patients are conscious, fully able to care for their own airways, and within the physiological limits defined by their pre-operative evaluation.

Stage 3 recovery Following day procedures patients can be discharged into the care of a competent and informed adult who can intervene in the case of untoward events.

Stress Occurs when the body's homeostatic mechanisms deviate from normal. A strain is the event causing the stress.

Stroke-volume The volume of blood ejected with each heart beat.

Subluxation Occurs where spinal joints are loose, and move relative to one another and in doing so may press on the spinal cord.

Substance P A peptide released from injured tissue. The P is an abbreviation for pain.

Substantia gelatinosa Part of the dorsal horn in the spinal cord where first-order sensory neurons synapse with second-order nerve cells passing to the brain. It works like a gate directing impulses either to the brain or back along reflex arcs.

Succinyl choline A short-acting depolarizing muscle relaxant principally used for intubating patients. It is sometimes called suxamthonium (chloride), or simply 'sux'.

Surfactant A complex phospholipid detergent produced by cells in the alveolus that prevents surface tension causing the alveolus to collapse. Premature neonates who do not produce enough surfactant get neonatal respiratory distress syndrome.

Supraventricular arrhythmias arise in the atria.

Supraventricular tachycardia (SVT) A heart rate of between 150 to 250 bpm. On the ECG P-waves are usually, but not always, still visible. There are a number of causes.

Sympathetic nervous system (SNS) Roused into action by threats to homeostasis such as hypovolaemia, hypoxia, fear and pain.

Sympatheticomimetic A tongue-twisting word that means mimicking the effects of the sympathetic nervous system. Sympatheticomimetic drugs imitate the actions of adrenaline or noradrenaline.

Sympathetic response is to raise the blood pressure, increase the heart rate and cardiac output. It make the person hyperalert and vigilant.

Synapse A gap between two nerve cells. When stimulated by an **action potential** the end of one nerve cell releases a **neurotransmitter**, which drifts across the synapse, latches on to a **receptor** on the next nerve to trigger an action potential in the next nerve cell.

System Describes a group of interacting elements organized into a complex functioning whole. Systems can be closed to outside influences, or open to them. Your hospital is a system, and the recovery room is a subset of that system.

Systolic heart failure Characterized by a dilated floppy ventricle where the actin and myosin filaments do not overlap adequately. Therefore any increase in intraventricular pressure just stretches the filaments further, so cardiac output falls, especially at the beginning of inspiration.

Systolic pressure The maximum blood pressure in the arteries during the cardiac cycle.

T3 Triiodothyronine – a potent form of thyroid hormone.

T4 Thyroxine.

Tachycardia–bradycardia syndrome – see **Sick sinus syndrome**.

Tachycardia A heart rate greater than 100/min.

Tachyphylaxis Occurs where patients develop an acute tolerance to a drug over minutes or hours. This means patients require progressively higher doses to achieve the same effect.

Tamponade To dam-up or squash. Cardiac tamponade means the heart is squashed by fluid pressure in the pericardial sac.

Temperature Difficult to define. Temperature is a physical measurement used to determine whether two bodies are in thermal equilibrium. If two bodies, A and B are placed next to each other, and heat energy moves from A to B then the temperature of A is higher than the temperature of body B.

Terminal respiratory units Functional clumps of alveoli and the terminal airways served by a common pulmonary arteriole. They are about the size of a match head.

Thalamus A collection of nerves shaped like two pigeon's eggs sitting deep in the brain. It lies above the hypothalamus right on top of the brainstem at the core of the brain. It is the key relay station for sensory information flowing to the brain. From the constant mass of information pouring in, and like a protective secretary, it only passes on immediately relevant information.

Therapeutic index Reflects the difference between the blood concentrations of a toxic dose of a drug, and its therapeutic levels. The therapeutic blood level of theophylline is only a whisker away from its toxic dose.

Thermistors Measure temperature. A thermistor is a tiny electrical device made from metal oxides semiconductors moulded together. A current passed through the wires varies exponentially with the temperature.

Thermodynamic activity The total kinetic and potential energy of a substance that could be converted into heat. It excludes electromagnetic and nuclear energy. Atoms and molecules vibrate and jiggle about according to their temperature, the hotter they are they faster they jiggle. The more they jiggle the more space they occupy. That is why things expand as they are heated. Thermodynamic activity is a measure of this vibration. At $-273°C$ (absolute zero) they stop jiggling, stay quite still and have no thermodynamic activity.

Third space fluid Fluid that has been sequestrated in the bowel, peritoneum or pleural spaces because of either transudation or exudation. If the surgeon handles the bowel extensively during abdominal surgery, fluids will transudate into the lumen over the next 2–3 days. This can cause hypovolaemia, even though no fluid has been lost to the outside world. Although third space fluid forms part of the **total body water**, it is not available to boost the plasma or ECF volume.

Threshold potential A level of stimulus at which something becomes perceivable.

Thrombophilia The tendency to form spontaneous blood clots. It can be either inherited or acquired.

Thromboxane (TXA$_2$) A powerful chemical made by platelets that causes them to stick together (aggregate) and causes vasoconstriction. It works hand in hand with a prostaglandin produced by vascular endocytes called PGI2 to help form blood clots and stop bleeding.

Tidal volume (TV) The amount of air moved into or out of the lungs with each breath.

Tolerance Tolerance to a drug is the progressive need for higher doses to achieve a consistent effect.

Tonicity is A measurement that compares the osmotic pressures of two solutions. The tonicity of a solution determines how water flows across cell membranes. Formally it can be defined thus: if two solutions are separated by a membrane only permeable to water, and water flows from one solution to the other, then the latter has a higher tonicity than the former.

In practice, this means hypertonic solutions drag water out of cells, while hypotonic fluids allow water to flow into cells. If the solutions are **isotonic** then no fluid moves the across the cell membranes.

Torsades de pointes (twisting of the points) A very fast and particularly lethal polymorphic ventricular tachycardia. Each impulse arises in a different place in the ventricles so that the rapidly changing QRS trace on the ECG looks as though it is rotating about a baseline.

Total body water The total amount of fluid containing water in the body. It does not only include water, but also extracellular fluid, intracellular fluid, and cerebrospinal fluid. The volume of total body water is about 60% of lean body mass.

TURP syndrome occurs if the fibrous capsule around the prostate gland is breached during a *transurethral resection of the prostate* (TURP). The irrigation fluid used to dilate the bladder can leak into the circulation. It is possible for large amounts of water to dilute the electrolytes in the plasma to cause the typical symptoms of water overload.

Tranexamic acid A drug (similar to amino-caproic acid) that inhibits plasminogen activation and fibrinolysis. It is rapidly excreted by the kidneys. The dose is 0.5–1 gm tds IV slowly.

Transducer A transducer is a device for converting one form of energy into another. For instance a pressure transducer converts pressure energy into electrical energy that a monitor can process. Unless carefully calibrated, transducers introduce inaccuracies and errors into measurements.

Transient ischaemic attack (TIA) These transient attacks of cerebral ischaemia are caused by micro-emboli lodging in the small vessels in the brain causing symptoms that by definition resolve within 24 hours. The tiny clots often arise from the walls of the left atria in patients with atrial fibrillation. To prevent the formation of these micro-emboli, patients in atrial fibrillation usually take the anticoagulant warfarin.

Trans-oesophageal echocardiography (TOE) A technique where the patient swallows an ultrasound probe which does an echocardiogram from about two-thirds of the way down the oesophagus.

Transfusion threshold A nominated trigger point at which to give blood. In fit young people a **haematocrit** of 25% is the usual transfusion threshold, but in older and sicker patients it may be 30% or more.

Transudate Fluid that has leaked across membranes. It is lower in protein content, than **exudate**. Exudate is protein-rich fluid produced by inflammation.

Trifasicular block A combination of an atrioventricular block, a right bundle branch block, and a left anterior hemiblock. Trifasicular blocks are high-grade blocks indicating extensive myocardial damage. If they are causing symptoms the patient requires a temporary pacemaker for major operations.

Triglycerides The body stores fat in fat cells (lipidocytes) in two forms: triglycerides and glycerol. These are easily broken down by enzymes called lipases into free fatty acids (FFAs). FFAs act as fast food for the heart and liver where they are degraded by β-oxidation to form energy. The proper name for triglyceride is triacylglycerol (but almost nobody uses it).

Ultrafiltrate see **Filtrate.**

Uraemia The clinical and biochemical effects of an abnormal accumulation of waste products in the blood. It is a descriptive term describing the signs and symptoms of a patient with renal failure.

Urine The end-product of the renal tubules filtering, reabsorption, secretion, and concentration of tubular filtrate.

Vasopressin Also called **arginine vasopressin** (AVP). Another name for **antidiuretic hormone** (ADH).

Venothromboembolism (VTE) An umbrella term used to describe abnormal blood clots that are fixed in one place (**thromboses**) or those that have moved elsewhere (**emboli**).

Ventricular fibrillation (VF) In VF the cardiac impulse is chaotic and incapable of organizing coordinated ventricular contraction. If the chest is open you can see the heart muscle writhing like a bag full of earthworms, and there is no cardiac output.

Ventricular premature beats (VPBs) Wide, bizarre QRS complexes with a down-sloping ST segment, not preceded by a P-wave. They indicate an irritable myocardium, where the ventricle has contracted without the usual triggering sequence. Sometimes these are known as ventricular ectopics, or ventricular extrasystoles (VEs), or even premature ventricular contractions (PVCs). Suspect myocardial ischaemia – or too much coffee.

Ventricular tachycardia (VT) occurs when there are runs of more than three VPBs together.

Visceral pain comes from deep structures such as the gastrointestinal tract, bladder and other organs. It is difficult to localize with one finger, and is described in terms such as aching, nauseating, dull, or boring.

Vital centres The brainstem contain the grey matter neural connections responsible for controlling blood pressure, heart rate, the pattern and rate of breathing, temperature, plasma osmotic pressure, carbon dioxide levels, vomiting, thermal regulation, sweating, and the adrenergic and noradrenergic responses. The vital centres mostly interact with the autonomic nervous system.

Vital signs traditionally involve the measurement of blood pressure, pulse rate, respiratory rate and conscious state. In contrast *observations* seems to mean the addition of measurement of temperature and perhaps urine output. Neither term has a formal definition. They are often used interchangeably as a verbal short hand. Should 'observations' include oxygen saturation? Almost certain in the recovery room, the answer is yes.

Volume depletion Jargon for a loss of fluid from the body. Usually it refers to blood loss, but it may also refer to loss of extracellular fluid (ECF) or even intracellular fluid depletion. It is a better term than **dehydration**.

von Willebrand's disease A term that covers four subgroups of the most common inherited bleeding disorders. It is caused by a defect in the production of von Willebrand's factor (vWF) by the endothelium lining blood vessels. Unlike haemophilia it affects men and women equally.

Water intoxication occurs after prolonged irrigation with hypertonic fluids during urological surgery, or hysteroscopy. The patient becomes acutely water overloaded (*hyponatraemic*) and their brain cells swell. It can be fatal, particularly in premenopausal woman and children.

Water-soluble hormones see **Hormones.**

Whistle-tip catheters Made of soft silicon-plastic, they have holes on their side, and a moulded tip that will not damage delicate mucosa.

Wind-up The process by which a nerve cell becomes far more sensitive to stimuli that would previously have not had much effect.

Wolff–Parkinson–White (WPW) syndrome is one of the congenital syndromes, where the ventricle becomes prematurely activated when the cardiac impulse takes a shortcut through an accessory pathway to bypass the AV node. Consequently the PR interval is short (0.1–0.2 seconds), and there is a wider QRS complex.

Work is a physical measurement. Work (W) is done when a force (F) moves a mass (m) through a distance. Work = F × D. Its SI unit is the newton.metre.

Abbreviations

Abbreviations are frequently used by medical and nursing staff. They are sometimes specific to a particular area, and are a mystery to outsiders, but many are in common use. To avoid errors and mishaps use only abbreviations approved by your hospital. Even approved abbreviations can be misunderstood if they are not written clearly, and clear script is not a virtue of many doctors. Always explain abbreviations if there is the possibility they have more than one meaning, for example, DOA could mean dead on arrival, or date of admission; ARF could mean acute respiratory failure or acute renal failure; and Cx could mean cervical spine or cervix.

This is a list of common abbreviations used in many hospitals.

Never act on an abbreviation
unless you are absolutely sure what it means.

#	fracture
#	number
%	per cent
α	Greek letter alpha
β	Greek letter beta
γ	Greek letter gamma
π	Greek letter pi (pronounced pie)
/	per or each (breaths/min)
@	at
[X]	concentration of substance X
[Na⁺]	concentration of sodium ion
<	less than
>	greater than
±	plus or minus
«	much less than
»	much greater than
Δ	Greek letter upper case delta used to describe differences
≤	less than or equal to
≥	greater than or equal to
©	copyright
®	registered name

™	trademark
°C	degree centigrade
°C	degrees Celsius
°F	degree fahrenheit
μ	Greek letter, mu (pronounced mew)
μ	micro
μgm or less clearly μg	microgram
μmol	micromol
5-HT	5 hydroxytryptamine (also called serotonin)
a.c.	before food is given; it applies to medication.
a.m.	before noon
ABG	arterial blood gases
AC	alternating current
ACE	angiotensin converting
ACEI	angiotensin-converting enzyme inhibitor
ACLS	advanced cardiac life support
ACS	acute coronary syndrome
ACTH	adrenocorticotropic hormone
ADH	antidiuretic hormone

AE	atrial ectopic beats	BBV	blood-borne virus
AED	automated external defibrillator	BCC	basal cell carcinoma
AED	automatic external	BCG	Bacille Calmette-Guérin
AF	atrial fibrillation	Bd	twice daily
AIDS	acquired immune deficiency	BF	breast fed
AIMS	Australian Incident Monitoring System	BIP	bisthmus iodine paste
AMI	acute myocardial infarction	BiPAP	bi-level positive airway pressure
ANP	atrial-naturetic peptide	BKA	below knee amputation
ANS	autonomic nervous system	BLS	basic cardiac life support
APACHE	acute physiology and chronic health evaluation	BLS	basic life support
aPPT	activated partial thromboplastin time	BMR	basal metabolic rate
		BP	blood pressure
APS	acute pain service	bpm	heart rate in beats per minute
aPTT	activated partial thromboplastin time	BUN	bound urinary nitrogen
		BVM	bab valve mask unit
AR	aortic regurgitation	Bx	biopsy
ARB	angiotensin receptor blockers	C5	fifth cervical vertebra
ARDS	acute respiratory distress syndrome	Ca	carcinoma
		Ca^{++}	calcium ion
ARDS	adult respiratory distress syndrome	CABG	coronary artery bypass graft
ARF	acute renal failure	CABG	coronary artery bypass surgery
AS	aortic stenosis	CAD	coronary artery disease
ASAP	as soon as possible	CAM	complementary and alternative medicine
Assist	assistants	CAN	cardiac autonomic neuropathy
AST	alanine aminotransferase	CaO_2	arterial oxygen content
ATLS	advanced trauma life	CAPD	ambulatory peritoneal dialysis
ATN	acute tubular necrosis	CAVDH	continuous arterio-venous haemodialysis
ATP	adenosine triphosphate		
AUC	area under curve	CBF	cerebral blood flow
AV node	atrioventricular node	CCF	congestive cardiac failure
AV shunt	arteriovenous shunt	CDH	congenital dislocation of the hip
AV	atrioventricular	CE	continuing education
AVB	atrioventricular block	CETT	cuffed endotracheal tube
AVP	arginine vasopressin	CGRP	calcitonin gene-related peptide
AXR	abdominal x-ray	CI	cardiac index
b.d.	twice daily	CJD	Creutzfeldt–Jakob disease
B.S.	blood sugar	CK	creatinine kinase
BA	bowel action	CKD	chronic kidney disease
BAN	British Approved Names	CKMB	creatinine kinase isoenzyme - muscle band

Cl⁻	chloride ion	DOA	dead on arrival
cm	centimetre	DOB	date of birth
CMV	cytomegalovirus	DPG	diphosphoglycerate
CNS	central nervous system	dTC	tubocurare
CO_2	carbon dioxide	DVT	deep vein thrombosis
COAD	chronic obstructive airway disease	Dx	diathermy
		E/o	excision of
COPD	chronic obstructive pulmonary disease	EACA	epsilon amino caproic acid
		EBP	evidence-based practice
CPAP	continuous positive airway pressure	ECF	extracellular fluid
		ECG	electrocardiograpm
C-PAP	continuous positive airway pressure	ECT	electroconvulsive therapy
		ED	emergency department
CPK	creatinine phosphokinase	EDTA	ethyl diamine tetra acetic acid
CPR	cardiopulmonary resuscitation	EEG	electroencephalogram
CRF	chronic renal failure	EF	ejection fraction
CRI	cardiac risk index	eGFR	estimated glomerular
CRT	capillary return time	eGFR	estimated glomerular filtration rate
CSF	cerebrospinal fluid		
CT	computed tomography	EKG	electrocardiograph (alternative abbrev.)
CTZ	chemo-trigger receptor zone		
CVA	cerebrovascular accident	ELISA	enzyme-linked immunosorbent assay
CVC	central venous catheter		
CVD	cerebrovascular disease	EMB	early morning breakfast
CVL	central venous line	EMLA	eutectic mixture of local anaesthetics
CvO_2	mixed venus oxygen content		
CVP	central venous pressure	ENT	ear, nose and throat
CWMS	colour, warmth, movement, sensation		enzyme
		EPAP	expiratory positive airway pressure
Cx	cervical spine		
Cx	cervix	EPP	exposure-prone procedures
CXR	chest X-ray	ER	emergency room
D&C	dilation and curettage	ERCP	endoscopic retrograde cholangiopancreatography
D5W	5% dextrose in water		
D5W	dextrose 5% in water	ERSF	end stage renal failure
DB&C	deep breath and cough	ESKD	end stage kidney disease
DC	direct current	ESR	erythrocyte sedimentation rate
DCR	direct current cardioversion	ESU	electrosurgical unit (diathermy in the UK)
DDAVP®	desmopressin		
DIC	disseminated intravascular coagulation	ESWL	extracorporeal shock wave lithotripsy
		ETA	estimated time of arrival
DNA	de-oxyribose nucleic acid	ETT	endotracheal tube
DO2	oxygen delivery		

EUA	examination under anaesthesia
FB	foreign body
FBA	foreign body aspiration
FBC	fluid balance chart
FBE	full blood examination
FDA	Federal Drug Authority - a USA agency
FDA	Food and Drug Administration (USA)
FDP	fibrin degradation products
FDPs	fibrin degradation products
FES	fat embolism syndrome
FEV1	forced expiratory volume in one second
FF	free fluids
FHx	family history
FIO2	fractional inspired oxygen concentration
FIx	for investigation
FNAB	fine-needle aspiration biopsy
FNH	febrile non-haemolytic reactions
FNHTR	febrile non-haemolytic transfusion reaction
FRC	functional residual capacity
FRC	functional residual capacity
FS	frozen section
FSH	follicle stimulating hormone
FSPs	fibrin split products
FVC	forced vital capacity
FWD	full ward diet
FWT	full ward test of urine
G	gauge
GA	general anaesthesia
GABA	gamma aminobutyric acid
GAMP	general anaesthetic, manipulation and plaster
GCS	Glasgow coma scale
GFR	glomerular filtration rate
GGT	gamma-glutamyltransferase
gm or less clearly abbrev g.	gram
GOK	goodness only knows
GSC	Glasgow Coma Scale

GTN	glyceryl trinitrate (preferred abbrev)
Gyn	gynaecology
H^+	hydrogen ion
H_2O	water
HAFOE	high airflow oxygen entrainment masks
Hb	haemoglobin
HBA	herpes A virus
HBC	herpes C virus
HBV	herpes B virus
$HCO3^-$	bicarbonate ion
HCT	haematocrit
HCW	health care workers
HDU	high dependency unit
HFV	high frequency ventilation
Hg	mercury
HIC	head injury chart
HITs	heparin induced thrombocytopaenia
HIV	human immunodeficiency virus
HME	heat and moisture exchangers
HNPU	has not passed urine
HOCUM	hypertrophic obstructive cardiomyopathy
HPV	hypoxic pulmonary vasoconstriction
hr	hour
hrly	hourly
HRT	hormone replacement therapy
HSV	herpes simplex virus
HT	hypertension
HTLV	human T cell lymphotrophic virus
Htn	hypertension
HTR	haemolytic transfusion reactions
Hx	history
i.d.	internal diameter
I.U.	International Units
I/M	intramuscular
IBP	invasive blood pressure monitoring

IBW	ideal body weight	LBM	lean body mass
ICC	intercostal catheter	LDH	lactic dehydrogenase
ICF	intracellular fluid	LIF	left iliac fossa
ICP	intracranial pressure	LMA	laryngeal mask airway
ICU	intensive care unit	LMWH	low molecular-weight heparin
IDDM	insulin-dependent diabetes mellitus	LOC	loss of consciousness
IgA	immunoglobin A, (others are M, E.and G).	LOE	levels of evidence
		LP	lumbar puncture
		LUQ	left upper quadrant
IHD	ischaemic heart disease	LVF	left ventricular failure
IM	intramuscularly	m^2	square metre
IMV	intermittent manditory ventilation	MAC	minimum anaesthetic concentration
INR	International normalized ratio (see PTT)	mane	in the morning
		MAO	mono-amine oxidase
IPAP	inspiratory positive airway pressure	MAOI	mono-amine oxidase inhibitor
		MAP	mean arterial pressure
IPC	intermittent pneumatic compression	MAT	multifocal atrial tachycardia
		MBA	motor bicycle accident
IPPV	intermittent positive pressure ventilation	MCA	motor car accident
		mcgm	microgram
ISO	International Standards Organization	MDRTB	multiple drug-resistant tuberculosis
ISQ	in status quo (meaning "unchanged")	MEAC	mean effective anaesthetic concentration
ITP	idiopathic thrombocytopenic purpura	MET	metabolic exercise tolerance
		mg	milligram
IU	international units	MG	myasthenia gravis
IUD	intrauterine device	Mg^{++}	magnesium ion
IV	intravenous	MH	malignant hyperthermia
IVI	intravenous injection	MHAH	micro-angiopathic haemolytic anaemia
JVP	jugular venous pressure		
K^+	potassium ion	MI	myocardial infarction
Kcal	kilocalorie	MIC	minimum inhibitory concentration
KCl	potassium chloride		
Kg	kilogram	Min	minute
kPa	kilopasacal	Mm	millimetre
L	litre	mmHg	millimetre of mercury pressure
L3-4	interspace between 3rd and 4th lumbar vertebrae	mmol	milimol
		mOsm	milli-osmol
LA	local anaesthesia	MRI	magnetic resonance imaging
Lac	laceration	MRSA	multiple resistant staphylococcus aureus
LAHB	left anterior hemiblock		
LBBB	left bundle branch block		

Ms	millisecond
MS	multiple sclerosis
MSOF	multisystem organ failure
MTBF	mean time between failures
MUA	manipulation under anaesthetic
mV	millivolt
MVA	motor vehicle accident
MVPS	mitral valve prolapse syndrome
MVR	mitral valve regurgitation
N	normal (as in 0.9% Normal saline)
N/G	nasogastric
N/S	normal saline
N_2O	nitrous oxide
Na+	sodium ion
NAD	nothing abnormal detected
NBP	non-invasive blood pressure
Neg	negative
NFO	no further orders
NFR	not for resuscitation
NHS	National Health Service (U.K.)
NIBP	non-invasive blood pressure
NIDDM	non-insulin dependent diabetes mellitus
NMBD	neuromuscular blocking drugs
NMDA	N-methyl-D-aspartic acid
nmol	nanomol
NMS	neuroleptic malignant syndrome
NNH	number needed to harm
NNT	number needed to treat
NO	nitric oxide
nocte	at night
NOF	neck of femur
NPA	nasopharyngeal aspiration
NRL	natural rubber latex
NSAID	non-steroidal anti-inflammatory drug
NTG	nitroglycerine (see GTN)
NYO	not yet ordered
O	oral

O	oxygen
O/A	on admission
O/call	on call
O_2	oxygen
OD	overdose
OPD	out-patients department
OR	operating room
Ortho	orthopaedics
OSA	obstructive sleep apnoea
OT	operating theatre
OTC	over the counter
OXI	pulse oximetery
P	partial pressure as in PO_2
p.c.	after meals
PA	pulmonary artery
PACE	postoperative adverse cardiac events
$PaCO_2$	partial pressure of carbon dioxide in arterial blood
PACU	post anaesthetic care unit
Paed	paediatrics
PAG	periaquecductal grey matter
PaO_2	partial pressure of oxygen in the arterial blood
PAP	pulmonary artery pressure
PAT	paroxysmal atrial tachycardia
PAWP	pulmonary artery wedge pressure
PCA	patient controlled analgesia
PCA	patient-controlled anaesthesia
PCEA	patient controlled epidural analgesia
PCI	percutaneous intervention
PCNL	percutaneous nephrolithotomy
PCO_2	partial pressure of carbon dioxide
PCTA	percutaneous transluminal angioplasty
PCV	packed cell volume
PD	peritoneal dialysis
PDE	phosphodiesterase
PDQ	pretty darned quick
PE	pulmonary embolism

PEA	pre-emptive analgesia	QD	once daily (use of this is discouraged)
PEA	pulseless electrical activity	QID	four times daily
PEEP	positive ende expiratory pressure	RAS	reticular activating system
PERLA	pupils equal and reacting to light and accommodation	RBBB	right bundle branch block
PFD	positive fluid displacement	RBF	renal blood flow
PFR	peak flow rate	RCT	randomized controlled trial
pH	inverse logarithm of the hydrogen ion activity	Resps	Respirations
		RIA	radio-immuno assay
PHx	past history	RIB	rest in bed
PINDA	pain indicator and assessment	RIF	right iliac fossa
PM	post mortem	rINNs	recommended International Non-Proprietary Names
pm.	after midday		
PND	paroxysmal nocturnal dyspnoea	RNA	ribose nucleic acid
		ROP	retinopathy of prematurity
PO_2	partial pressure of oxygen	RPAO	routine post anaesthetic orders
PONV	post operative nausea and/or vomiting	RUQ	right upper quarrant
		RVF	right ventricular failure
POP	plaster of paris	S/B	seen by
PORC	post operative residual curarization	S/C	subcutaneous
		SA node	sino-atrial node
Pos	positive	SA	sino-atrial
PPF	plasma protein fraction	SAED	shock advisory external fibrillators
PPI	proton pump inhibitor		
Ppm	parts per million	SAL	sterility assurance level
PR	per rectum	SaO_2	haemoglobin's oxygen saturation
PRBC	packed red blood cells		
Premed	premedication	SAP	systemic arterial pressure
prn	when necessary (pro re nata)	SBE	subacute bacterial endocarditis
PS	pressure support	sec	seconds
PT	prothrombin time (also see INR)	SG	specific gravity
		SG	substantia gelatinosa
PTB	pulmonary tuberculosis	SIADH	Syndrome of inappropriate antidiuretic hormone secretion
PTH	post transfusion hepatitis		
PTSD	post traumatic stress disorder	SLE	systemic lupus erythematosus
PUD	peptic ulcer disease	SMR	submucosal resection
PUO	pyrexia of unknown origin	SNP	sodium nitroprusside
PV	per vagina	SNS	sympathetic nervous system
PVB	premature ventricular beat	SOF	shaft of femur
PVC	premature ventricular contraction	SOOB	sit out of bed
		Sp/A	spinal anaesthesia
PVR	pulmonary vascular resistance	SPN	specialist perioperative nurses
		SR	sinus rhthym

SSG	split skin graft
SSS	sickle cell syndrome
stat	statum (immediately)
STD	sexually transmitted disease
STOP	suction termination of pregnancy
STP	sodium thiopentone
Sux	suxamethonium chloride
SVR	systemic vascular resistance
SVT	supraventricular tachycardia
SWMA	systolic wall movement abnormality syndrome
T3	tri-iodothyronine
T4	thyroxine
T6	sixth thoracic vertebra
Tabs	tablets
TAH	total abdominal hysterectomy
TB	tuberculosis
TCP	transcutaneous pacemaker
tds	three times a day
TENS	transcutaneous electrical stimulation
TENS	transcutaneous nerve stimulation
THR	total hip replacement
TIA	transient ischaemic attacks
TIVA	total intravenous anaesthesia
TMJ	temporo-mandibular joint
TMOA	too many obscure abbreviations
TOF	train-of-four with a nerve stimulator
TOP	termination of pregnancy
TPN	total parenteral nutrition
TPR	temperature, pulse and respiration
TRALI	transfusion related lung injury
Ts & As	tonsillectomy and adenoidectomy

TTN	transient tachypnea of the newborn
TURBT	transurethral bladder tumour resection
TURP	transurethral resection of prostate
U&E	urea and electrolyte
UH	unfractionated heparin
URTI	upper respiratory tract infection
UTI	urinary tract infection
UTT	up to toilet
UWSD	under-water sealed drainage
V	volt
VAPS	visual analogue pain scale
VC	vital capacity
VC	vomiting centre
VE	ventricular ectopics
VEs	ventricular extrasystoles
VF	ventricular fibrillation
VO_2	oxygen consumption
VPBs	ventricular premature beats
VRE	vancomycin-resistant enterococcus
VT	ventricular tachycardia
VTE	venothromboembolic disease
VVs	varicose veins
vWD	von Willebrand's syndrome
WHO	World Health Organisation
WNL	within normal limits
WPW	Wolff-Parkinson-White syndrome
wt	weight
WYSWYG	What you see is what you get (a computer term).
XDP	fibrin d-dimer
X-match	cross match blood
Yr	year

Useful data

Resources

Acid-base
http://http://www.acid-base.com

Acupuncture
http://http://www.acupuncture.com

American Heart Association
http://www.americanheart.org/aha.html

American Pain Foundation
http://www.painfoundation.com

American Pain Society
http://www.ampainsoc.org

American Society of Pain Management Nursing
http://www.aspmn.org

American Society of Peri-anesthesia Nurses
http://www.aspan.org

Association of Peri-operative Registered Nurses
http://www.aorn.org

Australian and New Zealand College of Anaesthetists
http://www.anzca.edu.au

Australian College of Critical Care Nurses
http://www.acccn.com.au

Australian College of Operating Room Nurses
http://www.acorn.org.au

Australian Institute of Health and Welfare
http://www.aihw.gov.au

Australian Lung Foundation
http://www.lungnet.org.au

Australian Nursing Council
http://www.anci.org.au

Australian Pain Society
http://www.iasp-pain.org

Australian Resuscitation Council
http://www.resus.org.au

British Anaesthetic and Recovery Nurses' Association
http://www.barna.org.uk

British Medical Journal
http://www.bmj.com

Cancer Council of Australia
http://www.cancer.org.au

Capnography
http://www.capnography.com

Center for Disease Control and Prevention
http://www.cdc.gov

Cochrane Collaboration
http://www.cochrane.org

College of Emergency Nurses Australasia
http://www.cena.org.au

Epidural manual (Royal Marsden)
http://www.blackwellroyalmarsdenmanual.com/sample/mars29.htm

Johns Hopkins Center for Tuberculosis Research
http://www.Hopkins-tb.com

Journal of Perianesthesia Nursing
http://www.jopan.com

Malignant Hyperthermia Association of the United States
http://www.mhaus.org

National Association of Theatre Nurses
http://www.natn.org.uk

National Heart Foundation of Australia
http://www.heartfoundation.com.au

North American Nursing Diagnosis Association
http://www.nanda.org

Nurse-Beat Cardiac Electronic Journal
http://www.nurse-beat.com

Operating Room Association of Canada
http://www.ornac.ca

Perioperative Nurses' College of New Zealand
http://www.pnc.org.nz

Postoperative Pain
http://www.postoppain.org

Royal Australasian College of Surgeons
http://www.surgeons.org

Royal Children's Hospital
http://www.rch.unimelb.edu.au

Royal College of Nursing Australia
http://www.rcna.org

The Cardiac Society of Australia and New Zealand
http://www.csanz.edu.au

VirtualAnaesthetics
http://www.virtual-anaesthesia-textbook.com

World Anaesthesia
http://www.nda.ox.ac.uk

World Health Organization
http://www.who.int

Standardization

The Systeme Internationale d'Unites (SI system) is the standard against which to measure length in metres, mass in kilograms, and time in seconds, pressure in pascals, work in joules, volume in cubic metres and so on. Non-standard units are still widely used and include millimetres of mercury, litres, degrees Fahrenheit. It will be sometime before we drink 0.180×10^{-3} cubic metres instead of a tumbler (or glass) of water, or say today's temperature is 300 Kelvin (not 'degrees' Kelvin).

Factors

Factor	Prefix	Symbol
10^6	Mega	M
10^3	Kilo	K
10^{-1}	dec	D
10^{-2}	centi	C
10^{-3}	milli	M
10^{-6}	micro	μ
10^{-9}	nano	N
10^{-12}	pico	P

Conversion table for solution strengths

By definition a 1% solution contains 1 gram of substance in every 100 ml of solution. This can also be written as 1:100 or 10 mg/ml.

Dilution	Solution (%)	mg/ml
1:200 000	0.0002	0.002 mg/ml
1:100 000	0.001	0.01 mg/ml
1:10 000	0.01	0.1 mg/ml
1:5000	0.02	0.2 mg/ml
1:1000	0.01	0.1 mg/ml
1:500	0.2	2 mg/ml
1:200	0.5	5 mg/ml
1:100	1	10 mg/ml
1:50	2	20 mg/ml
1:10	10	100 mg/ml

Length

SI unit is the metre.

1 metre = 100 centimetres = 1000 millimetres
            = 1 000 000 microns = 1 000 000 000 nanometres
1 foot = 30.48 cm = 304.8 mm
1 inch = 2.54 cm = 25.4 mm

Volume

SI unit is the cubic metre.

1000 millilitres = 10 decilitres = 1 litre
1 teaspoon = 4.5 ml
1 tablespoon = 15 ml
1 teacup = 120 ml
1 tumbler = 240 ml
1 pint = 568 ml
1 fluid ounce = 28.42 ml

Temperature

When heat energy flows from body A to body B, then body A is at a higher temperature than body B. Temperature is measure of thermodynamic activity.
SI unit is the Kelvin (not 'degrees Kelvin')
Centigrade means the same as Celsius.
Fahrenheit is a temperature scale used in the USA.
Water forms ice at 0° Celsius and boils at 100°C.
Water forms ice at 32° Fahrenheit and boils at 212°F.
Water forms ice at 273 Kelvin and boils at 373.

$$C° = (F° -32) \times 5/9$$
$$F° = (C° \times 9/5) + 32$$

C°	30	32	34	35	36	37	38	39	40
F°	86.0	87.8	93.2	95.0	96.8	98.6	100.4	102.2	104.0

Pressure

Pressure is the force per unit area exerted by a substance perpendicular to its boundary with another substance.

SI unit is the pascal. A kilopascal is 1000 pascals.

Some places measure pressures in kilopascals (kPa), whereas others measure it in millimetres of mercury (mmHg).

7.6 mmHg = 1 kPa

1 mmHg ≈ 13 Pa

Occasionally pressure is measured in centimetres of water.

1.32 mmHg = 10 cm H_2O

SI unit	Old unit	Old to SI	SI to old
kPa	mmHg	× 0.133	× 7.60
	cm H_2O	× 0.098	× 10.20
	lb per inch^2	× 6.894	× 0.145

mmHg	kPa	mmHg	kPa	mmHg	kPa	mmHg	kPa	mmHg	kPa
1	0.13	21	2.76	41	5.39	61	8.03	81	10.66
2	0.26	22	2.89	42	5.52	62	8.16	82	10.79
3	0.39	23	3.03	43	5.65	63	8.29	83	10.92
4	0.53	24	3.16	44	5.79	64	8.42	84	11.05
5	0.66	25	3.29	45	5.92	65	8.55	85	11.18
6	0.79	26	3.42	46	6.05	66	8.68	86	11.32
7	0.92	27	3.55	47	6.18	67	8.82	87	11.45
8	1.05	28	3.68	48	6.32	68	8.95	88	11.58
9	1.08	29	3.82	49	6.45	69	9.08	89	11.71
10	1.32	30	3.95	50	6.58	70	9.21	90	11.84
11	1.45	31	4.08	51	6.71	71	9.34	91	11.97
12	1.58	32	4.21	52	6.84	72	9.47	92	12.11
13	1.71	33	4.34	53	6.97	73	9.60	93	12.24
14	1.84	34	4.47	54	7.11	74	9.73	94	12.37
15	1.97	35	4.60	55	7.24	75	9.87	95	12.50
16	2.11	36	4.73	56	7.37	76	10.00	96	12.63
17	2.24	37	4.87	57	7.50	77	10.13	97	12.76
18	2.37	38	5.00	58	7.63	78	10.26	98	12.89
19	2.50	39	5.13	59	7.76	79	10.39	99	13.03
20	2.63	40	5.26	60	7.89	80	10.53	100	13.16

Blood pressure

Blood pressure is the force per unit area exerted by blood at right angle to its direction of flow.

Pressures in mmHg	Range	Comments
Central venous pressure (CVP)	0–7	Zero reference at isophlebotic point
Right atrium	0–8	Mean = 5
Right ventricle	22/0	
Pulmonary artery	22/8	Mean = 14
Pulmonary artery wedge	2–8	Mean = 5
Left atrium	7	

Weight

1 000 000 microgram = 1000 milligram = 1 gram = 0.001 kg
1 ounce (oz) = 28.35 g
1 pound (lb) = 0.4536 kg
1 stone = 14 lb = 6.35 kg

Average blood requirement

Average blood requirement is the amount of blood usually needed for these operations. These figures help you work out whether the patient has received roughly the correct amount of blood for their operation, or that there is enough available to cover future needs. Smaller patients require relatively larger amounts of blood than more muscular people. For instance a 90 kg man would probably not need any blood for a total knee replacement, while a 50 kg old woman may need at least one unit.

Operation	Blood cross-match in 450 ml units
Abdominal lipectomy	2
Abdomino–perineal resection	3
Adrenalectomy	2
Amputation – above knee	Group and hold (G+H)
Amputation – below knee	G+H
Anterior resection	2
Aortic aneurysm – elective	3
Aorto-femoral bypass	4

Operation	Blood cross-match in 450 ml units
Aorto-iliac bypass	4
Appendicectomy	Nil
Apronectomy	2
Arthroscopy	Nil
Bowel resection	2
Burns debridement	Lots
Caesarean section	G+H
Carotid endarterectomy	G+H
Cholecystectomy – laparoscopic	G+H
Cholecystectomy – open	G+H
Colostomy	G+H
Cystectomy	4
Cystoscopy	Nil
D&C ± hysteroscopy	Nil
Ectopic – ruptured	4
Ectopic – simple	G+H
Femoral–popliteal bypass	2
Femoro–popliteal bypass	2
Gastrectomy	2
Gastric – high reduction	G+H
Gastric stapling	G+H
Gastrostomy	G+H
Haemorrhoidectomy	Nil
Harrington's rods	4
Hepatectomy – partial	6
Hiatus hernia – transthoracic	2
Hiatus hernia repair	G+H
Hip replacement	3
Hysterectomy – radical	2
Hysterectomy – abdominal	G+H
Hysterectomy – vaginal	G+H
Ileal conduit	4
Ileostomy	G+H
Ilio-femoral bypass	2
Incisional hernia	G+H

Operation	Blood cross-match in 450 ml units
Infra-inguinal vascular redo	2
Inguinal hernia	Nil
Inguinal hernia – laparoscopic	G+H
Ivor Lewis oesophagectomy	4
Knee replacement	1
Laminectomy	G+H
Laminectomy + fusion	4
Laparoscopy	G+H
Lumbar sympathectomy	G+H
Lung lobectomy	2
Mammoplasty – reduction < 1 kg	Γ+H
Mammoplasty – reduction > 1 kg	2
Mastectomy – radical	2
Mastectomy – simple	G+H
Mastectomy + axillary clearance	2
Menisectomy	Nil
Myomectomy	G+H
Nephrectomy – simple	2
Nephrectomy for cancer	4
Nephrolithotomy – open	4
Nephrolithotomy fibreoptic	G+H
Oesophagectomy	4
Ovarian cystectomy	G+H
Pancreatectomy – partial	4
Pancreatectomy – total	6
Pancreatic cyst	2
Parotidectomy	G+H
Pelvic clearance	4
Pleurectomy	2
Pneumonectomy	4
Portocaval shunt	4
Prostatectomy – open	2
Pyelolithotomy	2
Pyeloplasty	G+H
Renal artery repair	3

Operation	Blood cross-match in 450 ml units
Salphingoplasty	G+H
Shoulder-arthroplasty	G+H
Spinal fusion	2
Splenectomy	2
Splenectomy for ITP	4
Synovectomy – knee	G+H
Termination of pregnancy	G+H
Thymectomy	2
Thyroidectomy – simple	G+H
Thyroidectomy for cancer	G+H
Thyroidectomy for goitre	G+H
Tubal ligation	G+H
TURP	G+H
Ureto-lithotomy	G+H
Vaginal repair	G+H
Varicose veins	G+H
Vulvectomy-radical	4
Vulvectomy-simple	2
Whipple's operation	4

Alpha and beta receptors

Receptor	Heart	Arterioles	Lungs	Other
$\alpha 1$	–	Constricts	–	Reduces gut mobility
$\beta 1$	Increase rate increases strength	Dilates coronary arteries	–	Glycogenolysis
$\beta 2$	Increases rate increases strength	Dilates most arteries	Bronchodilation	Tremor, tocolysis, hypokalaemia
$\beta 3$	–	–	–	Lipolysis

Drugs entering breast milk

Factors to consider include:

- Older infants are less susceptible to drugs in breast milk than neonates or premature babies.
- Premature babies' ability to metabolize and excrete drugs is less than older infants.

- Consider other factors, such as liver or renal disease, which impair a baby's ability to deal with drugs.

Drug	In breast milk	Recommendation
Amethocaine	Yes	Avoid – significantly toxic
Atenolol	Yes	Safe in short term
Atracurium	Unknown	Avoid where possible
Atropine	Yes	Safe as a single dose
Bupivacaine	Yes	Safe for 36 hours
Cisatracurium	Probably	Avoid where possible
Clonidine	Yes	Safe as a single dose
Codeine	Yes	Probably safe as a single dose
Dalteparin	Yes	Wait 2 days before restarting feeding
Desflurane	Trace	Probably safe
Diamorphine	Yes	Best avoid
Diazepam	Yes	Safe in single dose
Diclofenac	Trace	Safe in short term
Dolasetron	Probably	Avoid
Droperidol	Yes	Best avoid
Enoxaparin	Unknown	Safe in anaesthetic setting
Ephedrine	Yes	Safe as a single dose
Ergometrine	Yes	Safe as a single dose
Esmolol	Unknown	Best avoid
Fentanyl	Yes	Safe in anaesthetic setting
Flumazenil	Yes	Avoid where possible
Frusemide	Yes	Postpone breastfeeding
Gentamicin	Yes	Probably safe
Glycopyrrolate	Yes	Probably safe
Granisetron	Unknown	Best avoid
Hydrocortisone	Unknown	Safe as a single dose
Insulin	Unknown	Safe
Isoflurane	Unknown	Considered safe
Ketamine	Yes	Safe in short term
Lidocaine	Yes	Considered safe as a single dose
Mannitol	Unknown	Best avoid
Metoclopramide	Yes	May cause infant diarrhoea

Drug	In breast milk	Recommendation
Metronidazole	Yes	Withhold feeds for 4 hours after single dose
Midazolam	Yes – small	Considered safe
Morphine	Trace	Considered safe in normal doses
Naloxone	Yes	Safe as a single dose
Naproxen	Yes	Avoid
Neostigmine	Negligible	Safe as a single dose
Ondansetron	Yes	Avoid
Oxycodone	Yes	Considered safe
Pancuronium	Trace – possibly	Safe in anaesthesia
Paracetamol	Yes	Safe – analgesic of choice
Pethidine	Yes	Morphine safer
Prochlorperazine	Unknown	Avoid
Propofol	Trace	Considered safe
Ranitidine	Yes	Avoid – use famotidine instead
Salbutamol	Yes	Considered safe in low dose
Sevoflurane	Unknown	Considered safe
Temazepam	Yes	Considered safe in single dose
Thiopentone	Yes	Considered safe in one dose
Tramadol	Yes	Avoid
Vecuronium	Unknown	Considered safe

Surgery grades

Major procedure (highly invasive surgery)

- expected to take more than 60 minutes;
- involves extensive tissue mass and trauma;
- major disruption to body physiology persists after 24 hours;
- requires a blood transfusion;
- involves a patient of ASA III grade or higher;
- all vascular surgery;
- major joint replacement;
- open abdomen or thorax including laparoscopy;
- intracranial or spinal operations;
- is an emergency.

Examples: aortic aneurysm repair, bowel resection, thoracotomy, major joint replacement.

Minor procedure (moderately invasive surgery)

- expected to take from 30–60 minutes;
- some tissue trauma;
- minor disruption to body physiology persists after 24 hours;
- patient is intubated;
- no blood transfusion;
- laparoscopic surgery;

Examples: inguinal hernia repair, laparoscopic cholecystectomy, prostatectomy.

Minimal procedure (minimally invasive surgery)

- expected to take less than 30 minutes;
- minimal tissue trauma;
- no disruption to body physiology persist after 24 hours.

Examples: arthroscopy, D&C, cystoscopy.

Postsurgical classification

Postsurgical classification ranks patients according to how incapacitated they are, and allows resources to be allocated to suit the situation.

Stable

Patients who are to return to the ward who:

- had observations that remained within normal limits during their stay in the recovery room;
- are receiving no more than maintenance intravenous fluids;
- whose biochemistry and haematology results were normal.

Labile

Patients who are to return to the ward:

- after an invasive procedure whose stay in the recovery room was uneventful, but who now require more than routine observations. For example if they have an epidural catheter.

- who, while in the recovery room, developed an abnormal observation that is explainable and is unlikely to need intervention or to deteriorate.
- who, while in the recovery room, were found to have an abnormal biochemical or haematology result.

Unstable

Patients who are to return to the ward who:

- have undergone an invasive procedure, but whose recovery is not proceeding as expected;
- while in the recovery room had abnormal observations that responded to corrective measures;
- have worsening abnormal biochemical or haematological results;
- required additional unexpected intervention e.g. insertion of a thoracic drain for a pneumothorax.

Critical

Critical patients are discharged to a high care unit. They remain in Stage 1 recovery.

These patients include those who, while in recovery room, have:

- worsening abnormal observations despite corrective intervention;
- been classified as unstable emergency cases;
- abnormal observations and the diagnosis remains obscure.

How to assign risk

In 1941 the American Society of Anesthesiologists developed a scale to quantify surgical and anaesthetic risk. It subsequently became known as the ASA scale. This scale has withstood the test of time; it is easy to remember and has over the years proved reliable in predicting postoperative trouble.

Not only does the ASA status provide a useful way of quickly conveying how sick a patient is, but also it correlates well with mortality, theatre cancellations, and unplanned emergency operations, and is useful when you are developing protocols. The ASA status's grave disadvantage is that in makes no assessment of the magnitude of surgery; a wart can be removed from an ASA IV patient without problems, but a hip replacement may kill them.

The ASA PS Class (American Society of Anesthesiologists' Grading of Physical Status) is ranked in order of how severely the patient is incapacitated, and the numbers are easy to remember:

ASA I — fit,

ASA II — minor diseases,

ASA III — major disease,

ASA IV —life threatening disease,

ASA V — near dead.

If the case is an emergency append an E to the physical grade eg. IV E.

A more detailed classification

ASA class	Disability	Mortality rate (est)
Class I	The patient is perfectly fit for their age. The patient has no organic physiological, biochemical or psychiatric disturbance. The surgical site is localized, and surgery does not entail systemic disturbance.	< 0.08%
Class II	The patient has a condition which does not limit their day-to-day activity. Mild to moderate systemic disturbance caused either by the surgical condition or by the pathophysiological process. For example: mild organic heart disease, non-insulin-dependent diabetes, mild hypertension (diastolic < 100 mmHg), anaemia, old age, mild obesity, mild asthma.	0.08–0.42%
Class III	The patient has a condition which limits their day-to-day activity. Severe systemic disturbance or disease from whatever cause, even though it may not be possible to define the degree of disability with any finality. Includes obesity (BMI > 35), angina (exercise- or emotion-induced but stable), healed myocardial infarction, insulin-dependent diabetes, peripheral vascular disease, cardiac failure (moderate systolic or diastolic dysfunction), moderate hypertension (diastolic 100115 mmHg), severe asthma, warfarin therapy.	0.4–4.3%
Class IV	The patient has a condition which severely limits their activity and is a constant threat to life. Severe systemic disturbances that are already life-threatening and not necessarily correctable by surgery. This includes marked obesity (BMI > 40), cardiac insufficiency (diastolic or systolic dysfunction), Hypertension with diastolic blood pressure > = 115 mmHg, persistent, frequent or unstable angina, active myocarditis, recent CVA or TIA (within last 16 weeks), advance pulmonary, renal or endocrine, or hepatic insufficiency.	4.4–23%
Class V	Moribund. Little chance of survival with or without surgery, but submitted to operation in desperation.	24–51%
Class VI	Brain dead patient whose organs are being harvested	100%

Emergency surgery

Add an E after the grade if the operation is an emergency.

Index